Emerging Technologies for Nutrition Research

Potential for Assessing Military Performance Capability

Committee on Military Nutrition Research

Food and Nutrition Board

Institute of Medicine

Sydne J. Carlson-Newberry and Rebecca B. Costello, Editors

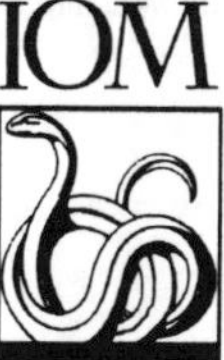

NATIONAL ACADEMY PRESS
Washington, D.C. 1997

NOTICE: The project that is the subject of this report was approved by the Governing Board of the National Research Council, whose members are drawn from the councils of the National Academy of Sciences, the National Academy of Engineering, and the Institute of Medicine. The members of the committee responsible for the report were chosen for their special competences and with regard for appropriate balance. Part I of this report has been reviewed by a group other than the authors according to procedures approved by a Report Review Committee consisting of members of the National Academy of Sciences, the National Academy of Engineering, and the Institute of Medicine.

The Institute of Medicine was established in 1970 by the National Academy of Sciences to enlist distinguished members of the appropriate professions in the examination of policy matters pertaining to the health of the public. In this, the Institute acts under both the Academy's 1863 congressional charter responsibility to be an adviser to the federal government and its own initiative in identifying issues of medical care, research, and education. Dr. Kenneth I. Shine is president of the Institute of Medicine.

This report was produced under grant DAMD17-94-J-4046 between the National Academy of Sciences and the U.S. Army Medical Research and Materiel Command. The views, opinions, and/or findings contained in chapters in Parts II through VIII that are authored by U.S. Army personnel are those of the authors and should not be construed as official Department of the Army positions, policies, or decisions, unless so designated by other official documentation. Human subjects who participated in studies described in those chapters gave their free and informed voluntary consent. Investigators adhered to U.S. Army regulation 70-25 and United States Army Medical Research and Development Command regulation 70-25 on use of volunteers in research. Citations of commercial organizations and trade names in this report do not constitute an official Department of the Army endorsement or approval of the products or services of these organizations. The chapters are approved for public release; distribution is unlimited.

Library of Congress Catalog Card No. 97-68316

International Standard Book Number 0-309-05797-3

Additional copies of this report are available from:

National Academy Press
2101 Constitution Avenue, N.W.
Lock Box 285
Washington, D.C. 20055

Call (800) 624-6242 or (202) 334-3313 (in the Washington metropolitan area), or visit the NAP's on-line bookstore at *http://www.nap.edu*.

Staff
REBECCA B. COSTELLO, Study Director (*from July 15, 1996*)
BERNADETTE M. MARRIOTT, Study Director (*through November 22, 1995*)
SYDNE J. CARLSON-NEWBERRY, Program Officer
SUSAN M. KNASIAK-RALEY, Research Assistant
DONNA F. ALLEN, Senior Project Assistant

Preface

This publication, *Emerging Technologies for Nutrition Research: Potential for Assessing Military Performance Capability,* is the latest in a series of reports based on workshops sponsored by the Committee on Military Nutrition Research (CMNR) of the Food and Nutrition Board (FNB), Institute of Medicine, National Academy of Sciences. Other workshops or symposia have included such topics as food components to enhance performance; nutritional needs in hot, cold, and high-altitude environments; body composition and physical performance; nutrition and physical performance; cognitive testing methodology; and fluid replacement and heat stress. These workshops form part of the response that the CMNR provides to the Commander, U.S. Army Medical Research and Materiel Command, regarding issues brought to the committee through the Military Nutrition Division (currently the Military Nutrition and Biochemical Division) of the U.S. Army Research Institute of Environmental Medicine (USARIEM) at Natick, Massachusetts.

HISTORY OF THE COMMITTEE

The CMNR was established in October 1982 following a request by the Assistant Surgeon General of the Army that the Board on Military Supplies of the National Academy of Sciences set up a committee to advise the U.S. Department of Defense on the need for and conduct of nutrition research and related issues. The committee was transferred to the FNB in 1983. The committee's current tasks are:

- to identify nutritional factors that may critically influence the physical and mental performance of military personnel under all environmental extremes,
- to identify deficiencies in the existing database,
- to recommend research that would remedy these deficiencies as well as approaches for studying the relationship of diet to physical and mental performance, and
- to review and advise on standards for military feeding systems.

Within this context, the CMNR was asked to focus on nutrient requirements for performance during operational missions rather than requirements for military personnel in garrison (the latter were judged to be not significantly different from those of the civilian population).

Although the membership of the committee has changed periodically, the disciplines represented consistently have included human nutrition, nutritional biochemistry, performance physiology, food science, and psychology. For issues that require broader expertise than exists within the committee, the CMNR has convened workshops or utilized consultants. The workshops provide additional state-of-the-art scientific information and informed opinion for the consideration of the committee.

FOCUS OF THE REPORT

The request for this review originated with scientists at USARIEM who were concerned that research, using traditional techniques, that focused on more complex issues of maintenance or enhancement of performance might not be sufficiently substantive to measure changes that may occur or might not be predictive of the effects of the stresses of operational environments. The request for this review also arose from a Science and Technology Objective to prevent soldier performance degradation under the stress of sustained field operations, as part of an overall initiative, "The Soldier as a System." This initiative recognized the importance of all aspects of the soldier's equipment and person for enhanced capabilities necessary for the future (Army Science Board, 1991).

Past reports of the CMNR usually have been focused on current issues of concern to the military. Traditional methods of research, data gathering, and analysis have provided the factual base for study of a problem and recommended solutions. This report looks further into the future at newer technologies that are being employed to identify and study basic issues that may be significant in nutrition research. Of specific interest are those techniques that can be applied to nutritional problems and that may result in improved performance by soldiers, particularly those exposed to the stress of military operations. The focus of this report is to identify those research techniques that may be applicable to maintaining or enhancing soldiers' performance and to suggest that those deemed most likely to be useful be incorporated into the nutrition research program and related areas at USARIEM.

Recognizing that there were a large number of technologies that could be reviewed and the need to limit the scope of this review to those areas of most interest to USARIEM, USARIEM personnel identified six relevant research areas for review. The primary criterion for inclusion was the possibility for application to field research. Those areas were body composition, tracer techniques to evaluate metabolism and energy expenditure, ambulatory methods to determine energy expenditure, molecular and cellular approaches to nutrition and immune function, and functional and behavioral measures of nutritional status. The factors that the CMNR was asked to consider in its evaluation of these research areas are summarized in Chapter 1.

The CMNR decided that the best way to review the state of knowledge in these disparate areas was through a workshop at which knowledgeable researchers could review published research and speculate with the committee on potential applications to the military environment. Such a workshop would enable the CMNR to review the state of the science and to identify the potential for application of the methods to the assessment of military performance capability.

A committee subgroup, USARIEM personnel, and CMNR staff participated in a series of conference calls to solicit suggestions for participants who were active in the research fields identified by USARIEM personnel as being of interest to them. Invited speakers were asked to prepare a paper for presentation and publication describing the techniques and their applications in the speakers' areas of expertise and making specific recommendations in response to several questions posed prior to the workshop. USARIEM scientists also participated in the workshop, which resulted in a well-rounded group. At the workshop, each speaker gave a formal presentation, which was followed by questions and a brief discussion period. The proceedings were tape recorded and professionally transcribed. At the end of each group of presentations, a general discussion of the overall topic was held. Immediately after the workshop, the CMNR met in executive session to review the issues, draw some tentative conclusions, and assign the preparation of draft reviews and summaries of specific topics to individual committee members. Committee members subsequently met with staff several times over the course of a year and worked separately and together using the authored papers, additional reference materials provided by the staff, and personal expertise and experience with the methods to draft the overview, summary, conclusions, and recommendations. A draft of the report was sent to a group of scientists, each of whom was identified as being an expert in one of the areas covered by the report. Their evaluations and suggestions were taken into consideration in preparing the final report, which was reviewed and approved by the entire committee.

ORGANIZATION OF THE REPORT

A project overview and summary, as well as the conclusions and recommendations of the CMNR, constitute Part I of this volume. Parts II through VIII include papers contributed by speakers at the workshop. Part I has been reviewed anonymously by an outside group with expertise in the topic areas and experience in military issues. For the most part, the authored papers in Parts II through VIII appear in the order in which they were presented at the workshop (see the Workshop Agenda in Appendix A). These chapters have undergone limited editorial changes, have not been reviewed by the outside group, and represent the views of the individual authors. Selected questions directed toward the speakers and the speakers' responses are included when they provide a flavor of the workshop discussion. The invited speakers also were requested to submit a brief list of selected background papers prior to the workshop. These recommended readings, relevant citations collected by CMNR staff prior to the workshop, and selected citations from each chapter are included in the Selected Bibliography (see Appendix D).

ACKNOWLEDGMENTS

It is my pleasure as chairman of the CMNR to acknowledge the contributions of the FNB staff, particularly the excellent technical and organizational skills of Bernadette M. Marriott. This is the last report in a series emanating from workshops sponsored by the CMNR for which Dr. Marriott was study director. She accepted a new and challenging position as the Director, Office of Dietary Supplements Research in the Office of the Director, National Institutes of Health, effective November 1995. She directed the planning for this workshop prior to accepting her new position. The CMNR past and present will sorely miss the quiet professionalism and utmost dedication that she brought to committee activities. The excellent series of published CMNR reports is testimony to her commitment to timely and quality publication of these proceedings. I wish to acknowledge as well the excellent contributions by the speakers and their commitment to participating in the workshop and preparing papers on their assigned areas with relatively short notice.

Sydne J. Carlson-Newberry joined the FNB staff as staff officer for the CMNR in September 1995 and had the leadership role in the publication of the workshop proceedings. Rebecca B. Costello joined the FNB staff in July 1996 as the study director of the CMNR. We are pleased to have her leadership in staffing CMNR activities.

Also, I wish to acknowledge the excellent editorial efforts and able assistance of Susan M. Knasiak-Raley, research assistant to the CMNR, and of Donna F. Allen, senior project assistant to the CMNR, in word processing and preparing the camera-ready copy for this report.

Finally, I express my appreciation to the members of the CMNR who have participated in the proceedings of the workshop and the discussions and preparation of summaries and recommendations in this report. Their continued dedication to providing sound, timely recommendations on issues brought to our attention is commendable. Thank you for your commitment to the success of this program.

ROBERT O. NESHEIM, Chair
Committee on Military Nutrition Research

REFERENCES

Army Science Board
1991   The Soldier as a System. 1991 Summer Study Final Report. Assistant Secretary of the Army Research, Development, and Acquisition. Washington, D.C.: U.S. Department of the Army.

Contents

III   TECHNIQUES OF BODY COMPOSITION ASSESSMENT

IV   TRACER TECHNIQUES FOR THE STUDY OF METABOLISM

V   AMBULATORY TECHNIQUES FOR MEASUREMENT OF
     ENERGY EXPENDITURE

VI   MOLECULAR AND CELLULAR APPROACHES TO NUTRITION

VII   ASSESSMENT OF IMMUNE FUNCTION

VIII   FUNCTIONAL AND BEHAVIORAL MEASURES OF NUTRITIONAL STATUS

Emerging Technologies for Nutrition Research

Potential for Assessing Military Performance Capability

I

Committee Summary and Recommendations

PART I OUTLINES THE TASK presented to the Committee on Military Nutrition Research (CMNR) by scientists at the Military Nutrition Division (MND) (currently the Military Nutrition and Biochemical Division), U.S. Army Research Institute of Environmental Medicine (USARIEM). This task was to identify and evaluate new technologies to determine whether these technologies will provide useful tools to help solve important issues in military nutrition research. As part of the charge to the CMNR, the Army posed the following six questions:

1. Will the technology be a significant improvement over current technologies?

2. How likely is the technology to mature sufficiently for practical use, and if so, how soon will it be available?

3. Consider the cost/benefit ratio of the new technology. How expensive (in both monetary and personnel terms) will it be to employ compared to the importance of the information it will provide?

4. Is the technology of such critical value that its development should be supported by DoD funds—such as can be provided by the SBIR (Small Business Innovative Research) program? If so, provide the necessary information to justify such support.

1

5. How practical is the technology? Will it require dedicated personnel and complex, exotic equipment? Will the data provided be difficult to analyze?

6. Is the technique applicable to field testing scenarios (could it be used in the field or used to analyze data collected in the field such as frozen plasma samples)?

In Chapter 1, the committee presents an overview of the project using relevant background materials and the workshop proceedings from May 22–23, 1995. The committee then summarizes the techniques under consideration with regard to their state of the art, maturity and availability, practicality, military relevance, and complicating factors and methodological questions. Considered were techniques of body composition assessment, tracer techniques for the study of metabolism, ambulatory techniques for determination of energy expenditure, molecular and cellular approaches to nutrition, assessment of immune function, and functional and behavioral measures of nutritional status.

Before presenting its conclusions and recommendations in Chapter 2, the CMNR frames its answers to the questions posed by the Army in terms of the 6 techniques reviewed. Body composition assessment is used for accession and retention standards; while anthropometric measurements are most applicable for evaluating compliance, more sophisticated methods (such as dual-energy x-ray absorptiometry, magnetic resonance imaging, and computerized axial tomography) should be used to refine the anthropometric measurements. Noninvasive tracer techniques for the study of metabolism, such as stable isotopes, are militarily relevant and applicable in the field; however, the costs associated with trained personnel and expensive equipment need to be considered. Ambulatory monitoring techniques allow for measuring energy expenditure in the field and are in use. At the present time, molecular and cellular approaches should be confined to already-established research laboratories, even for issues of military interest. Studies of immune function and the development of vaccines and antibodies are of particular military relevance when considering the stress of military operations in relation to performance. The development of monitoring devices for evaluating cognitive performance in the field are similarly important.

Emerging Technologies for Nutrition Research, 1997
Pp. 3–50. Washington, D.C.
National Academy Press

1

Project Overview and Committee Summary

PROJECT OVERVIEW

As the U.S. military faces the twenty-first century, it must contend with changes in the nature of warfare and deployment that have significant implications for individual performance. The more frequent redeployment of soldiers (necessitated by downsizing and by changing military strategies) mandates greater concern for their physical health and well-being and, therefore, the development of cutting-edge techniques for field assessment of health and nutritional status. Such assessment tools must demonstrate reproducibility and reliability in field tests, must be noninvasive, and must cause minimal interference with battlefield operations. Reliance upon techniques that are tied to laboratories must give way to ambulatory assessment. At the same time, the increasingly technological orientation of modern warfare raises the spectre of battles being waged by soldiers seated at computer terminals, with the capability for mass destruction at their fingertips, and necessitates great concern for the assessment and optimization of cognitive performance in those soldiers. Finally, budgetary constraints, coupled with the need to stay at the forefront of research, dictate that careful consideration be given to identifying the best available and emerging technologies and making priority decisions regarding which ones should be undertaken directly by the military, which deserve investment of funds to foster military applications, and which are best left to the private sector.

THE COMMITTEE'S TASK

As part of its responsibility to the Military Nutrition Division (MND) (currently the Military Nutrition and Biochemical Division) at the U.S. Army Research Institute of Environmental Medicine (USARIEM), the Committee on Military Nutrition Research (CMNR) on many occasions has provided evaluation of both research plans and ongoing research efforts funded by Department of Defense (DoD) appropriations. Examples include 1992 and 1996 reviews of research activities at the Louisiana State University's Pennington Biomedical Research Center, 1991 and 1993 reviews of a nutrition intervention project's results conducted during a U.S. Army Ranger training program, and a 1995 review of issues related to iron status of women enrolled in U.S. Army Basic Combat Training.

In 1994, the CMNR was asked by the MND to identify and evaluate new technologies to determine whether the technologies will provide useful tools to help solve important issues in military nutrition research in the areas identified by MND, USARIEM. The committee was requested: (1) to provide a survey of newly available and emerging techniques for the assessment and optimization of nutritional and physiological status and performance, and (2) to evaluate the potential of these techniques to contribute to future research efforts involving military personnel. In addition, the committee was asked to make recommendations regarding the practicality and the application of such techniques in field settings. The MND asked the CMNR to include in its response the answers to the six questions listed in Table 1-1.

To assist the CMNR in responding to these questions, a workshop was convened on May 22–23, 1995, in Washington, D.C., that included presentations from individuals with expertise in:

- techniques of body composition assessment,
- tracer techniques for the study of metabolism,
- ambulatory techniques for determination of energy expenditure,
- molecular and cellular approaches to nutrition,
- assessment of immune function, and
- functional and behavioral measures of nutritional status.

TABLE 1-1 Questions Posed by the Army

State of the Art

Will the technologies be a significant improvement over current technologies?

Maturity and Availability

How likely are the technologies to mature sufficiently for practical use?

Practicality

What is the cost/benefit ratio of the new technologies, and how expensive (in both monetary and personnel terms) will they be to employ compared with the importance of the information they will provide?

Military Relevance

Are the technologies of such critical value that their development should be supported by DoD funds—such as can be provided by the Small Business Innovative Research program?

Complicating Factors and Methodological Questions

How practical are the technologies? Will they require dedicated personnel and complex, exotic equipment? Will the data provided be difficult to analyze?

Possible Use in the Field

Can the technologies be used in the field (could they be used in the field or used to analyze samples collected in the field)?

As a background to these presentations, a representative of the MND provided an overview of the military nutrition program and its research activities. For the preparation of their presentations, the invited speakers were asked to address the questions posed by the Army. The speakers discussed their presentations with committee members at the workshop and submitted written reports based on their verbal presentations. The committee met after the workshop to discuss the techniques presented and the information provided. Later, the CMNR reviewed the workshop presentations, summarized the information pertinent to each technique, and drew heavily on its collective expertise and the scientific literature to evaluate the potential contribution of each technique to military nutrition research and make recommendations regarding development of capabilities in these areas. In preparing this report, the committee limited its evaluation to technologies discussed at the workshop. The committee's conclusions and recommendations, as well as the responses to the six questions posed by the Army, appear in Chapter 2.

THE CURRENT ARMY PROGRAM AND ITS FUTURE NEEDS

The Army's nutrition research program is driven by the need of the Armed Forces to maintain and enhance performance in all operational environments.

Key to the performance requirements is understanding how nutritional status affects physical and cognitive performance and long-term health. The research program to provide the knowledge about these relationships is discussed by James A. Vogel in Chapter 3 in this volume. Vogel indicates that this program is composed of four main areas:

- development of nutritional strategies,
- evaluation of operational rations,
- establishment of nutritional requirements under diverse field situations, and
- assessment of nutritional status of military populations.

In these areas of research, the technical requirements include methods for measurement of changes in body composition, plus the determination of lean mass and fat mass; measurement of protein metabolism; monitoring the metabolism of energy-yielding nutrients; measurement of energy expenditure under a wide variety of environmental conditions; measurement of molecular and cellular changes in nutrient utilization; measurement of immune function (status); measurement of physiological performance; and measurement of cognitive performance.

The unique requirements of the Armed Forces' nutrition research program are the need to make measurements in extremes of environmental conditions (high and low temperatures, high altitude, high and low humidity, noise, vibration, concussion, or combinations thereof) and stress (sleep deprivation, battle fatigue, prolonged physical exertion, dehydration, and underconsumption of nutrients) and the desire to extend performance while holding logistical requirements to a minimum. This research agenda makes consideration of new research technologies very attractive, especially in terms of cost and timeliness. At the same time, consideration must be given to the relative chances of successful outcome and cost or cost/benefit considerations. Relative to this latter consideration, Vogel suggests that attention be given to the relative potential for performance enhancement or the health benefit that is inherent in ration modification, ration supplementation, or other nutrition interventions. Although the relative military benefit of performance outcomes may be beyond the capacity of the CMNR to evaluate, some assessment can be made on the basis of improvement in the variability and certainty of research data.

COMMITTEE SUMMARY

TECHNIQUES OF BODY COMPOSITION ASSESSMENT

In Chapter 4 of this report, LTC Karl E. Friedl presents an overview of the use of body composition (BC) assessment by the military, the available technologies, and suggestions for future development. More detailed discussions of specific methods are provided by Steven Heymsfield and coworkers, Wendy M. Kohrt, and Wm. Cameron Chumlea and Shumei S. Guo (see Chapters 5, 6, and 7 in this volume).

The composition of the body reflects a number of factors, including the status of energy stores, training level, and other aspects of nutritional and hydration status. Characteristics that may be inferred indirectly from BC assessments include muscular strength, physical performance, and potential risk for musculoskeletal injury (Reynolds et al., 1994).

Body Composition Standards in the Military

The military utilizes the results of BC research and analysis to develop appropriate standards for selection (accession and retention) and for fitness. While the primary goal of military BC standards is to ensure military readiness (physical fitness, performance, and risk of chronic disease) (Friedl, 1992), a secondary goal is to maintain military appearance (Hodgdon et al., 1990), which is considered a part of readiness. The BC standards utilized by the military are specific to age, gender, and branch of military service. In addition to utilization in standards development, BC is used by the military to assess training programs and the risks and benefits of a wide variety of optimization strategies, including physical, nutritional, and pharmacological interventions. The first tier of BC analysis by the U.S. Army consists of a semiannual weight-for-height screen, based on body mass index (BMI, weight/height^2) (AR 600-9, 1986). Personnel who exceed the weight-for-height standards are permitted to undergo a second tier of analysis consisting of body fat assessment by anthropometric (circumference) measurement. As Friedl points out, the method of body fat assessment utilized by the Army must be part of a regulation and must be limited to one method that is accurate and does not inadvertently undermine the goals of classification by declaring those with the greatest muscle mass to be overweight or by requiring inappropriate energy restriction to "make weight."

BC standards utilized by the military are based primarily on the ability to predict body fat from BMI and secondarily on equations that estimate the percentage of body fat from anthropometric measurements (AR 600-9, 1986). Validation of the equations, which differ according to age, gender, and branch, traditionally has been accomplished by comparison with body fat estimations using hydrodensitometry, the "criterion" measure. Hydrodensitometric determination of body fat is based on a two-compartment model of BC (fat and fat-free mass) (Siri, 1961). This method may be unreliable for both technical and theoretical reasons. From a technical standpoint, residual air volume (air left in the body after voluntary expulsion) and body volume measurements are subject to significant error. From a theoretical standpoint, the method relies on assumptions regarding the two compartments' constancy of composition. These latter assumptions are based primarily on data collected either from men (Keys et al., 1950) or guinea pigs (Pace and Rathbun, 1945) and do not account for changes in hydration level or differences because of race (ethnicity) or gender. The military's equations tend to overestimate body fat in lean individuals and underestimate body fat in overweight individuals (Friedl and Vogel, 1992).

Recent attempts to validate the military's body fat equations have included the use of a four-compartment model combining hydrodensitometry with dual-energy x-ray absorptiometry (DEXA or DXA) to determine bone mineral density and soft tissue mass, according to Friedl (see Chapter 4 in this volume).

Body Composition Assessment Techniques Proposed to Replace Hydrodensitometry as the Criterion Method

Dual-Energy X-Ray Absorptiometry

The use of DXA for BC assessment is reviewed in Chapter 6 by Wendy M. Kohrt. According to Kohrt, the primary clinical application of DXA (which has replaced dual-photon absorptiometry) is the measurement of bone mineral content and bone mineral density (BMD) to assess risk for osteoporosis. As a tool for BMD assessment, DXA is considered highly reliable and precise; however, its validity, particularly for measuring changes in BMD, remains questionable because of interinstrument measurement discrepancies (see Kohrt, Chapter 6 in this volume), as well as intrainstrument errors resulting from changes in other tissue compartments (Schneider and Reiners, 1997).

The use of DXA to measure BC is based on the principle that the composition of an object can be determined by the attenuation of two distinct low- and high-energy x-ray beams. This technique can distinguish three compartments or materials: bone mineral, nonbone lean tissue, and fat (Nord and Payne, 1990). The x-ray attenuation of each pixel is compared to the known attenuation of reference materials (see Kohrt, Chapter 6 in this volume). As a means of measuring BC, DXA appears to be more precise, reproducible, and convenient than hydrodensitometry for both the patient and the investigator (Hansen et al., 1993). In addition, DXA yields information about regional BC (Jensen et al., 1995) and has the advantage of producing results that are independent of ethnic differences. Also, DXA allows measurement of bone, which is one of the compartments with the greatest interindividual variability. With DXA, less reliance needs to be placed upon assumptions regarding the consistency of the chemical composition of fat-free mass (FFM) than is the case with hydrodensitometry; thus, DXA could potentially replace hydrodensitometry as the criterion method for validation of anthropometric measurements of fat, according to Kohrt (see Chapter 6 in this volume).

Other investigators point out that, although DXA shows much promise in its ability to assess fat accurately (Haarbo et al., 1991), the susceptibility of DXA estimations of FFM to changes in hydration status (Formica et al., 1993; Horber et al., 1992) and protein content, and its inability to analyze the composition of soft tissues that lie close to bone (Tothill and Nord, 1995) demonstrate that more development is necessary. In addition, DXA is expensive (analyzer costs range from \$120,000 to \$150,000) and cannot be used in the field.

Bioelectrical Impedance Analysis and Other Techniques

Other techniques that have been utilized, particularly in the field, include near-infrared (NIR) spectroscopy, ultrasound, and bioelectric impedance analysis (BIA). Using hydrodensitometric determinations and anthropometric measurements as the standard, NIR spectroscopy has proven no better than simple height and weight measures (Israel et al., 1989), while ultrasound has proven no better than anthropometric measurements (Hodgdon and Fitzgerald, 1987; see Friedl, Chapter 4 in this volume).

BIA, reviewed in Chapter 7 by Wm. Cameron Chumlea and Shumei S. Guo, measures current flow through the body and was first used to assess hydration status (Nyboer, 1959). The measurements are based upon the assumption that the body is a water- and electrolyte-filled cylinder. When BIA is used to assess body composition, there is a requirement to generate mathematical equations that must be validated against some other criterion method of BC assessment.

BIA has the dual advantages of being noninvasive and relying upon equipment that is relatively portable. The use of BIA to assess body composition has, until recently, relied on measurements at a single frequency (of 50 Hz). Such estimates of body composition are often unreliable (Chumlea et al., 1996). Further, single-frequency BIA is not recommended for use in longitudinal studies since it is not a valid indicator of changes in BC within the same individual over time, particularly if the change is slow or is accounted for primarily by a change in fat content (Forbes et al., 1992).

An alternative method of BIA performs measurements at multiple frequencies. This method is an improvement over single-frequency methods in that data are fitted to a theoretical curve, and the frequencies that best fit the curve are used to estimate BC (Chumlea et al., 1996). A third alternative is the use of bioimpedance spectroscopy (BIS), which measures multiple components of impedance over a spectrum of frequencies and shows considerable promise for longitudinal assessment of body composition (Lukaski, 1996).

The placement of electrodes also influences the utility of BIA measurements. While electrodes are routinely placed on the distal extremities, proximal (toward the trunk) placement of electrodes has been shown to improve the precision of body composition assessment, although fluid accumulation in the extremities must be monitored (Lukaski, 1996). Segmental impedance measures, particularly when performed with BIS, have shown promise in the assessment of changes in body fat (Chumlea et al., 1996).

Because BIA is based on the assessment of total body water, its utility is affected by interindividual differences in hydrational status as well as any factors that influence intraindividual hydrational status, such as fluid intake, physical activity, nutritional status, illness, and environmental factors (Kushner et al., 1996). Among the recommendations of the 1994 National Institutes of Health Technology Assessment Conference on Bioelectrical Impedance Analysis in Body Composition Measurement (NIH, 1996) are that such variables be standardized and controlled and that additional research, validation, and standardization of procedures be performed.

Computerized Axial Tomography and Magnetic Resonance Imaging

The use of computerized axial tomography (CAT) and magnetic resonance imaging (MRI) (also known as nuclear magnetic resonance) for BC assessment is reviewed by Steven Heymsfield, Robert Ross, ZiMian Wang, and David Frager in Chapter 5 in this volume. CAT is based on the ability of tissues of varying composition to attenuate an x-ray beam to differing extents, with image reconstruction based on mathematical techniques such as Fourier analysis. MRI is based on the action of hydrogen nuclei in the presence of a strong magnetic field, which causes the nuclei to align either with or against the field in a predictable manner. Each orientation has a slightly different energy state; oscillation of the magnetic field at a designated frequency causes the nuclei to flip or precess between orientations with a resulting release or absorption of energy (Gadian, 1982). When the magnet is "turned off," the nuclei return to their original energy state (relax), and the released energy generates an image. The nuclear density and relaxation times are tissue-type dependent. Both CAT and MRI produce high-resolution, cross-sectional images of the whole body or body regions. These images are then analyzed by computer to estimate tissue- and organ-level body composition, and algorithms are applied to reconstruct and estimate the total volume of the tissue or system in question (see Heymsfield et al., Chapter 5 in this volume).

While both CAT and MRI permit clear visualization of the boundaries between adipose tissue, muscle, and bone and quantification of all major tissue components, CAT has the relative disadvantages of causing some radiation exposure and being extremely costly, according to Heymsfield and coworkers (see Chapter 5 in this volume). In contrast, MRI has no known health risks and has the added advantage of permitting the calculation of tissue volumes but is expensive. Both CAT and MRI have been validated using phantoms (composed of tissue or analogous materials), laboratory animals, and human cadavers and both appear to be accurate and reproducible, with MRI having the advantage of even greater precision. Because of its accuracy, its ability to provide cross-sectional imaging and make regional and whole-body measures, and its availability and apparent safety, MRI could provide criterion data for generation of equations to predict BC in diverse populations as well as permitting longitudinal and intervention studies that require multiple or serial measures.

According to Heymsfield and coworkers (see Chapter 5 in this volume), the primary disadvantage of MRI is the preclusion from study until recently of individuals with claustrophobia and the very obese. The availability of open MRI facilities will eliminate this problem. Other disadvantages include cost; sensitivity to motion artifacts, especially in the abdominal region; time required to analyze images; and a technical question regarding the (mathematical) conversion of adipose tissue volume to fat mass.

Included among the future trends for these technologies are CAT spiral imaging, which should permit better reconstruction of BC components and decrease required radiation dose (Fishman, 1994); linkage of MRI to magnetic resonance spectroscopy to permit the study of metabolic processes *in vivo*; and decrease in the time required to take and analyze MRI images because of technical advances (Jolesz, 1992).

Correlation between Body Composition, Health Status, and Physical Performance

The correlation of total body fat content or fat distribution with actual health, nutritional status, physical activity (fitness), and appearance measures is a major concern for the military (see Friedl, Chapter 4 in this volume).

The correlation between intra-abdominal fat stores, abdominal girth, and cardiovascular (CV) disease risk is well known (Larsson et al., 1984; Metropolitan Life Insurance Company, 1937); thus, there may be reason to assess fat content in that region rather than to assess total fat. In men, intra-abdominal fat deposition is highly correlated with abdominal girth (Despres et al., 1991), which is one of the anthropometric measures included in the Army's BC equation. No such relationship exists for women, however, except for the very heaviest women (Kvist et al., 1986; Vogel and Friedl, 1992; Weits et al., 1988). In women with the highest lean body mass (i.e., those with greatest physical strength), percentage of body fat tends to be overestimated by equations that include a measure of abdominal girth (Hodgdon and Beckett, 1984). Because such women also tend to exhibit male-type fat distribution with the same CV risk factors, the abdominal girth that correlates with greatest physical strength also may predispose these women to increased CV risk (Evans et al., 1983). Thus, women whose physical performance is greatest (as measured by lifting and carrying) are those most likely to exceed body fat standards and to carry the greatest health risk.

It is fairly well established that physical strength is independent of body fat (Sharp et al., 1994). The current military (Army) weight control programs do not select for physical performance nor do they predict strength. While the association between total or regional muscle mass and specific measures of physical performance remains unclear, FFM is the BC component most likely to correlate with physical performance as measured by lifting and carrying capacity (Fitzgerald et al., 1986; Johnson et al., 1994). However, an assessment of FFM is not currently a part of the military BC standards (AR 600-9, 1986).

Because the assessment of changes in nutritional and/or hydration status during military operational activities is one of the primary interests of the MND, considerable effort has been expended to explore the use of BC assessment techniques both in the field and in the laboratory using pre- and posttreatment (exercise) sampling designs to monitor such changes. Unfortunately, as Friedl points out, the standard anthropometric measures of body composition fail to reflect accurately the true changes in weight and composition over time (Ballor and Katch, 1989). In terms of performance, the real factor of interest, and the more practical measure in field settings, is rate of weight loss. While skinfold thickness appears to detect changes in fat mass with greater reliability than does BIA or hydrodensitometry, it is still relatively insensitive for detecting small changes in fat mass (Jebb et al., 1993). Because changes in body weight or exposure to environmental extremes tends to lead to measurable changes in body water content, the use of DXA or hydrodensitometry to assess changes in body composition under such conditions may result in serious measurement artifacts. BIA may provide relatively precise assessments of changes in body water, but interpretation of changes in body composition are problematic (Friedl et al., 1994a, b; Fulco et al., 1992; Westphal et al., 1995). Thus, there is a need for more than one type of measure to assess changes in BC over time.

Summary

Body composition assessment is performed by the military for several purposes. The primary purpose is to establish adherence to weight-for-height standards. All branches of the military maintain such standards for active-duty personnel. The reasons for these standards, while somewhat branch specific, include concerns about readiness, appearance, and health. Personnel who fall outside of the weight range for their height must undergo an assessment of body fat by circumferential measurement. The gender- and branch-specific equations that use these circumferential measures to calculate body fat have been validated with the criterion measurement of hydrodensitometry. Because hydrodensitometry is based on assumptions that are not valid in the field (constancy of body compartment composition) and is problematic to perform, other criterion methods are sought by which to validate and, if necessary, refine the military equations. A four-compartment model that relies on DXA to assess bone, soft lean tissue, and fat and requires measurement of body water as well appears to offer such a criterion method for validation of existing equations for routine body composition assessment. Validated BC equations requiring only circumferential measures continue to be used by the military because of practicality and cost.

Body composition measurement also is used by the military to assess the effects of field training exercises and fitness regimens on gain or loss of lean tissue and fat mass, in a pre- and posttreatment type of design. Although useful in the laboratory, the techniques of DXA, MRI, and CAT were acknowledged to be generally impractical for field use because of their cost and relative immobility. They are also almost as limited in their ability to detect and accurately measure small changes (< 5 kg or 11 lb) in body composition as is hydrodensitometry. The utility of BIA for assessing body composition is still limited by the need for technical improvements aimed at increasing its validity.

Muscle mass is the body compartment most closely predictive of physical performance. Many of the methods described could estimate muscle mass accurately enough to predict performance; however, at present the focus of military BC assessment remains on fat. Technology that would enable measurement of small changes in muscle mass has not yet been developed.

Finally, the military utilizes the measurement of abdominal girth to predict long-term risk for cardiovascular disease in active-duty men but not women.

TRACER TECHNIQUES FOR THE STUDY OF METABOLISM

In this section, the use of stable isotopes for evaluation of metabolic processes is discussed by Dennis M. Bier, Robert R. Wolfe, and V. R. Young and coworkers (see Chapters 8, 9, and 10 in this volume). Gerald I. Shulman's description of nuclear magnetic resonance as a tool to study metabolism follows (see Chapter 11 in this volume). While James P. DeLany uses the doubly labeled water technique to measure energy expenditure (see Chapter 12 in this volume), a more detailed summary of his presentation is included in the following section due to its extensive use in the field.

Use of Isotopic Tracers to Study Metabolism

Stable isotopes are naturally occurring forms of atoms that, by nature of the increased number of neutrons in their nuclei, can be "traced" with mass spectrometry. Because these atoms are found naturally and can be concentrated in major biological pools and fuels, this technology can be used to monitor quantitatively the rate and outcome of metabolic processes in the body precisely and accurately (see Wolfe, Chapter 9 in this volume). Specifically, by monitoring the steady-state tracer dilution curve of a given isotopically labeled molecule (precursor evaluation) within a metabolic pool or the accumulation of a labeled product such as urea, ammonia, or lactate, the processes contributing to the utilization or production of that molecule and the relative rate of those processes can be monitored. This technique currently is used routinely to monitor rate of protein turnover using ^{15}N-glycine or ^{13}C-leucine (both synthesis and breakdown, see Wolfe, Chapter 9 in this volume), absolute energy expenditure using doubly labeled water (water labeled with both ^{2}H and ^{18}O; see committee summary below and DeLany, Chapter 12 in this volume), and the rate and relative amount of metabolic substrate oxidation and gluconeogenesis using ^{13}C- and ^{2}H-labeled forms of glucose, glycerol, and fatty acids (see Bier and Wolfe, Chapters 8 and 9 in this volume).

The applicability of the use of stable isotopes in field situations depends upon the route of administration of label and the pool to be sampled. Oral administration of label followed by sampling of urine, as is done when monitoring protein turnover or energy expenditure, can be accomplished in the field, with samples saved for analysis in the laboratory. However, intravenous infusion and arterial or venous sampling of label, as is required for measurement of metabolic fuel oxidation, is better suited to the research laboratory.

Dennis M. Bier points out in Chapter 8 that the use of stable isotopes is somewhat more problematic than the use of radioactive isotopes. Because stable isotopes are naturally occurring, corrections must be made in calculations for the "preenrichment" composition of the pool being studied. In addition, the enriched sample may exchange its isotopic atoms for nonlabeled ones and complicate computation of the enrichment above baseline or specific activity (the tracer/tracee ratio or algebraic sum of tracer outflow to cells and unlabeled inflow to the pool from its various sources); recycling of label also is problematic, limiting the time course of most investigations. Finally, labeled molecules often must be derivatized before analysis, and these derivatizations are not trivial. The development of reliable and accurate methods requires dedicated staff and laboratory space.

The use of stable isotopes to study metabolism can be sensitive, however, allowing the monitoring of even single atoms, according to Bier (see Chapter 8 in this volume). Thus, it requires only small samples of the pool of interest for assessment. Further treatment of samples (derivatization and ionization) can increase sensitivity and precision. In addition, the use of multiple isotopes and separation of molecules labeled at more than one site (mass isotopomer distribution analysis) allow further elucidation of the product-precursor relationship, which maximizes the information gathered in any experiment.

The major advantages of the use of stable isotopes are associated with safety. There are no risks for persons involved in the transportation, storage, or hauling of the stable isotopes. It is also environmentally safe, and the high cost of waste management associated with radioisotopes is eliminated. The method is also safe because the isotopes present no health hazard to the subjects, and the sampling is primarily through easily accessed pools of blood, breath, or urine. In addition, as Robert R. Wolfe points out in Chapter 9, the method is less invasive than muscle biopsy or measurements of arteriovenous differences across an organ bed, which require catheterization of both the inflow and outflow to a particular organ. It should be noted, however, that the use of stable isotopes in conjunction with muscle biopsies or arteriovenous difference measurements allows the researcher to evaluate organ-specific metabolic processes (such as protein synthesis specifically in muscle rather than whole body or fuel utilization across an exercising limb) (Essen et al., 1992; Tessari et al., 1995; see

Young et al., Chapter 10 in this volume). In addition, the use of stable isotopes to monitor metabolic processes is safe to the environment, requiring no special disposal arrangements.

Stable isotope methodology requires highly sophisticated equipment for preparation and analysis of samples taken from body pools, with highly trained and attentive staff to do the derivatizations and run the equipment, as well as trained investigators to evaluate the validity of the data produced. Although the cost of the mass spectrometers used to analyze the derivatized products has decreased in recent years (gas chromatography mass spectrometer [GCMS] costs about $75,000), the initial outlay for setting up a facility is still expensive because more than one kind of spectrometer usually is required to analyze a variety of isotopic tracers in one experiment (GCMS may be used for ^{15}N or ^{2}H, but an isotope ratio mass spectrometer [$200,000] is required if ^{13}C or ^{18}O are to be used). Isotope prices themselves are no longer prohibitive, although not trivial (approximately $200–$500 per test per subject) (Personal communication, G. E. Butterfield, Palo Alto Veterans Affairs Health Care System, Palo Alto, Calif., 1996).

Future Directions

The continued development of the field is demonstrated by Bier, Wolfe, and Young and coworkers (see Chapters 8, 9, and 10 in this volume). Bier describes the use of high-energy bombardment to ionize high molecular weight molecules (matrix-assisted laser desorption ionization) so that fuel precursors, such as glycogen and protein, can be studied using very little product.

Wolfe (see Chapter 9 in this volume) describes the process of monitoring the naturally occurring ^{13}C to ^{12}C ratio in expired air in individuals "primed" with ^{13}C-glycogen to determine utilization of endogenous fuel stores (glycogen, fat, and protein), a methodology made possible by an increase in the sensitivity of mass spectrometers. Although this latter method may hold promise for field use because it requires only breath sampling, it still relies on indirect calorimetry for estimation of total fuel oxidation, necessitating the concomitant use of an additional technology for measurement of oxygen consumption and carbon dioxide production, according to Wolfe (see below, and also see DeLany, Chapter 12 in this volume) to give fruitful data.

Use of Positron Emission Tomography to Study Protein Metabolism

V. R. Young, Y-M. Yu, H. Hsu, J. W. Babich, N. Alpert, R. C. Tompkins, and A. J. Fischman (see Chapter 10 in this volume) describe the use of positron emission tomography (PET) as an emerging tool for the evaluation of protein metabolism. This method involves the use of radioactive atoms of carbon, nitrogen, oxygen, and fluorine that are made by bombarding naturally occurring nuclei with particles generated by a cyclotron. These atoms can be incorporated into a variety of biological fuels (glucose, oxygen, and fatty acids), and the organ- or organelle-specific metabolism of these fuels then can be followed using the noninvasive technique of PET. The use of this technique in conjunction with stable isotopes is proposed by Young and coworkers to evaluate the contribution of individual organs and body areas to whole-body protein metabolic processes. They describe a preliminary study in which ^{11}C-methionine was used to assess hind limb-muscle protein breakdown in dogs (Hsu et al., 1996), and good agreement with previously published values was found (Biolo et al., 1995). According to Young and coworkers (see Chapter 10 in this volume), the efficacy of this method in humans in the field is questionable due to the radioactive nature of the nuclei introduced, short half-life of those nuclei, and extreme cost of the facilities necessary to produce and monitor the nuclei (the approximate cost is $2,000,000 for a cyclotron facility, making this method purely a research tool at this time). Although the chapter focuses on the use of PET in evaluating protein metabolism, the technique can be useful for measuring the utilization of a range of metabolic components in a variety of organs.

Nuclear Magnetic Resonance as a Tool to Study Metabolism

Nuclear magnetic resonance (NMR), a measurement technology whose use in body composition assessment is discussed earlier (see page 10), also allows noninvasive investigation of intracellular processes. The theory behind the method is described by Gerald I. Schulman (see Chapter 11 in this volume), as well as Heymsfield and coworkers (see Chapter 5 in this volume).

NMR can be used to monitor water and fat in the whole body by activation of hydrogen nuclei (Jardetzky and Roberts, 1981) or can be used to evaluate more specific processes on an individual organ level using the naturally occurring ^{13}C or ^{31}P nuclei (Rothman et al., 1992). Because the natural abundance of these latter nuclei is so low, their measurement is less sensitive. However, because they are found in molecules of particular interest, such as glycogen and adenosine triphosphate (ATP), they are used to monitor, respectively, liver and muscle glycogen metabolism and muscle glycogen synthesis, as well as ATP production and utilization (Shulman et al., 1990). In addition, new techniques of editing signals, stronger magnets, and improved software recently have increased sensitivity (see Shulman, Chapter 11 in this volume).

The technique requires a large magnet into which a body or body part can be placed. Although mobile units are available and expand the utility of the method, other factors limit its applicability in the field. Extensive electronics, computer equipment, and software are required for analysis of signals produced; an electrical engineer or physicist is required as full-time attendant for maintenance and interpretation (Personal communication, J. Kent-Braun, San

Francisco Veterans Affairs Health Care System, San Francisco, Calif., 1996). Thus, the method is expensive (a good magnet may run $500,000 to $2,000,000).

Summary

Stable isotopes can be used to study turnover of protein, carbohydrates, and fats and thus allow monitoring of changes in energy expenditure, relative fuel utilization, and gluconeogenesis, as well as a wide variety of other aspects of metabolic substrate oxidation in response to various stimuli. The ability to adapt these techniques for field use depends upon the route of isotope administration and the pool to be sampled. A significant problem that must be overcome with the use of stable isotopes, particularly in the field, is the natural abundance of these isotopes, which differs from place to place. In addition, while the cost of analytical equipment limits the processing of samples to large, well-funded research facilities, the cost of the isotopes themselves limits to some extent the numbers of subjects who can be included in studies.

PET utilizes radioisotopes incorporated into biological fuels to study organ-specific substrate metabolism noninvasively. Use of this technique in the field is proscribed by its reliance upon radioisotopes and the size and immobility of the PET scanner. In addition, the cost of the equipment limits its use to that of a purely research tool.

The use of NMR to study body composition (MRI) and whole-body, organ-specific metabolism also is described. NMR is expensive, and its technical complexity makes it a technique that is of use primarily to the research laboratory. With the availability of more mobile units, this technique may offer a noninvasive way of measuring metabolic processes in real time.

AMBULATORY TECHNIQUES FOR
MEASUREMENT OF ENERGY EXPENDITURE

The measurement of energy expenditure and fuel utilization during military operations is of considerable importance to the MND. Total energy expenditure, as well as preferential fuel utilization, has been measured during special operations under a variety of environmental conditions (see IOM, 1993a, 1996), as well as in garrison, with the aim of optimizing the nutrient contents of military rations, designing supplemental rations for work in extreme conditions, and providing nutritional advice to soldiers. The need remains for optimizing these measurements with the best techniques available, for more accurately measuring total body protein turnover, and for determining energy expenditure in populations of female soldiers, among other groups.

This section reviews the discussion by: James P. DeLany on doubly labeled water for energy expenditure, Reed W. Hoyt and Peter G. Weyand on foot contact time for determining the metabolic cost of locomotion, and Donald Bodenner on near-infrared spectroscopy for measuring plasma metabolites (see Chapters 12, 14, and 15 in this volume).

Doubly Labeled Water for Energy Expenditure

The use of the doubly labeled water (DLW) method for the determination of energy expenditure, as described by James P. DeLany in Chapter 12 in this volume, is based on many of the principles described above regarding stable isotopes. It employs the differential excretion of two forms of water labeled with stable isotopes (^2H_2O and $H_2^{18}O$) as a means of estimating carbon dioxide production and inferring oxygen consumption (Lifson and McClintock, 1966; Lifson et al., 1975). Deuterated water (^2H_2O) leaves the body in the water compartment (measured via urine or saliva), and the rate of dilution of the ingested dose is a measure of the production of metabolic water, which is proportional to the energy expended and the dilution that occurs due to fluid intake. Water labeled with oxygen-18 leaves the body as both water and carbon dioxide (see DeLany, Chapter 12 in this volume). Thus, if the regression lines for the excretion in urine or saliva of the two isotopes are compared, the difference between the two lines represents the excretion in the breath of label as carbon dioxide. Knowing carbon dioxide excretion and the respiratory quotient (RQ = carbon dioxide produced/oxygen consumed), an estimate of oxygen consumption can be made and energy expenditure computed using the energy equivalent of oxygen at the RQ measured.

According to DeLany, the method has the advantage of being noninvasive because it requires only that the subject drink the labeled water and collect urine or saliva at the beginning and end of the testing period. It also requires no special dietary considerations on the part of the subject, thus increasing compliance. Also according to DeLany, the incorporation of additional sampling times other than start and end points does not increase the accuracy of the method, with the sample-to-sample variation being greater than the increased reliability obtained, although others do not agree with this assessment (Cole and Coward, 1992; Edwards et al., 1991).

Analysis of the data, in contrast, requires a great deal of care and attention. Calculations must be corrected for background enrichment, which may vary with the normal water supply and may change if the water supply itself changes (Dansgaard, 1964). Corrections must be made for fractionation of the deuterium in the body water compartments, such that evaporative losses from lung and skin have a greater deuterium content (Lifson and McClintock, 1966); correction must be made for the differential distribution of the two isotopes in total body water (N_D/TBW = 1.041; N_O/TBW = 1.007) (Coward et al., 1994; Racette et al., 1994). Sample analysis is problematic in that the isotopes may fractionate during preparation, or the sample matrix may interfere with measurements (as with saliva) (Ritz et al., 1994). Finally, the method gives only an integrated value for average daily energy expenditure over 4 to 21 days and cannot clearly differentiate energy requirements on individual days (Coward, 1990).

This method has been used successfully in several military field studies to determine energy expenditure and water turnover under a variety of circumstances (Moore et al., 1992). Situations of high water turnover have been found to flush out the isotope and require large initial doses or redosing on subsequent days to attain information over long study periods (such as 28 days) (DeLany et al., 1989).

The major disadvantage of the DLW method is its cost; according to DeLany, an isotope ratio spectrometer is required for analysis, and extensive laboratory facilities are required for preparation of samples for analysis. The isotopes are now easily obtained and cost about $400 per dose. These costs prohibit use in large-scale troop assessments, especially if repeated dosing is required due to the high rate of energy expenditure (DeLany et al., 1989).

Using Foot Contact Time to Estimate the Metabolic Cost of Locomotion

Determination of the metabolic costs of locomotion is of interest to the military in determining energy needs (and food supplies) for troops in the field. In Chapter 14 in this volume, Reed W. Hoyt and Peter G. Weyand describe a device and a microcontroller that can be inserted into the shoe of the soldier to record the time of foot contact on the ground with each step. This device, which is constructed of a sensor circuit and an analog-digital converter, is called a foot contact monitor (FCM). The information derived from such a device can be used in conjunction with body weight to determine the metabolic cost of locomotion. This device has been used in the laboratory setting to determine the validity of the measure of metabolic cost of locomotion from foot contact time and body weight, and has been found to produce data that vary less than 20 percent from measured cost (Hoyt et al., 1994).

The device has the ability to measure the energy cost of locomotion in free-living conditions and estimate absolute or relative fitness levels as they change with training (Blair et al., 1992). The authors further point out that the device could be used to clarify the relationship between walking or running and training injuries, and to provide a biofeedback tool (with a FCM attached to a display of real time energy expenditure) to weight control programs.

According to Hoyt and Weyand, the device has several advantages. It offers the potential to estimate accurately the expenditure of energy at a variety of activities of varying intensities without the need for indirect calorimetry and breath gas collection. Data are expressed in standard energy units, and there is no need for calibration beyond determination of body weight. In addition, the ease of use and lack of subject input make it suitable to large epidemiological and field studies. Finally, the cost is low, estimated to be $50 to $100 for each device.

The disadvantages of the device, according to the authors, include the failure to determine total energy expenditure or that for upper-body work; the need to incorporate body weight, which may change over time and while carrying heavy equipment; and the inability to account for up- and downhill movement.

Near-Infrared Spectroscopy for Measuring Plasma Metabolites

In Chapter 15 in this volume, Donald Bodenner discusses the development of techniques using NIR spectroscopy to measure the concentration of organic compounds in complex mixtures such as food and blood. These techniques could be used for the noninvasive measurement of plasma metabolite concentrations because most organic compounds exhibit unique absorption spectra when scanned over the range of NIR wavelengths. The wavelength at which peak height is proportional to concentration must be determined for the compound of interest. While concentrations of single compounds in solution traditionally are deduced from Beer's law, the use of multiple linear regression analysis to construct regression equations that correct for interfering peaks (Beebe and Kowalske, 1987; Haaland, 1992; Honigs et al., 1983) enables interfering substances to be taken into account. In addition, the use of complex mixtures with known concentrations of constituents as standards (sometimes the subjects' own blood) will increase accuracy.

In vitro, NIR spectroscopy has been used widely to measure food constituents, such as protein in flour and sugar in breakfast cereals (Baker and Norris, 1985; Hruschka and Norris, 1982). Of clinical relevance, NIR has been used for the measurement of serum cholesterol (Peuchant et al., 1987) and fecal fat (Peuchant et al., 1988). *In vivo,* NIR spectroscopy has been used as a noninvasive way to measure tissue oxygenation through fingertip monitoring of blood flow (Jobsis, 1977). Other applications have included monitoring hemoglobin saturation in the liver (Kitai et al., 1993), changes in protein and lipid in the brain (Carney et al., 1993), and blood flow and oxygen consumption in fetal brain (Faris et al., 1994). Measurement of plasma metabolites *in vivo* using this noninvasive technique is a more formidable problem because the composition of blood and tissue is in constant flux. Some success has been achieved measuring plasma glucose in diabetic patients (Robinson et al., 1992); however, each patient's samples require an individual calibration curve (Meehan et al., 1992; Vallera et al., 1991). In addition, the effect of changes in other metabolites, such as urea, is unknown.

Summary

Two newer techniques are available to measure energy expenditure in ambulatory individuals. Doubly labeled water, the older of the two, utilizes stable isotopes of water to measure average expenditure over a given time period. The technique is relatively expensive to employ, and analysis of the data requires considerable care. A newer technique utilizes a small device built into a shoe to estimate the metabolic cost of locomotion by measuring foot contact time. Although considerably less expensive, easier to interpret, and potentially able to monitor the effects of an imposed stimulus, this technique cannot as yet measure total energy expenditure or that resulting from upper body exertion. The technique of near-infrared spectroscopy has been used to monitor blood metabolites noninvasively. Its potential for field use awaits considerable technical improvement, according to the Bodenner (see Chapter 15 in this volume).

MOLECULAR AND CELLULAR APPROACHES TO NUTRITION

In Chapter 17 in this volume, Howard C. Towle provides an overview of the processes that contribute to gene expression and describes the techniques used to study the regulation of gene expression, drawing for examples upon genes involved in nutrient metabolism. In Chapter 16, Raymond K. Blanchard and Robert J. Cousins review what is known about genes whose expression is regulated or influenced by trace minerals, particularly iron and zinc. In Chapter 18, Donald B. McCormick describes the use of isolated cell techniques to study the cellular uptake and metabolism of naturally occurring glucosides of two water-soluble vitamins, riboflavin and pyridoxine. Guy Miller (see Chapter 19 in this volume) discusses the use of isolated cell systems to study the impact of hypoxia and oxidative stress on cellular function.

Regulation of Gene Expression by Nutrients and Metabolites

Gene expression is a multistep process involving transcription of DNA to RNA (ribosomal, transfer, and messenger), mRNA processing (capping, splicing, and polyadenylation), transport of the processed message to the cytoplasm, and attachment to ribosomes and translation of the message to protein. Control of gene expression can be exerted at many different sites in the process, but transcription is the most common site for regulation.

Howard C. Towle (Chapter 17 in this volume) cites several examples of metabolic pathways in which the role of nutrient- or metabolite-mediated regulation at the transcriptional level has been examined and transcription factors identified. One such pathway is that of biosynthesis of cholesterol in which the factors that mediate the cholesterol-sensitive regulation of transcription of the biosynthetic enzymes have been identified (Goldstein and Brown, 1990; Hua et al., 1993; Yang et al., 1994). Another example is the synthesis of triglyceride that is induced by feeding a diet high in carbohydrates; the genes for the enzymes whose transcription is induced share a common sequence in their promoter regions (Lefrancois-Martinez et al., 1994; Shih et al., 1995). In neither of these two examples are the exact mechanisms understood by which a nutrient or metabolite alters the binding of the transcription factors to the promoter regions. In contrast, Towle describes some members of the steroid receptor family, all of which are themselves transcription factors that are induced by dietary components or metabolites (Forman et al., 1995; O'Malley and Conneely, 1992).

Raymond K. Blanchard and Robert J. Cousins (Chapter 16 in this volume) describe the roles played by trace metals, such as zinc, in the control of gene expression. Three mechanisms have been identified by which metals may influence gene expression (Cousins, 1995). First, the metal may play a structural role, facilitating interaction among binding groups to alter their conformation. Alternatively, the metal may catalyze an enzymatic reaction required for gene expression. Finally, the metal may bind to a specific factor involved in the initiation of transcription. These zinc-containing transcription factors, known as zinc-finger proteins, exhibit what are called zinc-finger domains, which contain zinc and may assume one of four different conformations (Dawid et al., 1995; Klug and Schwabe, 1995; Vallee et al., 1991).

The metalloprotein-binding consensus sequences found in the promoters of metal-sensitive genes are termed metal-responsive elements. These may overlap or abut other sites, are orientation-independent, and can function in heterologous promoters (a property that has been exploited extensively, as described below) (Cousins, 1994; Stuart et al., 1984).

Applications for Techniques Used to Study Gene Expression

The ability of nutrients and their metabolites to influence metabolic processes by altering gene expression has been recognized for at least 20 years. While the techniques described both by Blanchard and Cousins and by Towle (see Chapters 16 and 17 in this volume) have permitted further elucidation of the mechanisms by which this occurs, understanding of the control of gene expression is still very basic and rudimentary and of limited immediate practical application.

Blanchard and Cousins describe several applications of the knowledge that has been gained from studying mechanisms of control of gene expression. Among them are the introduction of metal-responsive elements into heterologous genes of interest to produce metal-responsive transgenes, as exemplified by the creation of zinc-inducible growth hormone genes in mice and livestock (Palmiter et al., 1982). Another application involves synthesis of small peptides containing zinc-finger domains; because of their DNA sequence-specific binding capacity, they can inhibit the binding of actual zinc finger-containing transcription factors to promoter regions, thus preventing these factors from exerting their transcription-promoting effects (Rebar and Pabo, 1994; Wu et al., 1995). This is analogous to the use that has been proposed for antisense DNA (the noncoding or nonsense strand of DNA that is complementary to a region encoding a gene or its control sequence).

It is generally recognized that the synthesis of a protein may be influenced at a number of different stages, all of which may be roughly categorized as either transcriptional, translational, or posttranslational in nature. As Towle points out in Chapter 17 in this volume, the impact of nutrients and metabolites on the transcriptional control of gene expression, in terms of adaptation, is likely to be a long-term one, with the effects being observed over a matter of hours to days, rather than being a short-term adaptive response, such as the response of ferritin mRNA translation to increasing serum concentrations of iron. The implications of long-term adaptive responses presumably include allowing the organism to operate more efficiently in the face of changing nutritional status. Although the significance of the results of techniques such as "differential display" (that is, techniques that show which genes are being expressed under a specific set of conditions) (Kendall and Christensen, 1995; Liang et al., 1993; Orr et al., 1994) may be difficult to interpret, they may permit the identification of genes that would be beneficial to control during stressful situations. Blanchard and Cousins and Towle also raise the future possibility of combining nutritional therapy with gene modification, which might permit enhancement, for example, of the body's ability to counteract exposure to ionizing radiation, toxins, or oxidative conditions. It has been shown that high-level zinc supplementation provides protection against the cellular damage caused by exposure to ionizing radiation as well as a number of chemical toxins. It is believed that the mechanism responsible involves the prevention of free radical formation, although at what level(s) the zinc exerts control is unknown (Willson, 1989).

Isolated Cell Approaches

Isolated cell systems are being used increasingly to investigate physiological phenomena at the cellular level. In their two chapters, Donald B. McCormick (see Chapter 18 in this volume) and Guy Miller (see Chapter 19 in this volume) provides examples of current studies utilizing this approach. In addition to the more research-oriented applications described in Chapters 18 and 19, a number of potential clinical applications for isolated cell techniques are being evaluated. These include *in vitro* toxicity and allergy testing and drug-efficacy screening (Purcell and Atterwill, 1994).

According to Miller, the growing popularity of this approach stems from its relative ease of use (once requisite training is obtained and adequate facilities are in place) and the ability it confers on the investigator to isolate the experimental system, control variables rigidly, process a large number of samples within a short time frame, and generate data rapidly. While these are important advantages, it must also be verified that the *in vitro* test is a proper model for the *in vivo* question being asked. Miller enumerates the issues involved in the use of these techniques in general and the choice of cell types for investigations of particular questions. He emphasizes that cellular responses to stimuli, in his case to the stimulus of hypoxic stress, are dependent on the cell type, the nature of the stress, and the environment (cellular, exocrine, and endocrine) of the cells so that, if the purpose of using an isolated cell system is to model a more complex *in vivo* counterpart (which is almost always the case), the choice of cell system becomes critical. As a general rule, to maximize the utility of a particular cell model, the cell type chosen must display a pattern of response and sensitivity to the stimulus similar to the tissue or system of interest. An important challenge to the workers in this field will be to present convincing evidence that results obtained from such cell-based systems (in both the clinical and the research laboratory) are indeed applicable to intact organ systems.

Summary

Increased understanding of the mechanisms of gene expression has led to the development of techniques such as differential display that permit the identification of genes whose transcription markedly changes in response to a given stimulus. Such knowledge ultimately may lead to the development of preventive or enhancing treatments that work at the level of promoters or suppressers of transcription. The use of isolated cell systems enables researchers to examine the effects of stimuli at the organelle or cellular level where variables can be controlled that would not be possible to control *in vivo*. Great care must be taken to choose cell culture models that are as similar in response as possible to the entire organism and situation in question. Nevertheless, both gene expression and isolated cell approaches to nutritional problems are limited in their application and are largely restricted to basic research at this point.

ASSESSMENT OF IMMUNE FUNCTION

The role of nutrition in immune function has been of considerable interest to the military since it was established that the proinflammatory hormones secreted in response to infection were responsible for the anorexia, weight loss, redistribution of trace minerals, and shift in hepatic protein synthesis toward production of acute-phase proteins that are characteristic of this state (Beisel, 1980). Subsequent research has established that the hormones in question are the cytokines tumor necrosis factor-alpha (TNF-α), interleukin-1 (IL-1), and IL-6 (Dinarello, 1994). Earlier reports of the CMNR (IOM, 1992, 1993b) helped to identify the possible part played by acute undernutrition in the immune compromise suffered by Special Forces troops and helped pave the way for initiatives in optimization and assessment of immune function in the field. In addition, the military maintains a special interest in the development of improved methods of immunization, particularly oral vaccines directed against gastrointestinal and respiratory pathogens. In this section, Lyle L. Moldawer and Gabriel Virella, Candace Enockson, and Mariano La Via review techniques for assessment of abnormal immune function (see Chapters 20 and 21, respectively, in this volume), while COL Arthur O. Anderson focuses on the development of vaccines targeted toward mucosal immune function (see Chapter 22 in this volume).

New Approaches to the Study of Abnormal Immune Function

In Chapters 20 and 21 in this volume, Lyle L. Moldawer and Gabriel Virella and coworkers identify parameters of abnormal immune function that are valid and can be measured reproducibly in the field. This identification is complicated by the complexity of the immune system and by uncertainty as to how much assays of circulating factors or immune cells truly reflect the physiological state of organs responsible for the initiation and sustainment of immune responses.

Evaluation of Humoral Immunity (Production of Antibodies)

While humoral immune responses are easy to measure, the concentrations of circulating or secreted antibodies at any given time correlate poorly with the ability to mount an immune response to antigen (Virella, 1993a, b). In addition, wide variability exists in both primary and secondary humoral responses to an antigen challenge. For example, Virella showed that administration of fish oil over an 18-wk period to healthy subjects resulted in a decrease in circulating immunoglobulins by the sixth week relative to subjects receiving olive oil; while levels of IgA and IgM returned to normal by the eighteenth week, IgG remained suppressed. The considerable intersubject variability of the data nearly obliterated the effect of the treatment; however, longitudinal measurements demonstrated significant effects.

Two additional measures of *in vivo* humoral immune response are described by Virella and coworkers. The measurement of a primary response, that is the response to an initial vaccination, can be confounded by prior exposure to the antigen. The alternative is to measure the secondary response to a booster vaccination. When subjects who were receiving supplements of fish or olive oil were challenged with tetanus toxoid booster, no difference was observed between the two groups in their ability to mount a response, although this type of immune assessment has been used in the past to evaluate the influence of nutritional status.

In vitro tests of humoral immune function (using isolated cells), in contrast, may not be sufficiently sensitive, require viable cells, and demand skilled personnel to perform them (Virella et al., 1991). Finally, the use of whole blood for immunoassays adds confounding factors, such as inhibitors (Virella et al., 1988).

Evaluation of Cell-Mediated Immune Functions

Monoclonal antibody and flow cytometry technology permit the identification of a large number of subpopulations of lymphocytes in blood, based on membrane marker phenotype (Del Prete et al., 1995; Elson et al., 1994). However, due to the lack of strong correlations between membrane markers and cell function (Rahelu et al., 1993; Smyth and Ortaldo, 1993) and to the variability in the subpopulations (Hughes et al., 1994), the significance of changes in the distribution of lymphocyte subpopulations in peripheral blood is unclear. Furthermore, it is likely that the most significant changes occur not in blood but in lymphoid tissues, so that sampling peripheral blood may be irrelevant. Finally, changes in immunocompetence have not been related clearly to any documented change in lymphocyte profile (Virella et al., 1991).

Assays of Circulating Cytokines and Soluble Receptors. Thus far, at least 15 interleukins, a larger number of immunoreactive cytokines, and 3 types of interferon have been characterized and can be measured by enzyme-linked immunoabsorption assay. Of these, TNF-α, IL-1, and IL-6 have been the focus of much attention, primarily because they appear to be produced initially in response to inflammatory challenge and in turn induce secondary inflammatory mediators, such as IL-8 and some of the macrophage inflammatory proteins (see Moldawer, Chapter 20 in this volume). Hence, they have been viewed as the most proximal mediators of inflammation. Secondly, as cytokines, TNF-α, IL-1, and IL-6 are pluripotent. They were first identified (in the 1970s) as the activity called leukocyte endogenous mediator, induced after inflammatory challenge. In addition, they are the primary mediators responsible for the induction of the proinflammatory response to infection (Dinarello, 1994; Fong et al., 1990b; Powanda and Beisel, 1982).

A problem with discussing these cytokines is their dual nature: they can have both beneficial and detrimental effects (Beisel, 1975; Dinarello and Wolff, 1993). Thus, the challenge, according to Moldawer (see Chapter 20 in this volume), is how to interpret measurements of these cytokines when it is not clear whether they are playing a beneficial or an adverse role. The central questions are: (1) What is the diagnostic value of blood or urinary measurements of these cytokines for identifying the presence and magnitude of an inflammatory response? and (2) Can blood or urinary measurements be used to make decisions regarding therapy or performance in a field setting?

Under experimental conditions, cytokines are induced in response to the injection of certain bacteria (Fong et al., 1990a; Michie et al., 1988). In contrast, changes in the plasma concentrations of these cytokines are often not seen in patients with most types of acute inflammation, that is, in those exhibiting an acute-phase response (Waage et al., 1989). A poor correlation has been observed between TNF-α levels in blood and burn-induced sepsis, and there is not a strong correlation with survival or mortality. The likelihood of detecting TNF-α in the blood of septic burn patients is only slightly greater than that in healthy controls, with a tendency for values to be higher in those who died (Marano et al., 1990). The relationship was even less strong for IL-1 (Marano et al., 1990). In contrast, IL-6 values were correlated highly with the presence of and mortality from systemic inflammatory response syndrome (Moscovitz et al., 1994). Thus, IL-6 may be a reliable indicator of the presence of infection, while IL-1 and TNF-α clearly are not.

The failure to observe infection-associated elevations in blood IL-1 and TNF-α levels is attributable to a number of factors. First, both IL-1 and TNF-α are secreted episodically (Beutler et al., 1986). Second, they both have short half-lives. These two characteristics alone would decrease the likelihood of reliably observing increases in the circulating plasma concentrations of the cytokines following infection (Beutler et al., 1986).

The third reason for failing to observe infection-associated increases in TNF-α and IL-1 is that there are factors in the blood that bind, inactivate, and inhibit the assay of these cytokines (Engelberts et al., 1991). These binding factors consist primarily of receptors that are proteolytically cleaved from the cell membrane during inflammation but which bind to the TNF-α and IL-1 in circulation, preventing them from binding to functional receptors or to antibodies (Engelberts et al., 1991; Moldawer, 1994). Concentrations of these shed receptors as well as that of another circulating inhibitor, IL-1 receptor antagonist, may provide an indirect estimate of the presence and intensity of inflammation (Moldawer, 1994; Van Zee et al., 1992).

Finally, the primarily paracrine production of these cytokines (that is, the synthesis and secretion of these locally acting substances into the intercellular spaces of adjacent cells) (Suter et al., 1992) can account for the inability to observe a correlation between circulating TNF-α and IL-1 and the degree of infection since any of the cytokine that appears in the blood probably represents spillover from some paracrine compartment or direct production in plasma by immune cells in the blood (Suter et al., 1992). Data from several groups (Suter et al., 1992; Personal communication, G. Schultz and L. M. Moldawer, University of Florida, Gainesville, 1995) support the role of compartmentalization in controlling circulating levels of TNF-α. Concentrations of TNF-α in wound sites of patients with nonhealing wounds and in bronchioalveolar lavage of patients with acute respiratory distress syndrome were elevated significantly over values observed in healing wounds or in the circulation, respectively. The same pattern was observed for IL-1 (Colotta et al., 1993).

Field Measurements of Cytokines. The difficulty of collecting blood samples in the field necessitates validating the use of urinary cytokine values as a reflection of those in blood (or tissue). Because many of the cytokine inhibitors were originally identified and purified from urine, it is clear that they are present in urine (Prieur et al., 1987; Seckinger et al., 1987a, b, 1988), although urinary levels tend to be lower than those in blood (see Virella et al., Chapter 21 in this volume). As for the cytokines themselves, increases in both circulating concentrations and urinary production of IL-6 and TNF-α have been observed in conditioned athletes after a 20-km run, consistent with a nonspecific inflammatory response (Sprenger et al., 1992). The increases observed in urinary excretion were markedly greater than those in blood (Sprenger et al., 1992). In contrast to the conditioned athletes, normal volunteers and unconditioned athletes had no IL-6 excreted in their urine. Hence, urinary IL-6 excretion appears to respond to an inflammatory challenge, suggesting that elevated urinary IL-6 measurements could be detected in samples collected in the field. Consideration must be given, however, to any factors that might alter urinary output and concentration (renal function and hydration status), and data must be expressed relative to osmolarity or some other parameter (such as creatinine) that reflects changes in urinary volume. Furthermore, the questions that remain to be answered regarding the correlation between levels of circulating cytokines and immune status and the relevance of circulating lymphokines relative to their concentration in lymphoid tissues must be answered for urinary cytokine levels as well.

One application of cytokine measurements that is of potential interest to the military has been an attempt to determine if weight loss during spaceflight is related to a nonspecific inflammatory response. Data suggest that the psychological stress of spaceflight and adjustment to the decrease in gravitational force may induce a proinflammatory cytokine response, which is followed by a secondary (postflight) response during readjustment to normal gravitation (Stein and Schluter, 1994).

In Vitro *Assays of Lymphocyte Function*

In vitro assays of lymphocyte function can be performed in a variety of ways (for example, by measurement of incorporation of labeled DNA precursors or release of cytokines) and may provide a better reflection of immune status. The disadvantage of *in vitro* assays, according to Virella and coworkers (see Chapter 21 in this volume), is their requirement for freshly isolated cells.

Mitogenic assays (*in vitro*), in which the proliferation of lymphocytes in response to a known irritant is measured, are the classic test of lymphocyte responsiveness (see Virella et al., Chapter 21 in this volume). These assays are typically performed on monocytes and have the disadvantage of requiring the use of radioactivity (^{3}H-thymidine) or other expensive techniques. Furthermore, the assays are difficult to reproduce and are relatively insensitive. Recently, the trend has shifted to looking at more physiologically relevant end points, such as the release of one of the interleukins, IL-2. Because IL-2 release is often decreased even when mitogenic indices are normal or elevated, IL-2 release may be a sensitive index of regulatory abnormalities affecting initial stages of T-helper cell proliferation (Virella et al., 1993). IL-2 receptor (CD25) expression in response to mitogenic stimulation also is considered a useful end point in studies of the effect of stress on the immune system (La Via et al., 1996). However, the method requires access to a large number of flow cytometers to handle large numbers of samples in a short time.

Functional assays for helper or suppressor T-cell activity and cytotoxicity assays are complex, difficult to standardize, and rarely performed, according to Virella (Personal communication, Medical University of South Carolina, Charleston, 1997). Such techniques have given way to cytokine production assays (for example, assay of IL-10 as an indication of suppressor activity) on cells sorted by flow cytometry. The measurement of natural killer cell activity is not performed as its functional significance is unclear at this time.

Phagocytic Cell Assays

Phagocytic cell assays are usually carried out with polymorphonuclear leukocytes, but functional abnormalities involving phagocytes are rare compared to granulocytopenias in patients with less dramatic problems than severe trauma, such as burns and severe malnutrition (Virella, 1993b). These assays also require trained personnel, sophisticated equipment, and fresh cells and are difficult to perform on large numbers of individuals.

New Techniques for Producing Immunity via Oral Immunization

In Chapter 22, COL Arthur O. Anderson discusses several technical advances that have begun to influence the production of vaccines, in particular those targeted at enteric diseases, such as that produced by the biological warfare agent *Vibrio cholerae*. Because the effects of exposure to infectious agents and toxins can significantly impair the function of the military, safe and effective immunization becomes a major prerequisite of readiness.

The ability to immunize troops against the types of agents that they are likely to contact is influenced by many factors. The route of entry into the body for many pathogens is the gastrointestinal (GI) tract, respiratory tract, or epithelial lining of the reproductive tract. The mucosal immune system provides the first line of defense against most pathogens and the only one against agents such as cholera.

Stimulation of the mucosal immune system leads to the production of tetrameric secretory immunoglobulin A (Ma et al., 1995). In mammals, 75 percent of synthesized immunoglobulin is IgA, and two different types of cells are required for its synthesis and assembly (Mostov, 1994).

Whereas parenterally administered (injected) vaccines stimulate peripheral immunity but have very little effect on the mucosal immune system, oral vaccines tend to be relatively ineffective in stimulating peripheral immunity (a phenomenon referred to by Anderson as cross-regulation) (Koster and Pierce, 1983). Efforts to develop and administer oral vaccines against enteric agents have been hampered by the apparent need to use particulate antigens, such as live or killed intact microorganisms, and the ability of the GI tract to inactivate polypeptide antigens or to induce an immunologic tolerance (analogous to the process by which the GI tract is prevented from mounting an immunologic response to the antigens in food) (Chen et al., 1995). As outlined below, several lines of research have sought to overcome these problems by using different approaches.

Production of Recombinant Bacterial Antigen for Oral Immunization

Cholera bacteria (encountered as a biological warfare agent) and entero-toxigenic *E. coli* multiply in the small intestine, producing enterotoxins that bind to a glycoprotein, G_{M1} ganglioside, on the surface of the epithelial cells that form the lining of the GI tract, thus exerting a pharmacological (ADP-ribosylation) effect that results in massive hypersecretion of intracellular fluid (Sack, 1980; Sixma et al., 1991). Both cholera toxin (CT) and the heat-labile enterotoxin (LT) of *E. coli* consist of six subunits, one nonbinding but toxic A subunit and a pentamer of G_{M1}-binding but nontoxic B subunits (Sixma et al., 1991). Attempts to develop vaccines against these pathogens have utilized the B subunit because antibodies against the B subunit block the ability of the toxin to bind to cells (Clemens et al., 1990; Peltola et al., 1991). Utilizing an *Agrobacterium*-mediated plant transfection system, Arntzen and coworkers (Haq et al., 1995) constructed expression vectors containing the gene for the LT-B subunit and transfected tobacco and potato plants. Mice administered extracts of soluble tobacco leaf protein or potato tuber protein by gavage developed both serum and gut mucosal LT-B antibodies that inactivated the toxin *in vitro*. Oral immunity was conferred upon mice fed fresh transgenic potato tubers that expressed the B subunit.

Thus, the plant material provides both the expression and delivery systems, eliminating the need for trained medical personnel to administer the vaccine (Haq et al., 1995; see Anderson, Chapter 22 in this volume). Because the vaccine can be fed as part of a meal, deployment need not be delayed to allow for immunization of troops. Finally, the use of plant systems for the expression of heterologous genes (those not native to the species) permits almost limitless production of vaccine and may represent an economically feasible alternative use for the tobacco that is now grown for cigarettes (Haq et al., 1995).

Use of Enterotoxins as Vaccine Carriers and Adjuvants

As has been described, the binding subunits of enterotoxins such as CT and LT are potent antigens for both mucosal IgA production and peripheral IgG production, regardless of route of administration. Coadministration of a relatively weak antigen of interest with CT, or conjugation of the antigen with CT subunit B (CTB), enables the CT to function in an adjuvant capacity to promote the formation of antibodies to the weaker antigen (Elson and Dertzbaugh, 1994). Because conjugation of antigen to CTB can damage the tertiary structure, decreasing its adjuvant effect, efforts have been under way to utilize recombinant techniques to fuse antigenic constructs to the A subunit (Dickinson and Clements, 1995; Hajishengallis et al., 1995).

Use of Transgenic Plants to Generate Antibodies for Passive Immunotherapy

The ability to produce unlimited quantities of antigen-specific secretory antibodies would make it possible to induce passive mucosal immunity to a variety of organisms. Whereas two types of cells are required to synthesize and assemble secretory IgAs in mammals, researchers have demonstrated the ability to generate assembled, functional antibodies to a cell surface adhesion molecule of *Streptococcus mutans* (the bacteria responsible for tooth decay) in single cells of transgenic plants (Ma et al., 1995). By introducing the genes encoding each subunit of the immunoglobulin molecule into separate transgenic tobacco plants and performing the appropriate Mendelian crosses, plants synthesizing fully assembled, secretory IgA-G hybrid antibodies have been obtained. A product containing these antibodies in a toothpaste is undergoing testing.

Use of Polymerase Chain Reaction for Identification and Cloning of Antibodies

Unfortunately, the desire to produce an antibody in large quantities does not always have the advantage of a preexisting monoclonal antibody. The antibody molecule is composed of two pairs of polypeptide chains: one pair of light (low molecular weight) chains and one pair of heavy chains, all linked by disulfide bonds. The amino acid sequences of both light and heavy chains consist of alternating regions of variable and constant sequences. According to Anderson, the specificity of an antibody for its antigen is conferred by an area of the variable region known as the complementarity determining region (CDR). Following *in vivo* exposure to an antigen, clones of B-cells expressing specific antibodies undergo a process of "affinity maturation" in which single base pair mutations occur in the DNA of the CDRs, resulting in higher affinity of the antibodies for their antigens. Immunoelectrophoresis on frozen tissue slices and polymerase chain reaction amplification of the CDRs in cells that display high-affinity binding permits the identification and cloning of sequences responsible for that binding (Jacob et al., 1991, 1993; Marks et al., 1991). Following insertion of the sequences into heavy-chain variable regions, large-scale antibody production can occur using the recombinant plant system.

Microencapsulation of Antigens and Antibodies

Microencapsulation technology, first developed for delivery of pharmaceutical agents, has now been applied to the delivery of vaccines (Michalek et al., 1994). Administration of microencapsulated vaccines using polymers of lactic and glycolic acids confers several advantages, including the ability to protect the antigen from degradation in the GI tract (resulting in the need for less antigen); the ability to administer antigen in a timed-release manner; the adjuvant effect of the microencapsulation material itself, which boosts antibody production; and the ability of microparticles, when administered in a range of sizes, to undergo size-based migration to both mucosal and peripheral immune tissues and to induce both mucosal and peripheral immunity (Eldridge et al., 1990).

Summary

Assessment of Immune Function

A convincing rationale must exist to support the study of any given parameter of immune function. The choice of adequate end points is difficult because of the complexity of the immune response. Furthermore, the choice must be based on the availability and reproducibility of techniques.

Longitudinal studies of serum IgG concentrations, measurement of humoral responses to vaccines or boosters, and the determination of serum or urinary concentrations of select cytokines involved in inflammatory and immunoregulatory processes are parameters that are relatively easy to obtain and whose measurement can be supported by currently available basic and clinical research data. According to Moldawer (see Chapter 20 in this volume), plasma and urine levels of TNF-α and IL-1 are not reliable indicators of inflammation. Increased concentrations of the shed TNF-receptors and IL-1 receptor antagonists, however, are generally indicative of a local inflammatory response and may be used with caution as indicators of local TNF-α and IL-1 production.

Plasma and urinary IL-6 levels are elevated in a large number of inflammatory processes and seem to correlate with physiological parameters. Plasma and urinary measures of IL-6 receptor antagonist and shed TNF-receptors can be used to detect the presence of inflammation and metabolic stress.

Several of the *in vitro* functional assays, such as IL-2 release, IL-2 receptor (CD25) synthesis, or immunoglobulin synthesis in response to mitogenic stimulation appear to have the potential to reveal immunoregulatory abnormalities when other parameters (particularly cytokine concentrations in blood) appear normal. While such assays require freshly isolated cells, precluding collection of samples in the field, experiments could be designed around training exercises.

Techniques were described that have been applied successfully to assess the influence on immune response of factors such as dietary alteration, heavy exercise, emotional stress, surgical trauma, and other physical trauma, all of which are encountered in the military situation. The ability to obtain useful information is dependent on careful experimental design, elimination of as many variables as possible, taking into consideration the types of samples that can be obtained in the field, and, if possible, designing assessments around field exercises so that a wider variety of sample types can be obtained in a laboratory setting.

Techniques for Oral Vaccine Production

The gastrointestinal mucosa is the target for a significant number of pathogens that are encountered in the military situation and are directly or indirectly responsible for altered nutritional status. An increased understanding of mucosal immunology combined with progress in the fields of biotechnology and molecular genetics have led to a better understanding of how to optimize vaccine administration as well as significant advances in the production of antibodies and antigens for use as oral vaccines. These include the use of recombinant techniques to produce bacterial antigens for use as vaccines and antibodies for passive immunotherapy, both of which can be delivered in edible form. In addition, the polymerase chain reaction technique permits identification and amplification of antibodies. New encapsulation technologies permit the delivery of reduced doses of oral vaccines by protecting them from destruction in the GI tract and enable targeting of the vaccines to the mucosal or peripheral immune system.

FUNCTIONAL AND BEHAVIORAL MEASURES
OF NUTRITIONAL STATUS

In this section, James S. Hayes describes the use of involuntary muscle contraction to assess nutrition status, while Mary Z. Mays as well as Harris R. Lieberman and Bryan P. Coffey focus on cognitive assessment in the military (see Chapters 23, 24, and 25 in this volume). Summaries of the presentation by David F. Dinges on sleep and circadian rhythms and chapter by Ginger S. Watson and Yiannis E. Papelis on the use of simulators follow (see Chapter 26 in this volume).

Involuntary Muscle Contraction to Assess Nutritional Status

Skeletal muscle function has been studied by measuring both handgrip strength (voluntary contraction) and the response to electrical stimulation of the branch of the ulnar nerve that innervates the adductor pollicis (thumb) muscle (involuntary contraction). The use of the latter technique, referred to as muscle function analysis (MFA), to assess nutritional status is described by James S. Hayes (see Chapter 23 in this volume). According to Hayes, MFA has the advantage of being less susceptible to subject motivation than the measurement of voluntary contraction and, therefore, may be more sensitive and reliable. The stimulus is applied at various frequencies, and the pattern of involuntary contractions is measured and recorded. Although the basic technique was developed in 1954 (Merton, 1954), computerized data collection and analysis methods recently have been coupled to the MFA technique, making it much easier to apply.

The MFA response is thought to be associated with the nutritional status of the individual who is being assessed. There is some correlation between MFA results and total-body protein measurement; as the latter decreases, MFA relaxation rates also decrease (Brough et al., 1986; Russell et al., 1983a, b). The developers, therefore, contend that lower MFA relaxation rates indicate malnutrition or some other abnormality.

The advantages of MFA, according to Hayes, are its noninvasiveness and apparent sensitivity to early changes in muscle function due to malnutrition or to refeeding, the immediate availability of results, and the low cost of both the equipment and test administration.

The disadvantages, according to Hayes, include the difficulty of locating the ulnar nerve; discomfort; the size of the equipment; and the other mechanisms, such as voluntary muscle control and sodium potassium pump activity, that may influence the results. Therefore, the validity of the concept needs further testing.

In Chapter 23 of this report, Hayes describes studies currently under way on MFA. These include examining the ability of MFA to detect and monitor the nutritional status of HIV patients during nutritional intervention and throughout the course of the illness, evaluating the optimum type of protein supplement for trauma patients and the ability of nutritional support to improve the outcome and survival of renal dialysis patients, and determining the ability of MFA to assist in monitoring malnourished hospital inpatients. Because the results of such studies are as yet unavailable, the validity of the technique cannot be assessed.

Application of Cognitive Performance Assessment Technology to Military Nutrition Research

The field of military nutrition is based on the premise that readiness, hence physical and cognitive performance, are dependent, in part, on the nutritional state of soldiers. While it is known that cognitive performance in the military setting is influenced by nutrition (Consolazio et al., 1967, 1968; Johnson and Sauberlich, 1982; Johnson et al., 1971), the extent of this influence is not well understood. Traditionally, according to Mary Z. Mays (Chapter 24 in this volume), the Army's interest in the influence of nutrition on cognitive function has focused on three specific issues: food deprivation in the field, underconsumption of rations, and identification of performance-optimizing ration components. The lack of information concerning the role of nutrition in cognitive function is, in large part, the result of limitations in assessment technology. Assessments of cognitive performance attempt to identify and quantify measurable end points of complex intellectual behaviors. According to Mays, cognitive assessment has been accomplished largely through the use of one of three methods: observation of behavior, paper-and-pencil tests (or their computer counterpart), and tests of manual dexterity or hand-eye coordination (as part of a battery of tests). Increasingly, such tests have been replaced by assessment technologies that make use of computer games or performance tracking devices built into actual or simulated vehicles or other machinery.

As reviewed by Harris R. Lieberman and Bryan P. Coffey (see Chapter 25 in this volume), the measurement of cognitive performance in humans is associated with many problems. First, data collected using formal laboratory behavior tests may be difficult to relate to real-world performance. Second, circadian variation in performance occurs (Moore-Ede et al., 1982) and may overwhelm any differences caused by the nutritional alterations. Third, the underlying behavioral function that the performance test actually is assessing may be unclear, so it cannot be assumed that the limiting or critical factor being assessed can always be accurately defined. Finally, it may be difficult to identify the optimal test to evaluate the behavior of interest, so as to avoid the possibility of failing to detect treatment effects, especially when the effects of the manipulations are expected to be modest (which is the case for nutritional interventions).

The military's assessment of cognitive performance is of great importance, given the complexity of weaponry and the high level of performance and vigilance that is required under difficult working conditions. This assessment is further complicated, however, by a number of factors unique to the military situation. First, the desire to conduct testing in field settings limits the types of tests that are feasible. Field testing usually requires that subjects stop their ongoing activities to participate in the task, which is a particular problem if subjects are engaged in training exercises or actual operations. Studies performed in the field must be designed to be minimally intrusive on soldiers' time (see Lieberman and Coffey, Chapter 25 in this volume), and the tests used must be reliable under field conditions. Second, cognitive assessments of military personnel must employ tests that are psychometrically valid substitutions for critical military functions or tasks (see Mays, Chapter 24 in this volume). Third, because the primary nutritional deficits soldiers experience are likely to be the acute lack of energy intake, cognitive assessment must be extremely sensitive to any subtle performance decrement that may result. Fourth, the effects of battle stress , as well as boredom and frustration with the assessment task, can result in a decrease in the reliability of data collected. Finally, the process of identifying nutrients that will enhance performance in the field requires carefully controlled, clinical, dose-response evaluation that is best performed in a laboratory setting.

Technical Advances in Cognitive Performance Assessment

Computers and Miniaturization

Mays suggests that while the basic methods of cognitive assessment are unlikely to change significantly in the next 20 years, advances in computer software and hardware along with miniaturization should increase the ability of researchers to assess cognitive function in the field. The use of handheld computerized devices would decrease the invasiveness of performance assessment by permitting remote data collection and would allow repeated measures.

Lieberman and Coffey describe two electronic activity-monitoring devices designed to be worn on the wrist. The Motionlogger Actigraph, a commercially designed device, monitors sleeping and waking activity using a piezoelectric motion detector. Data collected by the monitor are downloaded to a computer that uses an algorithm validated to calculate sleeping and waking time. While the Actigraph does not provide as much information as polysomnography and cannot assess performance *per se*, it provides continuous assessment of physical activity behavior, which can be related to the physical and mental state (Lieberman et al., 1989; Tryon, 1991).

The Vigilance Monitor, developed at USARIEM, combines the measurement capabilities and characteristics of the Actigraph with vigilance assessment and intervention capability. Vigilance reflects the ability to process relevant information and to respond in a timely fashion (Koelega, 1989). Vigilance has been found to be sensitive to the effect of diet (for example, caloric restriction and caffeine intake), as well as a number of other factors (Clubley et al., 1979; Green et al., 1994; Lieberman, 1992). According to Lieberman and Coffey, the Vigilance Monitor functions by presenting an audible tone to the wearer and measuring response time. By repeating the stimulus presentation randomly and intermittently, vigilance is monitored on a more or less continuous basis. The Vigilance Monitor also is configured to collect data about environmental variables, such as air temperature, sound, and duration and amplitude of light exposure of the subject so that an attempt can be made to correlate the level of vigilance with these variables. The Vigilance Monitor has a number of advantages over traditional methods of cognitive assessment. These include its unobtrusiveness (it enables the wearer to continue with most activities while being monitored), its ability to be programmed to provide data on several variables concurrently, and its ability to monitor a number of subjects simultaneously over the course of many days. The device also has the novel attribute, although not yet validated in the field, of being able to maintain alertness in the wearer by functioning as an alarm. Finally, the cost of the monitor is relatively low, once the appropriate computer capabilities have been developed and implemented.

A similar method of psychomotor vigilance testing that utilizes a handheld device (the "psychomotor vigilance task") was described in a presentation by David F. Dinges (see Kribbs and Dinges, 1994). To perform this test, the subject is instructed to push a button on the device in response to the appearance of a light in the display window. The advantages of the test include its ability to test subjects of all intelligence levels on a basic cognitive skill (alertness or attention) that is required for almost all other cognitive functions, the absence of a learning curve for the task (which is known to confound much of the published data on cognitive performance [Dinges and Kribbs, 1991]), and high validity and reliability. The test utilizes an instrument that is portable and completely programmable with respect to interstimulus interval, auditory and visual feedback, and signal load rate. The use of a visual stimulus rather than sound is based on the finding that while auditory response time is faster than visual, visual response time is affected more quickly by fatigue (Dinges, 1992). The performance parameters (types of errors) that can be measured with the vigilance task include false starts, lapses (a long reaction time or a sudden period of nonresponse), decline in the optimal response capacity (response slowing), false response, and accelerated habituation (increase in the number of lapses with length of time on the task) (Dinges and Powell, 1985). Fatigue produces an increase in lapses and a decrease in the minimal ("best") response time, consistent with observations from traditional cognitive performance tests that, given the opportunity, people slow down to maintain accuracy (Dinges, 1992).

Improvement in Interface Technology

According to Mays, the design of natural interfaces will improve in the near future, permitting the use of identical assessment tools in the laboratory and in the field with no special training. One example of this may be the Iowa Driving Simulator (IDS), described in Chapter 26 in this volume by Ginger S. Watson and Yiannis E. Papelis, which also takes advantage of advances in computational methods to create a high-fidelity computational vehicle model set in a fully interactive, virtual environment. The IDS provides the subject with realistic motion and visual, auditory, and force feedback cues to simulate a wide range of driving conditions and scenarios (Kuhl et al., 1995). Thus far, military applications of the IDS have been limited to the development of a "virtual proving ground" that closely matches test courses at the Aberdeen Proving Ground, Maryland, for the design and testing of new Army vehicle prototypes (one simulator has been made to resemble the internal appearance and behavior of a high mobility multipurpose vehicle). Use of the IDS for research purposes is somewhat limited by the need for different degrees and types of fidelity for different performance measures (Alessi and Watson, 1994). In order for data to be valid, subjects must perceive that the experience is real and respond in a real way, and their perception must persist over time, with the novelty factor being eliminated or overcome. Research that has utilized the IDS has tended, thus far, to measure the effects of factors such as age, gender, and visual impairment on reaction time (Romano and Watson, 1994). To date, no studies have examined the effects of nutritional variables, and only one student-run study has examined the influence of sleep deprivation.

Summary

While there is evidence that cognitive performance is influenced by nutritional status, there are many problems associated with trying to evaluate this influence, particularly in the field. Two types of portable monitors have been described for the assessment of vigilance, one aspect of cognitive performance that is highly relevant to field situations. A third device, the IDS, was described that measures the multiple cognitive functions associated with driving. Each of these techniques can be used to assess the influence of some nutritional stimulus or change in status, but all await further validation.

The CMNR's overview and summary of emerging technologies for nutrition research set the stage for responding to the questions posed by the Army. The committee's responses, as well as its conclusions and recommendations, are presented in the next chapter.

REFERENCES

Alessi, S.M., and G.S. Watson
  1994   Driving Simulation Research at The University of Iowa. Proceedings of the 1994 Annual Meeting of the Association for the Development of Computer-Based Instructional Systems. 16–20 February 1994, Nashville, Tenn.
AR (Army Regulation) 600-9
  1986   *See* U.S. Department of the Army, 1986.

Baker, D., and K.H. Norris
   1985   Near-infrared reflectance measurement of total sugar content of breakfast cereals. Appl. Spec. 39(4):618–621.
Ballor, D.L., and V.L. Katch
   1989   Validity of anthropometric regression equations for predicting changes in body fat of obese females. Am. J. Hum. Biol. 1:97–101.
Beebe, K.R., and B.R. Kowalske
   1987   An introduction to multivariate calibration and analysis. Anal. Chem. 59:1007a–1017a.
Beisel, W.R.
   1975   Metabolic response to infection. Annu. Rev. Med. 26:9–20.
   1980   Endogenous pyrogen physiology. Physiologist 23:38–42.
Beutler, B., N. Krochin, I.W. Milsark, C. Luedke, and A. Cerami
   1986   Control of cachectin (tumor necrosis factor) synthesis: Mechanisms of endotoxin resistance. Science 232:977–980.
Biolo, G., R.Y.D. Fleming, and R.R. Wolfe
   1995   Physiologic hyperinsulinemia stimulates protein synthesis and enhances transport of selected amino acids in human skeletal muscle. J. Clin. Invest. 95:811–819.
Blair, S.N., H.W. Kohl, N.F. Gordon, and R.S. Paffenbarger, Jr.
   1992   How much physical activity is good for health? Annu. Rev. Public Health 13:99–126.
Brough, W., G. Horne, A. Blout, M.H. Irving, and K.N. Jeejeebhoy
   1986   Effects of nutrient intake, surgery, sepsis, and long-term administration of steroids on muscle function. Br. J. Med. 293:983–988.
Carney, J.M., W. Landrum, L. Mayes, Y. Zou, and R.A. Lodder
   1993   Near-infrared spectrophotometric monitoring of stroke-related changes in the protein and lipid composition of whole gerbil brains. Anal. Chem. 65(10):1305–1313.
Chen, Y., J. Inobe, R. Marks, P. Gonnella, V.K. Kuchroo, and H.L. Weiner
   1995   Peripheral deletion of antigen-reactive T-cells in oral tolerance. Nature 376:177–189.
Chumlea, W.C., S.S. Guo, D.B. Cockram, and R.M. Siervogel
   1996   Mechanical and physiologic modifiers and bioelectrical impedance spectrum determinants of body composition. Am. J. Clin. Nutr. 64 (suppl.):413S–422S.
Clemens, J.D., D.A. Sack, J.R. Harris, F. Van Loon, J. Chakraborty, F. Ahmed, M.R. Rao, M.R. Kahn, M. Yunus, N. Huda et al.
   1990   Field trial of oral cholera vaccines in Bangladesh: Results from three-year follow-up. Lancet 335(8684):270–273.
Clubley, M., C.E. Bye, T.A. Henson, A.W. Peck, and C.J. Riddington
   1979   Effects of caffeine and cyclizine alone and in combination on human performance, subjective effects and EEG activity. Br. J. Clin. Pharmacol. 7:157–163.
Cole, T.J., and W.A. Coward
   1992   Precision and accuracy of doubly labeled water energy expenditure by multipoint and two-point methods. Am. J. Physiol. 263 (26):E965–E973.
Colotta, F., F. Re, M. Muzio, R. Bertini, N. Polentarutti, M. Sironi, J.G. Giri, S.K. Dower, J.E. Sims, and A. Mantovani
   1993   Interleukin-1 type II receptor: A decoy target for IL-1 that is regulated by IL-4. Science 261:472–475.
Consolazio, C.F., L.O. Matoush, H.L. Johnson, R.A. Nelson, and H.J. Krzywicki
   1967   Metabolic aspects of acute starvation in normal humans (10 days). Am. J. Clin. Nutr. 20:672–683.

Consolazio, C.F., L.O. Matoush, H.L. Johnson, H.J. Krzywicki, G.J. Isaac, and N.F. Witt
  1968   Metabolic aspects of calorie restriction: Hypohydration effects on body weight and blood parameters. Am. J. Clin. Nutr. 21:793–802.
Cousins, R.J.
  1994   Metal elements and gene expression. Annu. Rev. Nutr. 14:449–469.
  1995   Trace element micronutrients. Pp. 898–901 in Molecular Biology and Biotechnology: A Comprehensive Desk Reference, R.A. Meyers, ed. New York: VCH Publishers.
Coward, A.
  1990   The doubly labeled water method for measuring energy expenditure. Technical recommendations for use in humans. Calculation of pool sizes and flux rates. Pp. 48–68 in NAHRES-4, A Consensus Report by the IDECG Working Group, A.M. Prentice, ed. Vienna: IAEA.
Coward ,W.A., P. Ritz, and T.J. Cole
  1994   Revision of calculations in the doubly labeled water method for measurement of energy expenditure in humans. Am. J. Physiol. 267 (30):E805–E807.
Dansgaard, W.
  1964   Stable isotopes in precipitation. Tellus 16:436–468.
Dawid, I.B., R. Toyama, and M. Taira
  1995   LIM domain proteins. C. R. Acad. Sci. Paris 318:295–306.
DeLany, J.P., D.A. Schoeller, R.W. Hoyt, E.W. Askew, and M.A. Sharp
  1989   Field use of $D_2{}^{18}O$ to measure energy expenditure of soldiers at different energy intakes. J. Appl. Physiol. 67(5):1922–1929.
Del Prete, G., M. De Carli, F. Almerigogna, C.K. Daniel, M.M. D'Elios, G. Zancuoghi, F. Vinante, G. Pizzolo, and S. Romagnani
  1995   Preferential expression of CD30 by human CD4+ T-cells producing Th2-type cytokines. FASEB J. 9:81–86.
Despres, J-P., D. Prud'homme, M-C. Pouliot, A. Tremblay, and C. Bouchard
  1991   Estimation of deep abdominal adipose-tissue accumulation from simple anthropometric measurements in men. Am. J. Clin. Nutr. 54:471–477.
Dickinson, B.L., and J.D. Clements
  1995   Dissociation of *Escherichia coli* heat-labile enterotoxin adjuvanticity from ADP-ribosyltranserase activity. Infect. Immun. 63(5):1617–1623.
Dinarello, C.A.
  1994   The biological properties of interleukin-1. Eur. Cytokine Netw. 5:517–531.
Dinarello, C.A., and S.M. Wolff
  1993   The role of interleukin-1 in disease. N. Engl. J. Med. 326:106–113.
Dinges, D.F.
  1992   Probing the limits of functional capability: The effects of sleep loss on short-duration tasks. Pp. 176–188 Sleep, Arousal and Performance, R.J. Broughton and R. Ogilvie, eds. Cambridge, Mass.: Birkhauser-Boston, Inc.
Dinges, D.F., and N.B. Kribbs
  1991   Performing while sleepy: Effects of experimentally induced sleepiness. Pp. 97–128 in Sleep, Sleepiness, and Performance, T.H. Monk, ed. New York: John Wiley & Sons, Ltd.
Dinges, D.F., and J.W. Powell
  1985   Microcomputer analyses of performance on a portable, simple visual RT task during sustained operations. Behav. Res. Meth. Instr. Comput. 17:652–655.
Edwards, J.S.A., E.W. Askew, N. King, C.S. Fulco, R.W. Hoyt, and J.P. DeLany
  1991   An assessment of the nutritional intake and energy expenditure of unacclimatized U.S. Army soldiers living and working at high altitude. Technical Report No. T10-91. Natick, Mass.: U.S. Army Research Institute of Environmental Medicine.

Eldridge, J.H., C.J. Hammond, J.A. Meulbroek, J.K. Staas, R.M. Gilley, and T.R. Tice
    1990   Controlled vaccine release in the gut-associated lymphoid tissues. I. Orally administered biodegradable microspheres target the Peyer's patches. Journal of Controlled Release 11:205–214.

Elson, C.O., and M.T. Dertzbaugh
    1994   Mucosal adjuvants. Pp. 391–401 in Handbook of Mucosal Immunology, P.L. Orga, J. Mestecky, M.E. Lamm, W. Strober, J.R. McGhee, and J. Bienestock, eds. New York: Academic Press, Inc.

Elson, L.H., S. Shaw, R.A. Van Liwer, and T.B. Nutman
    1994   T-cell subpopulation phenotypes in filarial infections: CD27 negativity defines a population greatly enriched for Th2 cells. Int. Immunol. 6:1003–1009.

Engelberts, I., S. Stephens, G.J. Francot, C.J. van der Linden, and W.A. Buurman
    1991   Evidence for different effects of soluble TNF-receptors on various TNF measurements in human biological fluids [letter; comment]. Lancet 338:515–516.

Essen, P., M.A. McNurlan, J. Wernerman, E. Vinnars, and P.J. Garlick
    1992   Uncomplicated surgery, but not general anesthesia, decreases muscle protein synthesis. Am. J. Physiol. 262:E253–E260.

Evans, D.J., R.G. Hoffmann, R.K. Kalkhoff, and A.H. Kissebah
    1983   Relationship of androgenic activity to body fat topography, fat cell morphology, and metabolic aberrations in premenopausal women. J. Clin. Endocrinol. Metab. 57:304–310.

Faris, F., M. Doyle, Y. Wickramasinghe, R. Houston, P. Rolfe, and S. O'Brien
    1994   A non-invasive optical technique for intrapartum fetal monitoring: Preliminary clinical studies. Med. Eng. Phys. 16(4):287–291.

Fishman, E.K.
    1994   Spiral imaging methods assure survival of CT. Diagn. Imaging. (November): 59–67.

Fitzgerald, P.I., J.A. Vogel, W.L. Daniels, J.E. Dziados, M.A. Teves, R.P. Mello, and P.J. Reich
    1986   The Body Composition Project: A summary report and descriptive data. Technical Report T5-87. Natick, Mass.: U.S. Army Research Institute of Environmental Medicine.

Fong, Y.M., M.A. Marano, L.L. Moldawer, H. Wei, S.E. Calvano, J.S. Kenney, A.C. Allison, A. Cerami, G.T. Shires, and S.F. Lowry
    1990a   The acute splanchnic and peripheral tissue metabolic response to endotoxin in humans. J. Clin. Invest. 85:1896–1904.

Fong, Y., L.L. Moldawer, G.T. Shires, and S.F. Lowry
    1990b   The biologic characteristics of cytokines and their implication in surgical injury. Surg. Gynecol. Obstet. 170:363–378.

Forbes, G.B., W. Simon, and J.M. Amatruda
    1992   Is bioimpedance a good predictor of body composition change? Am. J. Clin. Nutr. 56:4–6.

Forman, B.M., E. Goode, J. Chen, A.E. Oro, D.J. Bradley, T. Perlmann, D.J. Noonan, and L.T. Burka
    1995   Identification of a nuclear receptor that is activated by farnesol metabolites. Cell 81:687–693.

Formica, C., M.G. Atkinson, I. Nyulasi, J. McKay, W. Heale, and E. Seeman
    1993   Body composition following hemodialysis: Studies using dual-energy x-ray absorptiometry and bioelectrical impedance analysis. Osteoporos. Int. 3:192–197.

Friedl, K.E.
  1992　Body composition and military performance: Origins of the Army standards. Pp. 31–55 in Body Composition and Physical Performance, Applications for the Military Services, B.M. Marriott and J. Grumstrup-Scott, eds. A report of the Committee on Military Nutrition Research, Food and Nutrition Board, Institute of Medicine. Washington D.C.: National Academy Press.

Friedl, K.E., and J.A. Vogel
  1992　Looking for a few good generalized body-fat equations. Am. J. Clin. Nutr. 53: 795–796.

Friedl, K.E., R.J. Moore, L.E. Martinez-Lopez, J.A. Vogel, E.W. Askew, L.J. Marchitelli, R.W. Hoyt, and C.C. Gordon
  1994a　Lower limits of body fat in healthy active men. J. Appl. Physiol. 77:933–940.

Friedl, K.E., K.A. Westphal, L.J. Marchitelli, and J.F. Patton
  1994b　Effect of fat patterning on body composition changes in young women during U.S. Army basic training [abstract]. Int. J. Obes. 18(suppl. 2):69.

Fulco, C.S., R.W. Hoyt, C.J. Baker-Fulco, J. Gonzalez, and A. Cymerman
  1992　Use of bioelectrical impedance to assess body composition changes at high altitude. J. Appl. Physiol. 72:2181–2187.

Gadian, D.G.
  1982　Nuclear Magnetic Resonance and Its Application to Living Systems. New York: Oxford University Press.

Goldstein, J.L., and M.S. Brown
  1990　Regulation of the mevalonate pathway. Nature 343:425–430.

Green, M.W., P.J. Rogers, N.A. Elliman, and S.J. Gatenby
  1994　Impairment of cognitive performance associated with dieting and high levels of dietary restraint. Physiol. Behav. 55(3):447–452.

Haaland, D.M.
  1992　Multivariate calibration methods applied to the quantitative analysis of infrared spectra. Pp. 1–30 in Computer-Enhanced Analytical Spectroscopy, vol. 3, P-C. Jurs, ed. New York: Plenum Press.

Haarbo, J., A. Gotfredsen, C. Hassager, and C. Christiansen
  1991　Validation of body composition by dual energy x-ray absorptiometry (DEXA). Clin. Physiol. 11:331–341.

Hajishengallis, G., S.K. Hollingshead, T. Koga, and M.W. Russell
  1995　Mucosal immunization with a bacterial protein antigen genetically coupled to cholera toxin A2/B subunits. J. Immunol. 154:4322–4332.

Hansen, N.J., T.G. Lohman, S.B. Going, M.C. Hall, R.W. Pamenter, L.A. Bare, T.W. Boyden, and L.B. Houtkooper
  1993　Prediction of body composition in premenopausal females from dual-energy x-ray absorptiometry. J. Appl. Physiol. 75(4):1637–1641.

Haq, T.A., H.S. Mason, J.D. Clements, and C.J. Arntzen
  1995　Oral immunization with a recombinant bacterial antigen produced in transgenic plants. Science 268:714–716.

Hodgdon, J.A., and M.B. Beckett
  1984　Prediction of body fat for U.S. Navy women from body circumferences and height. Technical Report 84-29. San Diego, Calif.: Naval Health Research Center.

Hodgdon, J.A., and P.I. Fitzgerald
  1987　Validity of impedance predictions at various levels of fatness. Hum. Biol. 59:281–298.

Hodgdon, J.A., P.I. Fitzgerald, and J.A. Vogel
  1990   Relationships between body fat and appearance ratings of U.S. soldiers. Technical Report 12-90. Natick, Mass.: U.S. Army Research Institute of Environmental Medicine.

Honigs, D.E., J.M. Freelin, G.M. Hieftje, and T.B. Hirschfeld
  1983   Near-infrared reflectance analysis by Gauss-Jordan linear algebra. Appl. Spec. 37(6):491–497.

Horber, F.F., F. Thomi, J.P. Casez, J. Fonteille, and P. Jaeger
  1992   Impact of hydration status on body composition as measured by dual energy x-ray absorptiometry in normal volunteers and patients on haemodialysis. Br. J. Radiol. 65(778):895–900.

Hoyt, R.W., J.J. Knapik, J.F. Lanza, B.H. Jones, and J.S. Staab
  1994   Ambulatory foot contact monitor to estimate the metabolic cost of human locomotion. J. Appl. Physiol. 76:1818–1822.

Hruschka, W.R., and K.H. Norris
  1982   Least-squares curve fitting of near-infrared spectra predicts protein and moisture content of ground wheat. Appl. Spec. 36(3):261–264.

Hsu, H., Y-M. Yu, J.W. Babich, J.F. Burke, E. Livini, R.G. Tompkins, V.R. Young, N.M. Alpert, and A.J. Fischman
  1996   Measurement of muscle protein synthesis by positron emission tomography with L-[methyl^{11}C]methionine. Proc. Natl. Acad. Sci. USA 93:1841–1846.

Hua, X., C. Yokoyama, J. Wu, M.R. Briggs, M.S. Brown, J.L. Goldstein, and X. Wang
  1993   SREBP-2, a second basic-helix-loop-helix-leucine zipper protein that stimulates transcription by binding to a sterol regulatory element. Proc. Natl. Acad. Sci. USA 90:11603–11607.

Hughes, M.D., D.S. Stein, H.M. Gundacker, F.T. Valentine, J.P. Phair, and P.A. Volberding
  1994   Within-subject variation in CD4 lymphocyte count in asymptomatic human immunodeficiency virus infection: Implications for patient monitoring. J. Infect. Dis. 169:28–36.

IOM (Institute of Medicine)
  1992   A Nutritional Assessment of U.S. Army Ranger Training Class 11/91. A brief report of the Committee on Military Nutrition Research, Food and Nutrition Board. March 23, 1992. Washington, D.C.

  1993a Nutritional Needs in Hot Environments, Applications for Military Personnel in Field Operations, B.M. Marriott, ed. A report of the Committee on Military Nutrition Research, Food and Nutrition Board. Washington, D.C.: National Academy Press.

  1993b Review of the Results of Nutritional Intervention, U.S. Army Ranger Training Class 11/92 (Ranger II), B.M. Marriott, ed. A report of the Committee on Military Nutrition Research, Food and Nutrition Board. Washington, D.C.: National Academy Press.

  1996   Nutritional Needs in Cold and in High-Altitude Environments, Applications for Military Personnel in Field Operations, B.M. Marriott and S.J. Carlson, eds. A report of the Committee on Military Nutrition Research, Food and Nutrition Board. Washington, D.C.: National Academy Press.

Israel, R.G., J.A. Houmard, K.F. O'Brien, M.R. McCammon, B.S. Zamora, and A.W. Eaton
  1989   Validity of a near-infrared spectrophotometry device for estimating human body composition. Res. Q. Exerc. Sport 60:379–383.

Jacob, J., G. Kelsoe, K. Rajewsky, and U. Weiss
  1991   Intraclonal generation of antibody mutants in germinal centers. Nature 354:389–392.

Jacob, J., J. Przylepa, C. Miller, and G. Kelsoe
  1993   In situ studies of the primary immune response to (4-hydroxy-3-nitrophenyl)acetyl.
          III. The kinetics of V region mutation and selection in germinal center B-cells. J.
          Exp. Med. 178:1293–1307.
Jardetzky, O., and G.C.K. Roberts
  1981   NMR in Molecular Biology. New York: Academic Press.
Jebb, S.A., P.R. Murgatroyd, G.R. Goldberg, A.M. Prentice, and W.A. Coward
  1993   *In vivo* measurement of changes in body composition: Description of methods and
          their validation against 12-d continuous whole-body calorimetry. Am. J. Clin.
          Nutr. 58:455–462.
Jensen, M.D., J.A. Kanaley, J.E. Reed, and P.F. Sheedy
  1995   Measurement of abdominal and visceral fat with computed tomography and dual-
          energy x-ray absorptiometry. Am. J. Clin. Nutr. 61:274–278.
Jobsis, F.F.
  1977   Noninvasive, infrared monitoring of cerebral and myocardial oxygen sufficiency
          and circulatory parameters. Science 198:1264–1267.
Johnson, H.L., and H.E. Sauberlich
  1982   Prolonged use of operational rations: A review of the literature. Unnumbered
          technical report. Presidio of San Francisco, Calif.: Letterman Army Institute of Re-
          search.
Johnson, H.L., C.F. Consolazio, H.J. Krzywicki, G.J. Isaac, and N.F. Witt
  1971   Metabolic aspects of calorie restriction: Nutrient balance with 500-kilocalorie
          intakes. Am. J. Clin. Nutr. 24:913–923.
Johnson, M.J., K.E. Friedl, P.N. Frykman, and R.J. Moore
  1994   Loss of muscle mass is poorly reflected in grip strength performance in healthy
          young men. Med. Sci. Sports Exerc. 26:235–240.
Jolesz, F.A.
  1992   Fast spin-echo technique extends versatility of MR. Diagn. Imaging 14:78.
Kendall, S.D., and M.J. Christensen
  1995   Modified differential display identifies genes in rat liver differentially regulated by
          selenium [abstract]. FASEB J. 9:A158.
Keys, A., J. Brozék, A. Henschel, O. Mickelsen, and H.L. Taylor
  1950   The Biology of Human Starvation, vol. 1. Minneapolis: University of Minnesota
          Press.
Kitai, T., A. Tanaka, A. Tokuka, K. Tanaka, Y. Yamaoka, K. Ozawa, and K. Hirao
  1993   Quantitative detection of hemoglobin saturation in the liver with near-infrared
          spectroscopy. Hepatology 18(4):926–936.
Klug, A., and J.W.R. Schwabe
  1995   Zinc fingers. FASEB J. 9:597–604.
Koelega, H.S.
  1989   Benzodiazepines and vigilance performance: A review. Psychopharmacology
          98:146–156.
Koster, F.T., and N.F. Pierce
  1983   Parenteral immunization causes antigen-specific cell-mediated suppression of an
          intestinal IgA response. J. Immunol. 131:115–119.
Kribbs, N.B., and D. Dinges
  1994   Vigilance decrement and sleepiness. Pp. 113–125 in Sleep Onset Mechanisms, J.R.
          Harsh and R.D. Ogilvie, eds. Washington, D.C.: American Psychological Associa-
          tion.
Kuhl, J.G., D. Evans, Y.E. Papelis, R.A. Romano, and G.S. Watson
  1995   The Iowa Driving Simulator: An immersive environment for driving-related
          research and development. IEEE Comput. 28(7):35–41.

Kushner, R.F., G. Gudivaka, and D.A. Schoeller
1996 Clinical characteristics influencing bioelectrical impedance analysis measurements. Am. J. Clin. Nutr. 64(3S):423S–427S.

Kvist, H., L. Sjöström, and U. Tylen
1986 Adipose tissue volume determinations in women by computed tomography: Technical considerations. Int. J. Obes. 10:53–67.

La Via, M.F., J. Munno, R.B. Lydiard, E.A. Workman, J.R. Hubbard, Y. Michel, and E. Pauling
1996 The influence of stress intrusion on immunodepression in generalized anxiety disorder patients and controls. Psychosom. Med. 58:138–142.

Larsson, B., K. Svardsudd, L. Welin, L. Wilhelmsen, P. Björntorp, and G. Tibblin
1984 Abdominal adipose tissue distribution, obesity, and risk of cardiovascular disease and death: 13 year follow up to participants in the study of men born in 1913. Br. Med. J. 288:1401–1404.

Lefrancois-Martinez, A-M., M-J.M. Diaz-Guerra, V. Vallet, A. Kahn, and B. Antoine
1994 Glucose-dependent regulation of the L-type kinase gene in a hepatoma cell line is independent of insulin and cyclic AMP. FASEB J. 8:89–96.

Liang, P., L. Averboukh, and A.B. Pardee
1993 Distribution and cloning of eukaryotic mRNAs by means of differential display: Refinements and optimization. Nucl. Acids Res. 21:3269–3275.

Lieberman, H.R.
1992 Caffeine. Pp. 49–72 in Factors Affecting Human Performance. Volume II: The Physical Environment, D. Jones and A. Smith, eds. London: Academic Press.

Lieberman, H.R., J.J. Wurtman, and M.H. Teicher
1989 Circadian rhythms of activity in healthy young and elderly humans. Neurobiol. Aging 10:259–265.

Lifson, N., and R. McClintock
1966 Theory of use of turnover rates of body water for measuring energy and material balance. J. Theor. Biol. 12:46–74.

Lifson, N., W.S. Little, D.G. Levitt, and R.M. Henderson
1975 $D_2{}^{18}O$ method for CO_2 output in small mammals and economic feasibility in man. J. Appl. Physiol. 39(4):657–664.

Lukaski, H.C.
1996 Biological indexes considered in the derivation of the bioelectrical impedance analysis. Am. J. Clin. Nutr. 64(3S):397S–404S.

Ma, J. K.-C., A. Hiatt, M. Hein, N.D. Vine, F. Wang, P. Stabila, C. van Dolleweerd, K. Mostov, and T. Lehner
1995 Generation and assembly of secretory antibodies in plants. Science 268:716–719.

Marano, M.A., Y. Fong, L.L. Moldawer, H. Wei, S.E. Calvano, K.J. Tracey, P.S. Barie, K. Manogue, A. Cerami, G.T. Shires et al.
1990 Serum cachectin/tumor necrosis factor in critically ill patients with burns correlates with infection and mortality. Surg. Gynecol. Obstet. 170:32–38.

Marks, J.D., H.R. Hoogenboom, T.P. Bonnert, J. McCafferty, A.D. Griffiths, and G. Winter
1991 By-passing immunization. Human antibodies from V-gene libraries displayed on phage. J. Mol. Biol. 222:16007–16010.

Meehan, C.D., L.A. Bove, and A.S. Jennings
1992 Comparison of first-generation and second-generation blood glucose meters for use in a hospital setting. Diabetes Educ. 18(3):228–231.

Merton, P.A.
1954 Voluntary strength and fatigue. J. Physiol. 123:553–564.

Metropolitan Life Insurance Company
1937 Girth and death. Stat. Bull. 18:2–5.

Michalek, S.M., J.H. Eldridge, R. Curtiss, III, and K.L. Rosenthal
1994   Antigen delivery systems: New approaches to mucosal immunization. Pp. 373–380 in Handbook of Mucosal Immunology, P.L. Ogra, J. Mestecky, M.E. Lamm, W. Strober, J.R. McGhee, and J. Bienenstock, eds. Boston: Academic Press, Inc.

Michie, H.R., K.R. Manogue, D.R. Spriggs, A. Revhaug, S. O'Dwyer, C.A. Dinarello, A. Cerami, S.M. Wolff, and D.W. Wilmore
1988   Detection of circulating tumor necrosis factor after endotoxin administration. N. Engl. J. Med. 318:1481–1486.

Moldawer, L.L.
1994   Biology of proinflammatory cytokines and their antagonists. Crit. Care Med. 22:S3–S7.

Moore, R.J., K.E. Friedl, T.R. Kramer, L.E. Martinez-Lopez, R.W. Hoyt, R.E. Tulley, J.P. DeLany, E.W. Askew, and J.A. Vogel
1992   Changes in soldier nutritional status and immune function during the Ranger training course. Technical Report No. T13-92. Natick, Mass.: U.S. Army Research Institute of Environmental Medicine.

Moore-Ede, M.C., F.M. Sulzman, and C.A. Fuller
1982   The Clocks that Time Us. Physiology of the Circadian Timing System. Cambridge, Mass.: Harvard University Press.

Moscovitz, H., F. Shofer, H. Mignott, A. Behrman, and L. Kilpatrick
1994   Plasma cytokine determinations in emergency department patients as a predictor of bacteremia and infectious disease severity. Crit. Care Med. 22:1102–1107.

Mostov, K.E.
1994   Transepithelial transport of immunoglobulins Annu. Rev. Immunol. 12:63–84.

NIH (National Institutes of Health)
1996   Technology Assessment Statement on Bioelectrical Impedance Analysis in Body Composition Measurement, 1994 December 12–14. Am. J. Clin. Nutr. 64(suppl.):524S–532S.

Nord, R.H., and R.K. Payne
1990   Standards for body composition calibration in DEXA. Paper presented at the 2d Annual Meeting of the Bath Conference on Bone Mineral Measurement, Bath, U.K.

Nyboer, J.
1959   Electrical Impedance Plethysmography. Springfield, Ill.: Charles C Thomas.

O'Malley, B.W., and O.M. Conneely
1992   Orphan receptors: In search of a unifying hypothesis for activation. Mol. Endocrinol. 6:1359–1361.

Orr, S., T.P. Hughes, C.L. Sawyers, R.M. Kato, S.G. Quan, S.P. Williams, O.N. Witte, and L. Hood
1994   Isolation of unknown genes from human bone marrow by differential screening and single-pass cDNA sequence determination. Proc. Natl. Acad. Sci. USA 91:11869–11873.

Pace, N., and E.N. Rathbun
1945   Studies on body composition-III. The body water and chemically combined nitrogen content in relation to fat content. J. Biol. Chem. 158:685–691.

Palmiter, R.D., R.L. Brinster, R.E. Hammer, M.E. Trumbauer, M.G. Rosenfeld, N.C. Birnberg, and R.M. Evans
1982   Dramatic growth of mice that develop from eggs microinjected with metallothionein-growth hormone fusion genes. Nature 300:611–615.

Peltola, H., A. Sittonen, H. Kyronseppa, I. Simula, L. Mattila, P. Oksanen, M.J. Kataja, and M. Cadoz
1991 Prevention of travellers' diarrhoea by oral B-subunit/whole-cell cholera vaccine. Lancet 338(8778):1285–1289.

Peuchant, E., C. Salles, and R. Jensen
1987 Determination of serum cholesterol by near-infrared reflectance spectrometry. Anal. Chem. 59(14):1816–1819.
1988 Value of a spectroscopic "fecalogram" in determining the etiology of steatorrhea. Clin. Chem. 34(1):5–8.

Powanda, M.C., and W.R. Beisel
1982 Hypothesis: Leukocyte endogenous mediator/endogenous pyrogen/lymphocyte-activating factor modulates the development of nonspecific and specific immunity and affects nutritional status. Am. J. Clin. Nutr. 35:762–768.

Prieur, A.M., M.T. Kaufmann, C. Griscelli, and J.M. Dayer
1987 Specific interleukin-1 inhibitor in serum and urine of children with systemic juvenile chronic arthritis. Lancet 2:1240–1242.

Purcell, W.M., and C.K. Atterwill
1994 Human placental mast cells as an *in vitro* model system in aspects of neuroimmu-notoxicity testing. Hum. Exp. Toxicol. 13(6):429–433.

Racette, S.B., D.A. Schoeller, A.H. Luke, K. Shay, J. Hnilicka, and R.F. Kushner
1994 Relative dilution spaces of ^{2}H- and ^{18}O-labeled water in humans. Am. J. Physiol. 267 (30):E585–E590.

Rahelu, M., G.T. Williams, D.S. Kumararatne, G.S. Eaton, and J.S. Gaston
1993 Human CD4+ cytolitic T-cells kill antigen-pulsed target T-cells by induction of apoptosis. J. Immunol. 150:4856–4866

Rebar, E.J., and C.O. Pabo
1994 Zinc finger phage: Affinity selection of fingers with new DNA-binding specificities. Science 263:671–673.

Reynolds, K.L., H.A. Heckel, C.E. Witt, J.W. Martin, J.A. Pollard, J.J. Knapik, and B.H. Jones
1994 Cigarette smoking, physical fitness, and injuries in infantry soldiers. Am. J. Prev. Med. 10(3):145–150.

Ritz, P., P.G. Johnson, and W.A. Coward
1994 Measurements of ^{2}H and ^{18}O in body water: Analytical considerations and physiological implications. Br. J. Nutr. 72:3–12.

Robinson, M.R., R.P. Eaton, D.M. Haaland, G.W. Koepp, E.V. Thomas, B.R. Stallard, and P.L. Robinson
1992 Noninvasive glucose monitoring in diabetic patients: A preliminary evaluation. Clin. Chem. 38(9):1618–1622.

Romano, R.A., and G.S. Watson
1994 Assessment of Capabilities—Iowa Driving Simulator. Technical Report No. FHWA-IR-94. Washington, D.C.: U.S. Department of Transportation Federal Highway Administration.

Rothman, D.L., R.G. Shulman, and G.I. Shulman
1992 ^{31}P nuclear magnetic resonance measurements of muscle glucose-6-phosphate. Evidence for reduced insulin-dependent muscle glucose transport or phosphoryla-tion activity in non-insulin-dependent diabetes mellitus. J. Clin. Invest. 89:1069–1075.

Russell, D.M., L.A. Leiter, J. Whitwell, E.B. Marliss, and K.N. Jeejeebhoy
1983a Skeletal muscle function during hypocaloric diets and fasting: A comparison with standard nutritional assessment parameters. Am. J. Clin. Nutr. 37:133–138.

Russell, D.M., P.J. Prendergast, P.L. Darby, P.E. Garfinkel, J. Whitwell, and K.N. Jeejeebhoy
  1983b A comparison between muscle function and body composition in anorexia nervosa: The effect of refeeding. Am. J. Clin. Nutr. 38:229–237.
Sack, R.B.
  1980 Enterotoxigenic *Escherichia coli*: Identification and characterization. J. Infect. Dis. 142:279–296.
Schneider, P., and C. Reiners
  1997 Changes in bone mineral density in male athletes [letter in response to Klesges et al., 1996, 276:226–230]. J. Am. Med. Assoc. 277(1):23–24.
Seckinger, P., J.W. Lowenthal, K. Williamson, J.M. Dayer, and H.R. MacDonald
  1987a A urine inhibitor of interleukin-1 activity that blocks ligand binding. J. Immunol. 139:1546–1549.
Seckinger, P., K. Williamson, J.F. Balavoine, B. Mach, G. Mazzei, A. Shaw, and J.M. Dayer
  1987b A urine inhibitor of interleukin-1 activity affects both interleukin-1 alpha and -1 beta but not tumor necrosis factor alpha. J. Immunol. 139:1541–1545.
Seckinger, P., S. Isaaz, and J.M. Dayer
  1988 A human inhibitor of tumor necrosis factor alpha. J. Exp. Med. 167:1511–1516.
Sharp, M.A., B.C. Nindl, K.A. Westphal, and K.E. Friedl
  1994 The physical performance of female Army basic trainees who pass and fail the Army body weight and percent body fat standards. Pp. 743–750 in Advances in Industrial Ergonomics and Safety VI, E. Agezadeh, ed. Washington, D.C.: Taylor and Francis.
Shih, H-M., Z. Liu, and H.C. Towle
  1995 Two CACGTG motifs with proper spacing dictate the carbohydrate regulation of hepatic gene transcription. J. Biol. Chem. 270:21991–21997.
Shulman, G.I., D.L. Rothman, T. Jue, P. Stein, R.A. DeFronzo, and R.G. Shulman
  1990 Quantitation of muscle glycogen synthesis in normal subjects and subjects with non-insulin-dependent diabetes by ^{13}C nuclear magnetic resonance spectroscopy. N. Engl. J. Med. 322:223–228.
Siri, W.E.
  1961 Body composition from fluid space and density: Analysis of methods. Pp. 224–244 in Techniques for Measuring Body Composition, J. Brozek and A. Henschel, eds. Washington, D.C.: National Academy of Sciences/National Research Council.
Sixma, T.K., S.E. Pronk, K.H. Kalk, E.S. Wartna, B.A.M. vanZanten, B. Witholt, and W.G. Hol
  1991 Crystal structure of a cholera toxin-related heat-labile enterotoxin from *E. coli*. Nature (London) 351:371–377.
Smyth, M.J., and J.R. Ortaldo
  1993 Mechanisms of cytotoxicty used by human peripheral blood CD4+ and CD8+ T-cell subsets. The role of granule exocytosis. J. Immunol. 151:40–47.
Sprenger, H., C. Jacobs, M. Nain, A.M. Gressner, H. Prinz, W. Wesemann, and D. Gemsa
  1992 Enhanced release of cytokines, interleukin-2 receptors, and neopterin after long-distance running. Clin. Immunol. Immunopathol. 63:188–195.
Stein, T.P., and M.D. Schluter
  1994 Excretion of IL-6 by astronauts during spaceflight. Am. J. Physiol. 266:E448–E452.
Stuart, G.W., P.F. Searle, H.Y. Chen, R.L. Brinster, and R.D. Palmiter
  1984 A 12-base pair DNA motif that is repeated several times in metallothionein gene promoters confers metal regulation to a heterologous gene. Proc. Natl. Acad. Sci. USA 81:7318–7322.

Suter, P.M., S. Suter, E. Girardin, P. Roux Lombard, G.E. Grau, and J.M. Dayer
  1992 High bronchoalveolar levels of tumor necrosis factor and its inhibitors, interleukin-1, interferon, and elastase, in patients with adult respiratory distress syndrome after trauma, shock, or sepsis. Am. Rev. Respir. Dis. 145:1016–1022.

Tessari, P., S. Inchiostro, M. Zanett, and R. Barazzoni
  1995 A model of skeletal muscle kinetics measured across the human forearm. Am. J. Physiol. 269:E127–E136.

Tothill, P., and R.H. Nord
  1995 Limitations of dual-energy x-ray absorptiometry [letter]. Am. J. Clin. Nutr. 61:398–399.

Tryon, W.W.
  1991 Activity Measurement in Psychology and Medicine. New York: Plenum Press.

U.S. Department of the Army
  1986 Army Regulation 600-9. "The Army Weight Control Program." September 1. Washington, D.C.

Vallee, B.L., J.E. Coleman, and D.S. Auld
  1991 Zinc fingers, zinc clusters, and zinc twists in DNA-binding protein domains. Proc. Natl. Acad. Sci. USA 88:999–1003.

Vallera, D.A., M.G. Bissell, and W. Barron
  1991 Accuracy of portable blood glucose monitoring. Effect of glucose level and prandial state. Am. J. Clin. Pathol. 95(2):247–252.

Van Zee, K.J., T. Kohno, E. Fischer, C.S. Rock, L.L. Moldawer, and S.F. Lowry
  1992 Tumor necrosis factor soluble receptors circulate during experimental and clinical inflammation and can protect against excessive tumor necrosis factor alpha in vitro and in vivo. Proc. Natl. Acad. Sci. USA 89:4845–4849.

Virella, G., ed.
  1993a Diagnostic evaluation of humoral immunity. Pp. 275–285 in Introduction to Medical Immunology, 3rd ed. New York: Marcel Dekker.
  1993b Immunodeficiency diseases. Pp. 543–573 in Introduction to Medical Immunology, 3rd ed. New York: Marcel Dekker.

Virella, G., M.T. Rugeles, B. Hyman, M. La Via, J.M. Goust, M. Frankis, and B.E. Bierer
  1988 The interaction of CD2 with its LFA-3 ligand expressed by autologous erythrocytes results in enhancement of B-cell responses. Cell. Immunol. 116:308–319.

Virella, G., K. Fourspring, B. Hyman, R. Haskill-Stroud, L. Long, I. Virella, M. La Via, A.J. Gross, and M. Lopes-Virella
  1991 Immunosuppressive effects of fish oil in normal human volunteers: Correlation with the *in vitro* effects of eicosapentanoic acid on human lymphocytes. Clin. Immunol. Immunopath. 61:161–176.

Virella, G., C. Patrick, and J.M. Goust
  1993 Diagnostic evaluation of lymphocyte functions and cell-mediated immunity. Pp. 291–306 in Introduction to Medical Immunology, 3rd ed., G. Virella, ed. New York: Marcel Dekker.

Vogel, J.A., and K.E. Friedl
  1992 Body fat assessment in women—Special considerations. Sports Med. 13:245–269.

Waage, A., P. Brandtzaeg, A. Halstensen, P. Kierulf, and T. Espevik
  1989 The complex pattern of cytokines in serum from patients with meningococcal septic shock. Association between interleukin-6, interleukin-1, and fatal outcome. J. Exp. Med. 169:333–338.

Weits, T., E.J. van der Beek, M. Wedel, and B.M. Ter Haar Romeny
  1988 Computed tomography measurement of abdominal fat deposition in relation to anthropometry. Int. J. Obes. 12:217–225.

Westphal, K.A., N. King, K.E. Friedl, M.A. Sharp, T.R. Kramer, and K.L. Reynolds
   1995   Health, performance, and nutritional status of U.S. Army women during basic combat training. Technical Report T95-99. Natick, Mass.: U.S. Army Research Institute of Environmental Medicine.
Willson, R.L.
   1989   Zinc and iron in free radical pathology and cellular control. Pp. 147–172 in Zinc in Human Biology, C.F. Mills, ed. New York: Springer-Verlag.
Wu, H., W-P.Yang, and C.F. Barbas III
   1995   Building zinc fingers by selection: Toward a therapeutic application. Proc. Natl. Acad Sci. USA 92:344–348.
Yang, J., R. Sato, J.L. Goldstein, and M.S. Brown
   1994   Sterol-resistant transcription in CHO cells caused by gene rearrangement that truncates SREBP-2. Genes Dev. 8:1910–1919.

Emerging Technologies for Nutrition Research, 1997
Pp. 51–68. Washington, D.C.
National Academy Press

2

Committee Responses to Questions, Conclusions, and Recommendations

As outlined in Chapter 1, the Committee on Military Nutrition Research (CMNR) was asked to provide a survey of newly available and emerging technologies that may be of significant value to the military for assessing and optimizing nutritional, physiological, and cognitive status and performance in military personnel. The following six categories of technologies were identified and evaluated for their applicability to the military mission:

- assessment of body composition,
- tracer techniques for study of metabolic processes,
- improved measures of energy expenditure and respiratory exchange,
- molecular and cellular approaches for evaluating nutritional requirements and status,
- assessment of immune status and function, and
- functional and behavioral measures of nutritional status.

The Military Nutrition Division (MND) (currently the Military Nutrition and Biochemical Division) at the U.S. Army Research Institute of Environmental

Medicine (USARIEM) posed six questions for the CMNR to aid in its evaluation of the techniques reviewed and its provision of guidance to MND concerning their applications to the military.

In this chapter, the CMNR provides its answers to the questions posed by the Army, draws its conclusions on each of the six technologies reviewed, and makes its recommendations. The responses, conclusions, and recommendations were developed in discussion and prepared in executive session of the CMNR.

RESPONSES TO QUESTIONS POSED BY THE ARMY

This section is organized according to the six categories of technologies, with all of the Army's questions being answered under each technology.

Techniques of Body Composition Assessment

1. Will the technologies be a significant improvement over current technologies?

Anthropometric equations currently used by the military could be further refined with additional computer modeling, particularly with regard to their application to all ethnic groups. Computerized axial tomography (CAT) scanning, magnetic resonance imaging (MRI), and dual-energy x-ray absorptiometry (DXA) measurements can and have markedly improved compositional methodology in the clinic. These techniques could be used by the military to improve the accuracy and reliability of derived equations that use anthropometric measures to predict body fat content.

Single-frequency bioelectrical impedance analysis (BIA) is not a reliable measure of body composition, but the methodology may be helpful in answering specific questions concerning hydration status. Multiple-frequency bioelectrical impedance spectroscopy may hold promise for compositional measurement in the future.

2. How likely are the technologies to mature sufficiently for practical use?

Body composition (BC) methods are already quite mature, although multiple-frequency BIA requires some specific developmental work. The multifrequency method of BIA involves a simple and low-cost measurement system, but it is not sufficiently developed to provide accurate and reproducible estimates of changes in body composition. Its relative simplicity and low cost suggest that further development may be useful to see if current shortcomings can be overcome.

At present, CAT scanning, MRI, and DXA provide reliable measures of composition but are expensive. CAT requires exposure to x rays, although some

CAT scanners have been modified to reduce x-ray exposure, so this may no longer be a limitation. While all these techniques lack ease of use in the field, DXA at least appears to have the potential to serve as a new criterion measure to validate anthropometric equations.

3. What is the cost/benefit ratio of the new technologies, and how expensive (in both monetary and personnel terms) will they be to employ compared with the importance of the information they will provide?

Anthropometric measurements and BIA are low cost and reasonably noninvasive (although a period of training is required to perform the former measurements accurately). The equipment required for CAT scanning, MRI, and DXA are high cost ($100,000–$1,000,000), and the training required to utilize the equipment is considerable. These costs, as well as the time required to perform the measurements on an individual, are a major limitation. Therefore, these techniques have value primarily as research tools (criterion measures) to aid in refining practical anthropometric methods for everyday use.

4. Are the technologies of such critical value that their development should be supported by Department of Defense (DoD) funds—such as can be provided by the Small Business Innovative Research (SBIR) program?

Because fat-free mass (FFM) is the only BC component that appears to be correlated with physical performance capacity, technology is needed for the accurate estimation of muscle mass, lean body mass, or FFM.

To assess the effects of military operations on body composition in individual soldiers, improvement is needed in methods for assessment and prediction of modest longitudinal changes in body composition. While DXA might provide the most accurate, direct longitudinal assessment, its relatively limited practicality in the field makes it a more likely candidate to be the criterion against which new anthropometric equations can be validated.

Research with CAT, MRI, and DXA will continue in the private sector because of the medical applications of these technologies, including their potential to assess changes in body composition.

Multifrequency BIA represents a simple technology that, if it could be developed sufficiently to overcome its current shortcomings, may be a technology whose adaptation for military field use could benefit from additional development funding. Anthropometric measurements may need additional support from computer development in the refinement of predictive equations. Such fine tuning of anthropometric methods is low cost and would likely be performed in-house or with limited outside support.

5. How practical are the technologies? Will they require dedicated personnel and complex, exotic equipment? Will the data provided be difficult to analyze?

Anthropometric measurements and BIA are practical, although trained technicians should be utilized to perform these measurements. The large scanning devices are best used for developing predictive equations although mobile units are available. Cooperative work with medical or other institutions to utilize existing facilities and trained personnel appears to be the most practical and economical approach, as such facilities are experienced in collecting and analyzing data from these devices.

6. Can the technologies be used in the field (could they be used in the field or used to analyze samples collected in the field)?

Anthropometric measurements can be conducted in the field. Although BIA also can be performed in the field, it currently does not represent an improvement over anthropometric measures of BC. Because the interpretation of BIA predictions of body composition is influenced significantly by environmental factors, health status, and physical activity, its use in the field may provide a mechanism for easily monitoring these factors, which are of significant interest to the military. Although mobile units are available for DXA and MRI, their use in the field to measure small changes in body composition is costly in terms of technician time. Hence, the use of these latter instruments is limited to validation of currently used anthropometric equations.

Tracer Techniques for the Study of Metabolism

1. Will the technologies be a significant improvement over current technologies?

Major advances in the understanding and measurement of metabolic processes have been made by incorporating these methodologies into studies of substrate utilization, energy requirements, and muscle function. The methods provide a safe mechanism for monitoring metabolites that was not available previously.

2. How likely are the technologies to mature sufficiently for practical use?

Tracer methodology is developed and mature, although new labels, new techniques for separation of labeled metabolites (mass isotopomer distribution analysis), and more sensitive spectrometers are increasing its application. The doubly labeled water (DLW) technique has been used in field studies to estimate energy expenditure in troops. Other isotopic procedures have been used in laboratory settings to evaluate fuel use during exercise, and nuclear magnetic resonance (NMR) has been developed to assess intracellular metabolites and fuel stores. Reliable and reproducible data are best provided by laboratory groups with significant experience in the measurement and interpretation of the data obtained.

3. What is the cost/benefit ratio of the new technologies, and how expensive (in both monetary and personnel terms) will they be to employ compared with the importance of the information they will provide?

Compounds labeled with stable isotopes are moderately expensive and the mass spectrometers required for analysis are expensive ($100,000–$300,000), but the cost of such measurements can be reduced with batch processing of labeled compounds and the use of core facilities. There is significant variation in the cost of studies utilizing this technology.

When tracer isotopes can be administered and samples collected noninvasively in the field, cost is minimized. Samples and data can be analyzed in a core laboratory, and costs can be kept at a relatively low level for the value of the data obtained (an example being DLW studies of energy expenditure of troops in field operations). Incorporation of NMR or positron emission tomography (PET) greatly increases study expenses.

When invasive techniques are required for administration and collection of samples, the stable isotope methods described are largely confined to laboratory use. However, for the information obtained using these stable isotope methods, the amount of data acquired is immense.

NMR carries a large initial outlay for the magnet and the physicist to run it, but individual measurements are inexpensive to make, and the noninvasive nature increases its appeal.

PET is prohibitively expensive ($2,000,000), and its use is limited to those facilities where sufficient medical need warrants its purchase. The information on metabolic processes that can be derived from this method is, as yet, untapped.

4. Are the technologies of such critical value that their development should be supported by DoD funds—such as can be provided by the SBIR program?

The use of these techniques has developed in medical, nutrition, and physiology laboratories to improve the understanding of metabolic processes. It is a very active research field, heavily supported by federal funding. The MND should keep abreast of developments in the field to identify areas where the application to military nutrition is important. Funding for projects of specific interest to the military may be considered, but general funding is not necessary for this technology to develop rapidly.

5. How practical are the technologies? Will they require dedicated personnel and complex, exotic equipment? Will the data provided be difficult to analyze?

Studies using stable isotopes require trained personnel for design and implementation. The technique is not trivial, nor is data analysis, so that experienced personnel are required to ensure meaningful results. Within that framework, the ease of the technique depends on the mode of dosing and sampling. Oral dosing followed by urine sampling is practical and easy for subjects. Intravenous dosing and arterial sampling require medical personnel and facilities.

NMR and PET require little on the part of the subject, but highly trained personnel must run the equipment.

6. Can the technologies be used in the field (could they be used in the field or used to analyze samples collected in the field)?

Studies involving invasive procedures to deliver isotope and collect samples are inappropriate for field work at this time. Studies that require magnets or cyclotrons cannot be performed easily in the field at this time.

Ambulatory Techniques for Measurement of Energy Expenditure

1. Will the technologies be a significant improvement over current technologies?

The DLW technique is a major improvement over the use of portable indirect calorimetry for estimating energy expenditure in the field. However, the use of ambulatory monitoring devices is an evolving technology that shows promise for use in estimating energy expenditure in the field as well.

The application of near-infrared (NIR) spectroscopy, if perfected, could permit the noninvasive measurement of plasma metabolites, such as glucose, using a portable instrument with the accuracy and reliability of currently used blood-based methods. The difficulty in differentiating multiple metabolites in blood only may be overcome slowly.

2. How likely are the technologies to mature sufficiently for practical use?

The measurement of total energy expenditure with doubly labeled water is already practical for field use. Activity monitoring remains a fertile field of investigation as newer methods of measuring activity and energy expenditure are integrated.

NIR spectroscopy techniques and instrumentation are currently in use for routine food analysis and for blood flow monitoring of tissue oxygenation and are well developed. The measurement of a broad variety of other plasma metabolites, such as blood glucose, is an emerging technology that is not yet fully developed. Blood is a complex mixture of many organic compounds, each with overlapping spectra in the NIR range. In addition, blood flow is dynamic, and many plasma metabolites are in constant flux, particularly under conditions of stress. These represent formidable methodological obstacles not yet overcome, either by transcutaneous or reflectance NIR measurements. An additional obstacle is the unavailability, to date, of the portable equipment that would be required for field use. This is an area of considerable investigation.

3. What is the cost/benefit ratio of the new technologies, and how expensive (in both monetary and personnel terms) will they be to employ compared with the importance of the information they will provide?

Doubly labeled water carries a fairly high price tag due to the costs of isotope (about \$400–\$500 per dose) and analysis (about \$500 per dose). This cost is somewhat balanced by the ease of use, quantity of data produced, and safety of subjects. Portable oxygen consumption devices and ambulatory monitors are reasonably inexpensive and easy for subjects to use.

Although the equipment that is required for portable, noninvasive testing of plasma metabolites using NIR spectroscopy would be relatively inexpensive to build and operate, the cost of development of that equipment could be great.

4. Are the technologies of such critical value that their development should be supported by DoD funds—such as can be provided by the SBIR program?

The use of stable isotopes to measure energy expenditure is a well-developed method that requires no further support for development. Funds should continue to be appropriated to support the development of ambulatory monitoring, to refine the technology under development, and to validate the devices with field studies. The "foot strike" method is interesting and may be more useful if it can be applied to uneven terrain. This method is less expensive than isotopic methods and could be applied readily to significant numbers of individuals in the field.

The large potential market in the civilian sector for noninvasive, portable medical devices employing NIR spectroscopy for the measure of plasma metabolites should drive the development of suitable instrumentation. No investment should be required on the part of the military.

5. How practical are the technologies? Will they require dedicated personnel and complex, exotic equipment? Will the data provided be difficult to analyze?

The DLW method for determination of energy expenditure is fairly practical to administer in the field, although interpretation is complicated by changes in water supply and large changes in activity patterns. Thus, analysis is sometimes problematic, and sample handling and data interpretation require trained personnel.

Measures of oxygen consumption or ambulatory monitors are used more easily by individuals in the field but need further field testing. The data obtained are readily interpretable by computer analysis, but personnel who perform that interpretation require some training.

Noninvasive field applications of NIR spectroscopy will require simple, rugged, and portable equipment, while routine health screening of military personnel at their home bases would have less stringent equipment requirements. However, at the present time, neither the technology nor the necessary instrumentation are available for either of these applications.

6. Can the technologies be used in the field (could they be used in the field or used to analyze samples collected in the field)?

The performance of studies on energy expenditure in the field has a long history. The DLW technique has been widely used in the field and has yielded useful information in a variety of military studies. Studies of energy expenditure employing the DLW technique require oral dosing and urine sampling, and at present such studies are routinely conducted in the field; however, this method has only limited applicability due to cost. The foot strike method will benefit from more development and evaluation in a variety of field applications.

When simple, rugged, and portable NIR spectroscopy equipment is developed to measure blood flow, tissue oxygen saturation, and a variety of plasma metabolites, it is possible to see many important field applications both in training and in other operations.

Molecular and Cellular Approaches to Nutrition

1. Will the technologies be a significant improvement over current technologies?

At the present time, the use of molecular cloning techniques to elucidate the human genome, study the control of gene expression, and control the synthesis of particular desirable or undesirable gene products both *in vivo* and *in vitro* is rapidly advancing the front and the pace of research in many areas. The techniques described represent the state of the art for most applications of molecular biology and are widely used in both academic and industrial research laboratories.

In many respects, the use of isolated cell systems represents a significant advance over other methods (tissue culture and perfused organ systems, for example) for the study of cellular responses to external stimuli. The techniques await validation against appropriate *in vivo* measurements to demonstrate their true potential.

2. How likely are the technologies to mature sufficiently for practical use?

Apart from the use of molecular cloning techniques to facilitate *in vitro* production of cellular products, such as vaccines, and improve the food supply, the most promising application for these technologies at the present time and in the near future is basic research. By bringing the investigation down to the level of gene expression, it is becoming possible to elucidate completely the mechanisms, by which stimuli, such as environmental stresses or changes in nutritional status, exert their influence upon physiological systems.

Isolated cell techniques will find practical use largely, if not solely, in basic research settings. The likelihood that they will yield valid or useful information will depend on the effort that is expended to choose an appropriate model system and validate it properly. With the exception of the use of red cell hemolysis to assess vitamin E status, the use of isolated cells for determination of nutritional status is not an available technology at this time.

3. What is the cost/benefit ratio of the new technologies, and how expensive (in both monetary and personnel terms) will they be to employ compared with the importance of the information they will provide?

These are technical approaches that at the present time are almost exclusively limited in their application to the basic research setting. They require a considerable investment of capital for equipment and materials, time, and personnel to develop a well-conceived research plan. While the information obtained by the use of molecular cloning techniques could not be obtained in any other way, the potential benefit of obtaining such information must be evaluated by anyone considering undertaking such research.

Isolated cell approaches, in contrast, may be comparable in cost to molecular cloning techniques, yet the value of the information they can provide largely remains to be demonstrated (even within the scientific community).

4. Are the technologies of such critical value that their development should be supported by DoD funds—such as can be provided by the SBIR program?

This technology is under active investigation in a variety of settings and supported by federal and private industry funding. Unless a specific application to a military setting is recognized, the CMNR does not recommend DoD funding at this time. At some point, as the technology develops, DoD may wish to evaluate whether its support would help a specific area, such as the effect of oxidative stress on gene expression, in view of the number of military settings where oxidative stress may be of particular concern.

5. How practical are the technologies? Will they require dedicated personnel and complex, exotic equipment? Will the data provided be difficult to analyze?

At this time, techniques of molecular biology are not practical to answer nutritional questions of military significance. This type of work demands a considerable amount of equipment (although it is equipment that is currently available), extensive training, and the knowledge base to analyze the data. In addition, the development of the testing protocols alone for any product that emerges as a result of research conducted at the molecular biology level will require that a number of ethical and safety questions be taken into consideration.

If isolated cell techniques can be validated sufficiently, it is conceivable that they might be utilized to study samples drawn from individuals working in the field and transported to a laboratory in a remote location.

6. Can the technologies be used in the field (could they be used in the field or used to analyze samples collected in the field)?

While there is no reason to imagine conducting basic molecular biological or cell physiology research in the field, several field applications may become feasible in the future. One application that will become more appealing as the elucidation of the human genome progresses is the screening of cells taken from individuals recently exposed to extreme environmental conditions (stimuli) to determine the effects of these stimuli on gene expression. Such testing could be accomplished by sampling the tissues or cells of interest (if it can be done non-invasively) in the field setting and transporting them to a remote laboratory. Similar studies could be done to elucidate subcellular physiological processes using isolated cell approaches. A second application would involve techniques of gene transfer. These techniques, which are just now being developed and tested in humans who have been diagnosed with any of several rare genetic disorders or terminal cancers, may impart the ability to synthesize proteins not otherwise made by the body because of a missing or defective gene or some alteration in the regulatory process. The potential clearly exists to enhance the expression of particular genes or to place their expression under the control of nutrients (such as zinc) or some other dietary or environmental stimulus. Procedures of this sort await extensive testing, not to mention the solution of a myriad of ethical and practical questions, before realistic field applications can be considered.

Assessment of Immune Function

1. Will the technologies be a significant improvement over current technologies?

Improved methodologies for measuring functions of cell-mediated immunity and cytokine production are extensions of current methodologies. These generally are available in academic research institutions.

Novel approaches to the development of oral vaccines for active immunizations, and human antibodies for passive immunization, represent vastly important improvements over current technologies and give great promise for inducing better and more complete immunity than do current vaccines, and at a far lower cost.

2. How likely are the technologies to mature sufficiently for practical use?

Testing methodologies for evaluating immune system functions are constantly being studied and improved in academic centers. Whenever available, these improved methods will need to be adapted by military laboratories and modified for field use.

Exciting new methodologies and approaches for the development of oral vaccines are being pursued vigorously by many groups, and the first human testing of experimental new vaccines should occur shortly. Since the Army is already highly engaged in the development of uniquely important military vaccines, new technologies for vaccine development are of great potential importance.

The possible creation of specific, human-compatible antibodies by the development and use of transgenic plants represents an important medical advance which could be of great value to military medicine. Such antibodies could be used to confer weeks to months of prophylactic passive immunity, or they could be used as specific forms of therapy. The transgenic antibodies would replace and expand the diversity of the available and costly passive immunization practices, which require the gathering and processing of human serum or the much more dangerous use of serum obtained form horses or other animals.

3. What is the cost/benefit ratio of the new technologies, and how expensive (in both monetary and personnel terms) will they be to employ compared with the importance of the information they will provide?

The testing of immunological functions tends to be quite expensive, especially when these tests can only be done in research laboratories using costly reagents and equipment. Costs for field testing could be minimized (in terms of both money and loss of duty time by military personnel) if immunological studies could be limited to specific tests that prove to be most meaningful and reliable.

Tests based on cytokine assays, especially those of the proinflammatory cytokines and related molecules excreted in urine, have great potential for adding important new diagnostic measures at a relatively inexpensive cost/benefit ratio.

Costs of developing and testing potential new oral vaccines are likely to be comparable with those of conventional vaccines currently under development. However, oral vaccines have the potential for being far cheaper to produce (especially if effective antigens or antibodies can be produced in transgenic plants), and for being safer, more effective, and less costly to administer.

4. Are the technologies of such critical value that their development should be supported by DoD funds—such as can be provided by the SBIR program?

The occurrence of immune system dysfunctions, such as those induced by one episode of Ranger training and those that may arise in the course of basic combat training or any military operation, needs to be investigated further. Such investigations should be extended to other operational situations that involve extreme physical stress and weight loss. In conducting these investigations, the DoD should employ the best available testing methodologies and adapt them to field use whenever necessary.

Infectious diseases continue to have high DoD costs in terms of both medical care and lost time for military personnel. Infection-induced losses of body weight and essential nutrients can then impair physical performance for long periods of time. DoD use of immunizations to prevent (or minimize) the military impact of infectious diseases (including those due to biological warfare threat agents) has included the need for DoD funding and in-house research to develop, test, and procure all unique vaccines of military importance that are not available commercially. The potential for developing new families of oral vaccines that are more effective, less expensive, and easier to administer than currently available vaccines should not be ignored by the DoD. Creation of new families of transgenic plant-produced antibodies for passive protection against rare infections and toxemias of potential military importance represents a technological breakthrough that should be developed fully by the DoD in the immediate future. The CMNR supports the recommendation that a Science and Technology Objective be established for adaptation of militarily relevant vaccines for oral administration, and transgenic antibodies for passive protection, through the application of new technologies described in this report.

5. How practical are the technologies? Will they require dedicated personnel and complex, exotic equipment? Will the data provided be difficult to analyze?

Advanced methodologies for a wide assortment of immunological assessments are already available in research laboratories, but considerable effort may be required to adapt them for field use. This problem can be minimized by focusing on a small, select number of tests that will yield the greatest amount of clinical information.

Methodologies for developing a variety of effective new oral vaccines have already proven to be highly practical, and the first of such experimental vaccines are becoming available for human testing. Development and testing of new vaccines of unique military importance will still require time and money. The same is true for development of human antibodies in transgenic plants.

6. Can the technologies be used in the field (could they be used in the field or used to analyze samples collected in the field)?

Field studies of Rangers in training have helped to highlight the immune dysfunctions that may be a consequence of these types of extreme environmental stress. Further such studies are needed to elucidate the nature and course of these immune system dysfunctions. Measurements of proinflammatory cytokines (such as IL-6 and IL-6 receptor antagonists) may be performed on single urine specimens collected in the field, although caution must be exercised in the interpretation of results. Further development of noninvasive assays (i.e., those that would use saliva, urine, stool, or other available samples), as well as simple, rugged, portable equipment for analyzing plasma metabolites and blood cell counts, should increase the ease of performing field measurements.

Immunization is an important component of preparation for battlefield readiness. Refinement of vaccine production and improvement of delivery systems will greatly assist in increasing the effectiveness of, and compliance with, immunization programs.

FUNCTIONAL AND BEHAVIORAL MEASURES
OF NUTRITIONAL STATUS

1. Will the technologies be a significant improvement over current technologies?

These methods actually constitute a group of technologies that measure different aspects of physical and cognitive performance. For one of these techniques, Muscle Function Analysis (MFA), the basic premises underlying the association between collected data and lean body mass or other indicators of nutritional status remains to be validated. The effects of prior strenuous physical exercise on MFA readings are not clear nor is it possible as yet to eliminate the contribution of voluntary muscle contraction or changes in activity of the sodium potassium pump. Furthermore, although the MFA procedure is relatively noninvasive, it is considered painful. This technique has the advantage of providing data in a very short time.

Most of the methods of cognitive function assessment discussed in Chapters 24 and 25 represent the current state of the art. Some suggestions for new technologies, both those that were described in the chapters and those discussed during committee deliberations, were also considered. When miniaturization and interfaces are enhanced and portability is improved, such measures should have more field-relevant benefits for the military.

2. How likely are the technologies to mature sufficiently for practical use?

It is believed that within the next 5 years, studies validating the use of MFA for assessment of nutritional status should be completed and documented in the peer-reviewed literature. The device currently is being tested in healthy individuals, trauma patients, hemodialysis patients, HIV+ patients, and nutritionally compromised individuals in general hospital wards, both before and after realimentation. In subjects studied to date, contractile characteristics of healthy volunteers appear reliable, and the test appears to be capable of measuring rapid changes in nutritionally compromised patients following the initiation of refeeding.

Most of the cognitive assessment technologies discussed are already available. The inclusion of the ability to monitor or test cognitive function by incorporation of new technologies into existing equipment used by military personnel would be a significant step in nonintrusive testing. Such technologies should be readily available within 5 years, as required equipment is essentially available. Miniaturization may be required but should easily be developed.

3. What is the cost/benefit ratio of the new technologies, and how expensive (in both monetary and personnel terms) will they be to employ compared with the importance of the information they will provide?

The MFA apparatus is relatively inexpensive, as is the cost for use. Skilled technicians are required to perform the measurements. With proper validation, the cost/benefit ratio for this technique would be quite low, although personnel must leave their assigned tasks to be tested.

Some cognitive assessments, such as paper and pencil tests, are inexpensive but take personnel away from assigned tasks for short periods of time. Others, such as measures involving extensive computer hardware, other hardware (e.g., electroencephalogram monitors), or software programming have high start-up costs for equipment but are designed to monitor, rather than to interfere with, the functions and operations of personnel. The information gathered could be valuable for assessing the role of nutritional and other factors, such as sleep in the field. The use of devices such as simulators involves expensive equipment and also takes personnel away from their tasks to complete the tests.

4. Are the technologies of such critical value that their development should be supported by DoD funds—such as can be provided by the SBIR program?

Developments in the private sector need to be closely monitored by the DoD so that it may adapt what is already commercially available. Because most of the technologies are already developed, specific military field applications that involve miniaturization and increased portability should be financed by DoD.

5. How practical are the technologies? Will they require dedicated personnel and complex, exotic equipment? Will the data provided be difficult to analyze?

The practicality of the MFA device is problematic at present. Constant monitoring does not appear to be possible at this time. In addition, subjects must interrupt their tasks to be measured. Although the device is light enough to be transported to the field, it is somewhat cumbersome for continuous wear and restricts arm movement. Nevertheless, the measurement is noninvasive and in-expensive. The total measurement time is only 10 to 15 minutes, results are available immediately, and in the future, continuous monitoring may be possi-ble.

The cognitive assessment technologies are already in use. Dedicated per-sonnel needs are minimal except for data interpretation. The equipment is not complex or exotic, and most of it is already available. Analysis of these types of data has a long history, and few problems are anticipated; however, as with the MFA and many other assessment tools, personnel must leave their assigned tasks to participate in most tests of cognitive function.

6. Can the technologies be used in the field (could they be used in the field or used to analyze samples collected in the field)?

At present, the potential for use of MFA in the field appears to be low. Al-though the device is light and relatively portable, the validity of the technique remains to be demonstrated, and its use is associated with causing significant pain to the subject. Field use should be reevaluated in the future after existing problems are overcome.

The cognitive assessment techniques, with the exception of field simulators, are all applicable to field-testing scenarios. They await further improvements in miniaturization, portability, and durability.

COMMITTEE CONCLUSIONS

These conclusions were developed in executive session and represent the views of the CMNR.

* Methods of measuring body composition are relevant and important to the military to assure accuracy and fairness in the application of body composition measures to accession and retention of military personnel.
* Anthropometric measures are the most applicable methods for evaluating compliance with military standards of body fat. The more sophisticated technologies of CAT scanning, MRI, and DXA are useful tools for developing application equations from anthropometric measures to estimate body fat.
* BIA is a less-reliable method of measuring body fat at this time, but the methodology may be useful in answering specific questions concerning hydration state and function of cell membranes.
* Tracer methodology, particularly the use of stable isotopes, is an important technology for understanding and measuring metabolic processes (the doubly labeled water technique currently is used in studies of energy expenditure in the field and is a cost-effective technology for this purpose). Stable isotopes that can be administered and measured noninvasively through easily obtained samples offer important opportunities to estimate metabolic processes in the field. Central analysis of samples increases the practicality of their use in field studies.
* Ambulatory monitoring techniques, such as the foot strike measurement, also show good promise as field measures of work and energy expenditure.
* The various molecular and cellular technologies are interesting as research methods but are strictly laboratory research tools at present. Observing the development of these techniques and their application will be important for the MND at USARIEM, but investing in their in-house development is not recommended at this time. As questions develop that may be studied using these techniques, the DoD may wish to consider support for extramural research (for example, the effect of oxidative stress or malnutrition on gene expression).
* Studies of immune function are potentially very important to the military. An understanding of the effect of the various stresses of military operations on the body's immune function and how these may be modified to aid soldier performance is an important area for investigation.
* The development of vaccines that are effective against various infectious diseases of unique significance to the military population but not necessarily of significance to the civilian population may be very important in sustaining the ability of the soldier to operate effectively in the field. Oral vaccines may be most effective as they tend to mimic the route of exposure to the infectious agents that cause problems in the field.
* The development and production of human antibodies by transgenic plants create dramatic new possibilities for short-term (weeks-to-months) prophylaxis, or therapy, of unusual infectious diseases or toxemias of potential

military importance and for which no other forms of immunization currently are available.

• The ability to study the cognitive performance of individuals while they perform their duties has great potential for improving soldier performance under stress. Current developments in computerized and miniaturized technology appear to permit expanded studies of real-time cognitive behavior. Support for the development of specific monitoring devices that are compatible with field military equipment may be necessary to implement this technology.

COMMITTEE RECOMMENDATIONS

The following recommendations are based on the CMNR's review and evaluation of the workshop discussions.

• Fair and equitable implementation of body fat and BMI standards is important to the military. It is recommended that continued research be carried out to refine the anthropometric measures using the sophisticated measurements of body composition provided by DXA, MRI, and/or CAT scanning to assure that measures used to evaluate personnel are equitable for gender, ethnic, and body type characteristics.

• The development and use of scanning technologies for the measurement of changes in body composition (particularly changes in muscle mass) that may result from field exercises should be refined in controlled laboratory environments and in collaboration with the civilian sector.

• Currently, multifrequency BIA is not sufficiently precise to be a useful tool for body composition determination. However, its potential as a simple field measure of hydrational status suggests that research to improve its value should be encouraged.

• Research by the private sector on the use of stable isotopes should be carefully monitored so that issues of concern to the military that can be studied effectively by these methods may be identified and the technology applied to the military situation when the costs versus the benefits are favorable. Since the effective application of this technology requires well-trained personnel and expensive and sophisticated equipment, the collaboration with other government and private sector laboratories in these studies continues to appear most expedient. In addition, as much information as possible should be obtained in well-controlled laboratory environments.

• The various molecular and cellular techniques for the study of nutrition and other physiological processes are strictly laboratory research tools at present and are not ready for implementation by the MND. Military problems that would appear to be amenable to investigation with these tools are of sufficiently broad interest as to be under consideration by established private-sector research laboratories. Maintaining awareness of the activities of these laboratories now receiving significant support by federal and industrial funds should continue, and therefore, DoD investment is not recommended at this time.

• Since military operations are frequently stressful and may be carried out in very hostile environments, it is important to understand the role that the body's immune function plays in helping the soldier cope and to consider ways in which immune responses may be controlled or enhanced to maximize the individual's ability to perform. Awareness of this research field and investment in selected research of potential significance to the military mission should be continued. The military must keep apprised of research findings on the influence of nutritional status on immune function.

• Research on possible vaccine programs that may protect soldiers from infectious diseases frequently encountered in military operations should be supported, particularly when the potential infections are not usually a problem in the civilian sector. Oral vaccine development should be encouraged. Preliminary research at U.S. Army Medical Research Institute for Infectious Diseases to develop militarily important oral vaccines should be expanded. Research should be initiated or funded to develop transgenic plants that can produce antibodies against infections or toxins of unique military importance and to assess the influence of nutritional status on the response of military personnel to vaccinations.

• The development of techniques and equipment that would permit evaluation of cognitive performance of individuals while actually performing their operational tasks should be supported, with the caveat that such techniques must be validated and as much information gathered as possible in controlled laboratory environments prior to field testing. When special modification is required for use in military equipment, support should be given to such development (for example, miniaturization).

The Committee on Military Nutrition Research is pleased to have participated with the Military Nutrition Division (currently the Military Nutrition and Biochemical Division), U.S. Army Research Institute of Environmental Medicine, and the U.S. Army Medical Research and Materiel Command in progress relating to the nutrition, performance, and health of U.S. military personnel. The CMNR hopes that this information will be valuable to the U.S. Department of Defense in developing programs that continue to improve the performance and lifelong health and well-being of service personnel.

II

The Current Army Program and Its Future Needs

THE PAPERS PRESENTED AT THE WORKSHOP comprise parts II through VIII. These chapters have undergone limited editorial change, have not been reviewed by an outside group, and represent the views of the individual authors. Selected questions and the speakers' responses are included at the end of most chapters and sections to provide the flavor of the workshop discussion.

Part II provides an introduction to the workshop. In Chapter 3, an overview is presented of the military nutrition program at the U.S. Army Research Institute of Environmental Medicine. The main objectives of the program's activities are to maintain and to enhance physical and cognitive performance and overall health in all operational environments, particularly through ration enhancement and nutrition intervention. New technologies must be evaluated in terms of this research agenda.

Emerging Technologies for Nutrition Research, 1997
Pp. 71–78. Washington, D.C.
National Academy Press

3

Emerging Technologies in Nutrition Research for the Military: Overview of the Issues

James A. Vogel[1]

INTRODUCTION

Optimal garrison nutrition along with the use of nutritional interventions to maintain or enhance performance under demanding operational circumstances are important to the Armed Forces and are key features of the U.S. Department of Defense's Military Nutrition Research Program. While much of the program is applied in nature and field-trial oriented, the total program, including both intramural and extramural components, demands that the latest innovative technologies be utilized in order to find answers to highly complex issues that now confront the nutrition of today's military service member.

The Military Nutrition Research Program is broad in its scope as it addresses not only optimal nutritional intake and nutritional status of the service member, but also the issues of how nutritional status affects both physical and cognitive performance, as well as health issues that indirectly or directly affect

---

[1] James A. Vogel, P.O. Box 798, Springfield, VT 05156. *Formerly of* U.S. Army Research Institute of Environmental Medicine, Natick, MA 01760-5007

performance. The end result is a need for military nutrition researchers to utilize the latest available technologies in addressing a wide variety of applications to nutrition research, which is the focus of this workshop. This chapter describes the Military Nutrition Research Program in order to identify some of the technologies that are needed to support it.

ORGANIZATION OF THE MILITARY NUTRITION RESEARCH PROGRAM

The Army Surgeon General is responsible to the Department of Defense to conduct research on nutrition and related medical and performance issues for all services. This responsibility pertains both to operational rations and garrison feeding. The program is executed by the Military Nutrition Division (currently the Military Nutrition and Biochemical Division) at the U.S. Army Research Institute of Environmental Medicine at Natick, Mass., and comes under the management of the U.S. Army Medical Research and Materiel Command's Military Operational Medicine Directorate. The companion program for the formulation of operational rations, along with their packaging, field preparation, and delivery, is the responsibility of the Natick Research, Development and Engineering Center's Survivability Directorate under the U.S. Army Soldier Systems Command, also located at Natick, Mass. The requirements of these two research programs are identified by the Food Nutrition Research and Engineering Board, Office of the Secretary of Defense for Science and Technology.

PURPOSE OF THE PROGRAM

The Military Nutrition Research Program exists as an established Army Science and Technology Objective and is composed of four areas: (1) development of nutritional strategies to sustain and enhance military performance in operational environments; (2) evaluation of operational rations and field feeding systems for effects on nutritional status, health, and performance; (3) establishment of nutritional standards for operational rations; and (4) determination of nutritional status of military populations and improvement of garrison diets. Each of these program areas is described briefly.

Development of Nutritional Strategies

Nutritional strategies refer to steps taken, above and beyond providing for a well-balanced and nutritious garrison diet, to provide an enhanced capability to perform in hostile climatic or operational environments common to the Armed Forces. When a service member is subjected to the multiple stressors of these environments, such as caloric deprivation, sleep loss, and high work load, nutrients may become depleted, or their supplementation above usual levels may give a performance advantage in these unique settings. Research in this area is currently divided into three subtopics: (1) performance-enhancing ration components, (2) dietary treatments to counteract immunosuppression, and (3) dietary interventions to meet special requirements.

Performance-Enhancing Ration Components

The concept of adding specific nutrients to an already "optimal" field diet to maintain or enhance performance arose from the Special Operations Command's requirements for simple and safe ways to meet high performance requirements in demanding missions. These added nutrients include potential nutrient ergogenic aids as well as food additives that would counteract sleep loss and maintain alertness and cognitive function under severe stress. This program encompasses research ranging from basic studies on nutrient substrates for brain neurotransmitters to the actual field evaluation in simulated operational settings of proposed ration additives.

Two compounds proven as performance enhancers that can be incorporated within ration items are caffeine and extra amounts of carbohydrates. Caffeine is a proven ergogenic aid (Graham et al., 1994) and is also beneficial in maintaining alertness during sleep deprivation (Lieberman, 1992). Carbohydrate supplementation has proven beneficial for intense, sustained physical performance (Coyle, 1991). In both cases, further research is needed to determine optimal regimens customized to particular military tasks or missions.

Tyrosine (Banderet and Lieberman, 1989) and tryptophan (Segura and Ventura, 1988) are amino acid precursors for neurotransmitters that may aid in sustaining mental function under severe operational stress. Further research is needed to confirm their effect on humans in various militarily relevant environments.

Examples of additional nutrient-type ergogenic additives of recent interest to the military include choline (Wurtman and Lewis, 1991) and creatine (Harris et al., 1992). For the most part, these components have yet to be proven to have practical use in human performance settings.

Dietary Treatments to Counteract Immunosuppression

Recent research carried out as part of the Military Nutrition Research Program has shown that soldiers under the multiple stresses of simulated combat demonstrate an immunosuppressive state that places them at increased risk for infection. Original research on this topic carried out in Army Ranger trainees (Moore et al., 1992) focused on significant caloric deprivation as the primary stress leading to the immunosuppression. Subsequent research (Shippee et al., 1994) with lesser degrees of caloric deprivation suggests that other stressors that also are present—sleep deprivation, heavy work loads, and behavioral stress— may also be implicated. These findings have led to a search for nutritional countermeasures for immunosuppression. Glutamine, choline, antioxidant mixtures, and tyrosine have been studied or are currently under consideration for this purpose.

Dietary Interventions to Meet Special Requirements

In addition to supplementing diets with specific nutrients to enhance performance or correct performance deficits, the use of dietary manipulation also presents itself as a potential strategy to exploit. Topics that have been studied include adjusting the timing of food ingestion, using nutrition education to meet the particular needs of highly active personnel at high levels of performance, and customizing operational ration components to the individual service member and to his or her specific mission requirement. The latter concept stems from interest by the Special Forces in meeting the extreme demands of the individual and unique requirements of certain Special Forces missions.

Evaluation of Operational Rations and Field Feeding Systems

A major component of the Military Nutrition Research Program is the evaluation of the nutritional adequacy of newly developed operational rations to ensure that they meet the health and performance standards of military personnel under all operational conditions. Each new ration item or ration delivery system is tested under realistic field-operating environments to determine if it meets the goals of optimal nutritional delivery to service members in the field. Under this program the Meal, Ready-to-Eat, multi-serving tray packs, and the total field feeding system (USACDEC/USARIEM, 1986) have been tested under various operational and climatic conditions.

This research also has included the assessment of specialty operational rations such as the New Generation Survival Ration (Jones et al., 1992); the Ration, Lightweight (Askew et al., 1987); Long Life Ration Packet (King et al., 1992); and Ration, Cold Weather (Engell et al., 1987). The observed reduction in caloric consumption while eating operational rations also has been studied (Thomas et al., 1995).

Establishment of Nutritional Standards

Although the Military Recommended Dietary Allowances (MRDAs) are now generally well established, special or unique issues that require continued research still arise, particularly in relation to operational feeding. Some examples include: (1) the status of iron nutriture and the need for iron supplementation for female soldiers, (2) the composition and use of oral hydration (electrolyte-glucose) drinks for hot weather and heavy exercise, (3) nutrient requirements and delivery while wearing encapsulated protective clothing, and (4) energy requirements of various operational missions.

Determination of Nutritional Status of Military Populations

Another important component of the Military Nutrition Research Program is the periodic evaluation of the adequacy of military feeding, both in the field and in garrison, by the periodic assessment of the nutritional status of military populations and their dietary intakes. A major thrust of this program is to reduce the overall intake of total fat, cholesterol, and salt. Research in this area includes education (Torri and Baker-Fulco, 1992), menu assessments (Szeto et al., 1987), and menu modification to bring about these changes (Baker-Fulco et al., 1994).

Recent emphasis in this area has centered on nutritional status and dietary intake of women in the Army with particular focus on women entering the service and during initial entry training (King et al., 1994). Specific populations also are studied when questions arise regarding their intake; these include military academy cadets (Klicka et al., 1993), Ranger trainees (Moore et al., 1992; Shippee et al., 1994), and Special Forces candidates.

OTHER NUTRITIONALLY RELATED RESEARCH

Several areas of research are being conducted under the auspices of other military research initiatives, but they apply directly to military nutrition. One of these is body composition investigations. This research includes the development of body weight-for-height standards, body fat standards, and methodology for field estimation of body fat for the Army Weight/Body Fat Program (AR 600-9, 1986), and methodology for field estimation of how body fat and muscle mass relate to physical performance (Vogel and Friedl, 1992). Other research areas include the methodology of measuring caloric expenditure in the field and the relation of injuries and bone density to dietary intake.

AUTHOR'S CONCLUSIONS

The scope of military nutrition research has broadened considerably in recent years, well beyond that of nutritional status, requirements, and deficiencies and their impact on health. Modern warfare presents many new and unique challenges to feeding the fighting service member to maintain or enhance both health and performance. It is the latter factor—a focus on performance—that now frames much of military nutrition research.

The inability to maintain adequate nutritional intake at all times during combat, or the need to utilize nutrition to elicit supranormal performance in special operations, challenges the military nutrition researcher to seek new solutions to complex problems. The broad and varied Military Nutrition Research Program outlined in this chapter requires the best technology that can be assembled. It is displayed in the subsequent chapters.

REFERENCES

AR (Army Regulation) 600-9
  1986   *See* U.S. Department of the Army, 1986.
Askew, E.W., I. Munro, M.A. Sharp, S. Siegel, R. Popper, M.S. Rose, R.W. Hoyt, J.W. Martin, K. Reynolds, H.R. Lieberman, D. Engell, and C.P. Shaw
  1987   Nutritional status and physical and mental performance of Special Operations soldiers consuming the Ration, Lightweight or the Meal, Ready-to-Eat military field ration during a 30-day field training exercise. Technical Report T7-87. Natick, Mass.: U.S. Army Research Institute of Environmental Medicine.
Baker-Fulco, C.J., S.A. Torri, J.E. Arsenault, and J.C. Buchbinder
  1994   Impact of menu changes designed to promote a training diet [abstract]. J. Am. Diet. Assoc. 94(4 suppl.):A9.
Banderet, L.E., and H.R. Lieberman
  1989   Treatment with tyrosine, a neurotransmitter precursor, reduces environmental stress in humans. Brain Res. Bull. 22:759–762.
Coyle, E.F.
  1991   Carbohydrate feedings: Effects on metabolism, performance and recovery. Pp. 1–14 in Advances in Nutrition and Top Sport. Basel: Karger.
Engell, D.B., D.E. Roberts, E.W. Askew, M.S. Rose, J. Buchbinder, and M.A. Sharp
  1987   Evaluation of the Ration, Cold Weather during a 10-day cold weather field training exercise. Technical Report TR87/030. Natick, Mass.: U.S. Army Natick Research, Development and Engineering Center.
Graham, T.E., J.W.E. Rush, and M.H. van Soeren
  1994   Caffeine and exercise: Metabolism and performance. Can. J. Appl. Physiol. 19:111–138.
Harris, R.C., K. Soderlund, and E. Hultman
  1992   Elevation of creatine in resting and exercised muscle of normal subjects by creatine supplementation. Clin. Sci. Colch. 83:367–374.
Jones, T.E., S.H. Mutter, J.M. Aylward, J.P. DeLany, R.L. Stephens, D.M. Caretti, D.A. Jezior, B. Cheema, L.S. Lester, and E.W. Askew
  1992   Nutrition and hydration status of aircrew members consuming the Food Packet, Survival, General Purpose, Improved during a simulated survival scenario. Technical Report T1-93, AD A528 744. Natick, Mass.: U.S. Army Research Institute of Environmental Medicine.
King, N., S.H. Mutter, D.E. Roberts, E.W. Askew, A.J. Young, T.E. Jones, M.Z. Mays, M.R. Sutherland, J.P. DeLany, B.E. Cheema, and R. Tulley
  1992   Nutrition and hydration status of soldiers consuming the 18-Man Arctic Tray Pack Ration Module with either the Meal, Ready-to-Eat or the Long Life Ration Packet during a cold weather field training exercise. Technical Report T4-92. Natick, Mass.: U.S. Army Research Institute of Environmental Medicine.

King, N., J.E. Arsenault, S.H. Mutter, C. Champagne, T.G. Murphy, K.A. Westphal, and E.W. Askew
  1994   Nutritional intake of female soldiers during the U.S. Army basic combat training. Technical Report T17-94. Natick, Mass.: U.S. Army Research Institute of Environmental Medicine.

Klicka, M.V., D.E. Sherman, N. King, K.E. Friedl, and E.W. Askew
  1993   Nutritional assessment of cadets at the U.S. Military Academy: Part 2. Assessment of nutritional intake. Technical Report T1-94. Natick, Mass.: U.S. Army Research Institute of Environmental Medicine.

Lieberman, H.R.
  1992   Caffeine. Pp. 49–72 in Factors Affecting Human Performance, Volume II: Health and Performance, D. Jones and A. Smith, eds. London: Academic Press.

Moore, R.J., K.E. Friedl, T.R. Kramer, L.E. Martinez-Lopez, R.W. Hoyt, R.E. Tulley, J.P. DeLany, E.W. Askew, and J.A. Vogel
  1992   Changes in soldier nutritional status and immune function during the Ranger training course. Technical Report No. T13-92. Natick, Mass.: U.S. Army Research Institute of Environmental Medicine.

Segura, R., and J.L. Ventura
  1988   Effect of L-tryptophan supplementation on exercise performance. Int. J. Sports Med. 9:301–305.

Shippee, R., K. Friedl, T. Kramer, M. Mays, K. Popp, E.W. Askew, B. Fairbrother, R. Hoyt, J. Vogel, L. Marchitelli, P. Frykman, L. Martinez-Lopez, E. Bernton, M. Kramer, R. Tulley, J. Rood, J. Delaney, D. Jezior, J. Arsenault, B. Nindl, R. Galloway, and D. Hoover
  1994   Nutritional and immunological assessment of Ranger students with increased caloric intake. Technical report T95-5. Natick, Mass: U.S. Army Research Institute of Environmental Medicine.

Szeto, E.G., D.E. Carlson, T.B. Dugan, and J.C. Buchbinder
  1987   A comparison of nutrient intakes between a Fort Riley contractor-operated and a Fort Lewis military-operated garrison dining facility. Technical Report T2-88. Natick, Mass.: U.S. Army Research Institute of Environmental Medicine.

Thomas, C.D., K.E. Friedl, M.Z. Mays, S.H. Mutter, R.J. Moore, D.Z. Jezior, C.J. Baker-Fulco, L.J. Marchitelli, R.T. Tulley, and E.W. Askew
  1995   Nutrient intakes and nutritional status of soldiers consuming the Meal, Ready-to-Eat (MRE XII) during a 30-day field training exercise. Technical Report No. T95-6. Natick, Mass.: U.S. Army Research Institute of Environmental Medicine.

Torri, S.A., and C.J. Baker-Fulco
  1992   Sports nutrition in the military. Scan's Pulse: Sports and Cardiovascular Nutritionists Newsletter 11(4):16–17.

USACDEC/USARIEM (U.S. Army Combat Developments Experimentation Center and U.S. Army Research Institute of Environmental Medicine)
  1986   Combat Field Feeding System-Force Development Test and Experimentation (CFFS-FDTE). Technical Report CDEC-TR-85-006A. Vol. 1, Basic Report; vol. 2, Appendix A; vol. 3, Appendixes B through L. Fort Ord, Calif.: U.S. Army Combat Developments Experimentation Center.

U.S. Department of the Army
  1986   Army Regulation 600-9. "The Army Weight Control Program." September 1. Washington, D.C.

Vogel, J.A., and K.E. Friedl
  1992 Army data: Body composition and physical capacity. Pp. 89–103 in Body Composition and Physical Performance, Applications for the Military Services, B.M. Marriott and J. Grumstrup-Scott, eds. A report of the Committee on Military Nutrition Research, Food and Nutrition Board, Institute of Medicine. Washington, D.C.: National Academy Press.
Wurtman, R.J., and M.C. Lewis
  1991 Exercise, plasma composition, and neurotransmission. Med. Sports Sci. 32:94–109.

III

Techniques of Body Composition Assessment

PART III BEGINS WITH AN OVERVIEW in Chapter 4 of the military's use of body composition standards to enhance readiness, promote fitness, and maintain appearance. Body fat standards vary by age, gender, and branch. The military relies primarily on body mass index to predict percentage body fat. Equations incorporating anthropometric measurements are then used to determine percentage body fat in those who fail the initial screen. While hydrodensitometry has been the criterion method for validating these equations, other assessment techniques are being explored.

Imaging methods for studying body composition at the tissue-system level are explored in Chapter 5. Computerized axial tomography and magnetic resonance imaging/spectroscopy measure total-body skeletal muscle mass and adipose tissue. They allow clear visualization of the boundaries between adipose tissue, muscle, and bone and quantification of all major tissue-system level components: adipose tissue, skeletal muscle, bone, visceral organs, and brain. The images of these components are analyzed to estimate tissue- and organ-level body composition, and algorithms are applied to estimate total tissue-system volume.

Dual-energy x-ray absorptiometry, discussed in Chapter 6, measures bone mineral content and bone mineral density. As a means of body composition measurement, x-ray attenuation distinguishes bone mineral, nonbone lean tissue, and fat and can be used to evaluate regional body composition. While soft tissue measurements are not accurate, this method may become the criterion method of assessing body composition because of the precise data it produces and its independence from underlying assumptions.

As presented in Chapter 7, bioelectrical impedance analysis measures current flow through the body noninvasively to generate equations that are validated against other body composition assessment methods. This method is based on the assessment of total body water, so its utility is affected by differences in hydrational status.

Emerging Technologies for Nutrition Research, 1997
Pp. 81–126. Washington, D.C.
National Academy Press

4

Military Application of Body Composition Assessment Technologies

Karl E. Friedl[1]

Excess fat is viewed as the prime factor governing the level of specific gravity. Precise measurements, however, of this excess fat will necessarily await a knowledge of the relative percentage variation of the weight of the skeleton in lean persons.

> Technical limitations of using body density for estimation of body fat, noted in the U.S. Navy study that established the method of underwater weighing ("The specific gravity of healthy men: Body weight divided by volume as an index of obesity," Behnke et al., 1942)

Military operational medicine research focuses on sustainment of the warfighter. Body composition is a critical aspect of this research, reflecting energy stores and other aspects of nutritional status, hydrational status, muscular strength potential, and risk for musculoskeletal injury. Changes in body fat indicate shifts in energy balance, and changes in lean mass suggest adaptive or mal-

---

[1] Karl E. Friedl, Army Operational Medicine Research Program, U.S. Army Medical Research and Materiel Command, Fort Detrick, MD 21702-5012

adaptive responses to environmental stressors. Some of these maladaptive changes in body composition are mediated through endocrine stress responses also associated with increased susceptibility to traumatic stress and reduced immunocompetence.

Service members may be pregnant women concerned about trade-offs between appropriate weight gain for the health of their newborns and a prompt return-to-duty status following delivery.

Adolescent recruits are still physically immature and have not yet reached peak bone mineral accretion or peak muscle mass, yet these youngest soldiers are exposed to some of the Army's most physically demanding training.

Overweight individuals need scientifically based guidance in their attempts to comply with military fat standards through sensible fat weight reduction, enhancing (instead of inadvertently impairing) physical readiness.

An understanding of physiological mechanisms to maximize fat oxidation and to increase nitrogen and calcium recycling can lead to interventions to minimize muscle and bone loss in special operations. For example, long-range surveillance teams may be in a detraining state, with loss of Type II muscle fibers as a result of remaining virtually motionless for prolonged periods of time in forward positions. At the opposite extreme, direct action missions may require intense sustained performance without recovery from a catabolic state for several days.

Thus, body composition technologies are important to enhance military readiness. Research on body composition and metabolism helps the military to develop appropriate standards for selection and fitness; to assess military training programs; and to assess the risks and benefits of optimizing strategies, including exercise, pharmacological, and nutritional interventions.

This chapter will review the current body fat standards utilized by the military. It also will cover expedient methods that have been developed to categorize soldiers as overfat or within standards; improved criterion methods (including multicompartment models and dual-energy x-ray absorptiometry [DEXA or DXA]) to revalidate the expedient methods and to determine validity in weight loss settings with and without hydrational changes; and regional aspects of fat, muscle, and bone mineral distribution that identify physical and metabolic risks and advantages more precisely.

ARMY BODY COMPOSITION STANDARDS: GOALS AND METHODS

Army body composition standards are intended to enhance combat readiness (Friedl, 1992). Except for exclusion of grossly obese individuals, body composition standards are not designed to *select* for physical capabilities; instead, the standards promote fitness and prevent the development of obesity. Due to the absence of obese soldiers, studies of the relationship between adiposity and physical performance in Army studies demonstrate only weak to nonexistent relationships (i.e., within this restricted range of adiposity) (Vogel and Friedl, 1992a). Body fat standards also directly support a secondary objective of military appearance (Hodgdon et al., 1990).

The Army fat standards are derived from the average fatness of physically fit young men and women, averaging 15 and 25 percent, respectively (U.S. Department of Defense, 1981). These represent mean body fat levels corresponding to an *average* maximal aerobic capacity of approximately 50 and 39 ml/kg/min for military men and women, respectively. The upper limit of allowable body fat has an additional allowance for a normal distribution around the average and to allow for error in assessment methods; thus, young men and women are allowed up to 20 and 30 percent body fat, respectively. These levels of fatness correspond to break points where mean aerobic fitness declines to less than average fitness (Vogel and Friedl, 1992a), and military appearance for most individuals declines from "good" to "fair" (Friedl and Vogel, 1989). Line commanders and selection boards have been consistent in their complaints that the body fat standards are too lax, because many soldiers still *look* too fat. This is at least partly a problem of enforcement of the existing standards by some commanders (Friedl et al., 1987).

Above their body fat limit, soldiers must lose weight in a sensible weight loss program, or face elimination from the Army. Although it is referred to as the Army Weight Control Program, only recently has the regulation (AR 600-9, 1986) been modified to provide more positive assistance to soldiers exceeding the standards and to discourage inappropriate weight loss habits. Very little Army research has been performed in this area of weight loss and maintenance. One difficulty for Army researchers has been recruiting and retaining as experimental subjects individuals whose careers are at risk; most overweight soldiers wish to evade special attention. This research may become more important as the prevalence of obesity in the U.S. population continues to increase.

It is important to reiterate that there are gender-appropriate differences in body fat distribution and proportion because these differences still are not universally accepted by military policymakers. In recent Congressional testimony, one of the military services was quoted as claiming that "the higher percentage body fat in American women [is] not physiological, but because they are less fitness conscious. In short, American women are fatter than men and must be held to a higher standard until they get their act together" (U.S. Congress, House, 1992, 117). A ludicrous reversal of this concept, but one favoring women, would be to hold all service members, including men, to a narrow waist circumference standard based on the average for young women. Even in the twelfth century, a gender difference in body fat content was sufficiently well recognized that there was a policy in England that no woman would be put to the ordeal of cold water submersion; women were not likely to pass the test by sinking (they were given the test of the hot iron instead) (Kerr et al., 1992).

Qualitative differences in body fat due to gender-specific distributions also make direct quantitative comparisons inappropriate; there can be no direct linkage between male and female fat standards. The Army fat standards allow a constant difference of 10 percent body fat between men and women in each age category only by arbitrary design; this does not translate into a 10 percent physiological equivalency across the range of adiposity. For example, at the extreme low end of body fat, men and women can both achieve 4 to 6 percent body fat (Friedl et al., 1994a; Garg et al., 1992; Mazess et al., 1990a). At the higher end, a male with 30 percent body fat is not equivalent to a female with 40 percent body fat, because the male fat is primarily intraabdominal, with still greater health risks to the male than that to the female, whose fat is distributed to sites with other physiological roles (Lemieux et al., 1993).

The standards accommodate apparent but still poorly defined, age-related increases in relative fatness (Table 4-1). The upper end of this sliding scale is anchored by a health-related rather than an aerobic fitness relationship. Health-risk thresholds occur at higher fatness than do reductions in aerobic fitness. Male and female soldiers over age 40 are held to an upper limit of 26 and 36 percent body fat. These body fat levels approximate the body mass index (BMI) defined by the Surgeon General as obesity, the threshold of increased health risks including cardiovascular disease, insulin resistance, and gall bladder disease (DHHS, 1988). The fat standards for the military have been related to the male and female obesity definition using regression equations from a large sample of Army basic trainees, with body fat determined by the Army circumference equations (Friedl et al., 1989).

TABLE 4-1 Body Composition Standards[*]

Age (years)	Male		Female	
	BMI (kg/m^2)	Body Fat (%)	BMI (kg/m^2)	Body Fat (%)
< 21	25.9	20	23.5	30
21–27	26.5	22	24.3	32
28–39	27.2	24	25.0	34
≥ 40	27.6	26	25.5	36

NOTE: Body mass index (BMI) and equations in this table are the basis for the height-weight tables and body fat computation tables in AR 600-9 (1986) and updated female weight tables in the pending revision of AR 600-9.

[*] Soldiers exceeding the screening weight threshold (based on BMI) are then assessed for percentage body fat (%BF) using the Army circumference equations. Males: %BF = 43.74 − (68.68 · LOG(HT)) + (76.46 · LOG(ABDOMINAL CIRC − NECK CIRC)). Females: %BF = (105.3 · LOG(WT)) − (0.200 · WRIST CIRC) − (0.533 · NECK CIRC) − (1.574 · FOREARM CIRC) + (0.173 · HIP CIRC) − (0.515 · HT) − 35.6. Height (HT) is measured in cm; weight (WT) in kg; circumference (CIRC) in cm.

Maturational changes in body composition are still poorly understood, although there are suspected relationships to changes in anabolic hormones that occur with age, parity, menopause, and other aspects of the life cycle. In addition to physiologically regulated changes, there are increases in fatness and declines in muscle mass that reflect increasingly sedentary behavior as careers progress and many soldiers become more "desk bound." Superimposed on physiology and physical activity are the cumulative effects of long-standing health and nutrition habits, including smoking and excessive alcohol consumption (Björntorp, 1990). The only age stratification in the Army regulation (AR 600-9, 1986) that has firm data support is a steady increase in weight (not necessarily fat weight) of young males up to age 21; this is observed irrespective of modern nutritional advantages and lifestyle, in data from Civil War soldiers as well as in data from soldiers nearly a century later (Gould, 1869; Karpinos, 1961).

In the Biometric Survey of Army Officers, Reed and Love (1932) analyzed annual physical and medical records of 5,000 officers across a 29-y span. They concluded that there was a physiological increase in body weight and chest measurements that occurred between the late twenties and the forties; however, they also classified approximately 10 percent of the group as remaining at stable low weight over 25 to 30 years. New longitudinal studies of career male and female soldiers held to the current body composition standards using state-of-the-art body composition technologies would be valuable in determining the influence of military lifestyle and fitness on changes typically attributed to normal maturation.

All soldiers are assessed for compliance with body composition standards every 6 months throughout their careers. These standards are applied using weight-for-height screens (based on BMI). The weight screen is designed to identify soldiers who *may* be overfat and should be further assessed using the body fat equations. Adiposity and BMI are only roughly related ($r = \sim 0.7$ in most military samples) (Friedl and Vogel, 1997; Vogel et al., 1990), and the relationship is particularly susceptible to influences of physical activity, gender, and age. The weight screen is an important step in the assessment. It is not practical to perform body fat assessments on all soldiers every 6 months, nor is it desirable to apply the less precise body fat estimation directly when the weight screen can provide a first-tier assessment to the majority of the force (Table 4-1). The principal change in the administration of the weight control program in this decade has been the addition of an objective second-tier assessment, the measurement of relative body fat, which is an important improvement over the previous reliance on weight tables alone (or a subjective final decision by a physician). This is intended to protect some of the best performers, soldiers who are large but not fat (i.e., those men and women most suited to many military tasks requiring high physical work capacity).

As an example of how the weight screen is used, Figure 4-1 shows the distribution of fatness of young male recruits (ages 21–27) divided by results of the

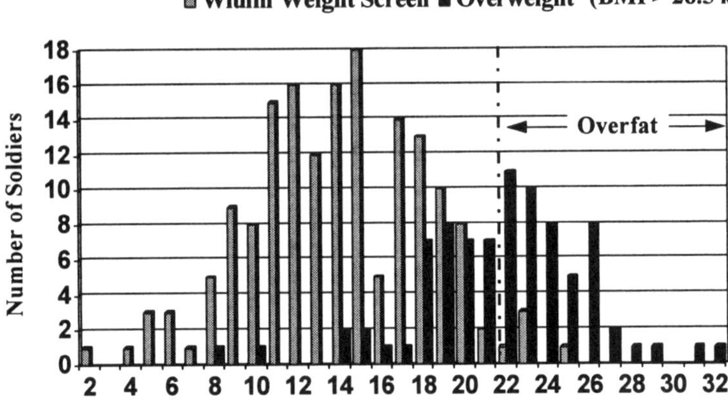

FIGURE 4-1 Distribution of soldiers by fatness predicted by the male Army equation, divided by those men within and exceeding the weight screen. Data are shown for 251 men aged 21 to 27. The screening weight thresholds for this age group are based on a body mass index (BMI) of 26.5 kg/m^2, and the upper limit of allowable body fat is 22 percent. AR 600-9, Army Regulation 600-9 (1986). SOURCE: Plotted data from the 1988 Accession Body Weight Standards Study (Friedl et al., 1989).

weight screen for this age group. These soldiers are held to an upper limit of 22 percent body fat after they leave basic training. Two overlapping distributions of fatness, one for men who are below the weight screen and one for large soldiers who exceed it, illustrate that adiposity and BMI are only roughly related. It also illustrates how the BMI cutoff points have been set for the screening tables. Few overfat soldiers are misclassified as within standards by the weight screen; approximately half of those *exceeding* the weight screen are determined to be overfat, with the remainder of "overweight" soldiers classified as within fat standards.

After more than a decade of enforcing weight control standards in the Army, some military posts with only a small influx of new recruits report that most soldiers exceeding weight standards are within fat standards (Personal communication, S. Newcomb, Office of the Deputy Chief of Staff for Personnel, Washington, D.C., 1995), instead of the 50 percent split in new recruits (Friedl et al., 1989). These reports from the field suggest that the Army weight control program has been effective in eliminating obesity from the Army. There are no data to indicate whether this is reflective of early discharge, prematurely ending careers of soldiers who do not comply with the standards, or if many soldiers are successfully modifying habits and better regulating body weight through their careers. Shortly after the major revision of the Army Weight Control Program (1983–1984), the individual progress of 174 overfat soldiers was quietly surveyed, and it was found that more than one-third did not make weight loss progress within 6 months in the program and that nearly half of these soldiers were lost from record or left the service. Of those soldiers who were initially successful in achieving their weight goals, 13 percent were formally returned to the program within another 6 months (Friedl et al., 1987). Although soldiers operating under these standards are more conscious of nutrition and fitness behaviors than ever before, there are no data on actual nutrition habits and whether these standards are any different from those of the general U.S. population.

The current method of body fat estimation is part of the Army regulation (AR 600-9, 1986) and cannot be substituted with any other method. This is a practical consideration that prevents soldiers from shopping around for the most favorable body fat measurement. By having only one approved method of measurement for the Army regulation, the regulation is enforceable and equitable; however, because of the potential impact to an individual's career, there are several requirements that must be satisfied with careful validation.

The first critical requirement is the accurate *classification* of soldiers and the absence of gross errors for any individual. (This is different from a research application, where a method needs to be quantitatively accurate across a range of adiposity; if the equations tend to overestimate at low body fat and underestimate at the high end, as most anthropometric equations do, they may still be fully adequate in classifying soldiers as fat and/or within standards.) The second requirement is that the classification must not inadvertently contradict the goals of the regulation, such as with body fat equations that penalize soldiers with the greatest strength fitness, or with overly stringent standards (i.e., based on the measurement of fat sites that are not readily modifiable) requiring physiologically inappropriate energy restriction that impairs readiness. The adequacy of the current Army body fat equations in satisfying these requirements is considered in the next two sections.

VALIDATION OF MILITARY EQUATIONS AGAINST CRITERION METHODS

Shortcomings of Underwater Weighing

Although all of the current military body fat equations were developed against relative body fat as determined by underwater weighing, the equations utilized by each service produce different results. A part of this difference is related to differences in the techniques used in underwater weighing, and another part of the variation is explained by fundamental shortcomings in this two-compartment model of body composition and by the manner in which the characteristics of the different military study sample behaved, or were interpreted, within the assumptions of this method. Thus, the technique of underwater weighing is not well standardized, and deviations from the assumptions of the two-compartment model can produce sizable errors. In addition, there are practical problems that affect reproducibility. Central to this problem of reproducibility is a subject's performance of the underwater breathing maneuvers. This is a big problem for Army sampling since half of the Army cannot swim, and many potential research subjects will not be comfortable with full submersion and underwater exhalation (Fitzgerald et al., 1986).

The effects of variations in methodology and calculations are not trivial. A survey of four journals covering a 5-y period, revealed a diversity of techniques used in underwater weighing (Table 4-2). In the face of this variety, it is discouraging to note from this tabulation that nearly a quarter of research articles, including some where body composition is central to the study, provide little information about how the underwater weighing was performed and no reference to a published method.

The most commonly provided information is the method of residual volume measurement (Table 4-2), and the reported variations in the methodology used introduce large differences to the measurement of body density. Fixed values and estimates based on vital capacity simply do not provide accurate density measurements (Morrow et al., 1986; Withers and Ball, 1988) but are found in the literature. The expedient oxygen dilution method developed by Wilmore et al. (1980) is the most frequently cited, perhaps because of the wide availability of oxygen monitors associated with exercise labs, whereas helium dilution and nitrogen washout devices are more likely to be found in clinical research labs. In a comparison of the three techniques, Forsyth et al. (1988) reported that helium equilibrium produced higher values than nitrogen washout or oxygen dilution. The mean difference between the helium and oxygen methods was 360 ml, producing calculated differences of greater than 2 percent body fat. If a body plethysmograph is available, total thoracic gas volumes can be measured. This becomes important in smokers and others who may have obstructive disease, (which would otherwise result in an underestimate of body density). However, this still does not account for gastrointestinal gas (which could be measured by plethysmography using an intragastric balloon).

It is most common to ignore gastrointestinal gas or to ask subjects to report to the lab for testing after an overnight fast and/or after a walk; whether or not this reduces variability is only assumed (Durnin and Satwanti, 1982). Less commonly, fixed volumes of 100 ml are subtracted along with residual volumes in the calculation of body density, an average volume measured by Bedell et al. (1956). However, in Bedell's study (1956), some normal individuals had measured volumes as high as 500 ml, and earlier studies suggested mean volumes as high as 1 liter (Blair et al., 1947). The difference between 0 and 500 ml of additional abdominal gas volume results in errors of 2 percent body fat or more.

Replication of the conditions for measurement of residual volume and exhalation under water is particularly challenging. Experienced swimmers tend to hold back air under water, and nonswimmers are inconsistent in their underwater performance, compared to maximal exhalation out of the water. To avoid these problems, some studies include measurement of the residual volume si-

TABLE 4-2 Variations of Underwater Weighing Methodology Reported in 150 Peer-Reviewed Journal Articles over a 5-y Span[*]

Approach/Technique	Number of Studies
Subject preparation	
Fasted	16
Not reported	134
Position for underwater weighing	
Sitting	14
Prone or kneeling	2
Not specified	134
Trials and selection	
Average of highest 2–3 of 10 trials	31
Average of all of 6–10 trials	7
Average of last 3 after 6–10 trials	7
Other method of selection	4
Not specified	101
Residual volume—timing of the measurement	
Underwater	16
In water, head out	1
Separate from underwater weighing[†]	88
Residual volume—method	
Oxygen dilution	63
Helium equilibration	25
Nitrogen washout	16
Estimated from vital capacity	6
Fixed value	1
Whole body plethysmography	1
Not specified	38
Method cited	
Brozék et al., 1963	20
Behnke and Wilmore, 1974	11
Siri, 1961	11
Akers and Buskirk, 1969	8
Katch et al., 1967	7
Goldman and Buskirk, 1961	7
Other specified	42

[*] Four journals were examined: *American Journal of Clinical Nutrition, International Journal of Obesity, Journal of Applied Physiology*, and *Medicine and Science in Sports and Exercise*; 192 articles reported results based on underwater weighing; 42 of these gave no description of (or reference to) methodology used.

[†] Specified or assumed.

                                            KARL E. FRIEDL

multaneously with the underwater weight, but corrections for the attached hoses may introduce other inconsistencies. Another technical variation, the use of a snorkel for subjects uncomfortable with underwater exhalation (used in the 1984 Army Body Composition Study [Vogel et al., 1988]), has been empirically determined to add approximately 1 percent body fat to final estimations (Siconolfi et al., 1987). Some investigators claim that a prone position in the water allows subjects to produce a better maximal exhalation, and this may be accompanied by measurement of residual volume outside of the tank in the prone position.

There is little consistency in how trials are selected and averaged. The most common approach is to perform two to three residual volume measurements and average the most consistent efforts. Repeated underwater weighing trials (10 trials are common) are usually performed, with an average taken of the highest two or three weights within some level of reproducibility (e.g., within 50 g of each other). However, an average of all of a smaller number of trials is also used. Since the first several trials tend to produce lower weights than subsequent trials (Katch et al., 1967), this approach will tend to give higher body fat estimations than a selection of highest or later trials.

The two most commonly used equations for estimating percentage body fat from density, the equations of Siri (1961) and of Brozék et al. (1963), produce different values, with 2 percent body fat difference at the higher end of adiposity (~40% body fat). Thus, it is apparent that a wide range of percentage body fat values could be obtained for any one individual across different laboratories simply because of differences in technique.

Errors Produced by Assumptions in the Interpretation of Body Density

Even within the same laboratory, errors in the way individuals are assessed by underwater weighing can be sizable because of the assumptions of the two-compartment models that are used to interpret density. Small relative changes in body water can have a large effect because it is by far the largest single constituent of human body composition; "bags-of-mostly-water" was the descriptive name for humans used by a Star Trek silica-based lifeform. Bone mineral content also has a prominent effect on variability of the fat-free mass (FFM) because of its high density compared to other constituents. Thus, these two components, which are lumped into the FFM, introduce variations to the assumed density of 1.100 g/cm^3. Lesser contributors to variation in FFM, such as glycogen stores and nonosseous minerals, may also be important in military environmental stress studies.

Although 73.2 percent is a commonly used value for the assumed hydration of the FFM, this value represents an average from six experiments with nonhuman mammalian species where the species averages ranged between 69.9 and 74.5 percent (Pace and Rathbun, 1945, 689). Physiological variations outside of this range in humans, such as those that have been encountered in semistarved

Ranger students (Friedl et al., 1994a), make this a risky assumption in military field studies.

In some military settings, changes in body water may not have a very marked effect. For example, a modest dehydration of 3 percent of body weight in a typical 70 kg, 15 percent body fat male soldier can be calculated to produce a relatively small underprediction of fatness (14.3% body fat) by underwater weighing. However, larger variations in body water may occur physiologically. In young women with complaints of water retention, Bunt et al. (1989) measured mean fluctuations in total body water of 1.5 liters over the course of single menstrual cycles. Mean body densities were 1.0434 and 1.0374 g/cm^3 at low and high weights through the menstrual cycle, corresponding to body fat estimations of 24.4 and 27.2 percent, respectively. With adjustments for actual body water measures, the true body fat was estimated to be 25.6 percent.

In studies of Ranger students with high rates of weight loss, an excess hydration of FFM has been observed, where decreases in fat and body cell mass were not accompanied by a concomitant reduction in total body water (Friedl et al., 1994a). Keys et al. (1950) observed this hydrational derangement in the semistarved men of the Minnesota Starvation Study and attempted corrections to the body fat estimates obtained from body density measured by underwater weighing. They found that corrections for the disproportionately high thiocyanate space (a measure of extracellular water) were approximately canceled by the increased contribution to density of the estimated bone mineral content (which was assumed not to have changed markedly within the period of the study, even as body cell mass diminished). However, whole body densities of greater than 1.100 g/cm^3 were still obtained for a few individuals.

Errors from variations in the fractional bone mineral contributions to the density of FFM have presented problems in several settings. Estimates of skeletal weights and bone mineral content differences suggest that the average bone mineral content is 20 percent greater in black compared with white subjects. Thus, it is not surprising that in the 1984 Army Body Composition Study, of the lean young men who had whole body densities of greater than 1.100 g/ml (i.e., for which a meaningful percentage body fat could not be calculated), five were black and one was Hispanic (Friedl and Vogel, 1992).

Osteopenic subjects (subjects with low bone density), particularly young amenorrheic white women, deviate from a reference man in the opposite direction. The effects of bone mineral differences can be demonstrated by measurements on two women at opposite extremes of total-body bone mineral densities, measured in a study by Cote and Adams (1993). These two young women were assessed with total-body bone mineral densities of 1.060 and 1.392 g/cm^2 (for reference, normal young female soldiers average ~1.15 g/cm^2); body fat by underwater weighing (and the Siri [1961] equation) was estimated at 21.4 and 16.7 percent, respectively. However, more accurate body fat estimates using measurements of bone mineral and body water in a four-compartment model, yielded values of 18.7 and 20.7 percent, respectively (Cote and Adams, 1993). In other words, the differences in bone mineral content produced individual errors of +2.7 and –4.0 percent body fat in a two-compartment model.

These problems with underwater weighing do not automatically invalidate the military body fat equations that were developed and "calibrated" against underwater weighing. Anthropometric estimates of fatness are less influenced by variations in bone density or hydration of the FFM, which confound the criterion measurement; thus, the military equations may actually be fairer to individuals than underwater weighing (Friedl and Vogel, 1992). The circumference equations also have superior reproducibility, with half of the variance in repeated measurements (0.5% body fat) of the underwater weighing method (1.0%).

Regardless of criterion method parentage, the military equations must be revalidated against the best, most practical criterion methods available so that they can be improved if biological accuracy is a concern and to ensure that the equations are not unintentionally biased (such as by ethnicity). Instead of two-compartment models, which are influenced by ethnic, gender, and various environmental factors, the four-compartment model that includes measurements of total body bone mineral and total body water along with hydrodensitometry is accurate, practical, and achievable (Heymsfield et al., 1990a).

Improved Criterion Measure with a Four-Compartment Model

Early attempts at multicompartment models of body composition were limited by technological barriers, primarily in the accurate assessment of bone mineral (Allen et al., 1959; Selinger, 1977). Three-compartment models, which include measurement of total body water (TBW), have been practical in military studies almost since the development of underwater weighing (Behnke et al., 1942; Freeman et al., 1955; Siri, 1961); however, a key factor in the variability of the FFM has been the fractional contribution of bone mineral. In studies with Army basic trainees, Best and Kuhl (1955) tried to improve on available methods with the use of x-ray outlines of soft tissue and quantification of nonbone tissues. What they lacked was modern computing power and the ability to quantify density of the tissue, now available with soft-tissue analyses by DEXA (Mazess et al., 1990b). The currently available DEXA soft tissue body composition analysis is a side benefit of the development of safer and more practical bone mineral measurement devices. Most importantly, with the advent of dual-photon absorptiometry (DPA) and further improvements with DEXA, four-compartment models, which include measurement of bone mineral content, have finally become practical. Heymsfield and his colleagues (1990a) have demonstrated the accuracy of such a four-compartment model that is safer and more convenient than the current *in vivo* gold standard of neutron activation analysis and tritiated water dilution.

The comparison of values from the Heymsfield four-compartment model for five male and five female soldiers selected for a range of adiposity with values obtained by two- and three-compartment model methods is shown in Table 4-3. Each of these methods provides estimates similar to the four-compartment model, and each of them is superior to field methods such as bioelectrical impedance analysis (BIA) or skinfold equations. Underwater weighing and total body water two-compartment models are related to the four-compartment model with shared components of the calculations (density and body water). DEXA soft tissue analysis is fairly independent since the bone mineral content used in the four-compartment model is measured in the bone-containing pixels that are excluded from the soft tissue analysis of body fat. This also makes the DEXA body composition analysis essentially a three-compartment model involving bone and fat and soft lean tissues.

It is this latter factor that makes DEXA a significant improvement for U.S. military studies, as will be discussed in the next section. It is critical to demonstrate the independence from ethnic bias of any proposed methods, and clearly two-compartment models are not independent because of the effect of bone mineral differences, whether between black and white subjects (Schutte et al., 1984) or even across different ethnic groups (Seidell et al., 1990). It will never be useful for the U.S. Army to develop race- or ethnicity-specific standards,

TABLE 4-3 Percentage Body Fat Estimated by Various Standard Methods in 10 Nonsmoking Young (Age < 40) Male and Female Soldiers Representing a Range of Fatness

Subject Characteristics			Body Fat (%)					
Ethnicity	Age	BMI	4-C	DEXA	UWW	TBW	BIA	DW
Males								
W	28	24.6	**5.9**	4.7	7.6	6.4	12.1	9.9
W	20	22.8	**10.1**	12.9	8.8	9.4	20.0	16.2
H	35	20.5	**15.2**	14.4	10.8	15.1	16.0	17.2
H	19	24.0	**19.5**	18.2	16.2	22.0	21.3	18.6
A	24	27.4	**26.6**	25.9	26.4	27.1	27.5	19.1
Females								
B	22	23.3	**15.7**	18.2	15.5	14.5	24.3	19.5
B	19	18.8	**18.8**	20.0	19.1	17.3	21.1	23.1
W	20	20.9	**25.0**	26.8	28.3	21.5	29.0	26.3
W	23	20.1	**29.4**	27.5	27.8	28.6	30.6	25.3
H	20	24.5	**34.7**	34.1	34.6	33.4	33.0	34.1

NOTE: BMI, body mass index (kg/m^2); 4-C, four-compartment; DEXA, dual-energy x-ray absorptiometry; UWW, underwater weighing; TBW, total body water; BIA, bioelectrical impedance analysis; DW, Durnin and Womersley (1974); W, white; H, Hispanic; B, black; A, Asian.

SOURCE: K. E. Friedl (Unpublished data, U.S. Army Research Institute of Environmental Medicine, Natick, Mass., 1993); methods described in Friedl et al. (1992).

equations, or tables; they must be independent of race and ethnic effects, either through inclusion of the measurements that account for known sources of variation, or it must be demonstrated that they are unaffected by these factors.

DEXA Soft Tissue Analysis as a Practical Improvement over Underwater Weighing

As a criterion method, DEXA[2] provides an improvement in precision, and probably in accuracy, over underwater weighing. More importantly, it is more convenient in large-scale military field research studies and has better reproducibility than underwater weighing (±0.5% vs ±1.0% body fat) (Friedl et al., 1992). Accuracy of the DEXA soft tissue analysis compares well with the four-compartment model for male and female soldiers (Figure 4-2). These data were obtained from fasted, young, nonsmoking soldiers, according to methods previ-

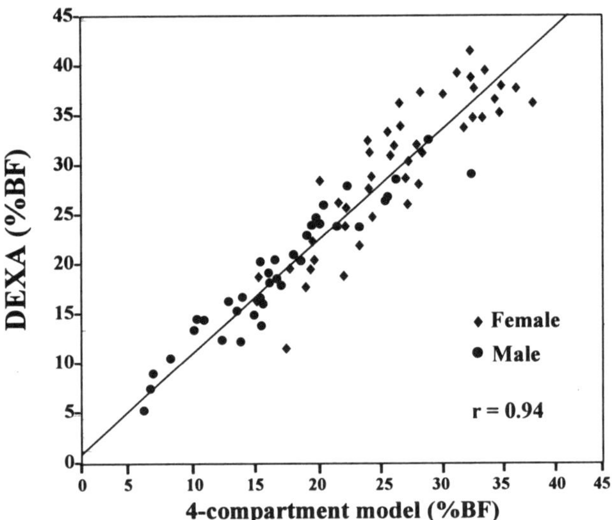

FIGURE 4-2 Percentage body fat (%BF) from dual-energy x-ray absorptiometry (DEXA) analysis compared to a four-compartment model for 37 male and 45 female soldiers. These data were obtained exactly as described in Friedl et al. (1992). SOURCE: Adapted from K. E. Friedl (Unpublished data, U.S. Army Research Institute of Environmental Medicine, Natick, Mass., 1993); methods described in Friedl et al. (1992).

---

[2] In this paper, DEXA refers to dual-energy x-ray absorptiometry using the DPX device (Lunar Corporation, Madison, Wis.), unless otherwise specified. Norland and Hologics manufacture similar devices but devices manufactured by these companies still appear less frequently in published research. There are differences in body composition results obtained from various devices, presumably related to the choice of energies, the software algorithms, and the design of the scanners.

ously described (Friedl et al., 1992). A comparison of DEXA to underwater weighing yielded similarly high correlations but a larger error of the estimate (0.90, standard error of the estimate [SEE] = 3.0), reflecting the greater variability introduced by the calculation of percentage body fat from uncorrected density. Other studies comparing the LUNAR DEXA with underwater weighing report high correlations for men and women (Haarbo et al., 1991; Hansen et al., 1993). However, even with good correlations, other studies have produced inexplicably low values (differences of 4–10% body fat units) for DEXA assessments of fatness compared with underwater weighing for lean, young men (Johansson et al., 1993; Van Loan and Mayclin, 1992). Comparison of DEXA results with body fat estimates from anthropometry or total body potassium also produced good results (Jensen et al., 1993; Svendsen et al., 1991).

Assessment of known combinations of lard and lean muscle yield good agreement and a linear relationship to the ratio of attenuation coefficients (on which percentage body fat is based) across the full range of fatness (Haarbo et al., 1991; Jensen et al., 1993; Svendsen et al., 1993). Chemical analysis after postmortem homogenization of seven pigs (35–95 kg weights) demonstrated excellent agreement with DEXA percentage fat, following the line of identity, correlation coefficient of 0.98, and SEE of 2.9 percent (Svendsen et al., 1993). However, earlier versions of the software did not properly adjust total-body bone mineral measures for overlying tissue thickness in heavy individuals (Jebb et al., 1993a; Laskey et al., 1992; Svendsen et al., 1993); the software algorithms have been revised to better take this into account (Mazess et al., 1992). Variations in hydration status may still be a problem for DEXA interpretation of lean mass, as discussed later in this chapter.

DEXA also yields information about regional distribution differences. For limbs, the soft tissue lean measurement is a direct measure of muscle (Heymsfield et al., 1990b). Thus, in the Ranger-I study, a differential catabolism of arm and leg muscle during heavy work with hypocaloric diet could be demonstrated (Friedl et al., 1993a). There was a larger proportion of arm muscle sacrificed, although in absolute terms the legs provided the greatest source of stored energy, both muscle and fat. This was further demonstrated in the Ranger-II study, where the arm fat also was preferentially consumed in the fattest soldiers (Nindl et al., 1996). Even when matched for fatness, these soldiers had a lower proportion of truncal (abdominal) fat than a group of more sedentary soldiers, leading to the conclusion that there is a "fit-fat" distribution pattern represented by a reduced proportion of fat energy stored in the abdominal region.

Other Technologies for Expedient Body Fat Assessment

Some of the expedient methods that have been considered for field research include anthropometry using skinfold measurements and imaging techniques such as ultrasound, BIA, and infrared interactance. Body composition prediction from skinfolds has a long history in Army research (e.g., Newman, 1955; Pascale et al., 1956). James Vogel brought the skinfold equation of Durnin and Womersley (1974) to U.S. military studies, and it has become the standard of comparison for body composition (Vogel and Crowdy, 1979). The Durnin and Womersley (1974) equations were used as an interim method for body fat assessments in the Army Weight Control Program until the circumference equations were developed. The method has proven reliable even in a setting of extreme weight loss and low body fat, as in the case of studies of Ranger students (Friedl et al., 1994a). Although developed on an ethnically homogeneous sample of Scottish men and women, no ethnic or racial bias has been found in the performance of this equation. However, as evident from even the limited data in Table 4-3, skinfolds are not as accurate as criterion lab methods. As with most anthropometric equations developed against underwater weighing, these equations tend to overestimate body fat in lean individuals and underestimate body fat in fat individuals.

Bioelectrical impedance analysis has also been extensively investigated and was the subject of the National Institutes of Health (NIH) Technology Assessment Conference on Bioelectrical Impedance Analysis in Body Composition Measurement in December 1994 (NIH, 1996). In brief, the conference concluded that the method is about as good as anthropometry but is not a "gold standard" for body composition analysis and is particularly susceptible to variations in hydration status. BIA has been tested for body composition assessment, with emphasis on measurement of FFM in a variety of Army and Navy studies and has not demonstrated significant advantage over skinfold measurements (Hodgdon and Fitzgerald, 1987; Hodgdon et al., 1996). In contrast, the NIH Technology Assessment Conference panel suggested that BIA provides a reasonable measure of total body water. Body fat assessment by BIA has not been tested in field settings where skin temperature and other factors may affect the measurement (Lukaski, 1987).

Ultrasound methods provide measurements that do not substantially improve on anthropometric estimates. This may be due to the regional dependence of ultrasound measurements on the subcutaneous fat layer, making ultrasound a technical approach that is really just a more precise method of measuring what is captured with a doubled-layer skinfold thickness in a caliper.

A trial with a commercially available infrared device in this laboratory demonstrated values that were no better than would be predicted from height and weight (required inputs to the device) (Unpublished data, K. E. Friedl, U.S. Army Research Institute of Environmental Medicine, Natick, Mass., 1993). In fact, when the device was held over a plastic wall covering and entries were made for a real individual, a reasonable readout of 15 percent body fat was obtained. More problematic is the recommendation from manufacturer representatives that entries be made at "high exercise habits" to obtain more appropriate values for black subjects, apparently because of confounding influences of skin pigmentation. A small study with lean white athletes demonstrated that the optical density data from a single biceps site, with or without other subject characteristics, did not provide values comparable to skinfold equations or underwater weighing (Israel et al., 1989). Except for the two original studies, which demonstrated the potential for this technology (performed with a research grade spectrophotometer and using only spectral data inputs in the regression equations) (Conway and Norris, 1987; Conway et al., 1984), this method has not been further developed technically or against credible criterion measures.

Such devices attract the interest of the lay public because they appear to be "high tech." This leads to the conclusion that if the Army circumference method of body fat estimation could be performed with a technologically complex instrumented tape measure, especially if it included a printout with "customized" diet recommendations, the same results would be more readily accepted.

SIGNIFICANCE OF BODY FAT TOPOGRAPHY AND MUSCLE MASS DISTRIBUTION

Abdominal Girth: Male Body Fat Predictor and Marker of Personal Readiness Goals

Although it would be convenient if circumference-based equations could be proven to be accurate predictors of total fatness, this skirts the main issue for the military, which is to identify a measure of excess fat that consistently relates to military appearance, health or nutrition, and exercise habits. The best physical predictor for any of these outcomes may not be total fatness. Differences in regional fat distribution have physiological significance in terms of regulation and metabolic consequences, particularly for women. Thus, assessment of specific regions may be preferential because it targets fat sites related to military goals, a theme that will be developed in this section.

Nearly every published anthropometric equation for males has included an assessment of the abdominal region. In one of the early anthropometric correlates with underwater weighing, Brozék and Keys (1951) demonstrated that the waist circumference and the chest-waist difference increased with increasing percentage body fat. The abdominal circumference used in the Army equation for males is adjusted with a neck circumference (instead of the earlier comparisons with chest circumference), a variable that appears to correct abdominal girth for total body volume (Personal communication, J. A. Hodgdon, Naval Health Research Center, San Diego, Calif., 1995). The Navy equation is essentially the same, with only the choice of coefficients changing the values produced (Table 4-4). The Marine Corps method, one of the first circumference equations produced, neglects only the correction for height, which is used by the Army and Navy equations. An equation developed on overweight civilian males goes even further than the military equations for males in the assessment of the abdomen, including measurement of three separate abdominal circumferences (at the waist, the navel, and above the iliac crests) (Tran and Weltman, 1988).

TABLE 4-4 Circumference, Weight, and Height Measurements Used in the Various Service Equations

	Equation Term	Army	Navy	Marines
Male	Add	Abdomen	Abdomen	Abdomen
	Subtract	Neck	Neck	Neck
		Stature	Stature	
Female	Add	Hips	Hips	Thigh
		Weight	Waist	Abdomen
				Biceps
	Subtract	Neck	Neck	Neck
		Forearm		Forearm
		Wrist		
		Stature	Stature	

NOTE: "Waist" is the minimal abdominal girth; "abdomen" is the girth taken at the navel. The Air Force uses the Navy equations.

Even before methods of body fat estimation had been worked out, the Metropolitan Life Insurance Company was advising that excessive abdominal girth (especially in excess of a chest girth) was associated with significantly increased health risk (Metropolitan Life Insurance Co., 1937). Abdominal girth is highly predictive of intraabdominal fat stores (Despres et al., 1991; Lemieux et al., 1996), the fat depot that is presumed to increase metabolic health risks, as a labile source of fats entering the hepatic portal blood flow and increasing insulin resistance and hepatic cholesterol regulation. The association between large abdominal fat stores and increased cardiovascular risk has been intensively explored and verified in more recent studies (e.g., Ducimetiere et al., 1986; Larsson et al., 1984; Leenen et al., 1992). Abdominal fat (or increased waist-to-hip ratio) also may reflect adverse health habits and stressors, such as excess alcohol consumption (Björntorp, 1990) and cigarette smoking (Shimokata et al., 1989).

Clearly, the abdominal site is associated with the prediction of both total body fat and physiological consequences (such as health end points) in males. Recently, data have been presented suggesting the use of abdominal fat as a marker of exercise habits, describing a fit-fat distribution as one of increasing adiposity without a predominant share in the abdominal region (Nindl et al., 1996). This relationship has been noted previously by other investigators, most notably those from Claude Bouchard's laboratory (Despres et al., 1985; Tremblay et al., 1990). The abdominal circumference used in the male Army equation is a practical marker of fatness that also is well suited to the goals of the Army Weight Control Program as a marker of fitness habits and appearance.

Army body fat evaluation can be performed reasonably by anyone following simple directions in the Army regulation (AR 600-6, 1986) and using only a stadiometer, calibrated floor scale, and tape measure. These circumference-based equations were developed from an active duty Army sample in the 1984 Army Body Composition Study (Vogel et al., 1988). The equation for males was derived from a sample of 1,126 male soldiers (with body fat ranging from 0 to 39.5% calculated from underwater weighing) at Fort Hood and the Army War College, with a correlation of 0.82 and SEE of ±4.0 percent body fat. Figure 4-3 illustrates the relationship between percentage body fat by the Army equation for males and DEXA in soldiers from three more recent studies. A more recent combined analysis of data from 496 men yielded a best correlation coefficient of 0.81 and SEE approaching 3 percent body fat (Friedl and Vogel, 1997).

Diversity of Female Body Fat Topography and Physiology

In marked contrast to the strong association between abdominal girth and adiposity in males, abdominal girth or any other circumference alone is a poor predictor of body fat in females, where excess fat will accrue in other estrogen-dependent sites such as the hips, triceps, thighs, and breasts. In the 1984 Army Body Composition Study, waist-to-hip ratio remained at a constant average

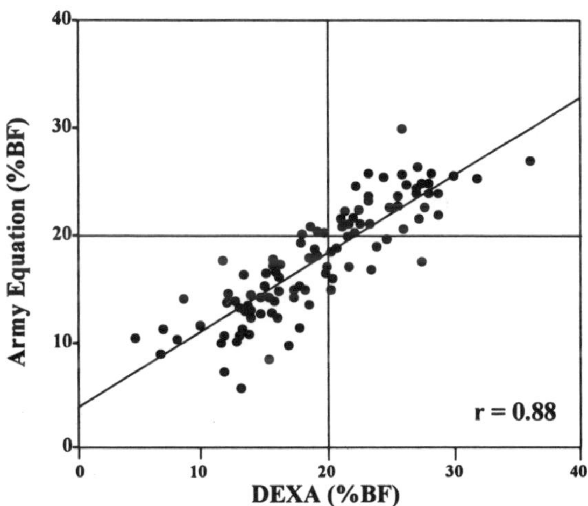

FIGURE 4-3 Percentage body fat (%BF) predicted from the Army equation for males compared to dual-energy x-ray absorptiometry (DEXA) for 100 male soldiers. The guidelines indicate the most stringent limit of body fat specified in the Army regulation. Note that the equation errs on the side of the soldier, slightly underestimating fatter men. SOURCE: Adapted from the 1991 Ranger study (Friedl et al., 1994a), the 1991 30-d Meal, Ready-to-Eat study (Thomas et al., 1995), and the 1993 Validation of Army Equations Study (based on methods in Friedl et al., 1992).

across the range of percentage body fat while it rose linearly with percentage body fat in men. Based on a computerized axial tomography scan at the umbilical level, Weits et al. (1988) demonstrated that an abdominal and hip circumference predicted 74 percent of the observed intraabdominal fat in males but only 56 percent of the variance in females. Kvist et al. (1986) have demonstrated that intraabdominal fat does not increase in women until a threshold level is achieved at approximately 30 kg of total body fat, while in men, abdominal fat increases linearly with increasing adiposity. Hattori et al. (1991) demonstrated an inverse relationship between subcutaneous fat and total percentage body fat in women, a relationship that could not be demonstrated in men. In their study, most fat was subcutaneous for lean women (i.e., those who were 15–25% body fat), but this decreased to less than half of the total fat in fatter women (~35% body fat). These data are consistent with the finding of this laboratory that abdominal girth is a discriminator of fatness in Army women only in the fattest 10 percent of the subjects of the 1984 Army Body Composition Study (Vogel and Friedl, 1992a). No single discriminator emerges for the remaining 90 percent of Army women in this sample (< 34% body fat), either because of the many choices of sites of fat deposition with precedence over the intraabdominal site, or because a general subcutaneous fat deposition occurs in advance of intraabdominal deposition. One conclusion from this is that an abdominal girth measurement is important in the assessment of fat women but may be less important to the prediction of adiposity in leaner women, possibly including the preselected Army population.

The equation for females was also derived in the 1984 Army Body Composition Study; ultimately the equation chosen was one based on a sample of 147 white women only (body fat range: 15.7–50.1%; $r = 0.82$; SEE = ±3.6%). This was largely because of the great difficulty in obtaining satisfactory data by underwater weighing for Hispanic and black female volunteers, and because an acceptable correlation could not be achieved with the entire sample (Vogel et al., 1988). The equation compared reasonably well with other standard equations and in a cross-validation using the Navy body composition study data (Hodgdon and Beckett, 1984; Vogel et al., 1988). However, with the data from the 1984 Army Body Composition Study, all of the standard anthropometric equations, including the Army equation (using all female soldiers, regardless of ethnicity), gave correlations of less than 0.8 and SEEs in excess of 4.0 percent body fat (Vogel et al., 1990). This highlights the greater difficulty in utilizing anthropometry to assess adiposity accurately in women compared with men. Questions concerning differences among ethnic groups in fat distribution and health risks are also unresolved (e.g., Conway et al., 1995).

Compared with DEXA, the equations for females have better agreement than in the original derivation, which was compared to underwater weighing. Validated against DEXA, the equations have higher correlations and lower SEEs (Figure 4-4).Given the greater choice of sites from which to develop predictive equations in women, it is not surprising that there is far less agreement

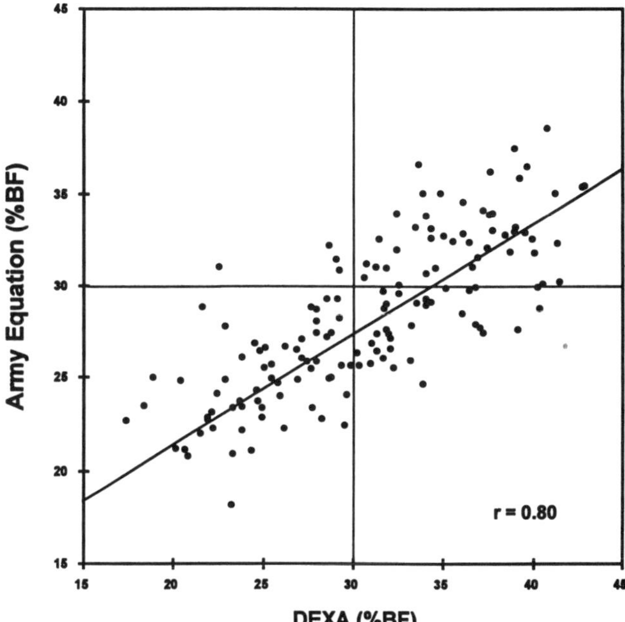

FIGURE 4-4 Percentage body fat (%BF) predicted from the Army equation for females compared with dual-energy x-ray absorptiometry (DEXA) for 170 female recruits. The guidelines indicate the most stringent limit of body fat specified in the Army regulation. Note that as with the male equation, this equation errs on the side of the soldier, slightly underestimating fatter women. Few women are misclassified by the Army equation as over the limit when they are within the limit of body fat standards. One extremely lean subject is off the scale of this graph. SOURCE: Adapted from the 1993 Fort Jackson Study (Westphal et al., 1995).

among methods of fat estimation in females compared with males (Table 4-4). These differences also produce relatively large differences in body fat predictions, unlike the military equations for males (Table 4-5). The five commonly considered sites of female fat deposition include hips (and gluteal), thighs (femoral), abdomen, upper arms, and breasts. Breast fat is usually discounted from anthropometric equations because of the personal nature of this measure, but this is of little consequence to total adiposity. Breast fat represents only a small proportion of total fat for most women, averaging 3.5 percent of total fat mass, irrespective of total adiposity (Katch et al., 1980). Circumferential measures of the other four sites are all strong correlates of total adiposity and appear in multiple regression analyses in various combinations. Of the three military equations, the Army equation emphasizes hip girth and total body weight as fat markers; the Navy equation emphasizes waist and hip; and the Marine equation uses arm, thigh, and waist (Table 4-4).

TABLE 4-5 Median Percentage Body Fat Estimation Using Different Equations on the Same Sample of Male and Female Soldiers[*]

Males, Age	n	DW	JP7	USA	MC	USN
17–20	155	16.4	14.0	13.5	13.3	12.5
21–27	371	18.3	15.2	15.0	14.1	14.2
28–39	299	23.3	20.3	19.8	18.2	19.3
40+	301	26.3	22.0	20.1	19.8	19.7
Females, Age	**n**	**DW**	**JP7**	**USA**	**MC**	**USN**
17–20	58	27.2	23.0	28.0	19.5	25.5
21–27	155	26.4	21.7	27.3	19.1	24.9
28–39	50	30.1	25.0	29.6	20.5	27.8
40+	n/a					

NOTE: Note the wider range of body fat estimates produced by the equations for females. DW, Durnin and Womersley (1974); JP7, men from Jackson and Pollock (1978), women from Jackson et al. (1980); USA, U.S. Army equations; MC, U.S. Marine Corps equations; USN, U.S. Navy equations (see Hodgdon, 1992 for military equations and primary sources).

[*] Calculated from data from the 1984 Army Body Composition Study (Fitzgerald et al., 1986).

As a practical consequence of these differences, the service equations are an integral part of each service's standards and are not readily interchangeable with other equations or even with other methods of fat assessment. For example, the Marine Corps equation for females gives a median value of 19.5 percent body fat for the same population of women that have a median value of 28.0 percent body fat by the Army equation (Table 4-5). Female Marines are held to an upper limit of 26 percent body fat while these young Army women are held to an upper limit of 30 percent body fat by the Army equation. Thus, the Marine Corps body fat standard is actually somewhat more liberal for young women, with a smaller proportion of this sample considered overfat by Marine standards than by Army standards (the standards become more stringent for older Marines because there is no allowance for age in the Marine standards). The Navy female equation yields average values that are in between those of the Army and Marine Corps equations. The mean values produced by the Navy equation tend to come closest to criterion methods (underwater weighing or DEXA). However, individuals are treated differently by each of these equations.

If only the strong women (lift capacity > 100 lb) from the previous plot (Figure 4-4) are considered, a similar regression line is plotted for the Army equation prediction of percentage body fat (Figure 4-5). However, percentage body fat for the same women, estimated from the Navy equation (Hodgdon and Beckett, 1984), demonstrates a tendency to overestimate fatness in just these strong women. These women are bigger and have more FFM than the weaker soldiers, but the groups had the same relative adiposity (~28% body fat) (Table 4-6). At least a part of the difference in the performance of the Army and Navy equations is attributable to the larger abdominal measurement in the stronger Navy women (about 5% greater than in the weaker soldiers), although this is only slightly greater than the increase in hip measurement. However, another reason for the difference may be the many factors in the more complicated Army equation that help to adjust for greater muscularity.

This discrepancy with a select population of strong women highlights a quandary in female body fat standards: the strongest women tend to share the male characteristics of fat distribution to the trunk and may experience a greater

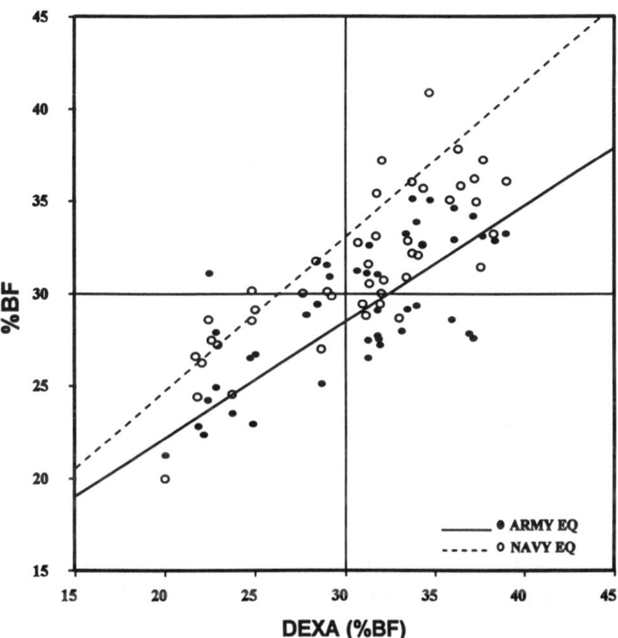

FIGURE 4-5 Percentage body fat (%BF) predicted from the Army equation for females and from the Navy equation for females, compared with dual-energy x-ray absorptiometry (DEXA) for 57 strong female recruits. These recruits all lifted greater than 100 lb in a maximal lift test. The same group of women tended to be overestimated by the Navy equation, which includes an abdominal circumference, compared with the Army equation, which does not. The Army equation also includes more factors (wrist and forearm circumference) to adjust for large body proportions. SOURCE: Adapted from the 1993 Fort Jackson study (Westphal et al., 1995).

TABLE 4-6 Physical Characteristics of Strong Women Compared with Those Who Cannot Lift 100 lb

	< 100 lb (n = 71)	≥ 100 lb (n = 57)
BMI (kg/m^2)	23.0 ± 2.4	24.5 ± 2.1[**]
Stature (cm)	161.5 ± 5.9	164.5 ± 6.6[*]
Body weight (kg)	59.9 ± 8.2	66.2 ± 7.3[**]
DEXA (%BF)	28.0 ± 6.2	28.3 ± 5.4
Army equation (%BF)	27.5 ± 4.0	28.5 ± 3.3
Navy equation (%BF)	29.1 ± 4.9	31.5 ± 4.1[**]
Neck circ (cm)	31.5 ± 1.2	32.7 ± 1.3[**]
Abdominal circ (cm)	75.3 ± 6.8	79.3 ± 6.0[**]
Hips circ (cm)	96.0 ± 5.8	99.5 ± 4.9[**]
Fat-free mass (kg)	42.9 ± 4.0	47.3 ± 4.4[**]
Push ups (count)	18.5 ± 9.3	23.6 ± 11.2[*]

NOTE: Although percentage body fat (%BF) is similar for the two groups, the strong women were significantly larger, and this includes many of the body circumferences. BMI, body mass index; DEXA, dual-energy x-ray absorptiometry; circ, circumference.

[*] $p < 0.05$, [**] $p < 0.01$ significance for differences between groups, compared by t-test.

SOURCE: Based on data from Sharp et al. (1994).

risk of cardiovascular disease (Evans et al., 1983; Hartz et al., 1984). Thus, if health concerns are the key objective, abdominal girth should be a prominent feature of the fat assessment for men and women (as in the Navy equation that is appropriate to Navy health goals); whereas, for an emphasis on combat readiness with importance placed on strength capacity, an abdominal assessment might be better avoided in women (as in the Army equation).

The reason for this difference in regional fat physiology appears to center in large measure on relative androgenicity of the individual woman (Friedl and Plymate, 1985). Even differences among ethnic groups, and among individuals within ethnic groups, correspond to differences in free testosterone levels (Evans et al., 1983; Hediger and Katz, 1986; Kirschner et al., 1990; Seidell et al., 1990). For example, in the European Fat Distribution Study (Seidell et al., 1990), serum free testosterone correlated with waist-to-hip circumference ratio (WHR); Mediterranean women had the highest free testosterone, highest WHR, and lowest triceps-to-subscapular skinfold ratios compared with northern European women who had lower androgenicity and a greater extremity fat distribution.

The extent to which male pattern adiposity translates into increased androgenicity and a consequent upper body muscularity and strength is unresolved. Krotkiewski and Björntorp (1986) reported a relationship between upper body fat distribution and the proportion of fast-twitch skeletal muscle (a male characteristic). They also found muscle mass increases more like males in abdominally fat women in a training program, compared with women of lower body fat. Ross and Rissanen (1994) also concluded that weight loss in overweight women was most frequently reflected in abdominal (both visceral and subcutaneous) fat.

It is interesting to note that thigh fat may also be a marker of cardiovascular health risks in women, in the opposite direction of abdominal fat (Terry et al., 1991). Thus, if long-term health is the primary consideration, reliance on thigh fat as a marker of adiposity would confound the goals of the standard because it is inversely correlated with serum lipid derangements. Assessment of thigh fat may also be undesirable in an equation that will be used to follow progress in fat reduction, until it is better established that thigh fat can be readily mobilized by exercise and dietary restriction in comparison with other sites. There is some evidence that thigh fat is primarily mobilized in postpartum women under the influence of specific lactational hormones (Rebuffe-Scrive et al., 1985; Steingrimsdottir et al., 1980) and may not be readily mobilized compared with other sites, even in men (Rognum et al., 1982).

Future Standards Development with Lean Mass Assessments

Eventually the military body composition standards may include a regional assessment of FFM, perhaps a flexed biceps or forearm circumference (Martin et al., 1990; Vanderveen et al., 1974), to ensure a minimum muscle mass in low-weight soldiers. One suggestion for a simple approach is a sliding scale that allows for greater relative body fat for heavier soldiers (Vogel, 1992). This would target small soldiers to ensure a minimum FFM (e.g., for a minimum FFM standard of 50 kg, a 60-kg soldier could have no more than ~15% body fat, while a 70-kg soldier could be allowed up to ~20% body fat). This is important because most jobs in the Army and Navy require strength for lifting and carrying (Beckett and Hodgdon, 1987; Harman and Frykman, 1992). The relationships among body weight, percentage body fat, and lifting strength, measured by incremental dynamic lift, is illustrated for males in Figure 4-6. It is evident that the typical 200-lb soldier, even one whose body fat exceeds 24 percent, can lift as much as the 150-lb soldier at 20 percent body fat. Clearly the relationship is explained by FFM, and strength is independent of the overlaying fat. In fact, maximal aerobic capacity is inversely correlated with BMI while maximal lift capacity is positively correlated (Gordon and Friedl, 1994). Women who exceed the weight-for-height allowed by the Army weight screening tables are stronger than smaller women, but there is no relationship between muscular strength and adiposity as assessed by the Army equation (Sharp et al., 1994). This re-empha-

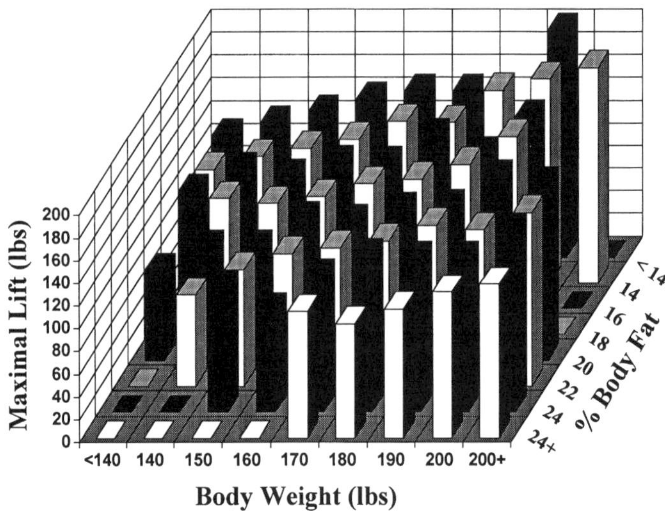

FIGURE 4-6 Mean lift capacity for male soldiers ($n = 998$) divided into body weight and percentage body fat categories. SOURCE: Plotted from data from the 1984 Army Body Composition Study (Fitzgerald et al., 1986).

sizes the point that the current Army weight control program is not intended to select for physical performance and would be especially unsuited to predicting strength performance (Vogel and Friedl, 1992b). Eventually, FFM might be a factor to include in military body composition standards, in order to provide some lower limit beneath which excessively thin individuals who cannot perform typical lifting and load-carrying tasks would be penalized or given special help. An immediately foreseeable problem with such a standard is that if it is related to job requirements, the standard must be gender neutral (i.e., the same for men and women). This means that a high proportion of women would be identified as failing to meet the standard. If the goal is to identify soldiers for special physical training rather than to have punitive effects, such a screening tool might be practical and useful. The connection between specific strength tests and regional or total muscle mass is far from clear (Johnson et al., 1994) and requires more research before any screening tests could be proposed.

ASSESSMENT OF CHANGES IN NUTRITIONAL AND HYDRATIONAL STATUS

Validity of Anthropometric Equations Derived from Cross-Sectional Data When Applied to Predict Changes in Body Composition

All of the standard anthropometric equations currently in use have been developed from studies of cross-sectional population data. There are no equations that have been derived from anthropometric changes in a longitudinal study. Many previous reports on weight loss of very large or small magnitude have suggested that anthropometry did not accurately reflect the true changes (Ballor and Katch, 1989; King and Katch, 1986; Moody et al., 1969; Scherf et al., 1986; Wilmore et al., 1970). However, these studies compared anthropometry with changes in total weight or in fat assessed by underwater weighing. As previously noted, the high variability in the underwater weighing technique introduces additional variance that confounds the results. Jebb et al. (1993b) compared changes in density (from underwater weighing), skinfold thickness, and BIA measures with continuous whole-body calorimetry during 12 days of underfeeding or overfeeding. They found that skinfold thicknesses better detected changes in fat mass than BIA; furthermore, skinfold thicknesses yielded a lower coefficient of variation in fat mass prediction than either density or resistance, results that are consistent with findings from this laboratory (Friedl et al., 1992). Within the choices of anthropometric methods, Bray et al. (1978) found that circumferences were superior to skinfolds in assessing progress in weight reduction, demonstrating lower coefficients of variation and better correlations. Nevertheless, the relative insensitivity of any anthropometric method to relatively small changes in fat mass makes it difficult to chart satisfactory progress in fat loss for military regulations. The current Army regulation (AR 600-9, 1986) requires that progress in weight loss or fat loss be demonstrated until body fat goals are achieved.

In the 1993 study of the health and performance of women in basic training (Westphal et al., 1995), extensive anthropometric measurements and DEXA measurements were performed on 150 women at the beginning and end of 8 weeks of basic training, in order to assess the effect of weight change, including fat loss with concurrent lean mass gain, on predictions by the Army anthropometric equation. Body water, as indicated by BIA, increased in proportion to the increase in lean mass, and at both the beginning and the end of training, DEXA-assessed body weight closely matched the measured scale weights, suggesting that the measurement artifacts observed earlier in the two Ranger school studies (Friedl et al., 1994a) were not present in the current setting of modest weight change. By DEXA measurements, the women demonstrated a mean gain of 2.0 kg of FFM, regardless of initial fatness. Change in body fat, however, was related to initial fatness, with the fattest soldiers demonstrating the largest losses, and soldiers below 25 percent body fat demonstrating increases in body fat content (Friedl et al., 1994b).

Figure 4-7 shows the changes in body fat predicted by the Army equation for females with respect to changes in fat as measured by DEXA. The equation shows a tendency to underestimate fat weight loss within a range of approximately 2 kg of actual fat loss as measured by DEXA; this is reflected by an apparent gain of up to 2 kg of fat using the Army equation. Higher rates of fat loss (> 2 kg/8 wk) did register correctly as fat loss in the Army equation. This is only

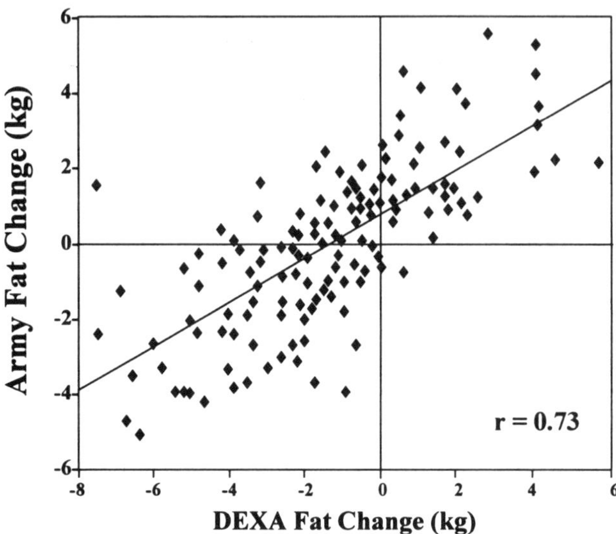

FIGURE 4-7 Change in fat weight predicted by Army equations for females compared with change assessed by dual-energy x-ray absorptiometry (DEXA) for 150 women assessed at the start and finish of basic training (8 weeks). Nearly 20 percent of the sample lost fat weight that was not reflected as a net loss by the Army equation. SOURCE: Adapted from Westphal et al. (1995).

a slightly better prediction of change than that reported by Ballor and Katch (1989) for commonly used equations (compared with underwater weighing), applied to a sample of somewhat fatter women (average 37% body fat) losing an average body weight of 3.0 kg over 8 weeks.

An earlier study by Pascale et al. (1955) from the Army Medical Nutrition Laboratory illustrates the need for more than one method of body composition assessment for interpretation of modest body composition changes in some field studies. Unlike the study of female recruits conducted by this laboratory (Westphal et al., 1995), there appear to be more confounding variables, particularly with hydrational derangements, in studies involving environmental extremes or strenuous activity levels. The study of Pascale et al. (1955) was conducted on a dozen selected, lean (< 10% body fat) soldiers going through airborne training of 3 weeks duration. Mean weight loss was 0.6 kg, which underwater weighing partitioned into a 0.8 kg fat loss and a 0.2 kg gain in FFM. However, by deuterium oxide dilution, a loss of 2.7 kg fat and a gain of 2.1 kg FFM were indicated. There were clearly substantial changes in fluid balance. Detailed analyses of fluid balance using deuterium oxide, radiosulfate, and thiocyanate dilutions indicated total body water increases of 1.6 liters (including +2.0 liters intracellular and –0.4 liters extracellular water). Changes in skinfold measurements indicated a decrease change of 1 percent in body fat, supporting the values obtained by underwater weighing. Thus, intensive training, even in approximate energy balance, appears to produce hydrational changes that still confound accurate detection of modest body composition changes.

It may be extraordinarily complicated to measure weight loss and apparent body composition changes in other specialized field settings. For example, in situations of a deployment to altitude to defend border regions, dramatic hydrational derangements could mask changes in body cell mass. Soldiers are at high risk for dehydration with elevated ventilatory rates in a cold, dry environment, but hypoxia promotes a hyperhydration, particularly in the maladaptors who will suffer acute mountain sickness (Singh et al., 1990). Identifying changes in body composition in this setting presents special problems that require measurement of fluid spaces and a critical interpretation of the results that purportedly identify body composition changes. For example, skinfold thicknesses, which are relatively robust indicators of changes in adiposity, are inadequate in the face of altitude-induced fluid shifts that also include regional subcutaneous differences (Gunga et al., 1995; Zachariah et al., 1987). BIA is one method that appears to identify gross hydrational changes reasonably in a field setting (Fulco et al., 1992) and could potentially be used to predict risk of illness.

Confounding Effects of Large Weight Losses in Ranger Training: Increases in Hydration and Questionable Criterion Measures

Small acute changes in TBW, induced by body water manipulations (~1–1.5 kg of water gain or loss) are assessed accurately as changes in total weight by DEXA (or the older dual-photon absorptiometry devices), but tend to misplace the specific components of weight change between the fat and soft-tissue FFM (Going et al., 1993; Lands et al., 1991). This effect can be illustrated by the following pilot study that was conducted by this laboratory (Friedl et al., 1993b). DEXA measurements were obtained in duplicate before and after a 6-h furosemide-induced (40 mg p.o.) diuresis in a 37-year-old, 80 kg, 17 percent body fat male. Weight loss totaled 2.4 kg, BIA predicted a water loss of 2.6 liters, and DEXA measurements indicated a reduction in soft-tissue weight of 2.5 kg. However, the DEXA measurement misplaced the change, indicating a loss of 3.0 kg from the soft-tissue FFM and a gain of 0.5 kg in fat mass; thus, body fat appeared to increase by more than 1 percent. This error was much greater than the variation between duplicate measurements (bone mineral content measurements remained constant) (Friedl et al., 1993b).

Large reductions in body weight appear to produce substantial increases in hydration (Deurenberg et al., 1989; Keys et al., 1946), and these changes produce large errors in the estimate of FFM. In the study by Deurenberg et al. (1989), a group of obese women lost an average of 10 kg of body weight during 8 weeks. The nature of this loss was estimated by underwater weighing as 2.3 kg of FFM but an improbable 0.6 kg of FFM (only 6% of the total weight loss) by BIA. Increased hydration would account for this discrepancy, with an expected underestimate of FFM loss based on BIA measurements but an overestimate of the changes in FFM when measured by underwater weighing. Thus, the true FFM loss is a value between these two. In the studies of semistarvation in Ranger students, similar changes were observed, with a 10 kg average weight loss during 8 weeks and a substantial underestimate by BIA of FFM loss (Hodgdon et al., 1996). Possibly also the result of hydrational changes (Roubenoff et al., 1993), DEXA overestimated the total mass present at the end of the Ranger I study by an average of 2.8 kg, an observation that was confirmed in Ranger II (Friedl et al., 1994a). This overestimate by DEXA occurred across all body weights, with a parallel overestimation of mass compared to scale weight (Friedl et al. 1994a) (Figure 4-8). In the second study (Nindl et al., 1996), fat stores were better preserved yet the artifactual error was similar in magnitude, suggesting that the primary error was not a result of deficiencies of the device algorithm at the lower end of the body fat range. Measurements of hydration by isotope dilution in a small subsample of Ranger students demonstrated that total body water did not decrease with the loss of body weight. This was supported by BIA measurements of the whole sample of men (Figure 4-9). An average 10 kg decline in body weight in 50 men included 4 kg of FFM loss but no change in the 50 liters of total body water (as estimated by BIA). This use of BIA to assess total body water during hydrational changes has been validated by Deurenberg et al. (1993).

Roubenoff et al. (1993) have suggested that overhydration causes errors in the DEXA estimate of FFM. Underwater weighing is sensitive to deviations in hydration but in the opposite direction from DEXA, with hydration greater than

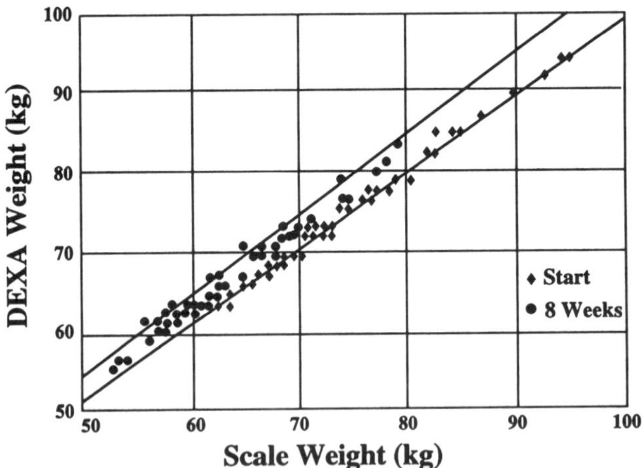

FIGURE 4-8 Comparison of body weight of 55 male soldiers assessed by dual-energy x-ray absorptiometry (DEXA) with that obtained with an electronic scale at the start and at the end of Ranger training (8 weeks). The values obtained are virtually identical at the start of training, but tissue mass was significantly overestimated by DEXA at the end of the course. SOURCE: Adapted from Friedl et al. (1994a).

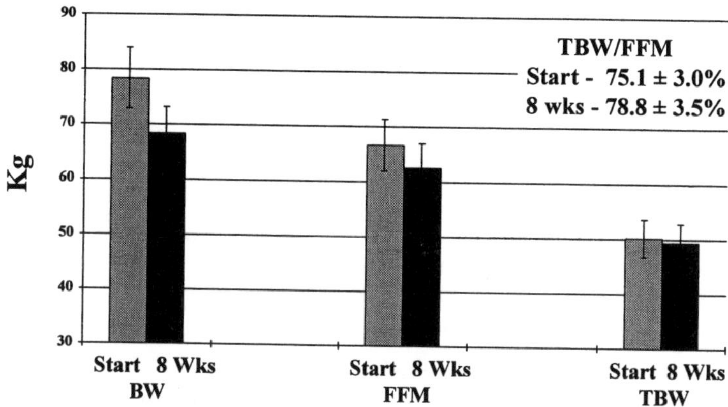

FIGURE 4-9 Body weight (BW), fat-free mass (FFM), and total body water (TBW) for 50 male soldiers at the start and end of Ranger training (8 weeks). The TBW data were predicted from resistance values obtained at 50 KHz by bioelectrical impedance analysis. SOURCE: Adapted from the 1992 Ranger study (Hodgdon et al., 1996; Nindl et al., 1996).

the assumed 73 percent of FFM leading to overestimates of fat in two-compartment models. DEXA overestimates total FFM while underwater weighing underestimates FFM in this setting; percentage body fat from the DEXA and actual scale weight give more plausible but still uncertain values. These data indicate that most of the commonly used methods of body composition measurement are affected by hydration status. At a minimum, military studies requiring precise assessments of body composition change (e.g., using DEXA) must also include some estimate of TBW. Body water appears to be suitably estimated from BIA with a high level of precision, although stable isotope dilution may be more accurate (Friedl et al., 1992). When a higher level of precision is not required or practical in a field study, the skinfold equations of Durnin and Womersley (1974) repeatedly have proven their value, as demonstrated by their measurement of fat loss in Ranger students (Friedl et al., 1994a). An understanding of the physiology of hyperhydration during rapid weight loss will be important to optimizing energy metabolism in intensive military scenarios. As Francis Moore noted in a much earlier Army symposium, "The ideal weight reduction program might be defined as one which would result in oxidation of body fat without erosion of body cell mass on the one hand, or excessive accumulation of extracellular water on the other" (Moore, 1966, 120).

Considerations in the Assessment of Nutritional Compromise

Low body fat is not, by itself, a marker of nutritional compromise. For example, at the end of Ranger training, the sum of skinfold measurements (at the four sites used for the Durnin and Womersley [1974] equation) had declined substantially, at a time when muscle catabolism and endocrine stress markers were substantially elevated (Moore et al., 1992). However, the same skinfold measurements were obtained in a group of weight-stable, elite, Kenyan runners in training who were approaching peak performance (Unpublished data, J. Staab and K. Friedl, U.S. Army Research Institute of Environmental Medicine, Natick, Mass., 1993) (Figure 4-10). In other words, body fat does not distinguish the very different nutritional status of these two groups, one in energy deficit and the other in energy balance. The practical distinguishing characteristic for these two lean groups is recent weight history. The Ranger students experienced large weight losses, with nearly every individual in the Ranger I study losing more than 10 percent of body weight within 8 weeks (Friedl et al., 1994a), while the Kenyan runners remained at stable weight.

There was also a large variation in responses of individuals to the stressors of Ranger training. For example, two individuals who began training with low body fat and other physical similarities later demonstrated weight loss and muscle mass catabolism at opposite ends of the range for the group (Friedl et al., 1994a). This is presumably related to cytokine and other stress hormonal responses, which can be adaptive or maladaptive (e.g., Stouthard et al., 1995). For example, the highest serum cortisol levels (1,200 nmol/liter) and the lowest concentration of serum interleukin-6 in the Ranger I study were measured in the individual who lost the most FFM (Moore et al., 1992). This may have been a

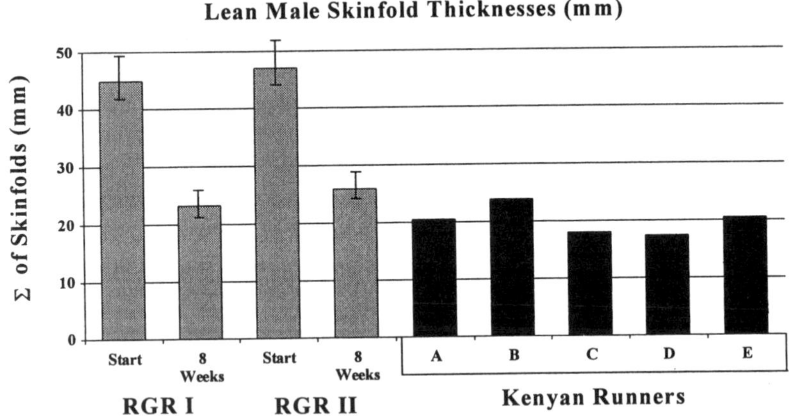

FIGURE 4-10 Mean sum of four skinfolds at the start and end (8 weeks) of the 1991 Ranger study (RGR I, $n = 55$) and 1992 Ranger study (RGR II, $n = 50$), compared with skinfolds of five elite Kenyan runners in training. Note that the skinfold thicknesses of the Kenyan runners are very similar to those of students at the end of Ranger training, even though nutritional status is remarkably different. SOURCE: Adapted from the Ranger I study (Friedl et al., 1994a), Ranger II study (Nindl et al., 1996), and elite Kenyan runners study (Unpublished data, J. Staab and K. Friedl, U.S. Army Research Institute of Environmental Medicine, Natick, Mass., 1993).

contributing factor to the catabolism, or it may have been a marker for an increasingly tenuous metabolic status. The critical marker of metabolic compromise in soldiers is the rate of weight loss. Conveniently, this is also the most practical measure in field settings or for nonresearch monitoring applications.

Oritsland (1990) concluded that 10 percent body fat is optimal for the longest period of survival (with declining survival times above and below this level), with or without the customary starvation-induced depression of basal metabolism. His model was based on data from the 1950 Minnesota Starvation Study (Keys et al., 1950) and data from field studies in Holland at the end of World War II (Burger et al., 1948). However, in some circumstances, such as cold combined with energy restriction, there may be a compromise of competing survival mechanisms. For example, Ranger students become hypothyroid in summer courses as a result of the energy restriction; this is also reflected in reduced body temperatures, as in other semistarvation studies (e.g., Fliederbaum et al., 1979, 18; Hehir, 1922). Cold exposure superimposed on energy restriction in Ranger classes during the winter would either produce extra risks to thermoregulation or it would compromise the attempt to reduce metabolic costs, which conserves body tissues. Individuals with a normal energy balance who are very lean (< 10% body fat) require a higher energy expenditure to stay warm during cold exposure through shivering thermogenesis (Glickman-Weiss et al., 1991). Thermogenesis is blunted by energy deficit, and these soldiers operate at a lower body temperature; however, aerobic fitness and the high exercise levels may help to sustain thermogenesis (Pi-Sunyer and Segal, 1992). The issue of special susceptibility of lean, undernourished soldiers in the cold has not been adequately addressed with research into the endocrine and metabolic responses.

AUTHOR'S CONCLUSIONS

This chapter has emphasized some of the methodological problems in the assessment of body composition for military fat standards and for field research. The Army's current approach to field study assessments is heavily dependent on DEXA, with confirmatory data obtained from skinfold thicknesses and hydrational information obtained by BIA. Ultimately, the most important component of body composition in military studies is muscle mass or nitrogen balance, but assessment of this still awaits the development of new enabling technologies such as a DEXA-like scanner for total body nitrogen or identification of suitable biochemical markers.

The evaluation of intervention strategies to prevent the loss of FFM during physically demanding military operations is dependent on a valid measurement of FFM (which must work in the face of other potential confounders). It also demands a better understanding of the biochemical correlates of overtraining, including markers of the breakdown of specific tissues such as collagen, bone, and muscle and a better understanding of cytokine regulation of the balance of muscle and fat tissues. Hydration status may be useful in monitoring of related aspects of nutritional status (e.g., as part of an automated soldier status monitoring system).

The study of female recruits in basic training has provided a robust test of the adequacy of the female fat equations (with an increase of FFM concurrent with loss of excess fat weight) (Westphal et al., 1995). The data indicate a clear need for further development of methods that predict modest changes in body composition.

A single set of equations and standards for all services that relate body composition, fitness goals, and physical performance requirements is a desirable goal. Research to support and demonstrate reasonable approaches to achieving and maintaining the standards would make this more defensible as a regulation that enhances readiness. It also would be of interest to know the long-range consequences of these military standards, in terms of both the health risks for those who gain weight after leaving the service following long-term weight suppression, and the benefits of preventing changes currently attributed to aging. Finally, the methods developed for use in surveillance or maintenance of standards need to be simple, with high reproducibility and a suitable relationship to the intended use (i.e., accurate compared to a multicompartment criterion method, or highly correlated with a military end point).

ACKNOWLEDGMENTS

The author wishes to thank Ms. Sherryl Kubel for her careful tabulation of the data on methods of underwater weighing and Ms. Lorraine Farinick for creation of each of the figures. Much of the new data reported here on DEXA and four-compartment models were collected with the expert assistance of Mr. Lou Marchitelli, Mr. Bob Mello, SPC Marjorie Harp, SPC Sherryl Kubel, SPC Sabrina Carson, and SPC Sonya Moore; the author is grateful to all of these individuals for their dedicated work.

REFERENCES

Akers, R., and E.R. Buskirk
  1969 An underwater weighing system utilizing "force cube" transducers. J. Appl. Physiol. 2:649–652.
Allen, T.H., B.E. Welch, T.T. Trujilo, and J.E. Roberts
  1959 Fat, water and tissue solids of the whole body less its bone mineral. J. Appl. Physiol. 14:1009–1012.
AR (Army Regulation) 600-9
  1986 *See* U.S. Department of the Army, 1986.
Ballor, D.L., and V.L. Katch
  1989 Validity of anthropometric regression equations for predicting changes in body fat of obese females. Am. J. Hum. Biol. 1:97–101.

Beckett, M.B., and J.A. Hodgdon
  1987   Lifting and carrying capacities relative to physical fitness measures. Technical Report No. 87-26. San Diego, Calif.: Naval Health Research Center.
Bedell, G.N., R. Marshall, A.B. DuBois, and J.H. Harris
  1956   Measurement of the volume of gas in the gastrointestinal tract. Values in normal subjects and ambulatory patients. J. Clin. Invest. 35:336–345.
Behnke, A.R., and J.H. Wilmore
  1974   Evaluation and Regulation of Body Build and Composition. Englewood Cliffs, N.J.: Prentice-Hall, Inc.
Behnke, A.R., Jr., F.G. Feen, and W.C. Welham
  1942   The specific gravity of healthy men: Body weight divided by volume as an index of obesity. J. Am. Med. Assoc. 118:495–498.
Best, W.R., and W.J. Kuhl
  1955   Physical, roentgenologic and chemical anthropometry in basic trainees. Technical Report No. 157. Denver, Colo.: Medical Nutrition Laboratory.
Blair, H.A., R.J. Dern, and P.L. Bates
  1947   The measurement of volume of gas in the digestive tract. Am. J. Physiol. 149:688–707.
Björntorp, P.
  1990   Obesity and adipose tissue distribution as risk factors for the development of disease. Infusiontherapie 17:24–27.
Bray, G.A., F.L. Greenway, M.E. Molitch, W.T. Dahms, R.L. Atkinson, and K. Hamilton
  1978   Use of anthropometric measures to assess weight loss. Am. J. Clin. Nutr. 31:769–773.
Brozék, J., and A. Keys
  1951   The evaluation of leanness-fatness in man: Norms and interrelationships. Br. J. Nutr. 5:194–206.
Brozék, J., F. Grande, J.T. Anderson, and A. Keys
  1963   Densitometric analysis of body composition: Revision of some quantitative assumptions. Ann. N.Y. Acad. Sci. 110:113–140.
Bunt, J.C., T.G. Lohman, and R.A. Boileau
  1989   Impact of total body water fluctuations on estimation of body fat from body density. Med. Sci. Sports Exerc. 21:96–100.
Burger, G.C.E., J.C. Drummond, and H.R. Sandstead
  1948   Malnutrition and Starvation in Western Netherlands, Part I. The Hague, Netherlands: General State Printing Office.
Conway, J.M., and K.H. Norris
  1987   Non-invasive body composition in humans by near infrared interactance. Pp. 163–170 in *In Vivo* Body Composition Studies, K.J. Ellis, S. Yasumura, and W.D. Morgan, eds. London: The Institute of Physical Sciences in Medicine.
Conway, J.M., K.H. Norris, and C.E. Bodwell
  1984   A new approach for the estimation of body composition: Infrared interactance. Am. J. Clin. Nutr. 40:1123–1130.
Conway, J.M., S.Z. Yanovski, N.A. Avila, and V.S. Hubbard
  1995   Visceral adipose tissue differences in black and white women. Am. J. Clin. Nutr. 61:765–771.
Cote, K., and W.C. Adams
  1993   Effect of bone density on body composition estimates in young adult black and white women. Med. Sci. Sports Exerc. 25:290–296.
Despres, J-P., C. Bouchard, A. Tremblay, R. Savard, and M. Marcotte
  1985   Effects of aerobic training on fat distribution in male subjects. Med. Sci. Sports Med. 17:113–118.

Despres, J-P., D. Prud'homme, M-C. Pouliot, A. Tremblay, and C. Bouchard
   1991   Estimation of deep abdominal adipose-tissue accumulation from simple anthropometric measurements in men. Am. J. Clin. Nutr. 54:471–477.
Deurenberg, P., J.A. Weststrate, and J.G.A.J. Hautvast
   1989   Changes in fat-free mass during weight loss measured by bioelectrical impedance and by densitometry. Am. J. Clin. Nutr. 49:33–36.
Deurenberg, P., F.J.M. Schouten, A. Andreoli, and A. de Lorenzo
   1993   Assessment of changes in extracellular water and total body water using multifrequency bio-electrical impedance. Pp. 129–132 in Human Body Composition, K.J. Ellis and J.D. Eastman, eds. New York: Plenum Press.
DHHS (U.S. Department of Health and Human Services)
   1988   The Surgeon General's Report on Nutrition and Health—Summary and Recommendations. DHHS (PHS) Publ. No. 88-50211. Public Health Service, U.S. Department of Health and Human Services. Washington, D.C.: U.S. Government Printing Office.
Ducimetiere, P., J. Richard, and F. Cambien
   1986   The pattern of subcutaneous fat distribution in middle-aged men and the risk of coronary heart disease: The Paris Prospective Study. Int. J. Obes. 10:229–240.
Durnin, J.V.G.A., and Satwanti
   1982   Variations in the assessment of the fat content of the human body due to experimental technique in measuring body density. Ann. Hum. Biol. 9:221–225.
Durnin, J.V.G.A., and J. Womersley
   1974   Body fat assessed from total body density and its estimation from skinfold thickness: Measurements on 481 men and women aged from 16 to 72 years. Br. J. Nutr. 32:77–97.
Evans, D.J., R.G. Hoffmann, R.K. Kalkhoff, and A.H. Kissebah
   1983   Relationship of androgenic activity to body fat topography, fat cell morphology, and metabolic aberrations in premenopausal women. J. Clin. Endocrinol. Metab. 57:304–310.
Fitzgerald, P.I., J.A. Vogel, W.L. Daniels, J.E. Dziados, M.A. Teves, R.P. Mello, and P.J. Reich
   1986   The Body Composition Project: A summary report and descriptive data. Technical Report T5-87. Natick, Mass.: U.S. Army Research Institute of Environmental Medicine.
Fliederbaum, J., A. Heller, K. Zweibaum, and J. Zarchi
   1979   Clinical aspects of hunger disease in adults. Pp 13–36 in Hunger Disease–Studies by the Jewish Physicians in the Warsaw Ghetto, M. Wynick, ed. New York: John Wiley and Sons.
Forsyth, R., M.J. Plyley, and R.J. Shephard
   1988   Residual volume as a tool in body fat prediction. Ann. Nutr. Metab. 32:62–67.
Freeman, S., J.H. Last, D.T. Petty, and I.L. Faller
   1955   Total body water in man: Adaptation of measurement of total body water to field studies. Technical Report EP-11. NTIS AD-067 598. Natick, Mass.: Quartermaster Research and Development Center.
Friedl, K.E.
   1992   Body composition and military performance: Origins of the Army standards. Pp. 31–55 in Body Composition and Physical Performance, Applications for the Military Services, B.M. Marriott and J. Grumstrup-Scott, eds. A report of the Committee on Military Nutrition Research, Food and Nutrition Board, Institute of Medicine. Washington D.C.: National Academy Press.

Friedl, K.E., and S.R. Plymate
  1985 Effect of obesity on reproduction in the female. J. Obes. Weight Regul. 4(2):129–145.
Friedl, K.E., and J.A. Vogel
  1989 The basis of current Army body fat standards. Unpublished technical report. Natick, Mass.: U.S. Army Research Institute of Environmental Medicine.
  1992 Looking for a few good generalized body-fat equations. Am. J. Clin. Nutr. 53:795–796.
  1997 Validity of percent body fat predicted from circumferences: Classification of men for weight control regulations. Mil. Med. 162:194–200.
Friedl, K.E., C.M. DeWinne, and R.L. Taylor
  1987 The use of the Durnin-Womersley generalized equations for body fat estimation and their impact on the Army Weight Control Program. Mil. Med. 152:150–155.
Friedl, K.E., J.A. Vogel, M.W. Bovee, and B.H. Jones
  1989 Assessment of body weight standards in male and female Army recruits. Technical Report 15-90. Natick, Mass.: U.S. Army Research Institute of Environmental Medicine.
Friedl, K.E., J.P. De Luca, L.J. Marchitelli, and J.A. Vogel
  1992 Reliability of body-fat estimations from a four-compartment model by using density, body water, and bone mineral measurements. Am. J. Clin. Nutr. 55:764–770.
Friedl, K.E., J.A. Vogel, L.J. Marchitelli, and S.L. Kubel
  1993a Assessment of regional body composition changes by dual-energy x-ray absorptiometry. Pp. 99–103 in Human Body Composition, K.J. Ellis and J.D. Eastman, eds. New York: Plenum Press.
Friedl, K.E., L.J. Marchitelli, S. Carson, K.A. Westphal, and W. Berkowitz
  1993b Validity of body water estimations by dual-energy x-ray absorptiometry and by bioelectrical impedance spectroscopy before and after isotonic dehydration. Research Protocol A-5827. Natick, Mass.: U.S. Army Research Institute of Environmental Medicine.
Friedl, K.E., R.J. Moore, L.E. Martinez-Lopez, J.A. Vogel, E.W. Askew, L.J. Marchitelli, R.W. Hoyt, and C.C. Gordon
  1994a Lower limits of body fat in healthy active men. J. Appl. Physiol. 77:933–940.
Friedl, K.E., K.A. Westphal, L.J. Marchitelli, and J.F. Patton
  1994b Effect of fat patterning on body composition changes in young women during U.S. Army basic training [abstract]. Int. J. Obes. 18(suppl. 2):69.
Fulco, C.S., R.W. Hoyt, C.J. Baker-Fulco, J. Gonzalez, and A. Cymerman
  1992 Use of bioelectrical impedance to assess body composition changes at high altitude. J. Appl. Physiol. 72:2181–2187.
Garg, A., J.L. Fleckenstein, R.M. Peshock, and S.M. Grundy
  1992 Peculiar distribution of adipose tissue in patients with congenital generalized lipodystrophy. J. Clin. Endocrinol. Metab. 75:358–361.
Glickman-Weiss, E.L., F.L. Goss, R.J. Robertson, K.F. Meets, and D.A. Cassinelli
  1991 Physiological and thermal responses of males with varying body compositions during immersion in moderately cold water. Aviat. Space Environ. Med. 62:1063–1067.
Going, S.B., M.P. Massett, M.C. Hall, L.A. Bare, P.A. Root, D.P. Williams, and T.G. Lohman
  1993 Detection of small changes in body composition by dual-energy x-ray absorptiometry. Am. J. Clin. Nutr. 57:845–850.

Goldman, R.F., and E.R. Buskirk
  1961   Body volume measurement by underwater weighing: Description of a method. Pp. 78–89 in Techniques for Measuring Body Composition, Proceedings of a Conference, Quartermaster Research and Engineering Center, Natick, Mass., January 22–23, 1959, J. Brozék and A. Henschel, eds. Washington D.C.: National Academy of Sciences/National Research Council.

Gordon, C.C., and K.E. Friedl
  1994   Anthropometry in the U.S. Armed Forces. Pp. 178–210 in Anthropometry: The Individual and the Population, S.J. Ulijaszek and C.G.N. Mascie-Taylor, eds. Cambridge, U.K.: Cambridge University Press.

Gould, B.A.
  1869   Investigations in the Military and Anthropological Statistics of American Soldiers. New York: Hurd and Houghton. (Also available in reprint from Arno Press, New York, 1979).

Gunga, H-Chr., K. Kirsch, F. Baartz, H-J. Steiner, P. Wittels, and L. Röcker
  1995   Fluid distribution and tissue thickness changes in 29 men during 1 week at moderate altitude (2,315 m). Eur. J. Appl. Physiol. 70:1–5.

Haarbo, J., A. Gotfredsen, C. Hassager, and C. Christiansen
  1991   Validation of body composition by dual energy X-ray absorptiometry (DEXA). Clin. Physiol. 11:331–341.

Hansen, N.J., T.G. Lohman, S.B. Going, M.C. Hall, R.W. Pamenter, L.A. Bare, T.W. Boyden, and L.B. Houtkooper
  1993   Prediction of body composition in premenopausal females from dual-energy x-ray absorptiometry. J. Appl. Physiol. 75:1637–1641.

Harman, E.A., and P.N. Frykman
  1992   The relationship of body size and composition to the performance of physically demanding military tasks. Pp. 105–118 in Body Composition and Physical Performance, Applications for the Military Services, B.M. Marriott and J. Grumstrup-Scott, eds. A report of the Committee on Military Nutrition Research, Food and Nutrition Board, Institute of Medicine. Washington, D.C.: National Academy Press.

Hartz, A.J., D.C. Rupley, and A.A. Rimm
  1984   The association of girth measurements with disease in 32,856 women. Am. J. Epidemiol. 119:71–80.

Hattori, K., N. Numata, M. Ikoma, A. Matsuzaka, and R.R. Danielson
  1991   Sex differences in the distribution of subcutaneous and internal fat. Hum. Biol. 63:53–63.

Hediger, M.L., and S.H. Katz
  1986   Fat patterning, overweight, and adrenal androgen interactions in black adolescent females. Hum. Biol. 58:585–600.

Hehir, P
  1922   Effects of chronic starvation during the siege of Kut. Br. Med. J. 1:865–868.

Heymsfield, S.B., S. Lichtman, R.N. Baumgartner, J. Wang, Y. Kamen, A. Aliprantis, R.N. Pierson, Jr.
  1990a   Body composition of humans: Comparison of two improved four-compartment models that differ in expense, technical complexity, and radiation exposure. Am. J. Clin. Nutr. 52:52–58.

Heymsfield, S.B., R. Smith, M. Aulet, B. Bensen, S. Lichtman, J. Wang, and R.N. Pierson, Jr.
  1990b   Appendicular skeletal muscle mass: Measurement by dual-photon absorptiometry. Am. J. Clin. Nutr. 52:214–218.

Hodgdon, J.A.
  1992 Body composition in military services: Standards and methods. Pp. 57–70 in Body
        Composition and Physical Performance, Applications for the Military Services,
        B.M. Marriott and J. Grumstrup-Scott, eds. A report of the Committee on Military
        Nutrition Research, Food and Nutrition Board, Institute of Medicine. Washington
        D.C.: National Academy Press.
Hodgdon, J.A., and M.B. Beckett
  1984 Prediction of body fat for U.S. Navy women from body circumferences and height.
        Technical Report 84-29. San Diego, Calif.: Naval Health Research Center.
Hodgdon, J.A., and P.I. Fitzgerald
  1987 Validity of impedance predictions at various levels of fatness. Hum. Biol. 59:281–
        298.
Hodgdon, J.A., P.I. Fitzgerald, and J.A. Vogel
  1990 Relationships between body fat and appearance ratings of U.S. soldiers. Technical
        Report 12-90. Natick, Mass.: U.S. Army Research Institute of Environmental
        Medicine.
Hodgdon, J.A., K.E. Friedl, M.B. Beckett, K.A. Westphal, and R.L. Shippee
  1996 Use of bioelectrical impedance analysis measurements as predictors of physical
        performance. Am. J. Clin. Nutr. 64(suppl.):463S–468S.
Israel, R.G., J.A. Houmard, K.F. O'Brien, M.R. McCammon, B.S. Zamora, and A.W. Eaton
  1989 Validity of a near-infrared spectrophotometry device for estimating human body
        composition. Res. Quart. Exerc. Sport 60:379–383.
Jackson, A.S., and M.L. Pollock
  1978 Generalized equations for predicting body density of men. Br. J. Nutr. 40:497–504.
Jackson, A.S., M.L. Pollock, and A. Ward
  1980 Generalized equations for predicting body density in women. Med. Sci. Sports
        Exerc. 12:175–182.
Jebb, S.A., G.R. Goldberg, and E. Marinos
  1993a DXA measurements of fat and bone mineral density in relation to depth and adi-
        posity. Pp. 115–119 in Human Body Composition, K.J. Ellis and J.D. Eastman,
        eds. New York: Plenum Press.
Jebb, S.A., P.R. Murgatroyd, G.R. Goldberg, A.M. Prentice, and W.A. Coward
  1993b In vivo measurement of changes in body composition: Description of methods and
        their validation against 12-d continuous whole-body calorimetry. Am. J. Clin.
        Nutr. 58:455–462.
Jensen, M.D., J.A. Kanaley, L.R. Roust, P.C. O'Brien, J.S. Braun, W.L. Dunn, and H.W.
        Wahner
  1993 Assessment of body composition with use of dual-energy x-ray absorptiome-
        try: Evaluation and comparison with other methods. Mayo Clin. Proc. 68:867–
        873.
Johansson, A.G., A. Forslund, A. Sjodin, H. Mallmin, L. Hambraeus, and S. Ljunghall
  1993 Determination of body composition–a comparison of dual-energy x-ray absorpti-
        ometry and hydrodensitometry. Am. J. Clin. Nutr. 57:323–326.
Johnson, M.J., K.E. Friedl, P.N. Frykman, and R.J. Moore
  1994 Loss of muscle mass is poorly reflected in grip strength performance in healthy
        young men. Med. Sci. Sports Exerc. 26:235–240.
Karpinos, B.D.
  1961 Current height and weight of youths of military age. Hum. Biol. 33:335–354.
Katch, F., E.D. Michael, and S.M. Horvath
  1967 Estimation of body volume by underwater weighing: Description of a simple
        method. J. Appl. Physiol. 23:811–813.

Katch, V.L., B. Champaigne, P. Freedson, S. Sady, F.I. Katch, and A.R. Behnke
 1980   Contribution of breast volume and weight to body fat distribution in females. Am.
        J. Phys. Anthropol. 53:93–100.
Kerr, M.H., R.D. Forsyth, and M.J. Plyley
 1992   Cold water and hot iron: Trial by ordeal in England. J. Interdisciplin. History
        22:573–595.
Keys, A., H.L. Taylor, O. Mickelsen and A. Henschel
 1946   Famine edema and the mechanism of its formation. Science 103:669–670.
Keys, A., J. Brozék, A. Henschel, O. Mickelsen, and H.L. Taylor
 1950   The Biology of Human Starvation, vol. 1. Minneapolis: University of Minnesota
        Press.
King, M.A., and F.I. Katch
 1986   Changes in body density, fatfolds and girths at 2.3 kg increments of weight loss.
        Hum. Biol. 58:709–718.
Kirschner, M.A., E. Samojlik, M. Drejka, E. Szmal, and G. Schneider
 1990   Androgen and estrogen metabolism in women with upper body versus lower body
        obesity. J. Clin. Endocrinol. Metab. 70:473–479.
Krotkiewski, M., and P. Björntorp
 1986   Muscle tissue in obesity with different distribution of adipose tissue: Effects of
        physical training. Int. J. Obes. 10:331–341.
Kvist, H., L. Sjöström, and U. Tylen
 1986   Adipose tissue volume determinations in women by computed tomogra-
        phy: Technical considerations. Int. J. Obes. 10:53–67.
Lands, L.C., G.J.F. Heigenhauser, C. Gordon, N.L. Jones, and C.E. Webber
 1991   Accuracy of measurements of small changes in soft tissue mass by use of dual-
        photon absorptiometry. J. Appl. Physiol. 71:698–702.
Laskey, M.A., K.D. Lyttle, M.E. Flaxman, and R.W. Barber
 1992   The influence of tissue depth and composition on the performance of the Lunar
        dual-energy x-ray absorptiometer whole-body scanning mode. Eur. J. Clin. Nutr.
        46:39–45.
Larsson, B., K. Svardsudd, L. Welin, L. Wilhelmsen, P. Björntorp, and G. Tibblin
 1984   Abdominal adipose tissue distribution, obesity, and risk of cardiovascular disease
        and death: 13 year follow up to participants in the study of men born in 1913. Br.
        Med. J. 288:1401–1404.
Leenen, R., K. van der Kooy, J.C. Seidell, and P. Deurenberg
 1992   Visceral fat accumulation measured by magnetic resonance imaging in relation to
        serum lipids in obese men and women. Atherosclerosis 94:171–181.
Lemieux, S., D. Prud'homme, C. Bouchard, A. Tremblay, and J-P. Despres
 1993   Sex differences in the relation of visceral adipose tissue accumulation to total body
        fatness. Am. J. Clin. Nutr. 58:463–367.
 1996   A single threshold value of waist girth identifies normal-weight and overweight
        subjects with excess visceral adipose tissue. Am. J. Clin. Nutr. 64:685–693.
Lukaski, H.C.
 1987   Bioelectrical impedance analysis. Pp. 78–81 in Nutrition '87, O. Levander, ed.
        Bethesda, Md.: American Institute of Nutrition.
Martin, A.D., L.F. Spenst, D.T. Drinkwater, and J.P. Clarys
 1990   Anthropometric estimation of muscle mass in men. Med. Sci. Sports Exerc.
        22:729–733.
Mazess, R.B., H.S. Barden, and E.S. Oldrich
 1990a Skeletal and body-composition effects of anorexia nervosa. Am. J. Clin. Nutr.
        52:438–441.

Mazess, R.B., H.S. Barden, J.P. Bisek, and J. Hanson
1990b Dual-energy x-ray absorptiometry for total-body and regional bone-mineral and soft-tissue composition. Am. J. Clin. Nutr. 51:1106–1112.

Mazess, R.B., J. Bisek, J. Trempe, and S. Pourchot
1992 Effects of tissue thickness on body composition measurement using dual-energy x-ray absorptiometry. Annual Meeting of the American College of Sportsmedicine, May 1992.

Metropolitan Life Insurance Company
1937 Girth and death. Stat. Bull. 18:2–5.

Moody, D.L., J. Kollias, and E.R. Buskirk
1969 The effect of a moderate exercise program on body weight and skinfold thickness in overweight college women. Med. Sci. Sports 1:75–80.

Moore, F.D.
1966 Energy stores as revealed by body compositional study. Pp. 110–121 in Energy Metabolism and Body Fuel Utilization, with Particular Reference to Starvation and Injury, A.P. Morgan, ed. Proceedings of the Committee on Metabolism in Trauma of the U.S. Army Research and Development Command. Cambridge, Mass.: Harvard University Printing Office.

Moore, R.J., K.E. Friedl, T.R. Kramer, L.E. Martinez-Lopez, R.W. Hoyt, R.E. Tulley, J.P. DeLany, E.W. Askew, and J.A. Vogel
1992 Changes in soldier nutritional status and immune function during the Ranger training course. Technical Report No. T13-92, September 1992. Natick, Mass.: U.S. Army Research Institute of Environmental Medicine.

Morrow, J.R., A.S. Jackson, P.W. Bradley, and G.H. Hartung
1986 Accuracy of measured and predicted residual lung volume on body density measurement. Med. Sci. Sports Exerc. 18:647–652.

Newman, R.W.
1955 Skin-fold changes with increasing obesity in young American males. Hum. Biol. 27:53–64.

NIH (National Institutes of Health)
1996 Technology Assessment Statement on Bioelectrical Impedance Analysis in Body Composition Measurement, 1994 December 12–14. Am. J. Clin. Nutr. 64(suppl.):524S–532S.

Nindl, B.C., K.E. Friedl, L.J. Marchitelli, R.L. Shippee, C. Thomas, and J.F. Patton
1996 Fat placement in fit males and regional changes with weight loss. Med. Sci. Sports Exerc. 28:786–793.

Oritsland, N.A.
1990 Starvation survival and body composition in mammals with particular reference to *Homo sapiens*. Bull. Math. Biol. 52:643–655.

Pace, N., and E.N. Rathbun
1945 Studies on body composition. III. The body water and chemically combined nitrogen content in relation to fat content. J. Biol. Chem. 158:685–691.

Pascale, L.R., T. Frankel, M.I. Grossman, S. Freeman, I.L. Faller, E.E. Bond, R. Ryan, and L. Bernstein
1955 Changes in body composition of soldiers during paratrooper training. Technical Report 156. Denver, Colo.: Physiology Division, U.S. Army Medical Nutrition Laboratory.

Pascale, L.R., M.I. Grossman, H.S. Sloane, and T. Frankel
1956 Correlations between thickness of skinfolds and body density in 88 soldiers. Hum. Biol. 28:165–176.

Pi-Sunyer, F.X., and K.R. Segal
  1992   Relationship of diet and exercise. Pp. 187–210 in Energy Metabolism—Tissue Determinants and Cellular Corollaries, J.M. Kinney and H.N. Tucker, eds. New York: Raven Press.
Rebuffe-Scrive, M., L. Enk, N. Crona, P. Lonroth, L. Ambrahmasson, U. Smith, and P. Björntorp
  1985   Regional human adipose tissue metabolism during the menstrual cycle, pregnancy, and lactation. J. Clin. Invest. 75:1973–1976.
Reed, L.J., and A.G. Love
  1932   Biometric studies on U.S. Army officers—Somatological norms, correlations, and changes with age. Hum. Biol. 4:509–524.
Rognum, T.O., K. Rodahl, and P.K. Opstad
  1982   Regional differences in the lipolytic response of the subcutaneous fat depots to prolonged exercise and severe energy deficiency. Eur. J. Appl. Physiol. 49:401–408.
Ross, R., and J. Rissanen
  1994   Mobilization of visceral and subcutaneous adipose tissue in response to energy restriction and exercise. Am. J. Clin. Nutr. 60:695–703.
Roubenoff, R., J.J. Kehayias, B. Dawson-Hughes, and S.B. Heymsfield
  1993   Use of dual-energy x-ray absorptiometry in body composition studies: Not yet a "gold standard." Am. J. Clin. Nutr. 58:589–591.
Scherf, J., B.A. Franklin, C.P. Lucas, D. Stevenson, and M. Rubenfire
  1986   Validity of skinfold thickness measures of formerly obese adults. Am. J. Clin. Nutr. 43:128–135.
Schutte, J.E., E.J. Townsend, J. Hugg, R.F. Shoup, R.M. Malina, and C.G. Blomqvist
  1984   Density of lean body mass is greater in blacks than in whites. J. Appl. Physiol. 56:1647–1649.
Seidell, J.C., M. Cigolini, J. Chorzewska, B.M. Ellsinger, and G. Di Brase
  1990   Androgenicity in relation to body fat distribution and metabolism in 38-year-old women—The European Fat Distribution Study. J. Clin. Epidemiol. 43:21–34.
Selinger, A.
  1977   The body as a three-component system. Doctoral Dissertation. University of Illinois at Urbana-Champaign, Champaign, Ill.
Sharp, M.A., B.C. Nindl, K.A. Westphal, and K.E. Friedl
  1994   The physical performance of female Army basic trainees who pass and fail the Army body weight and percent body fat standards. Pp. 743–750 in Advances in Industrial Ergonomics and Safety VI, E. Agezadeh, ed. Washington, D.C.: Taylor and Francis.
Shimokata, H., D.C. Muller, and R. Andres
  1989   Studies in the distribution of body fat. III. Effects of cigarette smoking. J. Am. Med. Assoc. 261:1169–1173.
Siconolfi, S.F., D.A. Coleman, and J. Staab
  1987   Determination of percent fat by hydrostatic weighing and functional residual capacity. Annual Meeting of the Eastern Region, American College of Sportsmedicine, 5 November.
Singh, M.V., S.B. Rawal, and A.K. Tyagi
  1990   Body fluid status on induction, reinduction and prolonged stay at high altitude of human volunteers. Int. J. Biometerorol. 34:93–97.

Siri, W.E.
  1961   Body composition from fluid spaces and density: Analysis of methods. Pp. 223–244 in Techniques for Measuring Body Composition, Proceedings of a Conference, Quartermaster Research and Engineering Center, Natick, Mass., January 22–23, 1959, J. Brozék and A. Henschel, eds. Washington D.C.: National Academy of Sciences/National Research Council.

Steingrimsdottir, L., M.R. Greenwood, and J.A. Brasel
  1980   Effect of pregnancy, lactation, and a high-fat diet on adipose tissue in Osborne-Mendel rats. J. Nutr. 110:600–609.

Stouthard, J.M.L., J.A. Romijn, T. van der Poll, E. Endert, S. Klein, P.J.M. Bakker, C.H.N. Veenhof, and H.P. Sauerwein
  1995   Endocrinologic and metabolic effects of interleukin-6 in humans. Am. J. Physiol. 268:E813–E819.

Study of the Military Services Physical Fitness
  1981   *See* U.S. Department of Defense, Office of the Assistant Secretary of Defense for Manpower, Reserve Affairs and Logistics, 1981.

Svendsen, O.L., J. Haarbo, B.L. Heitmann, A. Gotfredsen, and C. Christiansen
  1991   Measurement of body fat in elderly subjects by dual-energy x-ray absorptiometry, bioelectrical impedance, and anthropometry. Am. J. Clin. Nutr. 53:1117–1123.

Svendsen, O.L., J. Haarbo, C. Hassager, and C. Christiansen
  1993   Accuracy of measurements of body composition by dual-energy x-ray absorptiometry in vivo. Am. J. Clin. Nutr. 57:605–608.

Terry, R.B., M.L. Stefanick, W.L. Haskell, and P.D. Wood
  1991   Contributions of regional adipose tissue depots to plasma lipoprotein concentrations in overweight men and women: Possible protective effects of thigh fat. Metabolism 40:733–740.

Thomas, C.D., K.E. Friedl, M.Z. Mays, S.H. Mutter, R.J. Moore, D.Z. Jezior, C.J. Baker-Fulco, L.J. Marchitelli, R.T. Tulley, and E.W. Askew
  1995   Nutrient intakes and nutritional status of soldiers consuming the Meal, Ready-to-Eat (MRE XII) during a 30-day field training exercise. Technical Report No. T95-6. Natick, Mass.: U.S. Army Research Institute of Environmental Medicine.

Tran, Z.V., and A. Weltman
  1988   Predicting body composition of men from girth measurements. Hum. Biol. 60:167–175.

Tremblay, A., J-P. Despres, C. Leblanc, C.L. Craig, B. Ferris, T. Stephens, and C. Bouchard
  1990   Effect of intensity of physical activity on body fatness and fat distribution. Am. J. Clin. Nutr. 51:153–157.

U.S. Congress, House
  1992   Gender Discrimination in the Military. Hearing before the Defense Policy Panel, Committee on Armed Services, July 29–30. 102d Congress, 2d Session. Washington, D.C.: U.S. Government Printing Office.

U.S. Department of the Army
  1986   Army Regulation 600-9. "The Army Weight Control Program." September 15. Washington, D.C.

U.S. Department of Defense. Office of the Assistant Secretary of Defense for Manpower, Reserve Affairs and Logistics.
  1981   Study of the Military Services Physical Fitness. April 3. Washington D.C.

Vanderveen, J.E., C.F. Theis, R.J. Fuchs et al.
  1974   The use of a three-scale nomogram to predict lean body mass in men. Aerospace Med. Assoc. Ann. Proc :38–39.

Van Loan, M.D., and P.L. Mayclin
  1992   Body composition assessment: Dual-energy x-ray absorptiometry (DEXA) compared to reference methods. Eur. J. Clin. Nutr. 46:125–130.
Vogel, J.A.
  1992   Obesity and its relation to physical fitness in the U.S. military. Armed Forces Soc. 18:497–513.
Vogel, J.A., and J.P. Crowdy
  1979   Aerobic fitness and body fat of young British males entering the Army. Eur. J. Appl. Physiol. 40:73–83.
Vogel, J.A., and K.E. Friedl
  1992a   Body fat assessment in women–Special considerations. Sports Med. 13:245–269.
  1992b   Army data: Body composition and physical capacity. Pp. 89–103 in Body Composition and Physical Performance, Applications for the Military Services, B.M. Marriott and J. Grumstrup-Scott, eds. A report of the Committee on Military Nutrition Research, Food and Nutrition Board, Institute of Medicine. Washington, D.C.: National Academy Press.
Vogel, J.A., J.W. Kirkpatrick, P.I. Fitzgerald, J.A. Hodgdon, and E.A. Harman
  1988   Derivation of anthropometry-based body fat equations for the Army's weight control program. Technical Report T17-88. Natick, Mass.: U.S. Army Research Institute of Environmental Medicine.
Vogel J.A., K.E. Friedl, and P.I. Fitzgerald
  1990   Generalized prediction of body fat in young U.S. females. Med. Sci. Sports Exerc. 22 (suppl.):S672.
Weits, T., E.J. van der Beek, M. Wedel, and B.M. Ter Haar Romeny
  1988   Computed tomography measurement of abdominal fat deposition in relation to anthropometry. Int. J. Obes. 12:217–225.
Westphal, K.A., N. King, K.E. Friedl, M.A. Sharp, T.R. Kramer, and K.L. Reynolds
  1995   Health, performance, and nutritional status of U.S. Army women during basic combat training. Technical Report T95-99. Natick, Mass.: U.S. Army Research Institute of Environmental Medicine.
Wilmore, J.H., R.N. Girandola, and D.L. Moody
  1970   Validity of skinfold and girth assessment for predicting alterations in body composition. J. Appl. Physiol. 29:313–317.
Wilmore, J.H., P.A. Vodak, R.B. Parr, R.N. Girandola, and J.E. Billing
  1980   Further simplification of a method for determination of residual lung volume. Med. Sci. Sports Exerc. 12:216–218.
Withers, R.T., and C.T. Ball
  1988   A comparison of the effects of measured, predicted, estimated and constant residual volumes on the body density of female athletes. Int. J. Sports Med. 9:24–28.
Zachariah, T., S.B. Rawal, S.N. Pramanik, M.V. Singh, S. Kishnani, H. Bharadwaj, and R.M. Rai
  1987   Variations in skinfold thickness during de-acclimatisation and re-acclimatisation to high altitude. Eur. J. Appl. Physiol. 56:570–577.

DISCUSSION

JOHN VANDERVEEN: Karl, a result of our workshop on body composition, as I recall, was that body fat is a lousy predictor of performance, that lean body mass is a predictor, and I think we recommended that you look at lean body mass.

KARL FRIEDL: That is exactly right, and that would be one of our goals. Eventually what we need is the technology—I guess it is going to take faster computers so we can do these full-body MRI scans, and we will come up with a muscle volume, and then we will be looking at the right thing. Because if you look at the same data, for example, from that Army body composition study, with increasing body weight we have a big increase in lift capacity in these 1,000 or so male soldiers, and some of the fattest soldiers out here can still lift— If you are 200 lbs with 24 percent body fat, you have 150 lbs or more of lean body mass, which is more than the leanest guy back in the corner here.

So at a minimum, maybe what we need right now, just using simple techniques that are available, is a minimum body weight for soldiers. You are exactly right that there is this sort of reverse relationship, and lean body mass is much more important for predicting performance, if we wanted to predict performance. But remember, we are trying to motivate soldiers, too. We do not want obese soldiers. That is the bottom line in the Army, and it is for appearance reasons and some other things, too.

JOHANNA DWYER: Just a compliment. Karl, it was a wonderful presentation, and to point out, again, this research is very valuable because of all the groups in society, I think the Armed Forces are the only ones who have been able to decrease obesity over the past 10 or 15 years. So we civilians have a lot to learn from the techniques you are doing.

KARL FRIEDL: One of my questions is how much are we decreasing it or getting soldiers to maintain appropriate weights, and how much are we just making people who are not successful hit the street? And we do not really have data on that. There is a balance of the two. But we see a lot of soldiers running at noontime, which we did not used to see. I have to do it and there are a lot of us who have to do it just to maintain an appropriate weight.

DOUGLAS WILMORE: Karl, have you looked at the geometry of the body in the DEXA system, which is probably accounting for your errors of the DEXA?

KARL FRIEDL: Yes, especially at the upper end, there is still a body size problem.

DOUGLAS WILMORE: Even with the Rangers, just losing 12 kg, probably just the geometry of the body is—

KARL FRIEDL: We are concerned about that, and we need to look at it.

DOUGLAS WILMORE: And as you get into the systems that do more spherical kinds of counting, as DEXA really gets developed, I think you will minimize that error more and more. But what that means is you are going to have to go back and redefine your equations and redevelop your equations as the technology gets better.

KARL FRIEDL: We do not have to change them every time, but we need to keep checking on them to make sure that we are not doing something grossly inappropriate.

DOUGLAS WILMORE: You can make phantoms [models imitating body composition, used to calibrate instruments], though, and get into that without using people.

Emerging Technologies for Nutrition Research, 1997
Pp. 127–150. Washington, D.C.
National Academy Press

5

Imaging Techniques of Body Composition: Advantages of Measurement and New Uses

Steven Heymsfield,[1] Robert Ross, ZiMian Wang, and David Frager

INTRODUCTION

Few technical advances in medicine can claim greater importance than the development and clinical application of computerized axial tomography (CT or CAT) and magnetic resonance imaging/spectroscopy (MRI/MRS). Both CT and MRS led to Nobel Prizes for their inventors (Bloch et al., 1946; Hounsfield, 1973; Purcell et al., 1946), and rapid related advances such as functional MRI (Duyn et al., 1994) and spiral CT (Fishman, 1994) show great promise.

The opportunities presented by both CT and MRI for studying human body composition are no less important than they are for clinical medicine. The unique capabilities provided by modern imaging methods in studying body composition make them among the most important advances of the century. This review provides an overview of the historical development and current

[1] Steven Heymsfield, Weight Control Unit, Obesity Research Center, St. Luke's-Roosevelt Hospital, New York, NY 10025.

Supported by National Institutes of Health Grant RO1-AG 13021.

status of imaging methods; a final section provides suggestions for future research.

Historical Development

Students of human biology have expressed interest in body composition since the nineteenth century (Forbes, 1987; Lawes and Gilbert, 1859; von Bezold, 1857). Human shape, form, fatness, muscularity, and chemical composition were of interest to many investigators early in the twentieth century (Moulton, 1923; Spivak, 1915). Advances in radiographic methods led Stuart and colleagues (1940) to report the first use of standard x-ray films to capture fat and muscle "shadows." By the early 1960s, radiogrammetry was a well-developed method that provided investigators with estimates of subcutaneous adipose tissue (AT) layer thickness and muscle widths (Garn, 1957, 1961). Low image contrast and two-dimensional radiographs limited radiogrammetry to rough approximations of body composition components.

G. N. Hounsfield first introduced CT for brain imaging in 1971 and reported his findings in 1973. The theoretical framework and mathematical algorithms needed for image reconstruction were developed earlier by Raden (1917) and Cormack (1980). The historical roots for MRI appeared even earlier than for CT. Bloch et al. (1946) and Purcell et al. (1946) independently described the basic phenomena that ultimately gave rise to nuclear magnetic resonance spectroscopy in 1946. Differences between malignant tumors and normal tissue were first studied using magnetic resonance (MR) methods in 1971 by Damadian. That one could create images of phantoms using the signal from proton nuclear magnetic resonance was demonstrated in 1973 by Lauterber.

By the mid 1970s, CT scanners were being installed in many American medical centers, and by the early 1980s, MRI systems became available on a widespread basis. Unlike radiogrammetry, even early CT provided high-resolution cross-sectional images. Clear anatomic boundaries could be visualized between subcutaneous AT, skeletal muscle, visceral organs, brain, and skeleton. During this early era of CT technology, Heymsfield and colleagues were exploring the validity of anthropometric assessment methods as they applied to hospitalized patients. The installation of a CT scanner in the investigators' hospital provided an important opportunity to examine anthropometric assessment methods with CT as the "reference" standard. Their use of CT to quantify skeletal muscle mass was reported in 1979 (Heymsfield et al., 1979a), and subsequent reports by the group described methods of estimating visceral organ volumes (Heymsfield et al., 1979b) and visceral AT (Heymsfield and Noel, 1981).

The high radiation exposure of CT limited its use until the mid 1980s. Moreover, other methods with little or no radiation and lower cost appeared to provide adequate measures of components such as fat and fat-free body mass (Forbes, 1987; Lukaski, 1987). During this period, epidemiological studies began to appear that linked upper body AT distribution and visceral AT with obesity comorbidities (Björntorp, 1986). The need arose to quantify visceral AT, and CT quickly became the method of choice (Borkan et al., 1982). In addition, Sjöström and his colleagues (1986) introduced the concept of whole-body multicomponent CT. With this method, images are prepared at 22 or more predefined anatomic locations, and total body volumes of various body composition components are estimated by integrating appropriate slice areas. This approach allows the investigator to quantify total-body and regional AT, skeletal muscle, bone, and other organ and tissue volumes.

Use of MRI in body composition research lagged behind that for CT by several years. Foster et al. (1984) were the first to demonstrate that by comparison to cadaver samples, MRI could be used to discriminate between AT and adjacent skeletal muscle. Not until 1988 was MRI first used to characterize the distribution of subcutaneous AT in human subjects (Hayes et al., 1988). Since that time, numerous studies have utilized MRI technology to describe AT and/or lean tissue distribution in adolescents (de Ridder et al., 1992), normal males and females (Fowler et al., 1991; Ross et al., 1992; Sobel et al., 1991; Sohlström et al., 1993), obese males and females (Ross et al., 1993, 1994), diabetic patients (Gray et al., 1991), and elderly populations (Baumgartner et al., 1992). The observations within many of these studies were based on a single MR image. Because multiple images can be obtained without any known health risks to the subject, MRI is well suited for assessment of whole-body AT or lean tissue distribution using multislice models. A principal benefit of multislice acquisitions is that the volume measurement of various tissues can be derived, thereby eliminating the restrictions imposed by observations based on a single image. Four research groups have employed a multislice MRI protocol to evaluate whole-body AT distribution in human subjects. Fowler et al. (1991) acquired 28 MR images over the entire body, while Ross et al. (1992, 1993) reported using a multislice ($n = 41$ images) model to measure AT and lean distribution in normal male and obese female subjects. Sohlström et al. (1993) recently described AT distribution in normal, healthy women using a 30-image protocol. In addition to a characterization of body composition, multislice protocols are particularly useful when evaluating the efficacy of various interventions that induce changes in AT and lean tissue distribution (Ross and Rissanen, 1994; Ross et al., 1995a; Sohlström and Forsum, 1995).

Components Measured

Body composition can be considered as five levels of increasing complexity: atomic, molecular, cellular, tissue system (anatomical), and whole body (Wang et al., 1992). The first four levels of body composition and their respective components are shown in Figure 5-1. Both CT and MRI are measurement systems designed to quantify components at the tissue-system level of body composition. The major components at the tissue-system level are AT, skeletal

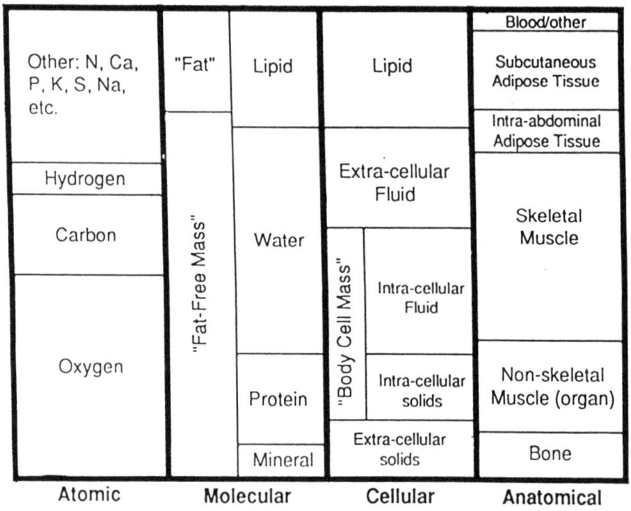

Atomic	Molecular	Cellular	Anatomical
Other: N, Ca, P, K, S, Na, etc.	"Fat"	Lipid	Lipid	Blood/other
				Subcutaneous Adipose Tissue
Hydrogen	"Fat-Free Mass"	Water	Extra-cellular Fluid	Intra-abdominal Adipose Tissue
Carbon				Skeletal Muscle
			Intra-cellular Fluid	
Oxygen		Protein	Intra-cellular solids	Non-skeletal Muscle (organ)
		Mineral	Extra-cellular solids	Bone

"Body Cell Mass"

FIGURE 5-1 First four levels of body composition and their main components. SOURCE: Baumgartner et al. (1995), used with permission.

muscle, bone, visceral organs, and brain (Figure 5-2). The AT component is further divided into subcutaneous, visceral, yellow marrow, and the interstitial AT that occurs between muscle fibers (Snyder et al., 1975).

Both CT and MRI can quantify all of the major components at the tissue-system level. Cross-sectional images are composed of picture elements or pixels, usually 1-mm squares. Slice thicknesses vary, and when considered in three dimensions, the image consists of volume elements or voxels. Each pixel or voxel has a gray scale that reflects the tissue's composition and gives contrast to the image. A later section in this chapter will expand on pixel contrast.

PHYSICAL BASIS OF METHODS

Overview

In vivo body composition methods involve measurement of some property of the human body. A simple formula that describes all *in vivo* body composition methods is the following (Wang et al., 1995),

$$C = f(Q),$$

(Equation 5-1)

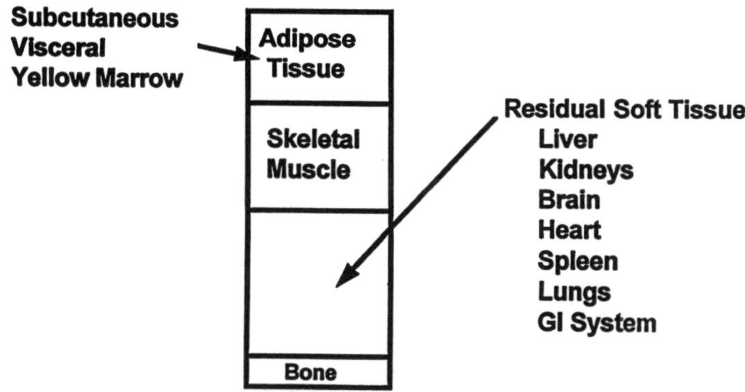

FIGURE 5-2 Main components of the tissue-system level of body composition. GI, gastrointestinal.

where C is an unknown component; Q, a measurable quantity; and f, the mathematical function that links Q to C. All *in vivo* methods are ultimately based on this general body composition methodology formula. The formula indicates that there are two parts to the equation that are used to estimate a body composition component. The first part is a measurable quantity, Q, and the second, a mathematical function, f. As a description of the physical basis of CT and MRI proceeds, this review is organized according to measurable quantity and mathematical function.

Computerized Axial Tomography

The basic CT system consists of an x-ray tube and receiver that rotate in a perpendicular plane to the subject. The measurable properties of CT are 0.1 to 0.2 amps, 60 to 120 kilovolt peak x rays that are attenuated as they pass through tissues (Sprawls, 1977). Attenuation is expressed as the linear attenuation coefficient or CT number. The CT number is a measure of attenuation relative to air and water. The CT numbers of air and water were defined as −1000 and 0 Hounsfield units (HU), respectively.

The x-ray beam attenuation is related to three factors: coherent scattering, photoelectric absorption, and Compton interactions[2] (Sprawls, 1977). Physical density is the main determinant of attenuation and thus CT number. There is a linear correlation between CT number and tissue density (Heymsfield et al.,

---

[2] The Compton effect occurs when high-frequency x rays eject an electron, and the resulting electron velocity and trajectory and x-ray frequency change and scatter are determined by the laws of energy and momentum conservation.

1979c; Wang et al., 1993). Each of the image's pixels or voxels has a CT number which gives contrast to the image.

Image reconstruction is usually done with mathematical techniques based on either two-dimensional Fourier analysis or filtered back-projection, or a combination of the methods.

Magnetic Resonance Imaging

Magnetic resonance imaging is based on the interaction among nuclei of hydrogen atoms, which are abundant in all biological tissues, and the magnetic fields generated, and is controlled by the MRI system's instrumentation. Protons, the nuclei of hydrogen, have a non-zero magnetic moment that causes them to behave like small magnets. In the earth's weak magnetic field, these magnetic moments are randomly oriented and they thus tend to cancel. When a subject is placed inside the magnet of an MRI scanner, however, the field strength is typically ten thousand times stronger than that of the earth, and the proton's magnetic moments align themselves with the magnet's field. The aligned protons are then pulsed with a radio-frequency (RF), and this causes some of the protons to absorb energy and flip. When the RF field is turned off, the protons gradually return to their original positions, releasing energy in the process. Relaxation times refer to the rate at which the absorbed energy is released. The measured relaxation times are used to generate proton (i.e., hydrogen) MR images by computer.

To increase the image contrast between AT and skeletal muscle, MRI data acquisition can be programmed to take advantage of the specific proton density and relaxation times of various tissue types. This is accomplished by varying two time parameters of the RF pulse, time to repeat (TR) and time to echo (TE). By manipulating TR and TE times, one varies the RF "pulse sequence." Using one such sequence called "spin-echo," the TR parameter can be adjusted to exploit the difference in T1 (Time 1) relaxation times of AT and muscle, which provides the tissue contrast required for high-quality MR images. With few exceptions, it is the spin-echo pulse sequence that has been selected to acquire MRI body composition data.

BODY COMPONENT RECONSTRUCTION

For both CT and MRI, there are two stages in component reconstruction. The first is to determine the amount of the specific tissue of interest in each image. The results from this stage of the analysis are usually expressed in area units (cm^2). The second stage is to assemble the area results from selected slices to compute total component volume in cm^3.

Computerized Axial Tomography

The cross-sectional CT image can be used to quantify the area of body composition components of interest (Chowdhury et al., 1994; Heymsfield et al., 1979a, b, c; Kvist et al., 1986; Seidell et al., 1990; Sjöström et al., 1986). There are two methods generally used to measure tissue area. The first is to trace visually the component's perimeter, and the CT scanner software then provides the component's cross-sectional area. Some technical concerns related to beam hardening[3] and partial volume effects[4] should be considered at this stage of the analysis (Chowdhury et al., 1994; Kvist et al., 1986).

Simple structures such as the liver and some skeletal muscles can be quantified using the tracing approach. A recent development is the automated tracing of specific tissue areas using specially designed CT software.

The validity of traced areas by CT is relatively easy to establish. For example, water-filled bottles of known diameter can be scanned and CT cross-sectional area compared to actual area. More complex structures can be created to test scan accuracy. A typical example is the construction of a mid-arm phantom from a human bone embedded in the center of a glycerol- (i.e., muscle) filled wax (i.e., fat) cylinder.

The second method also requires tracing the structure of interest. The CT scanner software can then be used to specify a pixel range for the component of interest. This approach assumes that the traced area consists of two or more components of interest. For example, the area of AT within an encircled region of skeletal muscle can be ascertained by selecting the pixels that range between −190 and −30 HU (Kvist et al., 1986; Sjöström et al., 1986). Most components have a characteristic range of pixel values that can be experimentally established (Sjöström, 1991).

This second approach is useful in separating complex structures that may include more than one tissue. For example, visceral AT is found anatomically between loops of intestine and other abdominal structures. It would be exceedingly difficult to trace visceral AT directly, thus necessitating use of the "pixel range" method. The details of quantifying tissues by CT are provided in the following references: Chowdhury et al., 1994; Heymsfield et al., 1979a, b, c; Kvist et al., 1986; Seidell et al., 1990; and Sjöström et al., 1986.

Kvist and colleagues (1988) developed improved methods of evaluating scans by taking into consideration beam hardening and partial volume effects.

---

[3] When polyenergetic x-ray photons pass through tissue, low-energy components are attenuated more rapidly than are higher-energy components. This phenomenon of selective "soft" photon removal and average photon energy increase is referred to as beam hardening. Hardening of the beam may cause changes in CT numbers and difficulties in tissue identification.

[4] The partial volume effect occurs when a voxel encompasses two components that differ in photon attenuation. The resulting CT number has a value intermediate between the two respective CT numbers for the homogeneous components. Errors can arise in component quantification if pixels are assigned to the incorrect tissue.

These and other similar studies over the past 15 years have gradually perfected the methods of evaluating body composition by CT.

Once the amount of tissue in a specific slice is known, the total volume of the component can be calculated by compiling data from multiple slices. This is usually done using the formula suggested by Sjöström et al. (1986),

$$C = d \times \sum_{i=1}^{n} [A_i \times (B_i + C_i / 2)], \qquad \text{(Equation 5-2)}$$

where C is the component of interest (kg) measured by CT or MRI; d, the assumed constant density (kg/cm^3) of the component; A_i, the distance (cm) between scans; and B_i and C_i, the component's area (cm^2) in adjacent scans. Other formulae are known, and additional discussion of this topic is presented in the next section.

Magnetic Resonance Imaging

To quantify the area of various tissues in a given image, MRI data are analyzed in a manner similar to that described for CT. Unfortunately, the quantification of MRI data is not as straightforward as it is for CT. Unlike CT where pixel values consistently represent specific tissues regardless of slice position or the individual being assessed, MRI pixel values for a given tissue (i.e., the emitted RF signal of the protons within a pixel) may vary from slice to slice or between individuals. This is because pixel values in MR images are dependent on excitation pulse sequences and a combination of proton density and tissue relaxation values, and these determinants may vary among individuals. Another more important cause of pixel variation is the variation in signal intensities that may occur for the same tissue within a set of images (i.e., seven images acquired at the same time). This variation may arise as a result of heterogeneities in the magnetic field or from other system imperfections.

Recent improvements to both MRI hardware and computer software have reduced artifacts and substantially improved the quality of MR images. However, artifacts still occur, and it is therefore useful to quantify a given tissue with image analysis software that permits visual verification of the results. In other words, the researcher must be able to correct manually for the tissue areas that are not counted by the initial pixel threshold selection. Although these procedures can be accomplished using straightforward image analysis techniques, they add a degree of subjectivity to the quantification of tissues on an MR image that is not usually required when quantifying a given tissue using CT.

The quantification of tissue areas on MR images thus cannot be accomplished by simply identifying the appropriate threshold and asking the software to count the pixels above or below that threshold. Until such time that MRI acquisition procedures improve, manual correction of MR component analyses is required. The reliability of these procedures is discussed later in this review.

The volume (cm^3) of a tissue for the whole body or a given region (i.e., legs, arms, etc.) is derived in two steps. First, the volume for each image is determined by multiplying the area (cm^2) of the tissue by the slice thickness. Whole-body or regional volume is then calculated using a mathematical algorithm similar to the one described earlier for CT.

VALIDATION STUDIES

Validation of both CT and MRI as body composition measurement systems can be organized into studies that establish the accuracy of a selected area or volume and those that examine the accuracy of whole-body component estimates. Validation experiments can be carried out in phantoms, animals, or humans. The following sections provide examples of previous CT and MRI validation studies in an effort to give an overall analysis of the various potential methods and to summarize the current relevant literature.

Computerized Axial Tomography

Phantoms and Cadavers

A number of studies have validated the accuracy of area and volume measurements by CT in systems ranging from water-filled balloons to *in situ* cadaver organs. As an example of a validation study, Heymsfield et al. (1979b) examined the accuracy of liver, kidney, and spleen volume and mass measurements by CT. The study was carried out in 4 water-filled balloons; in 12 excised human cadaver organs, including 6 kidneys, 3 livers, and 3 spleens; and in 2 human cadavers while the organs remained *in situ*. Reproducibility was determined in the first experiment by independent balloon weighing and calculation of CT mass. The coefficient of variation (CV) for weighing the balloon and for estimating CT mass was 1.6 percent and 3.9 percent, respectively. The absolute mean difference between the two methods was 2.6 percent. In the second experiment, the CV for weighing the organs and for estimating organ mass by CT was ±3 percent and ±5 percent, respectively. The mean absolute difference between the two methods was 4.6 percent. In the third experiment, the CV for weighing organs and for estimating organ mass by CT was ±3 percent and ±5 percent, respectively. The mean absolute difference between the two methods was ±5.6 percent. Thus in this study, CT volume and mass agreed with actual volume and mass within ±3 percent to 5 percent.

In a related experiment, Rossner and colleagues (1990) compared AT determinations by CT to those obtained by planimetry of 21 band-sawed slices of the corresponding sections from 2 male cadavers. Linear regression analyses indicated good agreement between CT-measured and cadaver AT areas and ratios (r values ranged from 0.77–0.94). The authors suggest that the excellent agreement between CT and cadaver AT measurements indicates that CT can be used as a body composition reference method.

Verification of Volume Measurements In Vivo

A simple method of evaluating the overall accuracy of total body CT scans is to compare CT-derived total-body volume to the subject's actual body volume. In one approach, Chowdhury and colleagues (1994) determined the volume of body subcompartments in eight males. A density was assigned to each compartment based on literature values, and compartment mass was then calculated from compartment volume. The mass of all compartments was then summed, and this was compared to actual body weight. The average of the difference between the two measures of body weight was 0.024 ± 0.65 kg, and the error calculated from the squared differences was 0.85 percent of body weight.

Wang and colleagues (1996) compared body volume calculated from 22 CT slices to body volume measured with a combination of underwater weighing and residual lung volume analysis. Whole-body volume derived by CT was highly correlated with body volume measured by underwater weighing ($r = 0.990$, $p = 0.0001$, standard error of estimate [SEE] = 1.9 liters, $n = 17$). The mean body volume measured by CT (74.8 ± 13.9 liters) agreed closely with mean body volume measured by underwater weighing (73.6 ± 13.7 liters), although there was a significant difference between the two results ($p = 0.02$). The slightly higher body volume estimate by CT was thought secondary to inclusion of trapped respiratory air, which is not included in the body volume estimate by underwater weighing.

Reproducibility

Some reproducibility studies for CT were mentioned earlier. In another study, Kvist et al. (1986) examined each of four subjects twice by CT. A total AT volume error of 0.6 percent was observed. Chowdhury et al. (1994) examined intraobserver "interpretation errors" in four subjects for a large number of CT-measured body composition components. Some examples are for skin, 2.4 percent; total AT, 0.4 percent; and heart, 3.4 percent. An earlier report by the research team (Brummer et al., 1993) indicated interobserver errors of 0.7 percent, 0.4 percent, and 2.1 percent for total AT, skeletal muscle, and visceral organs, respectively.

CT body composition analysis appears to be accurate and reproducible, although there is still a lack of careful human cadaver validation studies in samples of adequate size.

Magnetic Resonance Imaging

Phantoms

Few attempts have been made to validate MRI using phantoms. Ross et al. (1991) verified the surface area calculation of reconstructed images using two polyvinyl chloride tubes 38.1 cm long and 1.78 cm in diameter, filled to capacity with peanut oil and positioned on either side of rats during data acquisition. The mean cross-sectional area (cm^2) of the tubes was computed from a set of 12 transverse images and compared with the actual area. The mean area of the tubes obtained from image reconstruction was 2.47 cm^2, which differed from the actual value of 2.48 cm^2 by only 0.6 percent. The percent error ranged from 0.1 to 1.5 percent.

A comparison of MRI-measured whole-body volume with that obtained by underwater weighing was made in 14 women (Ross et al., 1995b). Good agreement between the methods was observed, as the correlation coefficient obtained was 0.99 ($p < 0.001$); the associated SEE was 1.5 liters or 1.8 percent.

Animals

Validation of MRI using animal models has been performed by two groups (Fowler et al., 1992; Ross et al., 1991). Using a rat model, Ross et al. (1991) reported a high correlation between chemically extracted carcass lipid and MRI-AT mass ($r = 0.97$, $p < 0.01$; SEE = 10.5%). Fowler et al. (1992) compared MRI-AT measurements with those obtained by dissection in a group of lean and obese pigs. The authors observed that the distribution of AT measured by MRI correlated strongly with AT distribution estimated by weighing dissected regional tissue samples ($r = 0.98$, mean square error [MSE] = 2.1%).

Cadavers

Engstrom et al. (1991) compared the cross-sectional area measurements of skeletal muscle determined from the proximal thigh in cadavers with corresponding MRI-measured cross-sectional areas and reported a correlation coefficient between the two that approached unity ($r = 0.99$, $p < 0.001$). Compelling evidence regarding the accuracy of MRI-AT measurements was reported by Abate et al. (1994), who compared MRI measures of abdominal subcutaneous and visceral AT in three cadavers with that obtained by direct weighing of the same AT compartments after dissection. In this study, the authors subdivided visceral AT into intraperitoneal and retroperitoneal depots. The mean difference between the two methods for the various compartments was 0.076 kg ($\sim 6\%$).

Comparison with CT

Attempts to validate MRI have been made by comparing MRI measurements of AT with those obtained by CT using both animal and human models (Table 5-1). Evaluation of the relationships between the two methods in humans generally has been performed by comparing measurements of subcutaneous AT and visceral AT area values obtained from a single abdominal image. The data presented in Table 5-1 reveal that, in general, the correlations obtained between MRI and CT for subcutaneous AT are quite high. Furthermore, given that measurements of the extremities are unaffected by the motion artifacts, it is likely that the CV between MRI- and CT-subcutaneous AT in the leg and arm regions is substantially less than the 5 to 12 percent reported for the abdomen region.

Although the difference between the two imaging modalities for subcutaneous AT is generally low, the CV for visceral AT is higher, ranging from 13 to 20 percent (Table 5-1). It has also been observed that the relationship between MRI- and CT-visceral AT improves with increasing visceral adiposity (Seidell et al., 1990). This may be explained by the increased signal to noise (i.e., from motion artifacts) ratio that results with increasing quantities of visceral AT. The ability of MRI to predict CT-visceral AT in lean subjects is likely poor, due to the low signal to noise ratio. Unfortunately, no data are available that would indicate the MRI-visceral AT area value (cm^2) below which substantial differences occur between MRI- and CT-visceral AT. Once again, the use of Fast Imaging protocols that avoid the problems associated with motion artifacts may enhance tissue contrast and improve the ability of MRI to measure visceral AT in lean subjects.

In summary, by comparison with limited cadaver and animal dissection data, it would appear that MRI measures total AT with a SEE in the range of 2 to 10 percent. Comparison with CT suggests that MRI provides images of the abdomen with similar anatomic detail and CVs for subcutaneous AT and visceral AT of about 5 percent and 15 percent, respectively.

Reliability

Adipose Tissue. Several studies have evaluated whether MRI measurements of subcutaneous AT and visceral AT are reproducible. The results presented in Table 5-2 show that for a single MR image in the abdominal region, the CV for repeated measures of subcutaneous AT ranges from 1 to 10 percent. For visceral AT, the CV for repeated measurements ranges from 6 to 11 percent. Taken together, these data suggest that when using MRI, the expected error for measurement of subcutaneous and visceral AT area is approximately 10 percent.

Unfortunately, there is little evidence regarding the reliability of MRI-measured lean tissue. Ross et al. (1994) recently reported that for a single MR image obtained at the level of the proximal thigh, the CV for repeated measurements of lean tissue (skeletal muscle and bone) was 1.2 percent. In addi-

TABLE 5-1 MRI Validation Studies

Reference	Subject (*N*)		IV	Correlation (SEE, %)			
				Subcut. AT	Visceral AT	Total AT	SM
			Comparison with CT				
Seidell et al., 1990	Human	(7)	Mid-abdomen	0.79 (4.9)	0.79 (12.8)	0.99 (4.4)	—
Sobel et al., 1991	Human	(11)	Umbilicus	0.98 (8)	0.93 (20)	—	—
Ross et al., 1991	Rat	(21)	Whole body	0.98 (12)	0.98 (13.6)	0.99 (8.7)	—
			Comparison with Cadavers				
Engstrom et al., 1991	Human	(3)	Thigh muscle CSA	—	—	—	0.99

NOTE: MRI, magnetic resonance imaging; SEE, standard error of estimate; IV, independent variable; AT, adipose tissue; SM, skeletal muscle; CT, computerized axial tomography; CSA, cross-sectional area.

TABLE 5-2 MRI Reliability Studies[*]

					Coefficient of Variation (%)			
Reference	Subject (N)	T	MRI Sequence	Anatomical Position	Subcut. AT	Visceral AT	Total AT	LT
Staten et al., 1989	Human (6)	0.5	SE	Mid-abdomen	5.0	10.0	3.0	—
Seidell et al., 1990	Human (7)	1.5	IR	Umbilicus	10.1	10.6	5.4	—
Garard et al., 1991	Human (4)	1.5	SE	6 abdomen images	3.0	9.0	—	—
Ross et al., 1991	Rat (11)	1.5	SE	Whole body	—	—	4.3	—
Ross et al., 1993	Human (3)	1.5	SE	L4–L5	1.1	5.5	—	—
				Whole body	—	—	2.5	—
Sohlström et al., 1993	Human (3)	0.02	SR	Whole body	1.7	5.3*	1.5	—
Ross et al., 1994	Human (11)	1.5	SE	Proximal thigh	—	—	—	1.2
Abate et al., 1994	Cadaver (3)	0.35	SE	Abdomen	2.2	6.0	—	—
Ross et al., 1995a	Human (19)	1.5	SE	L4–L5	—	—	—	1.0

NOTE: MRI, magnetic resonance imaging; T, strength of magnet in Teslas; AT, adipose tissue; LT, lean tissue; SE, spin-echo; IR, inverse recovery; SR, saturation recovery; L4–L5, lumbar vertebrae 4–5.

* Reported as nonsubcutaneous adipose tissue.

tion, the authors reported that for lean tissue volume in the leg, derived using 15 images, the CV was 3.9 percent. Although the issue of measurement reliability requires further investigation, these preliminary results are encouraging.

ADVANTAGES AND DISADVANTAGES

Early use of radiogrammetry with conventional x-ray systems was limited by poor image contrast and the availability of only two-dimensional images. Both CT and MRI offer the important opportunity for three-dimensional tissue volume quantification. Image contrast is sharp, and tissue boundaries are relatively clear. Competing technologies, such as ultrasound, cannot delineate tissue interfaces with the same level of accuracy as CT and MRI. No other currently available methods can assess body composition components at the tissue-system level with the same level of accuracy as CT and MRI.

A second major advantage of both CT and MRI is the capability of carrying out cross-sectional imaging. Conventional two-dimensional radiography cannot ascertain the area or volume of structures inside the body cavities. Visceral AT, brain, and heart volumes can all be quantified with CT and MRI. No other current body composition methods can accurately quantify visceral AT.

A third important aspect of CT and MRI is the capability of making regional and whole-body measurements. Ultrasound, which is also capable of estimating tissue-system level components, at present can only provide regional measurements.

A fourth important feature of CT and MRI is the availability of measurement systems. Almost every major medical research center in the United States has both a CT and MRI scanner that is capable of body composition analysis. Many systems are also available in developing countries.

With respect to body composition measurement, MRI offers an advantage over CT in not exposing subjects to ionizing radiation. Multiple MR images can therefore be obtained without known risk to the subject.

Magnetic resonance imaging has the potential to provide criterion data for the development of prediction equations on diverse subject populations. Examples are anthropometric prediction equations for visceral AT and whole-body skeletal muscle mass in which MRI-derived components serve as the reference component estimate.

The lack of radiation exposure with MRI also makes it suitable for longitudinal and intervention studies wherein multiple and/or serial measurements are required.

A disadvantage of some MRI systems is that the small bore magnet precludes study of claustrophobic and very overweight subjects. Open magnet MRI systems are available but are not in widespread use. The magnetic field generated with MRI also restricts study of patients with implanted metal objects.

Another disadvantage of MRI is that motion artifacts can affect tissue contrast in the abdominal region. Although improvements in MRI technology now permit the acquisition of multiple transverse images in a breath hold (i.e., ~20 seconds) (Ross et al., 1995a), reliable determination of AT in the abdominal region can be a problem (Seidell et al., 1990). A related disadvantage is that, due to the subjectivity associated with the determination of tissue areas on MR images, the time required to analyze MR images can be lengthy. The analysis of MRI data using specially designed software on computer workstations improves data analysis capabilities (Ross et al., 1992).

REFERENCE TECHNIQUE FOR HUMAN FAT MEASUREMENT?

Whether MRI or CT might serve as calibration techniques for other methods of body composition assessment is a question of considerable interest. In order to determine body fat by MRI or CT, two key issues must be resolved.

The first issue relates to the conversion AT volume of lipid or fat mass. Lipid is the total lipid solvent-extractable material from tissue. Fat in the current context is nonessential lipid, mainly triglycerides.

Adipose tissue is a body composition component at the tissue-system level, and total lipids and fat are components at the molecular level (Figure 5-1). Two steps are needed to convert AT volume to fat mass: AT volume conversion to AT mass, and AT mass conversion to fat mass. These conversions require knowledge of AT density and fat fraction: AT fat mass = measured AT volume × assumed AT density × assumed AT fat fraction. It has been shown that the normal physiological range for AT density and AT fat fraction is 0.91 to 0.98 g/ml and 0.5 to 0.9, respectively (Martin et al., 1994). Thus the conversion of AT volume to AT fat mass requires a factor that varies over the range of their product, approximately 0.5 to 0.8 g/ml. This variation is considerable and cannot be ignored; successful conversion of AT volume to fat mass requires a good estimate of this factor, which is valid across populations that differ widely in age, gender, and adiposity.

Although there are currently no *in vivo* methods for estimating either AT density or its fat fraction, it has been shown that these values are closely related to the degree of adiposity. The highest AT densities and fat fractions are observed in the leanest individuals, and the lowest AT densities and fat fractions are observed in the fattest individuals (Martin et al., 1994). Preliminary data in older men suggest that it may be possible to estimate AT fat fraction from overall adiposity, although this observation remains unconfirmed (Martin et al., 1994).

A second source of error when using CT or MRI to estimate total body fat is that once total body AT fat has been estimated, total body lipid is obtained by adding nontriglyceride lipids, a quantity that is variable and difficult to estimate.

Taken together, these observations suggest that the error inherent in the conversion of CT- and MRI-AT volumes to lipid mass precludes their use as a current reference measure of total body lipid. However, it is important to note that most clinical interest centers on total body fat, and thus this second source of error may not be of primary concern. It should be possible to estimate only total body fat from MRI or CT once the conversion factor(s) for AT volume to AT-fat mass are known.

FUTURE APPLICATIONS

There are many potential future areas of CT and MRI research, and only a few relevant topics are mentioned here.

Spiral (helical) imaging methods represent an important advance in CT technology (Fishman, 1994). Spiral CT was developed to help overcome technical problems with CT, such as patient movement and respiration during a single CT slice. The method allows rapid three-dimensional scanning of a large body segment or even the whole body. Although this capability is valuable in clinical radiographic studies, particularly with contrast agents, the possibility also exists that spiral CT can be used to reconstruct body composition components. It may be feasible to reduce radiation dosages with spiral CT as high image contrast is not needed in body composition research, as it is in clinical studies.

The eventual linkage of MRI and MRS systems will allow study of metabolic processes *in vivo*. There is already considerable research in this area, although access to large-bore magnets that can carry out both MRI and MRS is still limited. Magnets with high field strengths (up to 5 Teslas) are now either available for human studies or under construction. Imaging and spectroscopy can be carried out on these MR systems for protons (^{1}H), phosphorous (^{31}P), sodium (^{23}Na), carbon (^{13}C), and potentially other elements as well. The availability of combined MRI and MRS systems will allow for a union of body composition and metabolism studies.

Functional MR is an important development in the study of tissue metabolism, particularly of the brain (Duyn et al., 1994). As with MRS, metabolic processes can be evaluated in specific body composition components.

Another important area of future research involves MRI technical developments. What are the potential uses of coronal and saggital MR images in body composition studies? Spin-echo imaging is the traditional scanning sequence of choice for MRI-body composition studies (Table 5-2). This is due primarily to its inherent tissue contrast properties, robust signal strength, and relative insensitivity to artifacts that affect other MR sequences. The principal drawback of spin-echo is the time required for many of the preferred scanning routines. Recent developments in MR technology, however, have addressed this problem. Fast spin-echo pulse sequences can reduce conventional spin-echo by a factor of as much as 16 while maintaining excellent tissue contrast (Mansfield, 1977). Recent developments in Echo Planar Imaging (EPI) promise even greater reduction in the time required to obtain multiple images, as "snapshot" EPI boasts

20 to 100 µs acquisition rates (10 to 50 images per second) (Jolesz, 1992). At these rates, it would appear that MR applications in body composition measurement hold great promise for the future.

A final important research area is the use of both CT and MRI as reference standards against which useful and practical body composition methods can be developed. The uses of CT and MRI were mentioned earlier as measures of total body lipid and fat. Both CT and MRI may also be useful as reference standards for skeletal muscle, visceral AT, and other components. MRI has the advantage in this area over CT in that it poses no subject risk and thus populations, including children and young women, can be evaluated with little or no concern.

Some early work in this area has already been carried out by a number of investigators. For example, Sjöström (1991) used multislice CT as a reference method for estimating total body AT. The subjects were 19 women and 24 men whose weight ranged from approximately 70 to 130 kg for the women and 73 to 140 kg for the men. Anthropometric prediction equations were developed. Ross et al. (1992, 1994) similarly used MRI-measured visceral AT to develop anthropometric prediction equations.

AUTHORS' CONCLUSIONS

There are many important areas of potential future research that apply CT and MRI, not only in technology development, but also in the application of both imaging methods to the study of biological factors that influence human body composition. Advances in related technologies, such as MR spectroscopy, will also help bridge the gap between static body composition measurements and evaluation of dynamic metabolic and biochemical processes. Taken collectively, these capabilities of CT and MRI will undoubtedly allow both methods to play a central role in future body composition research efforts.

REFERENCES

Abate, N., D. Burns, R.M. Peshock, A. Garg, and S.M. Grundy
    1994   Estimation of adipose tissue mass by magnetic resonance imaging: Validation against dissection in human cadavers. J. Lipid Res. 35:1490–1496.
Baumgartner, R.N., R.L. Rhyne, C. Troup, S. Wayne, and P.J. Garry
    1992   Appendicular skeletal muscle areas assessed by magnetic resonance imaging in older persons. J. Gerontol. 47:M67–72.
Baumgartner, R.N., S.B. Heymsfield, and A.F. Roche
    1995   Human body composition and the epidemiology of chronic disease. Obes. Res. 3:73–95.
Björntorp, P.
    1986   Adipose tissue distribution and morbidity. Pp. 60–65 in Recent Advances in Obesity Research, V.E.M. Berry, S.H. Blundheim, H.E. Eliahou, and E. Shafrir, eds. London: John Libby.

Bloch, F., W.W. Hansen, and M.E. Packard
  1946   Nuclear introduction. Phys. Rev. 70:460–474.
Borkan, G.A., S.G. Gerzof, A.H. Robbins, D.E. Hults, C.K. Silbert, and J.E. Silbert
  1982   Assessment of abdominal fat content by computerized tomography. Am. J. Clin. Nutr. 36:172–177.
Brummer, R.J.M., L. Lonn, U.L. Grangard, B.A. Bengtsson, H. Kvist, and L. Sjöström
  1993   Adipose tissue and muscle volume determinations by computed tomography in acromegaly, before and one year after adenectomy. Eur. J. Clin. Invest. 23:199–205.
Chowdhury, B., L. Sjöström, M. Alpsten, J. Kostanty, H. Kvist, and R. Löfgren
  1994   A multicompartment body composition technique based on computerized tomography. Int. J. Obes. 18:219–234.
Cormack, M.M.
  1980   Early two-dimensional reconstruction and recent topics stemming from it. Med. Phys. 7:277–281.
Damadian, R.
  1971   Tumor detection by nuclear magnetic resonance. Science 171:1151–1153.
de Ridder, C.M., R.M. de Boer, J.C. Seidell, C.M. Nieuwenhoff, J.A.L. Jeneson, C.J.G. Bakker, M.L. Zonderland, and W.B.M. Erich
  1992   Body fat distribution in pubertal girls quantified by magnetic resonance imaging. Int. J. Obes. 16:443–449.
Duyn, J.H., V.S. Mattay, R.H. Sexton, G.S. Sobering, F.A. Barrios, G. Liu, J.A. Frank, D.R. Weinberger, and C.T. Moonen
  1994   Three-dimensional functional imaging of human brain using echo-shifted FLASH MRI. Magn. Reson. Med. 32:150.
Engstrom, C.M., G.E. Loeb, J.R. Reid, W.J. Forrest, and L. Avruch
  1991   Morphometry of the human thigh muscles. A comparison between anatomical sections and computer tomographic and magnetic resonance images. J. Anat. 176:139–156.
Fishman, E.K.
  1994   Spiral imaging methods assure survival of CT. Diagn. Imaging. (November): 59–67.
Forbes, G.B.
  1987   Human Body Composition. Growth, Aging, Nutrition and Activity. New York: Springer-Verlag.
Foster, M.A., J.M.S. Hutchison, J.R. Mallard, and M. Fuller
  1984   Nuclear magnetic resonance pulse sequence and discrimination of high- and low-fat tissues. Magn. Reson. Imaging 2:187–192.
Fowler, P.A., M.F. Fuller, C.A. Glasby, M.A. Foster, G.G. Cameron, G. McNiel, and R.J. Maughan
  1991   Total and subcutaneous AT distribution in women: The measurement of distribution and accurate prediction of quantity by using magnetic resonance imaging. Am. J. Clin. Nutr. 54:18–25.
Fowler, P.A., M.F. Fuller, C.A. Glasbey, G.G. Cameron, and M.A. Foster
  1992   Validation of the *in vivo* measurement of adipose tissue by magnetic resonance imaging of lean and obese pigs. Am. J. Clin. Nutr. 56:7–13.
Garard, E.L., R.C. Snow, D.N. Kennedy, R.E. Frisch, A.R. Guimaraes, R.L. Barbieri, A.G. Sorenson, T.K. Egglin, and B.R. Rosen
  1991   Overall body fat and regional fat distribution in young women: Quantification with MR imaging. Am. J. Radiol. 157:97–104.

Garn, S.M.
 1957 Roentgenogrammetric determination of body composition. Hum. Biol. 29:337.
 1961 Radiographic analysis of body composition. Pp. 36–58 in Techniques for Measuring Body Composition, Proceedings of a Conference, Quartermaster Research and Engineering Center, Natick, Mass., January 22–23, 1959, J. Broézek and A. Henschel, eds. Washington, D.C.: National Academy of Sciences/National Research Council.

Gray, D., K. Fujioka, P.M. Colletti, H. Kim, W. Devine, T. Cuyegkeng, and T. Pappas
 1991 Magnetic-resonance imaging used for determining fat distribution in obesity and diabetes. Am. J. Clin. Nutr. 54:623–627.

Hayes, P.A., P.J. Sowood, A. Belyavin, J.B. Cohen, and F.W. Smith
 1988 Subcutaneous fat thickness measured by magnetic resonance imaging, ultrasound, and calipers. Med. Sci. Sports Exerc. 20:303–309.

Heymsfield, S.B., and R. Noel
 1981 Radiographic analysis of body composition by computerized axial tomography. Nutr. Cancer 17:161–172.

Heymsfield, S.B., R.P. Olafson, M.H. Kutner, and D.W. Nixon
 1979a A radiographic method of quantifying protein-calorie undernutrition. Am. J. Clin. Nutr. 32:693–702.

Heymsfield, S.B., T. Fulenwider, B. Nordlinger, R. Balow, P. Sones, and M. Kutner
 1979b Accurate measurement of liver, kidney, and spleen volume and mass by computerized axial tomography. Ann. Intern. Med. 90:185–187.

Heymsfied, S.B., R. Noel, M. Lynn, and M. Kutner
 1979c Accuracy of soft tissue density predicted by CT. J. Comput. Assist. Tomogr. 3:859–860.

Hounsfield, G.N.
 1973 Computerized transverse axial scanning (tomography). Br. J. Radiol. 46:1016.

Jolesz, F.A.
 1992 Fast spin-echo technique extends versatility of MR. Diagn. Imaging 14:78.

Kvist, H., L. Sjöström, and U. Tylén
 1986 Adipose tissue volume determinations in women by computed tomography: Technical consideration. Int. J. Obes. 10: 53–67.

Kvist, H., B. Chowdhury, L. Sjöström, U. Tyler, and Å. Cederblad
 1988 Adipose tissue volume determination in males by computed tomography and ^{40}K. Int. J. Obes. 12:249–266.

Lauterber, P.C.
 1973 Image formation by induced local interactions: Examples employing nuclear magnetic resonance. Nature 242:190–191.

Lawes, J.B., and J.H. Gilbert
 1859 Experimental inquiry into the composition of some of the animals fed and slaughtered as human food. Philos. Trans. R. Soc. London 149:493–680.

Lukaski, H.C.
 1987 Methods for the assessment of human body composition: Traditional and new. Am. J. Clin. Nutr. 46:537–556.

Mansfield, P.
 1977 Multi-planar image formation using NMR spin-echoes. J. Phys. Chem. 10:L55.

Martin, A.D., M.Z. Daniel, D. Drinkwater, and J.P. Clarys
 1994 Adipose tissue density estimated adipose lipid fraction and whole body adiposity in male cadavers. Int. J. Obes. 18:79–83.

Moulton, C.R.
 1923 Age and chemical development in mammals. J. Biol. Chem. 57:79–97.

Purcell, E.M., H.C. Torrey, and R.V. Pound
1946   Resonance absorption by nuclear magnetic moments in a solid. Phys. Rev. 69:37–38.

Raden, J.
1917   On the determination of functions from their integrals along certain mainfolds. Math. Phys. Klasse. 69:262–277.

Ross, R., and J. Rissanen
1994   Mobilization of visceral and subcutaneous adipose tissue in response to caloric restriction and exercise. Am. J. Clin. Nutr. 60:695–703.

Ross, R., L. Léger, R. Guardo, J. de Guise, and B.G. Pike
1991   Adipose tissue volume measured by magnetic resonance imaging and computerized tomography in rats. J. Appl. Physiol. 70(5):2164–2172.

Ross, R., L. Léger, D. Morris, J. de Guise, and R. Guardo
1992   Quantification of adipose tissue by MRI: Relationship with anthropometric variables. J. Appl. Physiol. 72:787–795.

Ross, R., K.D. Shaw, Y. Martel, J. de Guise, and L. Avruch
1993   Adipose tissue distribution measured by magnetic resonance imaging in obese women. Am. J. Clin. Nutr. 57:470–475.

Ross, R., K.D. Shaw, J. Rissanen, Y. Martel, J. de Guise, and L. Avruch
1994   Sex differences in lean and adipose tissue distribution by magnetic resonance imaging: Anthropometric relationships. Am. J. Clin. Nutr. 59:1277–1285.

Ross, R., H. Pedwell, and J. Rissanen
1995a   Effects of energy restriction and exercise on skeletal muscle and adipose tissue in women as measured by magnetic resonance imaging. Am. J. Clin. Nutr. 61:1179–1185.

1995b   Response of total and regional lean tissue and skeletal muscle to a program of energy restriction and resistance exercise. Int. J. Obes. 19(11):781–787.

Rossner, S., W.J. Bo, E. Hiltbrandt, W. Hinson, N. Karstaedt, P. Santago, W.T. Sobol, and J.R. Crouse
1990   Adipose tissue determinations in cadavers—a comparison between cross-sectional planimetry and computed tomography. Int. J. Obes. 14:893–902.

Seidell, J.C., C.J.C. Bakker, and K. van der Kooy
1990   Imaging techniques for measuring adipose-tissue distribution—a comparison between computed tomography and 1.5-T magnetic resonance. Am. J. Clin. Nutr. 51:953–957.

Sjöström, L.
1991   A computer-tomography based multicompartment body composition techniques and anthropometric predictions of lean body mass, total and subcutaneous adipose tissue. Int. J. Obes. 15(suppl. 2):19–30.

Sjöström, L., H. Kvist, A. Cederblad, and U. Tylen
1986   Determination of total adipose tissue and body fat in women by computed tomography, ^{40}K, and tritium. Am. J. Physiol. 250:E736–E745.

Snyder, W.S., M.J. Cook, E.S. Nasset, L.R. Karhansen, G.P. Howells, and I.H. Tipton
1975   Report of the Task Group on Reference Man. Oxford: Pergamon Press.

Sobel, W., S. Rossner, B. Hinson, E. Hiltbrandt, N. Karstaedt, P. Santago, N. Wolfman, A. Hagaman, and J.R. Crouse, III
1991   Evaluation of a new magnetic resonance imaging method for quantitating adipose tissue areas. Int. J. Obes. 15:589–599.

Sohlström, A., and E. Forsum
  1995   Changes in adipose tissue volume and distribution during reproduction in Swedish women as assessed by magnetic resonance imaging. Am. J. Clin. Nutr. 61:287–295.
Sohlström, A., L-O. Wahlund, and E. Forsum
  1993   Adipose tissue distribution as assessed by magnetic resonance imaging and total body fat by magnetic resonance imaging, underwater weighing, and body-water dilution in healthy women. Am. J. Clin. Nutr. 58:830–838.
Spivak, C.D.
  1915   The specific gravity of the human body. Arch. Internal Med. 15:628–642.
Sprawls, P.
  1977   The Physical Principles of Diagnostic Radiology. Baltimore, Md.: University Park Press.
Staten, M.A., W.G. Totty, and W.M. Kohrt
  1989   Measurement of fat distribution by magnetic resonance imaging. Invest. Radiol. 24:345–349.
Stuart H.C., P. Hill, and C. Shaw
  1940   The growth of bone, muscle and overlying tissue as revealed by studies of roentgenograms of the leg area. Monogr. Soc. Res. Child Dev. 5 (no. 3, serial no. 26):1–190.
von Bezold, A.
  1857   Untersuchungen uber die vertheilung von Wasser, organischer Materie und anorganischen Verbindungen im Thierreiche. Z. Wissenschaftlische Zoologie, 8:487–524.
Wang, Z.M., R.N. Pierson, Jr., and S.B. Heymsfield
  1992   The five-level model: A new approach to organizing body-composition research. Am. J. Clin. Nutr. 56: 19–28.
Wang Z.M., S. Heshka, and S.B. Heymsfield
  1993   Application of computerized axial tomography in the study of body composition: Evaluation of lipid, water, protein, and mineral in healthy men. Pp. 343–344 in Human Body Composition: *In Vivo* Methods, Models, and Assessment, K.J. Ellis and J.D. Eastman, eds. New York: Plenum Press.
Wang, Z.M., S. Heshka, R.N. Pierson, Jr., and S.B. Heymsfield
  1995   Systematic organization of body composition methodology: Overview with emphasis on component-based methods. Am. J. Clin. Nutr. 61: 457–465.
Wang, Z.M., M. Visser, R. Ma, R.N. Baumgartner, D. Kotler, D. Gallagher, and S.B. Heymsfield
  1996   Skeletal muscle mass: Evaluation of neutron activation and dual-energy x-ray absorptiometry methods. J. Appl. Physiol. 80:824–831.

DISCUSSION

WENDY KOHRT: In the MRI procedure, besides the slice-to-slice variability in pixel intensity, isn't there also within-slice variability in pixel intensity?

STEVEN HEYMSFIELD: Yes, there is, and that is a problem. I am only now getting involved with MRI myself for the first time, but I find there is a certain amount of subjectivity involved in, for example, measuring visceral adipose tissue or subcutaneous adipose tissue and so on. We need very good reconstruction programs that people have developed to make these measurements, but there is subjectivity involved.

One first specifies, say, a certain range of relaxation times in subcutaneous adipose tissue. That might appear on the screen as different colors, but then you see there is a big blotch that has not been included, and then one has to, by hand, incorporate that into the area measurement.

WENDY KOHRT: Yes, since the area you know is fat does not necessarily always appear to be fat when you set a threshold.

STEVEN HEYMSFIELD: That is exactly right. It is a cause of concern, but the comparisons between CT and MRI, and a number of these have been done, are reasonably good.

DONALD McCORMICK: How far off are we from being able to use other nuclei?

STEVEN HEYMSFIELD: I think we are going to hear more. Gerry Shulman is going to talk about ^{13}C, I am sure, but there is a great proliferation of high field-strength magnets now. For example, I know at Columbia we have a 5 Tesla, and I heard that there is at Emory a 5 Tesla as well.

My understanding is that with those higher field-strengths magnets, you can do nuclei such as ^{23}Na, is that correct? So that, then, opens another whole set of interesting, not only physiological measurements, but body composition as well.

DOUGLAS WILMORE: Let me just mention for the group that the place that this really has economic value is for detection of animal composition. If you go to Europe, there are large research facilities in veterinary schools where you can vary food intake or feeding intake for large animals, such as goats and sheep and the like, and scan the animal and look at how much meat you are going to produce or how much fat will be on the meat and the like. That is technology that is growing and evolving and impacting everything in the veterinary schools in a real way.

WM. CAMERON CHUMLEA: Do the high-Tesla magnets have the problem of bore size? I mean the open magnets, as I understand it, are the low Tesla, and so basically we still cannot really get the people who need it most into the machine?

STEVEN HEYMSFIELD: I just know the Columbia magnet is also relatively small bore.

DOUGLAS WILMORE: They are getting up to 1 meter.

Emerging Technologies for Nutrition Research, 1997
Pp. 151–167. Washington, D.C.
National Academy Press

6

Dual-Energy X-Ray Absorptiometry: Research Issues and Equipment

Wendy M. Kohrt[1]

INTRODUCTION

The primary clinical application of dual-energy x-ray absorptiometry (DXA or DEXA) is the measurement of bone mineral content (BMC, g) and bone mineral density (BMD, g/cm^2) of the lumbar spine and proximal femur to assess risk for osteoporosis. Additional applications of DXA that are relevant to nutrition research include: (1) the determination of total body bone mineral content (TBBM, g), which can be used as an adjunct measure for the assessment of body composition using multicompartment models; (2) the independent assessment by DXA of a three-compartment model of body composition

[1] Wendy M. Kohrt, Department of Internal Medicine, Division of Geriatrics and Gerontology, Washington University School of Medicine, Saint Louis, MO 63110

Some of the research described here was supported by National Institutes of Health Research Grant AR40704, Research Career Development Award AG00663, and Program Project Award AG05562.

(TBBM, fat, and nonbone lean tissue); and (3) the evaluation of regional body composition.

EQUIPMENT

DXA instruments have been commercially available since 1987. Advantages of DXA compared to its predecessor, dual-photon absorptiometry (DPA), include reduced radiation exposure, stability of the energy source, faster data collection, and increased precision of measurements. The three major manufacturers of DXA instruments in the United States are Hologic (Waltham, Mass.), Lunar (Madison, Wis.), and Norland (Fort Atkinson, Wis.). Although the first generation of DXA instruments from these manufacturers was limited to the measurement of BMC and BMD of selected regions of the skeleton, all of the manufacturers now produce machines that can assess both total body and regional bone mineral and soft tissue masses. The principles of operation, methods of calibration, and other features of the various models of DXA instruments produced by each manufacturer have been reviewed by Lohman (1996).

ASSESSMENT OF BONE MINERAL DENSITY

Reliability and Precision

The short- and long-term reliability and precision of BMD measured by DXA have been shown to be excellent. Table 6-1 summarizes the findings of just a few of the studies that have assessed the short-term coefficient of variation (CV) in measuring BMD by DXA. It is apparent that there is good precision across manufacturers, instrument models, data collection modes, and measurement sites. Long-term precision of DXA, which is typically evaluated by measuring BMD of a spine phantom (a mechanical model for predicting irradiation dosage deep in the body), has been shown to be excellent, with CVs less than 1.0 percent (Lilley et al., 1991; Orwoll et al., 1993). The highly reproducible measurement of total body bone mineral content (Jensen et al., 1994; Mazess et al., 1990; Pritchard et al., 1993; Slosman et al., 1992; Snead et al., 1993; Svendsen et al., 1993) makes DXA particularly suitable for use in multicompartment models of body composition.

Validity

The validity of an instrument depends on how well it measures what it is intended to measure. In the case of the measurement of BMD by DXA, validity remains questionable because there is a wide disparity among BMD measures

TABLE 6-1 Coefficients of Variation of Measurement of Bone Mineral Density by Dual-Energy X-Ray Absorptiometry

Reference	Scanner	Manufacturer	Site/Object	CV (%)
Kohrt and Birge, Jr., 1995	QDR-1000W	Hologic	Total body	0.6
			PA spine	1.1
			Femoral neck	1.5
			Trochanter	1.1
			Ward's	3.2
			Ultradistal wrist	0.6
Jergas et al., 1995	QDR-2000	Hologic	PA spine	1.3
			Lateral spine	2.0
Mazess et al., 1992	DPX-L	Lunar	PA spine	
			Fast[*]	0.6
			Medium[†]	0.5
			Femoral neck	
			Fast	1.0
			Medium	1.4
			Trochanter	
			Fast	1.5
			Medium	2.0
			Ward's	
			Fast	2.6
			Medium	2.3
Sievanen et al., 1992	XR-26	Norland	PA spine	1.7
			Femoral neck	1.3
			Distal radius	1.9
Tothill et al., 1994a	QDR-1000W	Hologic	Nord phantom	0.9
	DPX	Lunar	(Nord, 1991)	1.1
	XR-26	Norland		1.2
Eiken et al., 1994	QDR-1000W	Hologic	Spine phantom	0.4
	QDR-2000 single-beam x-ray	Lunar		0.5
	QDR-2000 fan-beam x-ray	Lunar		0.5

NOTE: CV, coefficient of variation; PA, posterior→anterior.

[*] 2-min scan time.

[†] 4-min scan time.

obtained on different DXA scanners. *In vivo* assessments of the lumbar spine, proximal femur, and whole body and *in vitro* assessments of a number of different phantoms indicate that BMD values obtained from Lunar instruments are 12 to 24 percent higher (Genant et al., 1994; Horber et al., 1992; Lai et al., 1992; Pocock et al., 1992) than those from Hologic or Norland machines. Comparisons of Norland and Hologic instruments are variable, with differences in BMD ranging from −1 to 14 percent. Despite these differences, BMD values obtained on the three systems have consistently been shown to be highly correlated ($r \geq 0.88$).

The International DXA Standardization Committee has spearheaded efforts to standardize BMD measures across instruments (Genant et al., 1994). Using the European spine phantom, Genant et al. (1994) found that BMD values obtained on different machines were highly correlated ($r > 0.99$), but values were approximately 12 percent higher on Lunar than on Hologic or Norland machines. The differences in BMD values among the scanners were attributable both to differences in methods of calibration and to differences in the methods of edge detection (i.e., bone areas were smaller on Lunar instruments). This study indicated that Lunar overestimated the true BMD value of the phantom, while Hologic and Norland underestimated the true value. Equations were developed to predict true lumbar spine BMD from values measured on each instrument.

Although the attempt to standardize BMD values is laudable and the results are encouraging, investigators must be aware that features and options that emerge with each new generation of DXA may introduce additional sources of variance in BMD values. Some of the options currently available include x-ray beam configuration (single-beam vs. fan-beam), speed of data collection, the size of the collimator, and the software version used to analyze the scan. These factors have been shown to result in changes in BMD of up to approximately 4 percent (Blake et al., 1993; Eiken et al., 1994, 1995; Mazess et al., 1992). Table 6-2 illustrates the differences in BMD values obtained on different DXA models from the same manufacturer using either single-beam or fan-beam x-ray configurations. Obviously, controlling for these factors is of critical importance, particularly in prospective studies that involve serial assessments of BMD.

ASSESSMENT OF BODY COMPOSITION

Reliability and Precision

Because bone mineral, nonbone lean tissue, and fat have different x-ray attenuation properties, it is possible with some DXA instruments to acquire a three-compartment model of body composition. The measurement of total body BMC by DXA has a high degree of precision; CVs have been reported to be less than or equal to 1.5 percent (Jensen et al., 1994; Mazess et al., 1990; Pritchard et

TABLE 6-2 Comparisons of Bone Mineral Density and Body Composition Measures from Various Scanners and X-Ray Beam Configurations

	DXA Instrument and X-Ray Configuration		
	QDR-1000W (single-beam)	QDR-2000 (single-beam)	QDR-2000 (fan-beam)
Whole-body BMD (g/cm^2)	1.206	1.196[*]	1.164[*]
L_2–L_4 BMD (g/cm^2)	1.094	1.109[*]	1.077[*]
Total mass (kg)[†]	67.0	66.6[*]	66.4[*]
Body fat (%)[†]	17.7	20.6[*]	21.1[*]

NOTE: DXA, dual-energy x-ray absorptiometry; BMD, bone mineral density; L_2–L_4, lumbar vertebrae 2–4.

[*] Significantly different from the QDR-1000W; $p < 0.05$.

[†] Corresponding values measured by hydrodensitometry were 67.1 kg and 17.2 percent body fat.

SOURCE: W. M. Kohrt (Unpublished data, Washington University School of Medicine, St. Louis, Mo., 1995).

al., 1993; Slosman et al., 1992; Snead et al., 1993; Svendsen et al., 1993). The CVs of fat mass tend to be larger than those of total body mass or lean mass (Table 6-3), but this is largely due to the fact that the fat compartment has a smaller mass. In general, the standard deviations for repeat assessments of the total, fat, and lean compartments are approximately 0.4 to 0.7 kg.

Validity

The validity of the assessment of body composition by DXA remains questionable. Although some investigators have suggested that DXA is an accurate method of measuring body composition and that it can replace hydrodensitometry as the reference method for validating other techniques (Formica et al., 1993), others have suggested that this is premature (Kohrt, 1995; Roubenoff et al., 1993). There are a number of potential sources of error in the assessment of body composition by DXA, but the discussion of these errors requires at least a rudimentary understanding of the underlying principles.

TABLE 6-3 Coefficients of Variation of Body Composition Measurements by Dual-Energy X-Ray Absorptiometry

Reference	Scanner	Manufacturer	Total Mass (%)	Fat Mass (%)	Lean Mass (%)
Tothill et al., 1994b; *in vivo*	QDR-1000W	Hologic	0.1	1.9	0.6
	DPX	Lunar	0.1	2.6	1.1
	XR-26	Norland	1.2	2.7	1.4
Tothill et al., 1994b; phantom	QDR-1000W	Hologic	0.2	3.2	0.6
	DPX	Lunar	0.2	4.4	1.0
	XR-26	Norland	0.2	3.0	0.9
Pritchard et al., 1993	QDR-1000W	Hologic		2.1	0.6
Snead et al., 1993	QDR-1000W	Hologic	0.9	1.4	1.9
Svendsen et al., 1993	DPX	Lunar		4.6	1.5

Underlying Principles of Body Composition Assessment by DXA

The assessment of body composition by hydrodensitometry is based on the principle that the composition of an object can be determined if it comprises two materials that have different mass densities. Similarly, with DXA it is possible to determine the composition of an object if it comprises two materials that have different x-ray attenuation properties. In DXA, the x-ray attenuation of each pixel of the scan image is compared with that of the reference materials, which have x-ray attenuation properties similar to the biological tissues of interest (i.e., bone mineral, nonbone lean, and fat).

The x-ray attenuation coefficient of bone mineral is several orders of magnitude higher than that of either fat or lean soft tissue (Figure 6-1, Panel A) (Nord and Payne, 1990). Thus, bone pixels are readily distinguished from nonbone pixels, except when they contain a very small proportion of bone mineral (e.g., pixels that intersect the edges of bone). Because the x-ray attenuation coefficients of nonbone lean and fat tissues are also different (Figure 6-1, Panel B), the lean/fat composition of nonbone pixels can be quantified. Thus, in simplistic terms, the determination of body composition by DXA involves (1) the comparison of those pixels that contain bone mineral with the reference materials to determine bone mineral content, and (2) the comparison of nonbone pixels with the reference materials to determine lean and fat content.

Panel A

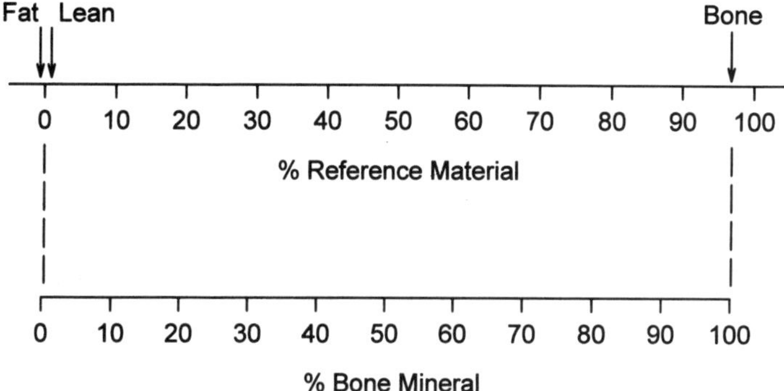

Panel B

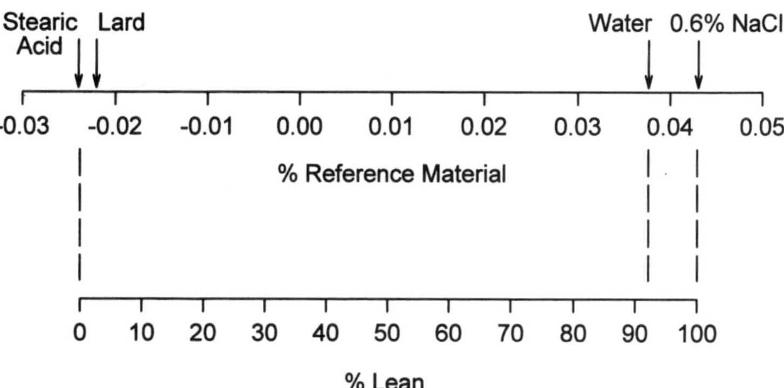

FIGURE 6-1 Overview of the general principles upon which the estimation of body composition by DXA is based. In those pixels that contain bone mineral, the x-ray attenuation is compared with attenuation characteristics of the appropriate reference materials for bone and nonbone tissue (Panel A). In those pixels that do not contain bone mineral, the x-ray attenuation is compared with attenuation characteristics of appropriate reference materials for nonbone lean and fat tissues (Panel B). SOURCE: Adapted from Nord and Payne (1990).

Sources of Error in the Assessment of Body Composition by DXA

Hydration Status. An acknowledged weakness in the assessment of body composition by hydrodensitometry is the requisite assumption that the fractional composition of the fat-free mass (i.e., percent water, protein, and mineral) is constant within and between individuals. Analogous to this is the assumption in DXA that nonbone lean tissue has fixed water and protein fractions. Thus, one source of error in the estimation of body composition by DXA is the hydration status of the subject.

The effects of hydration status have been studied in hemodialysis patients and in volunteers who ingest large volumes of fluid (Formica et al., 1993; Going et al., 1993; Horber et al., 1992). The removal of 0.9 to 4.4 kg or the ingestion of 0.4 to 2.4 kg of fluid were reflected by DXA as changes in nonbone lean mass; there were no significant changes in bone mineral or fat mass. These findings indicate that small fluctuations in hydration status were accurately assessed by DXA.

From a theoretical perspective, even large deviations from the assumed water fraction of fat-free mass should have a relatively small effect on body composition assessment by DXA. Based on x-ray attenuation properties, mineral-free water appears to be approximately 8 percent fat by DXA (Goodsitt, 1992) (as exemplified in Figure 6-1, Panel B). Thus, if the water content of fat-free mass was actually 83 percent rather than the assumed 73 percent, 8 percent of the "extra" 10 percent water would be measured as fat rather than as lean mass (i.e., $0.08 \times 0.10 \times$ fat-free mass). In most individuals, the magnitude of error in fat or fat-free mass would not exceed 0.5 kg, even under conditions of extreme physiological variance in hydration status.

Tissue Thickness. DXA is subject to beam-hardening errors, which occur as a result of the preferential attenuation of low-energy x rays (Goodsitt, 1992). The magnitude of error varies with the thickness of the tissue, with thicker tissues yielding a lower effective attenuation coefficient and, therefore, a higher apparent fat content.

The effect of tissue thickness has been evaluated under *in vitro* conditions with biological tissues of known composition or materials that simulate biological tissues (Haarbo et al., 1991; Heymsfield et al., 1989; Laskey et al., 1992). Using a spine phantom in combination with varying amounts of water and lard to simulate lean and fat tissues, respectively, Laskey et al. (1992) found that large errors in the assessment of fat and lean masses occurred at tissue depths less than 10 cm and greater than 20 cm. Using a mixture of ox thigh and porcine lard at a depth of 15 cm, Haarbo and colleagues (1991) found that DXA underestimated fat content, which was verified by chemical analysis. Thus, even under controlled *in vitro* conditions, there appear to be inaccuracies in the assessment of tissue composition by DXA.

In contrast, the marked reduction in bone mass that has been shown to accompany weight loss in obese individuals does not appear to be an error associated with changing tissue thickness. In a unique study design, Jensen and colleagues (1994) positioned up to 23 kg of lard, which has an x-ray attenuation coefficient similar to that of fat tissue, on nonobese individuals undergoing DXA scans, with portions of the lard gradually removed for subsequent scans to imitate the loss of fat weight. In these subjects, the apparent reduction in bone mineral content was only 0.5 g/kg lard removed. Conversely, in obese patients who lost approximately 12 kg in 15 weeks, the loss of bone mineral averaged

16.5 g/kg fat loss. The results of this study suggest that changes in tissue thickness have a minimal effect on the assessment of bone mineral and that large reductions in body weight may result in a significant loss of bone mass. The extent to which changes in tissue thickness affected the assessment of soft tissue composition was not reported and is an issue that requires further investigation.

Soft Tissue Composition in Bone Regions. A limitation of DXA is that soft tissue within bone pixels, which constitute approximately 40 percent of the total pixels (Tothill and Nord, 1995), cannot be evaluated. Another source of error in the assessment of body composition is, therefore, the means by which the composition of soft tissue over- and underlying bone is estimated. This is of particular concern for regional assessments of the thoracic and pelvic regions, where the majority of the pixels contain bone mineral.

Some investigators have positioned packets of lard (Figure 6-1, Panel B) over various regions of the body to evaluate the accuracy of soft tissue assessment by DXA (Lohman, 1996; Snead et al., 1993). In these experiments, DXA accurately assessed the increase in fat mass when packets of lard were positioned on the legs. However, only approximately 50 percent of the added mass was identified as fat when the packets were positioned on the chest and abdomen. These studies, which utilized Hologic and Lunar instruments, suggest that the algorithms used to estimate the composition of soft tissue in regions that cannot be measured (i.e., regions that contain bone mineral) may be a source of significant error.

The extent to which these three sources of error (i.e., hydration status, beam-hardening effects, and the estimation of the composition of soft tissue in bone mineral-containing pixels) affect the assessment of body composition cannot be succinctly summarized. It is likely that the strategies used to adjust for or correct known sources of error vary among DXA manufacturers. Moreover, for a given manufacturer, it is likely that the accuracy of assessing body composition changes as new features or options become available on the hardware and as revisions are made in the software used to analyze body composition data. The success of these strategies in improving the assessment of body composition by DXA must be methodically tested by independent investigators.

Comparisons of DXA and Hydrodensitometry

Because hydrodensitometry has long been regarded as the reference method for the assessment of body composition, it has been used to assess the validity of DXA. It must be noted, however, that since both DXA and hydrodensitometry are indirect measures of body composition, there is no definitive way of determining which, if either, is valid. Some of the studies that have estimated

                                          WENDY M. KOHRT

body fat content by DXA and by hydrodensitometry are summarized in Table 6-4. While estimates of body fat by DXA closely approximated those by hydrodensitometry in some study cohorts, wide discrepancies occurred in others. These inconsistencies are apparent both between and within the various DXA instruments; one factor may be the version of the software used to analyze the data, which was not always reported.

Even when there is apparently excellent agreement in the estimation of body composition by DXA and hydrodensitometry, results must be interpreted cautiously. For example, there were only small differences in the mean body fat levels estimated by DXA and hydrodensitometry in the relatively large cohorts studied by Hansen et al. (1993) and Wellens et al. (1994), and the correlations between the methods were strong (correlation coefficients > 0.86). However, the equations for the lines describing the relationships between percent body fat measured by DXA and hydrodensitometry (HW) were markedly different from the equation for the line of identity:

(Hansen et al., 1993)	$DXA = 1.29 \times HW - 9.0$
(Wellens et al., 1994)	$DXA_{men} = 0.63 \times HW + 7.5$
	$DXA_{women} = 0.87 \times HW + 5.8.$

The wide variance in comparisons of DXA with hydrodensitometry, coupled with the findings that DXA does not accurately assess fat (i.e., lard experiments) in some regions of the body (Lohman, 1996; Snead et al., 1993), suggest that DXA is not yet a valid method of assessing body composition. Nevertheless, since DXA is less reliant on assumptions regarding the consistency of fat-free mass than is hydrodensitometry, it holds great potential for becoming the criterion method.

TABLE 6-4 Comparisons of Body Fat Content Measured by Dual-Energy X-Ray Absorptiometry and by Hydrostatic Weighing

Reference	Subjects (*N*) Age (yr)	Scanner (software version)	Manufacturer	Body Fat (%)		
				DXA	HW	Δ
Johansson et al., 1993	23 males 37 ± 10	DPX-L	Lunar	9.5	18.1	−8.6
Withers et al., 1992	12 males 22 ± 5	DPX-L	Lunar	6.8	9.7	−2.9
Van Loan and Mayclin, 1992	26 males 37 ± 10	DPX	Lunar	19.4	23.5	−4.1
	23 females 36 ± 11			30.8	31.7	−0.9

Continued

TABLE 6-4 *Continued*

Reference	Subjects (*N*) Age (yr)	Scanner (software version)	Manufacturer	Body Fat (%)		
				DXA	HW	Δ
Penn et al., 1994	10 males 28 ± 4	DPX	Lunar	20.5	20.8	−0.3
Hansen et al., 1993	100 females 34 ± 3	DPX (3.1)	Lunar	29.7	29.9	−0.2
Wellens et al., 1994	50 males 39 ± 14	DPX (3.4)	Lunar	21.7	22.5	−0.8
	78 females 42 ± 14			34.6	33.2	+1.4
Clark et al., 1993	35 males 39 ± 14	XR-26 (2.0.1)	Norland	21.3	17.4	+3.9
Pritchard et al., 1993	14 males, and females 37 ± 13	DPX (3.4)	Lunar	24.1	19.4	+4.5
		QDR-1000W (5.35)	Hologic	20.7	19.4	+1.3
Tothill et al., 1994b	11 males and females	DPX (3.6)	Lunar	26.8	23.6	+3.2
		XR-26 (2.4)	Norland	29.5	23.6	+5.9
		QDR-1000W (5.51p)	Hologic	23.1	23.6	−0.5
Snead et al., 1993	33 males and females 29 ± 5	QDR-1000W (5.50)	Hologic	12.7	13.9	−1.2
	13 males 49 ± 6			19.0	22.3	−3.3
	26 males 68 ± 4			21.3	26.6	−5.3
	32 females 29 ± 5			22.7	21.3	+1.4
	19 females 48 ± 6			27.6	27.8	−0.2
	62 females 66 ± 3			34.5	38.2	−3.7

NOTE: DXA, dual-energy x-ray absorptiometry; HW, hydrostatic weighing.

ASSESSMENT OF REGIONAL BODY COMPOSITION

A distinct advantage of DXA over hydrodensitometry is that it can be used to assess the composition of specific regions of the body. However, until the validity of soft tissue assessment by DXA is established, this technique is not suitable for use in research. An exception to this is the comparison of regional assessment of body composition by DXA and some other method, such as magnetic resonance imaging (MRI) or computed tomography (CT), as a means of evaluating the validity of DXA.

In one such study, Jensen and colleagues (1995) evaluated whether DXA could be combined with anthropometry to estimate abdominal and visceral fat volumes, which also were measured by CT. Subcutaneous abdominal fat was estimated from circumference and skinfold thickness measurements. Visceral fat was assumed to be the difference between total abdominal fat measured by DXA and subcutaneous abdominal fat. The estimation of visceral fat by DXA was poor, yielding negative values in one-third of the study cohort. Estimates of total abdominal fat by DXA and CT were similar ($8,448 \pm 5,005$ ml vs. $8,066 \pm 5,354$ ml, respectively; $r = 0.98$). However, since CT incorporates the nonfat constituents of adipose tissue, whereas DXA does not, it was expected that total fat would be approximately 15 percent higher by CT. The authors suggested that DXA is not yet appropriate for use in research studies that require an accurate quantification of adipose tissue.

AUTHOR'S CONCLUSIONS AND RECOMMENDATIONS

For the measurement of both bone and soft tissue masses, there are several advantages of DXA: (1) it provides reliable and precise data; (2) the data acquisition process is fast, easy to perform, involves minimal radiation exposure, and is easily tolerated by subjects; (3) the data analysis process is fast, versatile, and easy to perform; and (4) the assessment of body composition by DXA appears to be less reliant on underlying assumptions than most other methods.

A major disadvantage of DXA is that currently there is a lack of standardization in bone and soft tissue measurements. There are large discrepancies in measurements obtained on instruments from the three major manufacturers of DXA machines. Moreover, for a given manufacturer, results may vary by the model of the instrument, the mode of operation (e.g., single-beam vs. fan-beam or normal speed vs. fast speed), or the version of the software used to analyze the data. Nevertheless, it is encouraging that bone measurements obtained on different machines or in different operation modes are consistently found to be highly correlated, suggesting that the standardization of results is possible. Although currently available data suggest that soft tissue measurements are not accurate, it seems likely, at least from a theoretical perspective, that DXA has the potential to become the reference method of assessing body composition.

Whether this will occur depends largely on the manufacturers and whether the demand for this application of DXA is sufficient to justify the costs of research and development.

Most of the expense associated with the use of DXA is in the cost of the instrument itself, which is likely to be in excess of $100,000. Although DXA is best suited for laboratory-based research, as opposed to field testing, transportable models of DXA instruments are available.

The following conclusions can be drawn regarding the advantages and disadvantages of DXA:

- For research that requires the assessment of bone mass, DXA is superior to any other available methodology.
- The highly reliable and precise measurement of total body bone mineral mass by DXA makes it an excellent adjunct for multicompartment modeling of body composition.
- Although DXA is an attractive means by which to obtain an independent, three-compartment model of body composition, there is considerable evidence that the results are not accurate.
- The regional assessment of body composition by DXA is inferior to MRI and CT.

REFERENCES

Blake, G.M., J.C. Parker, F.M.A. Buxton, and I. Fogelman
    1993   Dual x-ray absorptiometry: A comparison between fan beam and pencil beam scans. Br. J. Radiol. 66:902–906.

Clark, R.R., J.M. Kuta, and J.C. Sullivan
    1993   Prediction of percent body fat in adult males using dual energy x-ray absorptiometry, skinfolds, and hydrostatic weighing. Med. Sci. Sports Exerc. 25:528–535.

Eiken, P., O. Bärenholdt, L. Bjorn Jensen, J. Gram, and S. Pors Nielsen
    1994   Switching from DXA pencil-beam to fan-beam. I: Studies *in vitro* at four centers. Bone 15:667–670.

Eiken, P., N. Kolthoff, O. Bärenholdt, F. Hermansen, and S. Pors Nielsen
    1995   Switching from DXA pencil-beam to fan-beam. II: Studies *in vivo*. Bone 15:671–676.

Formica, C., M.G. Atkinson, I. Nyulasi, J. McKay, W. Heale, and E. Seeman
    1993   Body composition following hemodialysis: Studies using dual-energy x-ray absorptiometry and bioelectrical impedance analysis. Osteoporos. Int. 3:192–197.

Genant, H.K., S. Grampp, C.C. Glüer, K.G. Faulkner, M. Jergas, K. Engelke, S. Hagiwara, and C. Van Kuijk
    1994   Universal standardization for dual x-ray absorptiometry: Patient and phantom cross-calibration results. J. Bone Miner. Res. 9:1503–1514.

Going, S.B., M.P. Massett, M.C. Hall, L.A. Bare, P.A. Root, D.P. Williams, and T.G. Lohman
    1993   Detection of small changes in body composition by dual-energy x-ray absorptiometry. Am. J. Clin. Nutr. 57:845–850.

Goodsitt, M.M.
    1992   Evaluation of a new set of calibration standards for the measurement of fat content via DPA and DXA. Med. Phys. 19:35–44.

Haarbo, J., A. Gotfredsen, C. Hassager, and C. Christiansen
  1991   Validation of body composition by dual energy x-ray absorptiometry (DEXA). Clin. Physiol. 11:331–341.
Hansen, N.J., T.G. Lohman, S.B. Going, M.C. Hall, R.W. Pamenter, L.A. Bare, T.W. Boyden, and L.B. Houtkooper
  1993   Prediction of body composition in premenopausal females from dual-energy x-ray absorptiometry. J. Appl. Physiol. 75:1637–1641.
Heymsfield, S.B., J. Wang, S. Heshka, J.J. Kehayias, and R.N. Pierson, Jr.
  1989   Dual-photon absorptiometry: Comparison of bone mineral and soft tissue mass measurements *in vivo* with established methods. Am. J. Clin. Nutr. 49:1282–1289.
Horber, F.F., F. Thomi, J.P. Casez, J. Fonteille, and P. Jaeger
  1992   Impact of hydration status on body composition as measured by dual energy x-ray absorptiometry in normal volunteers and patients on haemodialysis. Br. J. Radiol. 65:895–900.
Jensen, L.B., F. Quaade, and O.H. Sorensen
  1994   Bone loss accompanying voluntary weight loss in obese humans. J. Bone Miner. Res. 9:459–463.
Jensen, M.D., J.A. Kanaley, J.E. Reed, and P.F. Sheedy
  1995   Measurement of abdominal and visceral fat with computed tomography and dual-energy x-ray absorptiometry. Am. J. Clin. Nutr. 61:274–278.
Jergas, M., M. Breitenseher, C.C. Glüer, W. Yu, and H.K. Genant
  1995   Estimates of volumetric bone density from projectional measurements improve the discriminatory capability of dual x-ray absorptiometry. J. Bone Miner. Res. 10:1101–1110.
Johansson, A.G., A. Forslund, A. Sjodin, H. Mallmin, L. Hambraeus, and S. Ljunghall
  1993   Determination of body composition—a comparison of dual-energy x-ray absorptiometry and hydrodensitometry. Am. J. Clin. Nutr. 57:323–326.
Kohrt, W.M.
  1995   Body composition by DXA: Tried and true? Med. Sci. Sports Exerc. 27(10):1349–1353.
Kohrt, W.M., and S.J. Birge, Jr.
  1995   Differential effects of estrogen treatment on bone mineral density of the spine, hip, wrist, and total body in late postmenopausal women. Osteoporos. Int. 5(3):150–155.
Lai, K.C., M.M. Goodsitt, R. Murano, and C.H. Chesnut III
  1992   A comparison of two dual-energy x-ray absorptiometry systems for spinal bone mineral measurement. Calcif. Tissue Int. 50:203–208.
Laskey, M.A., K.D. Lyttle, M.E. Flaxman, and R.W. Barber
  1992   The influence of tissue depth and composition on the performance of the Lunar dual-energy x-ray absorptiometer whole-body scanning mode. Eur. J. Clin. Nutr. 46:39–45.
Lilley, J., B.G. Walters, D.A. Heath, and Z. Drolc
  1991   *In vivo* and *in vitro* precision for bone density measured by dual-energy x-ray absorption. Osteoporos. Int. 1:141–146.
Lohman, T.G.
  1996   Dual energy x-ray absorptiometry. Pp. 63–78 in Human Body Composition, A.F. Roche, S.B. Heymsfield, and T.G. Lohman, eds. Champaign, Ill.: Human Kinetics.
Mazess, R.B., H.S. Barden, J.P. Bisek, and J. Hanson
  1990   Dual-energy x-ray absorptiometry for total-body and regional bone-mineral and soft-tissue composition. Am. J. Clin. Nutr. 51:1106–1112.

Mazess, R., C.H. Chesnut, III, M. McClung, and H. Genant
  1992 Enhanced precision with dual-energy x-ray absorptiometry. Calcif. Tissue Int. 51:14–17.
Nord, R.H.
  1991 Soft tissue composition phantom for DXA. Osteoporos. Int. 1:203.
Nord, R.H., and R.K. Payne
  1990 Standards for body composition calibration in DEXA. Paper presented at the 2nd Annual Meeting of the Bath Conference on Bone Mineral Measurement, Bath, U.K.
Orwoll, E.S., S.K. Oviatt, and J.A. Biddle
  1993 Precision of dual-energy x-ray absorptiometry: Development of quality control rules and their application in longitudinal studies. J. Bone Miner. Res. 8:693–699.
Penn, I-W., Z-M. Wang, K.M. Buhl, D.B. Allison, S.E. Burastero, and S.B. Heymsfield
  1994 Body composition and two-compartment model assumptions in male long distance runners. Med. Sci. Sports Exerc. 26:392–397.
Pocock, N.A., P.N. Sambrook, T. Nguyen, P. Kelly, J. Freund, and J.A. Eisman
  1992 Assessment of spinal and femoral bone density by dual x-ray absorptiometry: Comparison of Lunar and Hologic instruments. J. Bone Miner. Res. 7:1081–1084.
Pritchard, J.E., C.A. Nowson, B.J. Strauss, J.S. Carlson, B. Kaymakci, and J.D. Wark
  1993 Evaluation of dual energy x-ray absorptiometry as a method of measurement of body fat. Eur. J. Clin. Nutr. 47:216–228.
Roubenoff, R., J.J. Kehayias, B. Dawson-Hughes, and S.B. Heymsfield
  1993 Use of dual-energy x-ray absorptiometry in body composition studies: Not yet a "gold standard." Am. J. Clin. Nutr. 58:589–591.
Sievanen, H., P. Oja, and I. Vuori
  1992 Precision of dual-energy x-ray absorptiometry in determining bone mineral density and content of various skeletal sites. J. Nucl. Med. 33:1137–1142.
Slosman, D.O., J-P. Casez, C. Pichard, T. Rochat, F. Fery, R. Rizzoli, J-P. Bonjour, A. Morabia, and A. Donath
  1992 Assessment of whole-body composition with dual-energy x-ray absorptiometry. Radiology 185:593–598.
Snead, D.B., S.J. Birge, and W.M. Kohrt
  1993 Age-related differences in body composition by hydrodensitometry and dual-energy x-ray absorptiometry. J. Appl. Physiol. 74:770–775.
Svendsen, O.L., J. Haarbo, C. Hassager, and C. Christiansen
  1993 Accuracy of measurements of body composition by dual-energy x-ray absorptiometry *in vivo*. Am. J. Clin. Nutr. 57:605–608.
Tothill, P., and R.H. Nord
  1995 Limitations of dual-energy x-ray absorptiometry [letter]. Am. J. Clin. Nutr. 61:398–399.
Tothill, P., A. Avenell, and D.M. Reid
  1994a Precision and accuracy of measurements of whole-body bone mineral: Comparisons between Hologic, Lunar and Norland dual-energy x-ray absorptiometers. Br. J. Radiol. 67:1210–1217.
Tothill, P., A. Avenell, J. Love, and D.M. Reid
  1994b Comparisons between Hologic, Lunar and Norland dual-energy x-ray absorptiometers and other techniques used for whole-body soft tissue measurements. Eur. J. Clin. Nutr. 48:781–794.
Van Loan, M.D., and P.L. Mayclin
  1992 Body composition assessment: Dual-energy x-ray absorptiometry (DEXA) compared to reference methods. Eur. J. Clin. Nutr. 46:125–130.

Wellens, R., W.C. Chumlea, S. Guo, A.F. Roche, N.V. Reo, and R.M. Siervogel
  1994   Body composition in white adults by dual-energy x-ray absorptiometry, densitometry, and total body water. Am. J. Clin. Nutr. 59:547–555.
Withers, R.T., D.A. Smith, B.E. Chatterton, C.G. Schultz, and R.D. Gaffney
  1992   Comparison of four methods of estimating the body composition of male endurance athletes. Eur. J. Clin. Nutr. 46:773–784.

DISCUSSION

WM. CAMERON CHUMLEA: Wendy, you made a statement that DXA was less reliant on some of the underlying assumptions of body composition, but is it then more reliant on software assumptions, so that there is a wash, in a sense? I mean, Hologic went back in and massaged the software until they got the right answers for you, but does that just simply mean that the software package was sample specific?

WENDY KOHRT: Well, I will tell you, they did not do it just for me.

I am dealing with the software engineer at Hologic, who, in the very early stages of this work, went on the basic assumption that water was a minimal component of fat-free mass. We have had to go through all these transitions. I think they are really learning more about the biology of body composition. So, yes, validity is reliant on the technical aspects, but that is kind of a good feature, because those are things that are amenable to change. We can modify the hardware and the software to get it to where it is a valid measure of body composition.

DENNIS BIER: That is, if the biological basis of the software change is going to be open to the public. [You must] understand that this is a proprietary thing, and what you really have is a black box, and unless you can understand the biological basis for the calculations, you are left in the cold.

WENDY KOHRT: And that is a big problem. My experiences with Hologic have not all been favorable. When I was dealing with the software engineer, who had a vested interest in what he was doing and really wanted to know if it was right, my interactions were very useful, but in dealing with the people who wanted to sell machines, it was a different story.

DENNIS BIER: I can give you just a very practical example from mass spectrometry. We had an instrument from a company that met all of their specs until we took apart the software and found out that they calculated the numbers wrong so that they met their specs. We pointed that out to them, but if an investigator did not have the ability to do that, then he would not have discovered that discrepancy, so the machine functioned fine.

WENDY KOHRT: I think there are people working in this area who are trying to make the manufacturers much more accountable. Whether that will be successful, I do not know.

G. RICHARD JANSEN: If you took the initial cost and amortized it over a reasonable life of the machine and added in maintenance contracts, labor costs, and all the rest of it, and if you assume a certain level of use, have you calculated per analysis what it would cost?

WENDY KOHRT: I have not, but I will give you some idea. The new machines are in the neighborhood of $120,000. I think a full service contract on that is $9,000 a year. The cost to maintain it on a day-to-day basis is the normal cost of electricity, computer supplies, disks, and then the labor.

JAMES DeLANY: Have you had power problems with yours?

WENDY KOHRT: No.

JAMES DeLANY: Do you have a power conditioner on yours?

WENDY KOHRT: The DXA instrument is housed in a different hospital from where I am, so I am not sure about that.

DAVID SCHNAKENBERG: Just another thought for the Army people. Hologic has actually done a spec on a transportable machine, one that could be put in a large truck and taken around just as x rays were done for tuberculosis screening.

KARL FRIEDL: Yes, it has been taken to the field.

Emerging Technologies for Nutrition Research, 1997
Pp. 169–192. Washington, D.C.
National Academy Press

7

Bioelectrical Impedance:
A History, Research Issues, and
Recent Consensus

Wm. Cameron Chumlea and Shumei S. Guo[1]

A window on the biology of the human body has opened as a result of numerous studies utilizing bioelectrical impedance. The view from this window is affected by the previous and current works of human biologists and biomedical engineers and by the future potential of bioelectrical impedance. This article briefly describes the research history of bioelectrical impedance, the status of present research related to body composition and future research directions. The final section is an abbreviated summary of the 1994 National Institutes of Health (NIH) Technology Assessment Conference on Bioelectrical Impedance Analysis in Body Composition Measurement.

---

[1] Wm. Cameron Chumlea, Division of Human Biology, Department of Community Health, Wright State University School of Medicine, Yellow Springs, OH 45387
This work was supported by Ross Laboratories, Columbus, OH and by grants HD-12252 and HD-27063 from the National Institutes of Health, Bethesda, MD.

HISTORY

Impedance is the frequency-dependent opposition of a conductor to the flow of an alternating electric current. A measure of impedance (Z) is composed of the sum of two vectors, resistance (R) and reactance (Xc), measured at a particular frequency and is described mathematically by the equation $Z^2 = R^2 + Xc^2$. Resistance is the opposition of a conductor to the alternating current, and as the electric current travels through the body, resistance is basically the same as in nonbiological conductors (Kay et al., 1954; Nyboer, 1959). Reactance is produced by the additional opposition to the current from the capacitant (storage) effects of cell membranes, tissue interfaces, and structural features (Baker, 1989; Barnett and Bagno, 1936; Schwan and Kay, 1956). The occurrence of these capacitant effects produced by the bilipid cell membrane reaches a peak and then declines as the current changes from low to high frequency. The phase angle (see Figure 7-1), which has been found to be important for describing relationships between bioelectrical impedance and the body and for measuring physiological variables (Baumgartner et al., 1988; Lukaski and Bolonchuk, 1987; Subramanyan et al., 1980), is expressed in degrees as the arctangent of the ratio of Xc/R and changes with changes in the frequency of the current.

Early studies of bioelectrical impedance focused on the meaning of impedance measures in relation to the water and electrolyte content of the body and to physiological variables such as thyroid function, basal metabolic rate, estrogenic activity, and blood flow in human and animal tissues (Barnett, 1937; Lukaski, 1987; Spence et al., 1979). These explorations developed into some of the

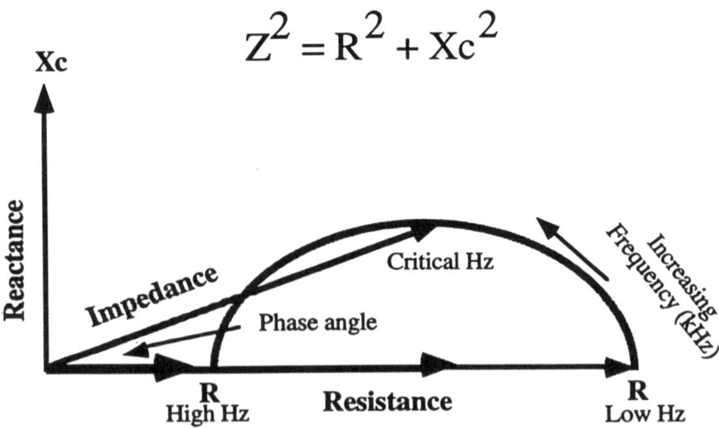

FIGURE 7-1 Impedance plot curve of resistance and reactance with frequency. Z, impedance; R, resistance; Xc, reactance; Hz, hertz; kHz, kilohertz. SOURCE: Chumlea and Baumgartner (1990), used with permission.

present-day areas of impedance cardiography, pulmonary impedance, brain impedance, and impedance imaging. The use of bioelectrical impedance to estimate body composition developed from more recent exploratory works in the areas of single-frequency and multiple-frequency impedance.

Nyboer (1959) and Hoffer et al. (1969) first used single-frequency measures of impedance at 50 kHz to estimate total body water (TBW) based upon a volumetric relationship of impedance and a conductor using the "impedance index." This volumetric relationship between resistance and a conductor is described by the formula $V = \rho L^2/R$ from which the "impedance index," body stature (S) squared divided by resistance (R) (or S^2/R), is derived (Table 7-1). This volumetric relationship is theoretically dependent upon conductors of uniform shape or of suspensions of cell solutions and upon a uniform current distribution throughout the conductor. However, the geometrical relationship in this formula between the value of resistance and the volume of the body is not adequately explained in its application to human body composition because uniformity is not a characteristic of the human body or of human populations.

The specific resistivity, or ρ, in this volumetric formula (Table 7-1) is an electrical property particular to the conducting medium and independent of its size or shape. For a homogeneous conductor, it is a constant physical property similar to specific gravity. Specific resistivity for the whole body is assumed to be a constant, but each tissue has a characteristic specific resistivity, and the observed specific resistivity for a body segment or the whole body is supposed to be the mean specific resistivity of all conductive tissues (Kay et al., 1954; Schwan and Kay, 1956).

Thomasset (1962) and coworkers (Bolot et al., 1977; Ducrot et al., 1970; Jenin et al., 1975) first used measures of impedance at more than a single frequency to describe the proportion of extracellular water in TBW. These investigators used a ratio of impedance at low and high frequencies to differentiate this extracellular total-body relationship. Multifrequency bioelectrical impedance analyzers measure resistance and reactance at a set of selected frequencies. Ana-

TABLE 7-1 Basic Principles of Bioelectrical Impedance

$$V = L \times A$$

$$A = V/L$$

$$R = \rho(L/A)$$

$$R = \rho L(L/V)$$

$$V = \rho L^2/R$$

NOTE: V, volume; L, length; A, area; R, resistance; ρ, specific resistivity.

SOURCE: Chumlea and Baumgartner (1990), used with permission.

lytical aspects of impedance plots of resistance and reactance (Figure 7-1) relate to physiological characteristics of the body (Boulier et al., 1990; Kanai et al., 1987; Rush et al., 1963). However, these graphic impedance analyses are limited in their ability to estimate body composition if the impedance information cannot be reduced to a few parameters for statistical analysis. With multifrequency bioelectrical impedance, large amounts of data are collected for each individual, and this creates a problem of how to analyze and interpret these data so as to estimate body composition.

These groups of investigators explored the basics of bioelectrical physiology that provide the foundation for much of the present research efforts in body composition with single- and multiple-frequency impedance. However, application of these groups' work was not fully recognized until the development of inexpensive, commercial, bioelectrical impedance body composition analyzers that did not require the expertise of a biomedical engineer. With the advent of the first single-frequency body composition impedance analyzer, and now the newer multifrequency analyzers, there has been a plethora of studies and subsequent reports on the use of impedance to estimate aspects of body composition (Chumlea and Baumgartner, 1990; Chumlea and Guo, 1994). However, these studies of bioelectrical impedance estimates of body composition have, to some extent, drifted from the mainstream of bioengineering impedance research, especially regarding the validity of the machine measurements from the body. The present confusion in using and interpreting single- and multiple-frequency impedance estimates of body composition, in light of its research potential, led NIH to conduct a technology assessment conference in December 1994 (NIH, 1996) to determine current conditions and develop future research goals and directions for bioelectrical impedance.

IMPEDANCE AND BODY WATER

The conduction of an alternating electric current in the body is through its water content or, more correctly, the solution of electrolytes in the body (Hoffer et al., 1969; Kushner and Schoeller, 1986). An alternating current is used for bioelectrical impedance analysis because it penetrates the body at low levels of voltage and amperage. In a complex electrical structure such as the human body, the part of the fluid volume or TBW measured by bioelectrical impedance is also a function of the current frequency. At low frequencies of less than about 5 kHz, the bioelectrical current travels primarily through extracellular fluids, but as the frequency increases, the current starts to penetrate body tissues, creating reactance, and the measure of this current flow starts to represent more of a measure of TBW. At high frequencies (above 100 kHz), the current is assumed to penetrate all conductive body tissues or all of the total body water in the conductor and supposedly overcomes the capacitant properties of the body, reducing reactance to zero. Electrical circuit diagrams (Figure 7-2) have been used

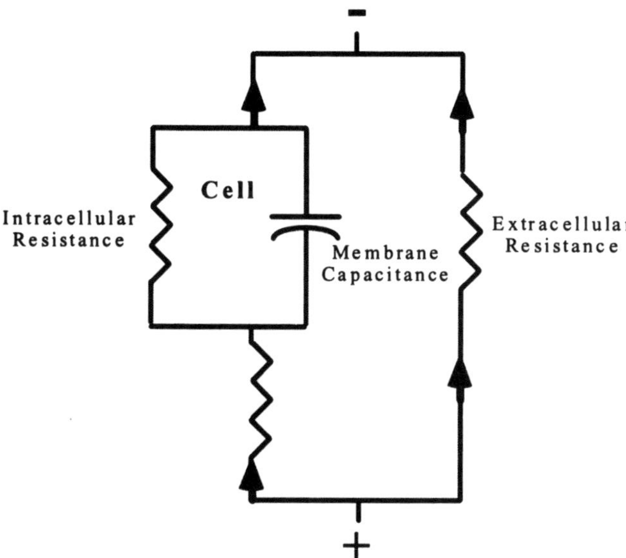

FIGURE 7-2 Intracellular and extracellular electrical circuit diagram.

to describe or model the electrical characteristics of the impedance-body intra-cellular-extracellular water relationships (Nyboer, 1959; Schwan and Kay, 1956).

The ability to quantify TBW and to differentiate it into intra- and extracellular body fluid compartments is important in order to describe fluid shifts and balance and to explore variations in levels of hydration and clinical and nutritional status (Chumlea and Guo, 1994). At present, most bioelectrical impedance analyzers operate at a single frequency of 50 kHz, where the resistance value is primarily for TBW. The quantification of TBW from single-frequency impedance measures has been reasonably accurate. However, the estimation of TBW that results from single-frequency analyzers is limited in its ability to distinguish among individuals the distribution of body water into its intra- and extracellular compartments. This limitation is due in part to the inability of body water estimates from 50 kHz-impedance analyzers to discriminate the relative proportions of extra- and intracellular fluids in the body. Some studies have used reactance at 50 kHz as an additional independent variable to help make this differentiation among individuals, but ratios of bioelectrical impedance measures at low and high frequencies have been more successful in differentiating the proportion of extracellular fluid volume (ECFV) in TBW than have single-frequency impedance and reactance measures (Bolot et al., 1977; Ducrot et al., 1970; Jenin et al., 1975; Thomasset, 1962). The accurate indirect estimation of TBW and ECFV could greatly expand the knowledge of these fluid spaces in normal and clinical conditions. Little further work in this area has occurred despite reports that the relative proportions of TBW and ECFV determined from multifrequency impedance are reasonably constant with deviations occurring in disease states (Bolot et al., 1977; Jenin et al., 1975). The availability of relatively inexpensive multifrequency body composition impedance analyzers should again spark interest in this significant aspect of body hydration.

IMPEDANCE AND BODY COMPOSITION

To estimate body composition from measures of bioelectrical impedance requires the generation of a mathematical equation that is validated against some criterion method for body composition determination. This is the only way to convert impedance values into estimates of body composition. The use of single-frequency bioelectrical impedance measures in a prediction equation assumes a two-compartment model of body composition, where the total conductive volume of the body is equivalent to TBW and where the hydration of adipose tissue is minimal. Fat-free mass (FFM) is then estimated from single-frequency impedance estimates of TBW based upon the percentage of TBW in FFM. This percentage has a reported mean value of 73 percent, which varies with age, gender, and possibly race and is altered by disease and some physiological conditions (Lohman, 1986; Moore, 1963). Single-frequency impedance estimates of body composition from a two-component model are not accurate for all ages and genders; however, a multicomponent model of body composition using impedance and including measures of bone density has not been developed.

Numerous studies have developed equations that predict body composition from bioelectrical impedance data, but such an impedance estimate will only be as accurate as the criterion method used to determine the dependent variable in the equation. In single-frequency impedance prediction equations, the dependent variable is most frequently derived from densitometry, TBW (as measured by deuterium oxide dilution), and dual-photon absorptiometry (or more recently dual-energy x-ray absorptiometry [DXA or DEXA]). These criterion methods, however, add further assumptions of questionable validity regarding clearance of chemicals and their distribution within the body and levels of hydration and density of the fat-free body. There are assumptions and limitations for almost all body composition methods, old and new, but among the best methods, mean differences of about 2.0 to 3.0 kg are reported for estimates of FFM. This is also true of bioelectrical impedance predictions in comparison with other body composition methods.

The performance of a single-frequency impedance equation with respect to its ability to predict body composition is evaluated by goodness-of-fit measures and measures of accuracy (Guo and Chumlea, 1996). Aspects of goodness of fit generally include the coefficient of determination (R^2), the root mean square error (RMSE), and the coefficient of variation (CV). The accuracy of an equation, when applied to independent samples, is determined by the pure error. Independent cross-validation of impedance prediction equations produces pure errors that are frequently more than twice the RMSE values of the original published equations. In predicting an individual's body composition for a clinical or nutritional assessment, there is a greater statistical uncertainty than there is for a group. The standard error for an individual is several times larger than the standard error of the estimate (for a group) that is provided with statistical program packages. Predictions for an individual have a reduced accuracy and large error bounds, which are exacerbated when an individual differs from the sample used to develop a prediction equation.

The performance of the prediction equation depends also on the selection and the number of independent variables (Guo and Chumlea, 1996). The independent variables used most often are the impedance index (S^2/R) from the volumetric equation and weight, followed by stature, arm and thigh circumferences, gender, and age. Arm circumference is an index of the cross-sectional area of muscle tissues and is highly correlated with FFM. Thigh circumference also has been reported as a predictor of FFM, and its inclusion in some equations relates to the amount of muscle tissue in the legs. These circumferences also are related to the geometrical aspects of current and conductor because resistance is inversely proportional to the circumference of the conductor. However, too many independent variables in an equation result in instability and too few result in large RMSE values, causing the equation to perform poorly when applied to independent samples. Independent variables included in an equation can also be interrelated, which causes the regression estimates to be unstable. As a result, a prediction equation may have independent variables that are not statistically significant, and its performance when applied to other samples will be unsatisfactory.

Estimates of body composition derived from single-frequency bioelectrical impedance that have been reported for samples of normal persons have been poor, and single-frequency impedance does not significantly improve estimates of body composition over anthropometry, especially in obese and thin individuals. In the obese and individuals with greater-than-normal amounts of adipose tissue, errors of measurement using whole-body single-frequency impedance and prediction overestimate FFM (Unpublished data, W. C. Chumlea, Wright State University School of Medicine, Dayton, Ohio, 1995). A possible reason for this reduced performance is that specific resistivities vary among body tissues and segments and among individuals because of intra- and interindividual differences in tissue composition and electrolyte concentrations. This variance contributes further to subsequent differences noted among individuals in single-frequency impedance estimates of body composition. Individual and group results also may be influenced by sampling effects, the validation method, and the limitations of $V = \rho L^2/R$ at a single frequency of 50 kHz.

QUANTIFICATION OF CHANGES IN BODY COMPOSITION

It is important to be able to estimate body composition at any age, but it is equally important that estimates of body composition for the same person at two different ages accurately reflect the change over time. From their analysis of the data from seven studies reporting body composition changes, Forbes and co-workers (1992) have justifiably questioned the basic assumptions of the impedance index (S^2/R) in determining the validity of repeated, single-frequency bioelectrical impedance estimates of body composition from the same individuals over time. Part of the problem is the limited sensitivity of the impedance index.

The value of resistance is proportional to the number of ions in a conductor, and a change in the composition that affects the number of ions should be reflected in the value of resistance. However, when the resistance value is used in the geometrical relationship of the index (S^2/R) and related to FFM, then changes in body weight or FFM must be sufficient to produce concurrent changes in the volume of conductor before significant changes are detectable in the impedance index. This raises the question as to the quantitative value of a change in body composition in relation to resistance. The relationship between changes in body weight and the proportion of FFM may be different depending upon whether the change is positive or negative. However, a measure of bioelectrical resistance can only account for the fat-free portion (that is, the water) in the change. Therefore, if a change in weight is predominantly fat, or is prolonged over time, it will not be detected by resistance easily until a sufficient change in the FFM (that is, TBW) has occurred. However, a measure of body weight can easily detect a change of 3.0 kg, irrespective of its composition.

The effect of the interrelationship of corresponding changes in volume and composition of the body upon the sensitivity of bioelectrical impedance at a single frequency is unknown. If there is a change in the ionic composition without a concurrent change in the volume of a biological conductor, then the ionic change will not be detected accurately without knowing the change in the value of the specific resistivity. It has not been determined if a measure of resistance in the human body is more sensitive to volume than to composition or of equal sensitivity to both. Accurate measures of changes in body composition are needed. Considering the complex structure and composition of the human body and the fact that the theory and axioms of impedance are based upon constancy of the conductor and a uniform current distribution, it may be asking too much of impedance at a single frequency or any frequency to assess changes in body composition.

SEGMENTAL BIOELECTRICAL IMPEDANCE

Patterson and coworkers (Patterson, 1989; Patterson et al., 1988) have reported that measures of changes in segmental impedance at a single frequency

are more sensitive to changes in body composition than are whole-body impedance measures. This use of a segmental approach to bioelectrical impedance
makes use of the work put forth by Settle et al. (1980) who noted that 85 percent
of total body impedance was accounted for by the sum of impedance for the arm
and the leg. The total conductive volume of the body is derived from impedance
indices, measures of the lengths of these body segments, and their single-frequency impedance values. This approach has been used to estimate total and
segmental body composition with good results. There is also increased clinical
use of segmental impedance in the assessment of diseases that affect body fluid
balance (Fuller and Elia, 1989; Scheltinga et al., 1991; Tedner et al., 1985;
Ward et al., 1992).

Whole-body impedance, measured from the wrist to the ankle, is less than
the sum of impedance values for corresponding body segments by an amount
approximately equal to the impedance of the trunk (Baumgartner et al., 1989).
This suggests that at 50 kHz, the trunk contributes little to whole-body impedance. Considering the amount of fat on and within the trunk in adults and the
relationship of trunkal adipose tissue to cardiovascular disease (CVD) risk factors, further study is needed to clarify this point with multiple-frequency impedance. This is especially important if impedance is to provide improved estimates
of or to be used to screen for levels of fatness among those persons at greatest
risk of obesity and CVD.

MULTIFREQUENCY BIOELECTRICAL IMPEDANCE

Impedance values measured at a spectrum of frequencies or at several discrete frequencies or some combination of frequencies may help to explain interindividual variations in body composition more precisely than an impedance
measurement at a single frequency can. Innovative uses of all data in an impedance spectrum should be considered through multivariate and curve-fitting statistical applications to estimate body composition. When impedance data are
collected at multiple frequencies, however, the amount of interpretable information per subject can be large, especially if numerous frequencies are measured.
What is the degree of redundancy and multicollinearity among these measurements? Also, at what frequencies should impedance be measured in order to
produce the best models of body composition? The most appropriate combination of frequencies and multivariate methods of using multifrequency impedance values in estimating body composition and changes in body composition
are just now being explored. Hopefully these studies are of sufficient size so that
adequate power is available for inferential interpretation of the results.

Pairs of multiple-frequency impedance values and ratios of low- to high-
frequency impedance have been used to explore variations in levels of hydration
(Jenin et al., 1975) and to differentiate disease conditions (Thomasset, 1962),
and more recently multiple-frequency impedance has been used to estimate

  WM. CAMERON CHUMLEA AND SHUMEI S. GUO

body composition (see Table 7-2). A comparison of these latter body composition studies is presented in Table 7-2. In the study by Segal and coworkers (1991), impedance was measured at 5, 50, and 100 kHz, and each determination used independently with anthropometry to estimate TBW and ECFV in prediction equations. In the study by Van Loan and Mayclin (1992), a spectrum of multifrequency impedance values at 25 frequencies was measured. However, Van Loan and Mayclin (1992) did not attempt to model the spectrum of frequencies but simply used regression analysis to select a single impedance value at 224 kHz to use in a prediction equation; Deurenberg and Schouten (1992) did the same. Only very recently have measures of impedance at four separate frequencies been used to predict body composition (Deurenberg et al., 1995; van Marken Lichtenbelt et al., 1994) (Table 7-2). However, these four measures were used separately as independent variables in prediction equations. In addition, none of the samples listed in Table 7-2 included minority subjects. There also have been reports of the use of multifrequency impedance in France

TABLE 7-2 Comparison of Frequencies Used with Frequencies Measured, in Published Studies of Multifrequency Bioelectrical Impedance

Reference	Frequencies Measured (kHz)	*N*	Frequencies Used in Models
Segal et al., 1991	5, 50, 100	36	Only a single frequency used with stature and weight
Van Loan and Mayclin, 1992	1, 2, 3, 4, 5, 6, 8, 10, 15, 20, 27, 37, 50, 64, 90, 100, 122, 167, 224, 300, 400, 548, 740, 1000, 1348	60	Only a single frequency used with stature, weight, and gender
Deurenberg and Schouten, 1992	1, 5, 10, 15, 20, 25, 50, 75, 100, 250, 750, 1000, 1250, 1350	12	Only a single frequency used with stature
Hannan et al., 1994	5, 50, 100, 500, 1000	43	One or two frequencies used with stature and weight
Sergi et al., 1994	1, 50	40	Only a single frequency used with stature, weight, gender, and health status
van Marken Lichtenbelt et al., 1994	1, 50, 100, 400	29	Four frequencies used with stature, gender, age, and body mass index
Visser et al., 1995	1, 5, 50, 100, 250, 500, 1000, 1350	117	Only a single frequency used with stature, weight, gender, and age
Deurenberg et al., 1995	0, 1, 5, 50, 100, 250, 500	48	Four frequencies used with stature and weight

(Boulier et al., 1990), but these investigators used a two-electrode (needle electrode) method rather than the tetrapolar electrode method used in the United States. Thus, published studies reporting the use or "model" of multifrequency impedance have been limited in terms of sample size, minority representation, and analytical methods.

From these published studies using multifrequency impedance (Table 7-2), there is little new in the analyses used from what has been reported with single-frequency 50-kHz impedance. Most models have simply used a single impedance value measured at some frequency with anthropometry in a prediction equation, and the performance of these equations is similar to that of 50-kHz impedance prediction equations. There has been little or no analytical consideration or modeling of the representative nature of the spectrum of multifrequency impedance and its relation to body composition. All of the published uses of multifrequency bioelectrical impedance have related whole-body impedance measures to total-body composition. None of the published multifrequency models are applicable to ethnic or minority groups.

Multifrequency Bioelectrical Impedance Spectral Analysis

The multifrequency bioelectrical impedance spectrum can be modeled through multivariate and curve-fitting statistical applications to develop summary parameters to estimate body composition. These models and their statistical applications appear to expand the use of the multifrequency bioelectrical impedance spectrum to quantify body fatness among individuals in clinical, epidemiological, and nutritional settings.

In a feasibility study conducted in this laboratory, the validity of multiple-frequency impedance spectra measured across 16 frequencies to estimate body composition measured by DXA was tested using a small sample of young adult, normal-weight, Caucasian men and women (Chumlea et al., 1996). The spectra of total body and segmental multifrequency impedance values plotted against frequency for each individual follow a similar set of curves as demonstrated in Figure 7-3. The general shape of these curves is described by the same mathematical function containing three components that allow for asymptotes as the frequency approaches zero and as the frequency increases. The function that best describes the shapes of the impedance spectrum for the ith individual is shown in Figure 7-3 where $f_{ik}(x_j)$ is the impedance value (total body, arm, leg, or trunk) for the ith individual measured at the jth frequency for the kth measure, where x_j is the jth frequency; a_{ik}, b_{ik}, and c_{ik} are the parameters for the kth impedance measure (total body, arm, leg, or trunk) of the ith individual; and ε_{ijk} is an error term assumed to be normally distributed with a mean of zero and variance of σ^2. The parameter a_i is the asymptote, b_i is the slope of the curve, and c_i is the acceleration or change in b_i with frequency for the ith individual. For an individ-

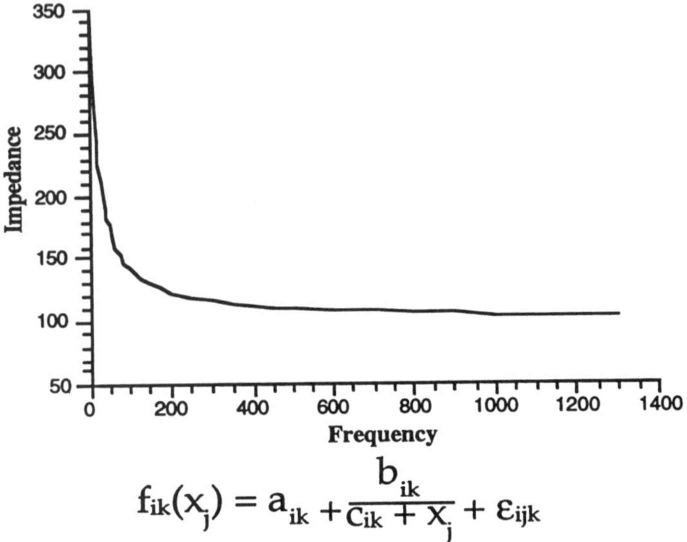

$$f_{ik}(x_j) = a_{ik} + \frac{b_{ik}}{c_{ik} + x_j} + \varepsilon_{ijk}$$

FIGURE 7-3 Spectrum curve and formula of impedance (expressed in ohms) against frequency (expressed in Hertz); $f_{ik}(x_j)$, impedance value; a_{ik}, asymptote; b_{ik}, slope; c_{ik}, acceleration; ε_{ik}, error. SOURCE: Adapted from Chumlea and Guo (1994).

ual, the parameters, a_i, b_i, and c_i, contain information derived from the individual measurements of impedance, summarized across the spectrum of current frequencies.

Models of these impedance spectrum parameters demonstrated gender and anatomical differences in their relation to the variance in body composition values. In regression models of the total body parameters a_i, b_i, and c_i on total body FFM, the R^2 values were higher in the men than in the women. In the regression models of segmental parameters on total-body FFM, the R^2 values were higher in the arms and legs of the men than in the women where the significant gender difference in muscle mass exists. Regression models of the total-body and segmental impedance spectrum parameters on total body fat (TBF) or percentage body fat (%BF) also demonstrate gender differences in body fatness and possible association with fat patterning in the variance associations. The total-body impedance spectrum parameters for TBF and %BF had higher R^2 values in the women than in the men. This pattern continued in the segmental analyses that corresponds to greater amounts of subcutaneous adipose tissue on the limbs in women than in men. However, the impedance spectrum parameters for the male trunk had higher R^2 values for TBF and %BF than occurred for the limbs, conforming to the pattern of greater adiposity on the trunk than the limbs in men.

The patterns of these R^2 values appear to demonstrate possible differences in fat patterning between men and women, in that a greater variance for amounts of adipose tissue on the trunk than the limbs occurs in the women than the men. Ratios of low- to high-frequency impedance measures of the trunk also were correlated significantly and negatively with levels of TBF and total body %BF ($r = -0.7$ to -0.9). These correlations with body fatness remained significant even after removing the effects of waist circumference or the waist/hip circumference ratio. Different placements of electrodes on the trunk might discriminate the location of trunkal adipose tissue more clearly between men and women, but it is doubtful that multifrequency impedance can discriminate levels of internal adipose tissue.

IMPEDANCE AND BLOOD CHEMISTRY

There are few if any significant associations reported among physiological variables and bioelectrical impedance, and possible associations of bioelectrical impedance to blood chemistry and electrolytes generally have not been considered in detail (Azcue et al., 1993; Cha et al., 1994a, b; Shirreffs and Maughan, 1994; Shirreffs et al., 1994). Factors that affect body fluid or electrical activity potentially affect measures of impedance. Total-body and segmental measures of multifrequency impedance were significantly correlated with blood chemistry variables, which included hemoglobin, hematocrit, serum sodium and potassium, serum creatinine, and serum osmolality (Chumlea et al., 1996). The values of the significant correlation coefficients ($p < 0.05$) ranged from 0.4 to 0.7. These correlations represent an association of multifrequency impedance with the physiological status of the body. Several of the blood variables represent electrolytes or ion levels in the body. Impedance measures the electrical conductivity of the body, so correlations with these types of variables is expected. The effect of interrelationships among blood chemistry values on the variance in impedance measures and subsequent estimates of body composition needs further study. Understanding the relationship of impedance and blood chemistry values might help improve estimates of body composition. Increased knowledge is needed about the relationship of multifrequency impedance measures to physiological factors, especially related to electrolytes or possibly viscosity in large normal and clinical samples.

ETHNICITY

Body composition studies of non-Caucasian ethnic groups have never equaled the application to samples from Caucasians. Studies of bioelectrical impedance in non-Caucasian samples are needed and should be cross-validated to help ensure their generalizability to other samples. There have been a limited number of reports on the use of single-frequency impedance with Native-American and African-American samples (Rising et al., 1991; Sparling et al., 1993; Stolarczyk et al., 1994; Zillikens and Conway, 1991). It is unknown whether there are published studies of bioelectrical impedance with Hispanic- or Asian-American groups. Because of the specificity of these ethnic samples, the results have been anecdotal or of limited application to other corresponding samples in the United States. Studies of impedance and body composition in non-Caucasian and mixed ethnic samples are seriously warranted.

NIH TECHNOLOGY ASSESSMENT CONFERENCE: BIOELECTRICAL IMPEDANCE ANALYSIS IN BODY COMPOSITION MEASUREMENT

Recently, Dr. Van Hubbard, Nutrition Sciences Branch, National Institute of Diabetes and Digestive and Kidney Diseases, and Dr. Elsa Bray, Office of Medical Applications of Research, NIH, conducted a technology assessment conference of bioelectrical impedance chaired by Dr. John Rombeau. This conference consisted of a panel of impartial scientists who listened to a series of expert presentations covering the area of bioelectrical impedance. The following is an abbreviated summary of the panel's comments from the final report (NIH, 1996). This 1994 conference assessed the present state of knowledge and technological development in the area of bioelectrical impedance so that some of what follows is redundant with what has already been presented. The conference addressed the five questions listed in Table 7-3.

What does bioelectrical impedance measure in terms of electrical and biological parameters?

Precise bioelectrical impedance measures of electrical and biological parameters are unknown and vary from person to person. The actual parameter measured with bioelectrical impedance is voltage produced between two meas-

TABLE 7-3 NIH Technology Assessment Conference Questions

1. What does bioelectrical impedance measure in terms of electrical and biological parameters, and how safe is it?

2. How should bioelectrical impedance be performed, and how can BIA measurements be standardized?

3. How valid is the bioelectrical impedance technology in the estimation of total body water, fat-free mass, and adiposity?

4. What are the appropriate clinical uses of bioelectrical impedance technology, and what are the limitations?

5. What are the future directions for basic science, clinical research, and epidemiological evaluation of body composition measurements?

uring electrodes. The current magnitude is small and not perceived by the subject, but it is large enough that the current produces voltages that are above the interfering electrical "noise" of the body. However, other detectable electrical "noise" may arise from myoelectric sources, such as muscles, or possibly from outside electromagnetic interference from such sources as heaters and radio transmissions.

The voltage or impedance measurement does not provide any direct information as to how much current travels through intracellular versus extracellular volumes, in blood versus muscle, or in fat versus fat-free tissues. Current paths in the body used by impedance will generally differ from person to person because of differences in body size, shape, electrolytes, fluid distribution, or other aspects of the body's composition. These characteristics vary within an individual, and almost any change in body size, shape, or composition will have at least a small effect on impedance. Relationships between impedance and other variables such as TBW, FFM, or body fat have been established as statistical associations with impedance for a particular population rather than on a biophysical basis. These relationships are not absolute because the current diffuses throughout the conducting volume and makes use of any and all conductive paths that are available at the time of measurement.

The assumptions underlying bioelectrical impedance, those of uniform cross-sectional and homogeneous conductivity, are not fulfilled in humans. No values for specific resistivity are identified or used in work with human subjects. Instead, an analogous statistical parameter (Ht^2/R), where height (Ht) replaces length, is used as an independent variable in a statistical regression procedure, and its degree of association with the output of interest, such as TBW, is evaluated. As used with humans, the bioelectrical impedance measurement does not directly measure any biological quantity of interest, such as fat, on the basis of a physical or biophysical model. Resistance is used as one element of a statistical evaluation, where it may or may not be found to be significant as related to a particular output variable in a particular population.

The bioelectrical impedance equations describe statistical relationships found for a particular population and are not derived from biophysical reasoning, and the measurement is affected by numerous variables. Such populations are chosen to be similar in many attributes so that the bioelectrical impedance result can then be correlated with the remaining attributes that are allowed to vary. Consequently, each equation is useful only for subjects that are a close match to the reference population used in the original derivation of the equation.

How safe is it?

Bioelectrical impedance is considered safe because: the current frequency of 50 kHz is unlikely to stimulate electrically excitable tissues, there is an absence of reports of untoward events induced by bioelectrical impedance after thousands of trials, the relatively small current magnitudes are below the threshold of perception, and batteries or low-voltage power sources are used. However, there are no formal safety standards for bioelectrical impedance instruments. In fact, the introduced current is larger in magnitude than leakage currents allowed for some medical devices, such as electrocardiograph machines. A systematic assessment of all safety-related issues is needed.

How should bioelectrical impedance be performed, and how can bioelectrical impedance measurements be standardized?

Standardization of procedures is essential. Proper electrode placement is crucial for accurate and reproducible bioelectrical impedance measurements. More information is needed to determine whether additional electrode placement sites offer improvement over present examination techniques.

Other variables that affect the validity, reproducibility, and precision of the measurements include body position, hydration status, consumption of food or beverages, ambient air and skin temperature, recent physical activity, and conductance of the examination table. Additionally, the accuracy of the determination of other measures that are used in the equations to predict TBW or fatness with bioelectrical impedance affects the accuracy of the estimate.

Measurements are made with the subject reclining, but evidence indicates that impedance values change sharply within the first 10 minutes after the subject assumes a supine position and continue to do so for several hours. Standardization of procedures should include the length of time the subject is recumbent before the measurement is performed. Measurements obtained several hours postprandially may also influence impedance values, depending on the volume change. This can be controlled by obtaining bioelectrical impedance measurements after a fast of at least 4 hours.

Different manufacturers of bioimpedance machines use various equations to convert the raw data of impedance to estimates of body composition. There has been difficulty in obtaining the actual equations in the software of the machines and the data upon which these equations were derived. The availability of this information would allow more application of bioelectrical impedance in research and clinical settings.

All instruments should report the directly measured resistance and reactance values. Computational algorithms and the characteristics of the validation population used to convert the fundamental electrical parameters to the instrument-reported biological ones should be provided with the instrument. In all cases, reported biological values should include an assessment of the precision of the *individual* (not the *population*) estimate based on propagated instrumental and measurement errors and on the statistical error limits of the computational algorithm.

How valid is the bioelectrical impedance technology in the estimation of body composition?

The common assumption that the current penetrates cell membranes and freely passes through all fluids is known to be false. The current is carried by extracellular fluid plus some component of intracellular fluid. The human body poorly approximates a cylinder, and the bioelectrical impedance measurement is disproportionately sensitive to limb versus trunk water content. The correlation between bioelectrical impedance resistance measurements and isotopic dilution TBW differs slightly in conditions where there are disturbances in extracellular versus intracellular water or limb versus trunk water distribution.

The ability to predict fatness from bioelectrical impedance in severely obese subjects (BMI > 32) should be interpreted with caution. The obese have a greater proportion of body mass and body water accounted for by the trunk in relation to the extremities than do leaner subjects. The trunk does, however, contribute a relatively minor amount to total body impedance, resulting in the overestimation of body fat from standard equations. The hydration of FFM is greater in the obese, and the ratio of extracellular to intracellular water is increased in the obese, resulting in the underestimation of body fat from standard predictive equations.

Additional research that links bioelectrical impedance measurements to the underlying physiological and biophysical structure will help to place bioelectrical impedance technology on a much stronger scientific basis. A major need in clinical research is the establishment of reference norms to improve data interpretation. There is little information on how trunkal obesity affects impedance measurements.

Additional studies are also needed for population-specific equations to predict adiposity in the elderly, the very lean, and the obese as well as to determine racial or ethnic predictions. These studies should include multifrequency impedance measurements and multicomponent criterion methods accounting for TBW and total body mineral as well as body density and should include statistically accepted cross-validation methods. Other clinical variables might be used to improve estimates of TBW if valid prediction equations are developed for specific demographic subgroups. Additional validation studies are needed using multicompartment models to test how well bioelectrical impedance-derived estimates of TBW predict body mass and adiposity.

What are the appropriate clinical uses of bioelectrical impedance technology, and what are the limitations?

The relationship between impedance and TBW is of necessity empirical. This constrains the derived value of TBW in that it must be altered in the torso and extremities in a fixed relationship in health and disease in order to retain predictive value. This relationship occurs in most normal subjects, as well as those with any one of a number of mild disease states or chronic illnesses that do not produce local fluid accumulation. It appears to be of value to assess nutritional status in early HIV infection. However, in conditions where water distribution is disturbed, such as during critical illness, the assumptions of body impedance analysis and TBW are invalid.

In the hospital setting, particularly among the critically ill, the role of bioelectrical impedance has not been clearly defined. Disturbances of intracellular water are known to be characteristic of protein calorie malnutrition, and direct or indirect measures of TBW do not reliably reflect FFM. This likely invalidates bioelectrical impedance as an assessment of the response to parenteral and enteral nutrition in such patients, at least in terms of changes in FFM that reflect protein accretion. There are clinical conditions for which knowledge of TBW may be helpful in monitoring the critically ill, but the role of bioelectrical impedance in this assessment remains to be defined.

Bioelectrical impedance does not appear to be useful to assess acute weight changes due to dieting in the obese. Neither acute changes in weight by infusion nor acute loss by the development of protein calorie malnutrition appear to be reliably detected by bioelectrical impedance. More gradual nutritional repletion may be accurately assessed by bioelectrical impedance in malnourished patients who are not critically ill.

For patients undergoing hemodialysis, bioelectrical impedance is useful in the prescription and monitoring of the adequacy of dialysis. Where urea kinetic modeling has become the common standard, bioelectrical impedance can provide the accurate assessment of TBW as this model requires. Bioelectrical impedance also can be of value in assessing volume status in the dialysis patient and may serve to improve interpretation of drug pharmacokinetics.

The third National Health and Nutrition Examination Survey (NHANES III) single-frequency bioelectrical impedance data may be useful for examining the relationship between body composition estimates from this technique and clinical risk factors such as blood pressure, blood lipids, and glucose intolerance. This could help determine whether bioelectrical impedance provides additional information on disease risks compared with other techniques of body composition assessment. The availability of the longitudinal follow-up of the NHANES III cohort would provide valuable information relating body composition data derived from bioelectrical impedance with clinical outcome.

AUTHORS' CONCLUSION

Bioelectrical impedance has an interesting history, and much research is currently underway for single- and multiple-frequency measures. The application of single- and multiple-frequency impedance to body composition is not proven yet. The recent NIH Technology Assessment Conference highlighted several areas where additional research is needed and indicated some of the directions this research should take. Persons interested in developing and exploring bioelectrical impedance and its technology are directed to the full report of the NIH Technology Assessment Conference (NIH, 1996).

ACKNOWLEDGMENTS

The assistance of Lisë Hall, Jean Payne, Leona Miller, Merita Moffitt, and Xiaoyin Wu is gratefully acknowledged.

REFERENCES

Azcue, M., D. Wesson, M. Neuman, and P. Pencharz
  1993   What does bioelectrical impedance spectroscopy (BIS) measure? Basic Life Sci. 60:121–123.
Baker, L.E.
  1989   Principles of the impedance technique. IEEE Eng. Med. Biol. Mag. 3:11–15.
Barnett, A.
  1937   The basic factors in proposed electrical methods for measuring thyroid function, III. The phase angle and the impedance of the skin. West. J. Surg. Obstet. Gynecol. 45:540–554.
Barnett, A., and S. Bagno
  1936   The physiological mechanisms involved in the clinical measure of phase angle. Am. J. Physiol. 114:366–382.
Baumgartner, R.N., W.C. Chumlea, and A.F. Roche
  1988   Bioelectric impedance phase angle and body composition. Am. J. Clin. Nutr. 48:16–23.
  1989   Estimation of body composition from bioelectric impedance of body segments. Am. J. Clin. Nutr. 50:221–226.
Bolot, J-F., G. Fournier, A. Bertoye, J. Lenior, P. Jenin, and A. Thomasset
  1977   Determination of lean body mass by the electrical impedance measure. Presse Med. 6:2249–2251.
Boulier, A., J. Fricker, A.L. Thomasset, and M. Apfelbaum
  1990   Fat-free mass estimation by the two electrode impedance method. Am. J. Clin. Nutr. 52:581–585.
Cha, K., E.F. Brown, and D.W. Wilmore
  1994a A new bioelectrical impedance method for measurement of the erythrocyte sedimentation rate. Physiol. Meas. 15:499–508.
Cha, K., R.G. Faris, E.F. Brown, and D.W. Wilmore
  1994b An electronic method for rapid measurement of haematocrit in blood samples. Physiol. Meas. 15:129–137.
Chumlea, W.C., and R.N. Baumgartner
  1990   Bioelectrical impedance methods for the estimation of body composition. Can. J. Sport Sci. 15(3):172–179.
Chumlea, W.C., and S.S. Guo
  1994   Bioelectrical impedance: Present status and future directions. Nutr. Rev. 52:123–131.
Chumlea, W.C., S.S. Guo, D.B. Cockram, and R.M. Siervogel
  1996   Mechanical and physiologic modifiers and bioelectrical impedance spectrum determinants of body composition. Am. J. Clin. Nutr. 64(suppl.):413S–422S.

Deurenberg, P., and F.J.M. Schouten
 1992   Loss of total body water and extracellular water assessed by multifrequency impedance. Eur. J. Clin. Nutr. 46:247–255.
Deurenberg, P., E. Van Malkenhorst, and T. Schoen
 1995   Distal versus proximal electrode placement in the prediction of total body water and extracellular water from multifrequency bioelectrical impedance. Am. J. Hum. Biol. 7:77–83.
Ducrot, H., A. Thomasset, R. Jolz, P. Jungers, C. Eyraud, and J. Lenior
 1970   Determination of extracellular fluid volume in man by measurement of whole body impedance. Presse Med. 51:2269–2272.
Forbes, G.B., W. Simon, and J.M. Amatruda
 1992   Is bioimpedance a good predictor of body composition change? Am. J. Clin. Nutr. 56:4–6.
Fuller, N.J., and M. Elia
 1989   Potential use of bioelectrical impedance of the "whole body" and of body segments for the assessment of body composition: Comparison with densitometry and anthropometry. Eur. J. Clin. Nutr. 43:779–791.
Guo, S.S., and W.C. Chumlea
 1996   Statistical methods for the development and testing of predictive equations. Pp. 191–202 in Human Body Composition: Methods and Findings, A.F. Roche, S.B. Heymsfield, and T.G. Lohman, eds. Champaign, Ill.: Human Kinetics Press.
Hannan, W.J., S.J. Cowen, K.C.H. Fearon, C.E. Plester, and J.S. Falconer
 1994   Evaluation of multi-frequency bio-impedance analysis for the assessment of extracellular and total body water in surgical patients. Clin. Sci. 86:479–485.
Hoffer, E.C., C.K. Meador, and D.C. Simpson
 1969   Correlation of whole-body impedance with total body water volume. J. Appl. Physiol. 27:531–534.
Jenin, P., J. Lenoir, C. Roullet, A. Thomasset, and H. Ducrot
 1975   Determination of body fluid compartments by electrical impedance measurements. Aviat. Space Environ. Med. 46:152–155.
Kay C.F., P.T. Bothwell, and E.L. Foltz
 1954   Electrical resistivity of living body tissues at low frequencies. J. Physiol. 13:131–136.
Kanai, H., M. Haeno, and K. Sakamoto
 1987   Electrical measurement of fluid distribution in legs and arms. Med. Prog. Technol. 12:159–170.
Kushner, R.F., and D.A. Schoeller
 1986   Estimation of total body water by bioelectrical impedance analysis. Am. J. Clin. Nutr. 44:417–424.
Lohman, T.G.
 1986   Applicability of body composition techniques and constants for children and youths. Exerc. Sports Sci. Rev. 14:325–357.
Lukaski, H.C.
 1987   Methods for the assessment of human body composition: Traditional and new. Am. J. Clin. Nutr. 46:537–556.
Lukaski, H.C., and W.W. Bolonchuk
 1987   Theory and validation of the tetrapolar bioelectrical impedance method to assess human body composition. Pp. 49–60 in *In Vivo* Body Composition Studies, K.J. Ellis, S. Yasumura, and W.D. Morgan, eds. London: The Institute of Physical Sciences in Medicine.
Moore, F.D.
 1963   The Body Cell Mass and Its Supporting Environment. London: W.B. Saunders.

NIH (National Institutes of Health)
  1996   Technology Assessment Statement on Bioelectrical Impedance Analysis in Body Composition Measurement, 1994 December 12–14. Am. J. Clin. Nutr. 64 (suppl.):524S–532S.
Nyboer, J.
  1959   Electrical Impedance Plethysmography. Springfield, Ill.: Charles C Thomas.
Patterson, R.
  1989   Body fluid determinations using multiple impedance measurements. IEEE Eng. Med. Biol. Mag. 3:16–18.
Patterson, R., C. Ranganathan, R. Engel, and R. Berkseth
  1988   Measurement of body fluid volume change using multisite impedance measurements. Med. Biol. Eng. Comput. 26:33–37.
Rising, R., B. Swinburn, K. Larson, and E. Ravussin
  1991   Body composition in Pima Indians—validation of bioelectrical resistance. Am. J. Clin. Nutr. 53:594–598.
Rush, S., J.A. Abildskov, and R. McFee
  1963   Resistivity of body tissues at low frequencies. Circ. Res. 12:40–50.
Scheltinga, M.R., D.O. Jacobs, T.D. Kimbrough, and D.W. Wilmore
  1991   Alterations in body fluid content can be detected by bioelectrical impedance analysis. J. Surg. Res. 50:461–468.
Schwan, H.P., and C.F. Kay
  1956   The conductivity of living tissues. Ann. N.Y. Acad. Sci. 65:1007–1013.
Segal, K.R., S. Burastero, A. Chun, P. Coronel, R.N. Pierson, and J. Wang
  1991   Estimation of extracellular and total body water by multiple-frequency bioelectrical-impedance measurement. Am. J. Clin. Nutr. 54:26–29.
Sergi, G., M. Bussolotto, P. Perini, I. Calliari, V. Giantin, A. Ceccon, F. Scanferla, M. Bressan, G. Moschini, and G. Enzi
  1994   Accuracy of bioelectrical impedance analysis in estimation of extracellular space in healthy subjects and in fluid retention states. Ann. Nutr. Metab. 38:158–165.
Settle, R.G., K.R. Foster, B.R. Epstein, and J.L. Mullen
  1980   Nutritional assessment: Whole body impedance and body fluid compartments. Nutr. Cancer 2:72–80.
Shirreffs, S.M., and R.J. Maughan
  1994   The effect of posture change on blood volume, serum potassium and whole body electrical impedance. Eur. J. Appl. Physiol. 69:461–463.
Shirreffs, S.M., R.J. Maughan, and M. Bernardi
  1994   Effect of posture change on blood volume, serum potassium and body water as estimated by bioelectrical impedance analysis (BIA). Clin. Sci. (London) 87:21.
Sparling, P.B., M. Millard-Stafford, L.B. Rosskopf, L.J. Dicarlo, and B.T. Hinson
  1993   Body composition by bioelectric impedance and densitometry in Black women. Am. J. Hum. Biol. 5:111–117.
Spence, J.A., R. Baliga, and J. Nyboer
  1979   Changes during hemodialysis in total body water cardiac output and chest fluid as detected by bioelectric impedance analysis. Trans. Am. Soc. Artif. Intern. Organs 25:51–55.
Stolarczyk, L.M., V.H. Heyward, V.L. Hicks, and R.N. Baumgartner
  1994   Predictive accuracy of bioelectrical impedance in estimating body composition of Native American women. Am. J. Clin. Nutr. 59:964–970.
Subramanyan, R., S.C. Manchanda, J. Nyboer, and M.L. Bhatia
  1980   Total body water in congestive heart failure. A pre- and post-treatment study. J. Assoc. Physicians India 28:257–262.

Tedner, B., L.E. Lins, H. Asaba, and B. Wehle
    1985   Evaluation of impedance technique for fluid-volume monitoring during hemo-dialysis. Int. J. Clin. Monit. Comp. 2:3–8.
Thomasset, A.
    1962   Bio-electrical properties of tissue impedance measurements. Lyon Med. 207:107–118.
Van Loan, M.D., and P.L. Mayclin
    1992   Use of multi-frequency bioelectrical impedance analysis for the estimation of extracellular fluid. Eur. J. Clin. Nutr. 46:117–124.
van Marken Lichtenbelt, W.D., K.R. Westerterp, L. Wouters, and S.C. Luijendijk
    1994   Validation of bioelectrical-impedance measurements as a method to estimate body-water compartments. Am. J. Clin. 60:159–166.
Visser, M., P. Deurenberg, and W.A. Van Staveren
    1995   Multi-frequency bioelectrical impedance for assessing total body water and extracellular water in the elderly. Eur. J. Clin. Nutr. 49:256–266.
Ward, L.C., I.H. Bunce, B.H. Cornish, B.R. Mirolo, B.J. Thomas, and L.C. Jones
    1992   Multi-frequency bioelectrical impedance augments the diagnosis and management of lymphoedema in post-mastectomy patients. Eur. J. Clin. Invest. 22:751–754.
Zillikens, M.C., and J.M. Conway
    1991   Estimation of total body water by bioelectrical impedance analysis in Blacks. Am. J. Hum. Biol. 3:25–32.

DISCUSSION

JOHANNA DWYER: In renal disease, in renal dialysis patients, you are measuring dry weight. Do you believe that you can really get reliable estimates of lean body mass and fat, as well as total body mass, using dual frequency?

WM. CAMERON CHUMLEA: I would seriously doubt that [you could get reliable estimates] with a commercial machine like the RJL or the Zytron. Much of the early work that was done with the renal patients was by a man named Tadnor, who I believe was in Scandinavia. He used multifrequency machines there and built his own machines. That work is at least 5 years old, if not older.

There have been some reports in the literature using the more recent commercial machines, and I do not think that those results have been outstanding. They tend to be too subject to error.

DOUGLAS WILMORE: I enjoyed your presentation. One of the things that you were directed to talk about was composition, but one of the things that you did not talk about was phase angle and the value that phase angle may have in assessing physiological function of individuals and determining whether they should go ahead and perform a task or not.

For example, in looking at a very, very large group of HIV patients in Europe, phase angle has been found to be the single best predictor of outcome in that population, more so than CD4 count, weight loss, serum albumin, food intake, and a whole variety of things, basically because phase angle is probably assessing either a membrane function or a partitioning of intracellular or extracellular water.

When you look at performance of the troops, for example, and you start to predict which people should go ahead with a task and which should not, this methodology, if somewhat refined, may really be very appropriate for that. I wonder if you would comment on that.

WM. CAMERON CHUMLEA: That is correct. Just for the information of the audience, phase angle is the ratio of reactance to resistance, and the arctangent is then taken to convert it into degrees, so it is the low angle that this vector traces as it goes around the semicircle [see Figure 7-1]. That is phase angle.

I agree with you. What I did not have a chance to report is that we have correlations of phase angle with blood chemistry values and we find that phase angle is correlated with hematocrit, serum sodium, and osmolality, so it has some potential there, and it does not surprise me that the Europeans have found this also.

I think it is a variable that is poorly related to body composition in the prediction-equation type of relationships, although some people have included it on occasion. It is a variable that may be sensitive to the physiological status of an individual. I am not surprised at that because it would appear that it does have that sensitivity.

As I said, we found correlations between phase angle and blood chemistry values. Those have only been considered anecdotally almost, in relationship to body composition. It is possible that it could be used in terms of body composition to explain some part of the variance that is included in the measurement, but it is more sensitive, I think. I agree with you.

DENNIS BIER: So this would be an in-field use?

WM. CAMERON CHUMLEA: It could be.

DENNIS BIER: Whereas blood chemistries would be more complex?

WM. CAMERON CHUMLEA: That is right. You could have a distribution of phase angles that would relate to sodium levels or something like that that could be important.

LYLE MOLDAWER: Are you implying that these phase angles or membrane potentials are indirect estimates of, say, skeletal muscle?

WM. CAMERON CHUMLEA: Well, the reactance is supposedly produced by some aspect of the membrane acting as a capacitor. Again, the theory is that the current eventually exceeds some magic number there, and it basically overpowers the capacitor effect. However, with the commercial machines, we still recorded reactance values up at over a megahertz. Now, I do not know if that is a function of the quality of the machine or the fact that the body was not doing what it was supposed to be doing.

But what we have found from theory and from using these commercial machines is that they do not always agree. Now, maybe the Hewlett-Packard or some of these more expensive ones would give us the correct answers.

DENNIS BIER: As you mentioned in your presentation, there are a variety of people here who are on the NIH Technology Assessment Conference panel, and I do not want to compete with them.

WM. CAMERON CHUMLEA: Dennis was on the panel.

DENNIS BIER: It was hung up on two things. As opposed to what we heard about this morning, where there was one black box (you have a measurement and you know what it is measuring, and an algorithm, which is a black box), here we have two black boxes. We have the algorithm, in which remains a black box, and then we have a measurement which we do not really know what it is measuring. So we have a lot of theories about what it should be measuring and calculations based on electrical principles in defined physical systems, but until we determine what it is actually measuring on a biophysical basis, we have real trouble understanding what we are doing.

WM. CAMERON CHUMLEA: The report of this panel, if I am correct, will be published in *The American Journal of Clinical Nutrition* (NIH, 1996) as a special issue some time later this year.

Emerging Technologies for Nutrition Research, 1997
Pp. 193–197. Washington, D.C.
National Academy Press

III

Discussion

DAVID SCHNAKENBERG: The Army has been using body composition estimates for a lot of reasons for many, many years. It is used most frequently on a cross-sectional basis, so I think what we realize now, in this era when we are trying to relate body composition to performance, is that it is critical for the technologies out there to detect change, in particular to detect change in the lean body mass, the muscle mass. If we feel somewhat comfortable from your earlier work, with a certain level of lean body mass loss you will have a loss of muscle strength.

So I think a promising technology would be one for assessing change in body composition in a relatively short period of time that could be used in the course of a field trial or where you are manipulating situations.

ROBERT NESHEIM: One of the things that occurred to me when Jim Vogel was talking about training injuries was that you could take a look at the body composition information and see whether you can get some predictability of those people who are going to be most susceptible to certain training injuries. For example, if you could look at things such as bone mass, muscle mass, and some of these things, then perhaps this could be used to implement some sort of a training regimen that would strengthen those individuals predicted to be susceptible before they really get into the usual training program, which may cause these injuries. In other words, do some pretraining build-up of some of these conditions. I do not know whether this is a practical use for many of these techniques or not.

VERNON YOUNG: I would like to go back to Karl Friedl's interesting presentation and ask you to elaborate a little further on the change in the hydration of the lean body mass and whether you think this is extracellular, interstitial, or from another site. I ask this question as a follow-up to Doug Wilmore's area of concern, and because there is a lot of interest now in the role of cell volume in metabolic regulation and the role of the osmotic status of cells in gene transcription, even.

I think it is a really interesting observation, and we should not leave it at that. We should try to understand what it means from a mechanistic as well as a metabolic and functional point of view. Can you elaborate a little further, Karl?

KARL FRIEDL: Well, I agree it is interesting. I am not sure that we can elaborate too much over what we presented. It is there, and Ancel Keys never could explain why they had that. They had lower extremity swelling, so it seemed likely to be interstitial, at least certainly extracellular. We have Rangers that end up with a lot of these knee problems. Dr. Vogel showed you a slide of four pairs of knees that looked like examples of cellulitis, but some of those may be bursitis. They may even just be related to this hydration, and they may have gotten swollen knees from this excess fluid.

There is a different look to these guys. There was one more slide I did not show you where we had looked at five Kenyan runners who had the same sum for skinfold thickness that we had at the end of Ranger training. There was a big difference between these guys and the Rangers. First of all, in the Kenyans' appearance, the skin is sort of tight, and the Rangers have almost a squishy look to them. Just subjectively, there are some differences there, and we cannot explain it further.

DOUGLAS WILMORE: Karl, do you have biopsies on any of those people?

KARL FRIEDL: No. People have been suggesting that we should try to get those.

DOUGLAS WILMORE: You could do the hydration coefficients from your biopsies.

KARL FRIEDL: Yes, and we would like to know about the glycogen status at the same time. I mean, is there something about glycogen, perhaps, that affects the DXA [dual-energy x-ray absorptiometry] when soldiers are glycogen deprived? We talked about our other body conformational differences, but we have people who have the dimensions of these Rangers, but whose weight measures appropriately on the DXA. The weight that we measure on the scale is the weight the DXA sees, with nutritional balance, so is there something different about Rangers who are nutritionally deprived?

ARTHUR ANDERSON: I have been very interested in some of these discussions because I am going to be talking later about immunity, and it will be a completely different subject area. We have discovered that the molecular signaling that takes place that allows coordination between lymphatic tissue and components of the body so that they can respond quickly to antigenic stresses depend on extracellular fluid passing through a structure that I call the fibroblastic reticular cell conduit. It is like a blood vessel, except that it is a fiber matrix structure that pumps fluid at the speed of arterial blood flow from the skin to the lymph node in microseconds, and carries antigen in peptide form. It carries cytokines, specifically the chemokines that control the type of inflammatory cells that migrate into tissue.[1]

It depends on a certain amount of extracellular fluid being present in the loose connective tissues of the body. In training situations, where individuals will be constantly pumping this fluid out by the passive pumping of lymphatics back to the blood, you deplete this extracellular fluid. This phenomenon could, in fact, underlie the comment that was made about training situations resulting in decrements in immunity; there is a certain amount of extracellular fluid that is absolutely essential for maintaining normal immune signaling functions as part of the afferent phase of the immune response.

I just wanted to insert that comment here because I am not going to talk about it during my presentation later on.

ROBERT WOLFE: I would just like to say that the thing I would encourage in terms of the investigation of these body composition methods, as we become more sophisticated, is exactly how direct the link is between these units of body

---

[1] A.O. Anderson and S. Shaw. 1993. T-cell adhesion to endothelium: The FRC conduit system and other anatomic and molecular features which facilitate the adhesion cascade in lymph node. Sem. Immunol. 5:271–282.

composition and performance. Particularly in Dr. Vogel's introduction, he referred to a lot of the trained soldiers as being like athletes.

I think that the presumption that there is a close relationship between lean body mass and performance is a considerable exaggeration. We have had experience in two different circumstances, one of which is that we studied the U.S. swimming team over the past few years, and there is almost no relation at all between muscle mass or lean body mass and performance.

Depending on the time of year and their intensity of training, the swimmers' performance varies tremendously, but their muscle mass does not change significantly. The fractional turnover rate of the muscle may change, but there are no changes in muscle mass to speak of.

We also have studied elite female triathletes and there, again, see no relation between body composition and performance. In the females, the group we studied had a range of percentage body fat of 7 to 26 percent, and yet there was no significant relation between performance and body composition.

I think when we are looking at a large population base, it is one thing to consider the general relation between body composition and performance, but within a more narrowly defined group of subjects who all have similar body composition, then body composition will not predict performance.

DONALD McCORMICK: Just a follow-up to Bob Wolfe's comment. None of these techniques that we have heard about, save one, has the potential to go into the qualitative aspect of what the composition of the material is. Fat is fat. There are a lot of different kinds of fat, as everybody here knows, but probably nothing is known about the micronutrient compositions. Only one method, nuclear magnetic resonance, with proper probes, may someday lead us to what, in fact, is the quality.

ROBERT NESHEIM: And I suppose there is another factor that gets in there and that has to do with a person's motivation. You might think all these soldiers are highly motivated, but I assume there are different degrees of high motivation, which can also be a factor.

HARRIS LIEBERMAN: I want to make a point here that there is sort of a disconnect in that we have our two extremes. Our ability to make biophysical measurements of the composition of particular substances is clearly highly refined, and as we get to more exotic and expensive technology, it becomes even better and reaches a molecular level.

On the other hand, when we try to measure performance outcomes, we have a great deal of difficulty specifying the meaning of even the simpler ones, and it is difficult even to find an appropriate metric that we can use to pin down a particular performance.

You were saying before that it is difficult to relate muscle mass in elite athletes to their performance. On the other hand, in the general population of soldiers I believe some would say there clearly was a relationship between muscle mass and performance. So we have kind of a breakdown. What is the performance we are interested in? How can we specify it at the level of sophistication, the level of accuracy at which we can make our physical measurements? I am not sure I have a solution for that problem, but it certainly is a significant problem.

REED HOYT: I think it is important to differentiate between endurance performance and strength-related performance. I think strength-related performance is where the relationship between lean mass and performance resides, in terms of lifting so many pounds and so forth. Lean mass clearly may not be related to endurance.

ROBERT WOLFE: But even there, they obviously have weight divisions in Olympic weightlifting, because if you have more muscle, you can lift more weight, but if you take subjects of a similar body weight, it is very difficult to show any relation between total lean body mass and strength.

Nonetheless, the point is valid that the type of work that is being evaluated is important.

IV

Tracer Techniques for the Study of Metabolism

THE AUTHORS IN THIS SECTION discuss various tracer techniques, stable isotopes, positron emission tomography, and nuclear magnetic resonance, for studying metabolic processes. Chapters 8 and 9 focus on stable isotopes, which can be used to study turnover of protein, carbohydrate, and fat, thus monitoring changes in energy expenditure, relative fuel utilization, gluconogenesis, and other aspects of metabolic substrate oxidation. For *in vivo* nutritional studies, stable isotope tracers are injected into accessible compartments in order to compile data on inaccessible compartments from the tracer dilution curve. Mass spectrometry is the analytical method used for measuring stable isotope samples. The problem of the natural abundance of stable isotopes, which differs from place to place, must be overcome if any meaningful data are to be collected, especially in the field.

Positron emission tomography (PET), a noninvasive technique for the evaluation of protein metabolism that traces radioactive atoms incorporated into biological fuels, is discussed in Chapter 10. This technique can be used in conjunction with stable isotopes to evaluate the contribution of individual organs and body areas to whole-body protein metabolic processes. Unfortunately, widespread use of PET is not possible at this time due to the limited number of specialized laboratories that are needed and the high cost of operation.

Chapter 11 describes the use of nuclear magnetic resonance (NMR) spectroscopy for the investigation of both liver and muscle glycogen synthesis as well as the pathogenesis of Type II diabetes mellitus. This technique is based on the action of nuclei in the presence of a strong magnetic field, which in the end generates an image from released energy. For the purposes described here, NMR is noninvasive and safe but is relatively insensitive and expensive when the costs of the magnet and staff are considered. The use of NMR imaging for body composition analysis is described in Chapter 5 of this volume.

Emerging Technologies for Nutrition Research, 1997
Pp. 203–213. Washington, D.C.
National Academy Press

8

Stable Isotope Tracers: Technological Tools That Have Emerged

Dennis M. Bier[1]

ISOTOPES IN NATURE

By and large, when one discusses biomedical applications of isotopic methods, the public, and often many scientists as well, conceptualize the notion as the use of radioactive counterparts of elements occurring in nature, which, in turn, are assumed to be nonradioactive. This ideation ignores what most everyone learned in high school chemistry (Table 8-1), namely that only a few biologically important elements are monoisotopic in nature (e.g., ^{31}P); there are trace amounts of naturally occurring radioactive isotopes of several common elements (e.g., ^{14}C and ^{40}K); and most of the common naturally occurring elements occur as a mixture of two or more stable, nonradioactive isotopic forms (e.g., ^{16}O, ^{17}O, and ^{18}O). Twenty-five years ago, the latter information was of limited use to the biomedical investigator since significant quantities of highly

---

[1] Dennis M. Bier, Children's Nutrition Research Center and Department of Pediatrics, Baylor College of Medicine, Houston, TX 77030-2600

TABLE 8-1 Natural Abundance of Elements Commonly Found in Biological Substances

Element	Mass	Abundance (%)
Hydrogen	1	99.985
	2	0.015
Carbon	12	98.89
	13	1.11
	14	*
Nitrogen	14	99.63
	15	0.37
Oxygen	16	99.76
	17	0.04
	18	0.20
Sodium	23	100
Phosphorus	31	100
Sulfur	32	95.02
	33	0.75
	34	4.21
	36	0.02
Chloride	35	75.77
	37	24.23
Potassium	39	93.258
	40	0.012
	41	6.730
Iodine	127	100

* Approximately 6.1 pCi/g carbon depending on carbon source. ^{14}C production rate = ~1.8 atoms/cm^2 sec.

enriched, minor, stable isotopic nuclides of the elements were generally unavailable, save for deuterium. This situation has changed dramatically over the last two decades. Now, except for enriched stable isotopic forms of the mineral elements, which remain in short supply and are prohibitively expensive, the stable isotopes of carbon, hydrogen, nitrogen, and oxygen and a wide variety of biochemicals containing these nuclides are commercially available in relative abundance. Similarly, analytical instrumentation for routine measurements of these isotopes is now widely available and, because of the advances in computer hardware and software, this instrumentation is more user friendly. For these reasons, the use of nonradioactive, stable isotope tracers as probes for *in vivo* nutrition and metabolic studies has increased enormously over the last 20 years.

ACCESS TO INACCESSIBLE COMPARTMENTS

Why are these isotopic probes needed? The answer is best illustrated by Figure 8-1. This schematic representation of an intricate biological system shows a multicompartmental complex, in which the compartments reflect constitutive entities that are discrete but otherwise not constrained. Thus, depending on the question, the compartments might be viewed anatomically (e.g., brain, liver, and kidney), functionally (e.g., respiration, circulation, and digestion), biochemically (e.g., glucose, lactate, and alanine), or otherwise.

For human nutritional studies *in vivo*, there are generally only a few compartments, such as the blood or urine, that are accessible for sampling information of relevance to nutrient dynamics or action. However, the direct answers to

Multipool System

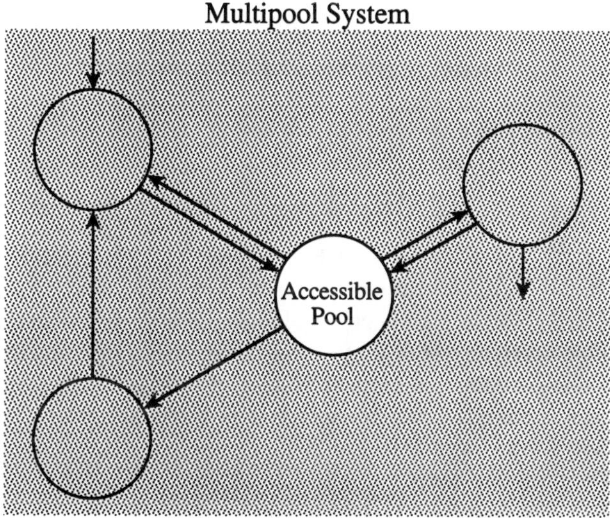

FIGURE 8-1 Schematic representation of a generic multipool system. Each pool or compartment reflects a relatively homogenous, well-mixed portion of the system. The arrows represent movement of materials between compartments. Compartments may be anatomical, functional, or biochemical. The uncovered central compartment, labeled accessible pool, is meant to reflect the fact that that portion of the entire system is available to the investigator for sampling. Thus, for an anatomical model, the accessible pool might be venous blood. The stippled, covered pools are meant to represent those hidden within the system and inaccessible for routine sampling. A tracer that is injected into the accessible pool and then traverses the system provides the necessary information to uncover the hidden structure of the system.

most biological questions lie at the site of the nutrient's metabolic effects, that is, within organs and cells. In some instances, this information can be obtained invasively by inserting sampling catheters into the site of interest. Nonetheless, this approach is generally not ethically acceptable for routine studies in otherwise healthy individuals. For this reason, alternative approaches that provide information about events within inaccessible compartments from data collected in the accessible ones must be used. An established approach to this problem is to inject an appropriate tracer into the accessible compartment and monitor the dilution of the tracer in the accessible pool by sampling the compartment repeatedly after introduction of the tracer. The shape of the tracer dilution curve is determined by the characteristics of the tracer outflow into the inaccessible compartments and the nature of the unlabeled substrate movement into the accessible compartment—in other words, by the structure of the system in question. Thus, by analyzing the attributes of the tracer dilution curve by the widely verified mathematical techniques of compartment analysis (Shipley and Clark, 1972), the previously hidden structure of the system can be uncovered. Stable isotope tracers are the optimal candidates for this analytical approach in humans, as discussed below.

EXPRESSION OF TRACER DILUTION

The similarities and differences in expressing the dilution of a radio isotope tracer and stable isotope tracer are shown in Figure 8-2 for carbon. In the context of a radiotracer experiment (B), the biological substance of interest (tracee, B1) is all unlabeled and composed of the major, naturally occurring, nonradioactive nuclide, ^{12}C, plus its minor stable isotope, ^{13}C. The radiolabeled tracer (B2) is the highly enriched isotope ^{14}C. Although there is a trace amount of naturally occurring ^{14}C in the tracee, its abundance is very low and its radioactivity negligible compared with that of the tracer. In an experiment, when the radiotracer probe is added to the tracee system and a sample taken subsequently (B3), the tracee is analyzed for its mass content by an acceptable method, and the radioactivity of the tracer is determined independently by counting the disintegrations. The resultant tracer to tracee ratio, commonly called the specific activity, represents the degree of tracer dilution.

For a stable isotope-tracer experiment (Figure 8-2, A), the situation is somewhat more complicated. The tracee (A1) remains composed of the two naturally occurring, stable isotopes of carbon, ^{12}C and ^{13}C. In contrast, (A2), unlike the "massless" radiotracer, a stable isotope "tracer" has a finite mass and, while composed principally of the enriched minor isotope ^{13}C, it also invariably contains some ^{12}C. When this stable tracer is injected or infused into the tracee system, a resultant sample (A3) is composed of a mixture of ^{12}C and ^{13}C contributed by both the tracee and the tracer. The analytical methods measure total ^{12}C and total ^{13}C in the sample directly. To calculate the unknown tracer-to-tracee ratio in the sample, the fractional contributions of the tracer and the tracee

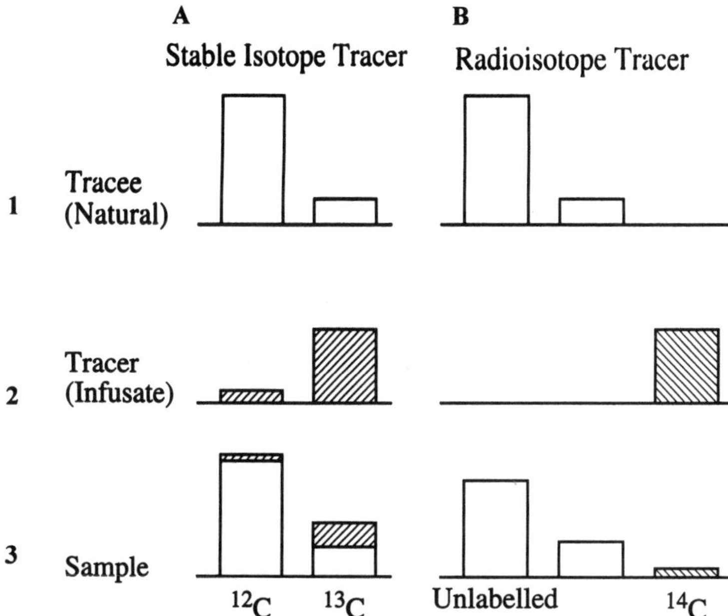

FIGURE 8-2 Generic representation of the isotopes of carbon and how they contribute to the determination of isotope content in a sample taken during a stable or radioisotope tracer experiment (see text). The clear bars represent the endogenous carbon (tracee) in the system that consists of the stable, nonradioactive nuclides of carbon, ^{12}C and ^{13}C. In a stable isotope experiment, these can be measured separately by mass spectrometry. In a radioisotope experiment, ^{12}C and ^{13}C are measured together as "unlabeled" carbon. Similarly, in a stable isotope tracer experiment, the stable carbon tracer itself (hatched bars in A) is composed primarily of ^{13}C but also contains a small amount of residual ^{12}C. The experimental sample consists of a mixture of these nuclides that are measured individually by mass spectrometry. In a radiotracer experiment, the ^{14}C tracer is distinct from the unlabeled tracee and measured by an entirely different approach. In both cases, the required ratio of tracer to tracee must be derived from the individual measurements.

to each of these isotopic totals must be derived mathematically from the known isotopic characteristics of the natural or fully "unlabeled" tracee and the corresponding known isotopic composition of the "labeled" tracer. The procedures for this process are well described (Cobelli et al., 1987, 1992).

Two additional reporting conventions of stable isotope-tracer dilution are available for specialized cases. During the constant infusion of a stable isotope tracer at steady state, tracer isotopic enrichment above natural abundance can be used appropriately (Cobelli et al., 1987; Segel, 1968). Further, in experiments in which tracer and tracee abundance or enrichment differ by several orders of magnitude, their relationships are often conveniently described with respect to international reference standards according to the so-called delta (δ) notation (Boutton, 1991).

ANALYTICAL CONSIDERATIONS

Although advances in magnetic resonance spectroscopy now permit limited noninvasive measurements of stable isotope tracers *in vivo* and a broad approach to *in vitro* measurements of selected stable nuclides in samples obtained during *in vivo* tracer experiments, mass spectrometry has been the most commonly used tool for quantifying samples containing stable, isotopically labeled substrates. This use is appropriate since mass spectrometry is the most rapid, sensitive, specific, and precise general analytical method available for this purpose. Since all biochemical substrates have mass, and since mass is the principle of mass spectrometric measurements, this approach is potentially applicable to all biochemical substrates. In practice, there are some obvious limitations, but these are relatively few for substances with molecular weights less than about 1,000 daltons. Mass spectrometry is also an extraordinarily sensitive method. Picomole analyses are commonplace, and attomole analyses can be accomplished with commercially available gas chromatography-mass spectrometry (GC-MS) instrumentation. With specialized instruments, single atoms can be detected. Analytical specificity is exceptionally high with the advent of separatory capabilities of capillary GC column inlets, as well as selective derivatization and ionization methods.

The characteristics of mass spectrometry approaches to stable isotope quantitation are shown in Table 8-2. This table demonstrates that while gas isotope ratio mass spectrometry has the ability to quantify the lowest tracer/tracee ratios, this advantage is at the expense of sample size. The additional disadvantage of gas isotope ratio mass spectrometry is that the sample nuclide must be converted to a purified gaseous form, a process that often adds considerably to analytical time and difficulty.

Recently, commercial GC-combustion-isotope ratio mass spectrometry systems have been introduced. This new alternative couples the separatory advan-

TABLE 8-2 Characteristics of Quantitative Mass Spectrometry Methods

Characteristics	Gas Chromatography-Mass Spectrometry	GC-Combustion-Isotope Ratio Mass Spectrometry	Gas Isotope Ratio Mass Spectrometry
Tracer/Tracee Ratio (%)	0.1–100	0.0005–0.5	0.00005–0.01
Sample Size	Picogram	Nanogram	Microgram
Preparation	Derivatization	Derivatization	Purified gas
Precision (%)	±0.2	±0.01	±0.001
Matrix	Plasma, urine	Plasma, tissue	Breath, urine

tages of capillary gas chromatography to the high isotope dilution and precision characteristics of gas isotope ratio mass spectrometry and is a valuable addition to the analytical repertoire (Goodman and Brenna, 1992; Yarasheski, 1992).

The high level of precision achieved by quantitative mass spectrometric methods also is demonstrated in Table 8-2. Tables 8-3 and 8-4 demonstrate the practical implications of this precision. Presented in Table 8-3 are the individual interlaboratory coefficients of variation for the measurement of eight common substances of clinical interest by various hospital pathology laboratories surveyed by the American College of Pathologists using standard clinical laboratory protocols. The best of these (for sodium) was ±1.3 percent, while the worst was ±11.1 percent (for creatinine). Table 8-4 shows the results for a similar multiple-laboratory survey of the measurements of four stable nuclides by gas isotope ratio mass spectrometry. The most analytically challenging measurement, which is that of deuterium, had an interlaboratory coefficient of variation of ±1.02 percent, better than the best measurement of variation in the clinical laboratory. Such precise measurements are of very great value in compartmental analysis of tracer data, since they permit more precise definition of the mathematical function fitted to the isotope decay curve and, therefore, to the model of the biological compartmental system derived from this curve.

ADVANTAGES OF STABLE ISOTOPE TRACER USE

The most salient advantage of stable isotope tracers for use in human experiments is their complete safety. In the nearly half century of their use, the most significant side effect reported in humans has been transient vertigo, result-

TABLE 8-3 Precision of Selected Routine Clinical Chemistry Methods

Analyte	Coefficient of Variation (%)
Calcium	3.1
Chloride	2.8
Cholesterol	5.8
Creatinine	11.1
Glucose	3.9
Potassium	2.9
Sodium	1.3
Urea	5.3

TABLE 8-4 Measurement Precision of Selected Stable Nuclides by Gas Isotope Ratio Mass Spectrometry[*]

Isotope	Substance	Atom % Excess	Coefficient of Variation (%)
Carbon-13	Glucose	1.2143	0.255
Deuterium	Water	0.02359	1.021
Nitrogen-15	Urea	0.45548	0.138
Oxygen-18	Water	0.25039	0.292

* Different laboratories than those reporting data in Table 8-3.

ing from the acute ingestion of relatively large quantities of deuterium oxide. Other than this relatively unique event that is apparently a consequence of alterations of cochlear fluid density, the other stable nuclides have been uniformly safe in human studies. Thus, stable isotope tracers can and have been used appropriately in both children and pregnant women.

Table 8-5 demonstrates several additional but perhaps less well-appreciated advantages of using a stable isotope tracer. In addition to the analytical and ethical advantages, there is the very practical advantage of not having the isotope disposal costs that are associated with the use of radiotracers. Depending on the magnitude of activity in a research laboratory, this may represent a significant savings. Additionally, with mass spectrometry, the position of the isotopically labeled nuclide within a molecule usually can be determined with relative ease. This approach, called mass isotopomer analysis because mass isotopomers are chemically identical molecules that differ in mass by virtue of the number and position of their isotopic constituents, is a valuable tool for dissecting precursor-

TABLE 8-5 Selected Advantages of Stable Isotope Tracer Methods

1. No practical radiotracer exists for certain elements.

2. There are no isotope disposal costs.

3. Some studies are not practical to perform using radiotracers.

4. Isotope effects are less than with corresponding radiotracer.

5. Substrate content and isotope enrichment are measured simultaneously.

6. Confidence in assay specificity is very high.

7. Intramolecular location of label(s) is determined easily.

8. Simultaneous and repeated use of several tracers is possible in the same subject.

product relationships in biological systems, as described more fully below. Lastly, because of their safety, several stable isotope tracers can be used simultaneously and repeatedly in the same subject, a luxury not available with radiotracers because of acceptable exposure limits. This advantage of using stable isotope tracers is extraordinarily valuable in human experiments since the use of multiple tracers maximizes the information content of each human study. Further, the ability to study the same individual repeatedly allows analysis of the results of various test interventions to be compared on the basis of paired statistics, with the subject serving as his own control. The combined use of several isotopes and paired analysis allows a reduction in the number of research subjects needed to accomplish multiple objectives, without sacrificing statistical power.

SELECTED RECENT EXAMPLES OF STABLE ISOTOPE USE

The stable isotope literature is now sufficiently large that innumerable examples of human kinetic studies that are of direct basic or applied nutritional importance are available (Bier, 1987). Further, the technology has been used successfully in military field studies (Hoyt et al., 1994). Most recently, however, the realization that the use of the full isotopic information content inherent within substrate mass isotopomers has opened up a highly productive new approach to stable isotope tracer research, called mass isotopomer distribution analysis (MIDA) (Hellerstein and Neese, 1992). MIDA is the process of quantifying precursor-product events from the distribution of mass isotopomer patterns in the labeled precursor and product. A simple example, depicted by the data in Figure 8-3, will illustrate this concept. Berthold and coworkers (1991) incorporated uniformly ^{13}C-labeled *Spirulina platenis* algal hydrolysate into the diet of a laying hen that was fed this mixture for 27 days. During that time, they measured the isotopic enrichment of each carbon atom of egg white protein phenylalanine and glutamine plus glutamate (GLX). Figure 8-3A shows that there was a gradual decline in the fraction of egg protein phenylalanine that was unlabeled (M) over the period of feeding with a corresponding fractional increment in phenylalanine that was fully labeled with carbon-13 (M+9). No egg white protein phenylalanine isotopomers were found with fewer labeled carbon atoms (M+1 to M+8). These data show convincingly that dietary algal [U-^{13}C]phenylalanine was incorporated fully intact into the egg protein; in other words, all egg protein was derived from the diet, confirming that phenylalanine is an essential amino acid with no evidence of endogenous synthesis. Figure 8-3B shows that the situation for glutamine plus glutamate is quite different. Thus, while the decline in unlabeled GLX(M) occurs as expected, carbon-13 labeling of egg protein GLX is distributed throughout the isotopomers having one to five labeled carbons (M+1 to M+5). These data show that dietary algal [U-^{13}C]GLX is metabolized extensively and there is *de novo* resynthesis before synthesis of egg white protein, confirming the nonessentiality of the amino acids

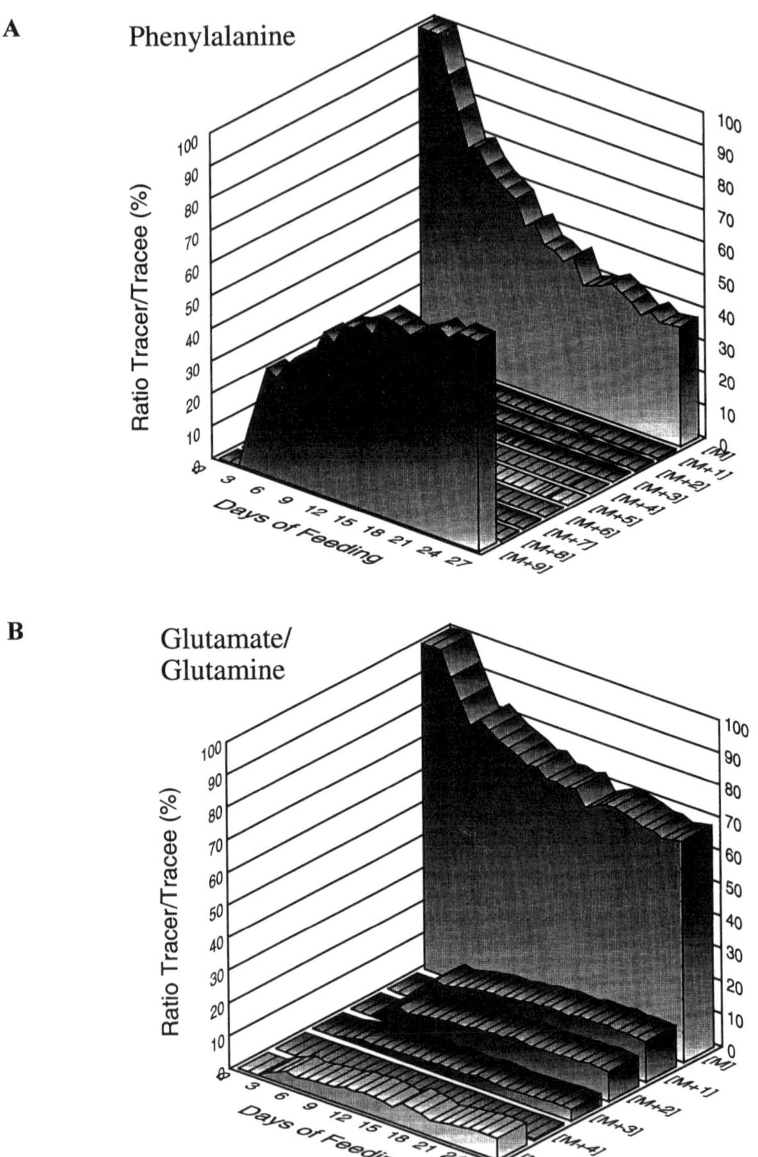

FIGURE 8-3 Mass isotopomer distribution patterns in egg white protein phenylalanine (A) and glutamine plus glutamate (B) obtained from eggs laid during a 27-d period when a chicken was fed [U-^{13}C]-labeled algal biomass. M represents the completely unlabeled isotopomer (i.e., all ^{12}C). The isotopomers at M+1 to M+n represent those molecules labeled with a single carbon-13 atom (i.e., ^{13}C$_1$) to molecules fully labeled with carbon-13 (i.e., ^{13}C$_n$), respectively. The vertical axes represent the percent label at the individual isotopomers. SOURCE: Berthold et al. (1991), used with permission.

glutamine and glutamate. Thus, this experiment illustrates the fact that careful consideration of the full isotopic information content of a synthesized product can contain significant information about the metabolism of its precursor.

Over the last several years, this principle has been applied successfully to the study of glycogenolysis and gluconeogenesis (Des Rosiers et al., 1995; Katz and Lee, 1991; Landau et al., 1995; Neese et al., 1995), lipogenesis (Hellerstein et al., 1996), contribution of *de novo* fatty-acid synthesis to very-low density lipoprotein triglyceride fatty acids (Leitch and Jones, 1993; Yang et al., 1996), and incorporation of dietary pyridimidine nucleosides into hepatic DNA (Berthold et al., 1995).

SIGNIFICANCE TO THE MILITARY

The basic mechanistic questions of nutritional relevance to military personnel cannot be answered convincingly or conclusively by indirect methods. Specifically, the quantitative aspects of interorgan metabolic fuel transport and the pathophysiological basis for alterations in fuel and energy balance because of physical activity, restricted rations, environmental and psychological stress, and injury cannot be answered by static substrate measurements or balance studies. These answers require quantitative assessments of fuel dynamics. In the context of safe, relatively noninvasive approaches to these issues in normal volunteers, stable isotope tracer studies are the only practical alternative. The results of such kinetic investigations will enhance significantly the functional data available for subsequent implementation of decisions important to the health of U.S. service members under both training and battle conditions.

Given this, it is impossible to escape the conclusion that this technology should be supported by Department of Defense funds. It is unclear what the precise role of the Small Business Innovative Research program might be in the funding process other than design of specialized analytical instrumentation useful in field circumstances or the development of new synthetic routes toward cost-effective production of stable, isotopically labeled substrates of interest to the military but not commercially available. The benefit/cost ratio is extremely high once the initial, one-time capital outlay for mass spectrometry equipment is satisfied.

Since NASA sent a mass spectrometer to Mars where it collected data during the Voyager mission, the technology is clearly applicable to any terrestrial "field" study. Further, many currently available mass spectrometers are now "bench top" size and could easily be operated in the field, given the appropriate power supply and environmental protection. Nonetheless, it is far more likely that samples collected in the field would be measured at a central core facility elsewhere. This approach has been utilized already in many stable isotope studies conducted in both industrialized and developing countries.

With modern instrumentation and commercial isotope availability, the technology is very practical to apply to human studies of all kinds. This has been amply demonstrated by the large and ever-increasing number of such studies over the last two decades. This technique is now a widely accepted, basic method for human investigation applied in laboratories worldwide by individuals of vastly different types and degrees of basic education, training, and accomplishment. Current software and data reduction routines facilitate sample analysis by mass spectrometers, the practical operation of which cannot be more difficult than many other kinds of high-tech digital equipment already utilized by appropriately trained service personnel. However, the scientific questions forming the basis for the subsequent sample analysis must be asked by highly competent military scientists. These questions and the studies designed therefrom are, in fact, the rate-limiting step to productive application of the technologies described.

REFERENCES

Berthold, H.K., D.L. Hachey, P.J. Reeds, O.P. Thomas, S. Hoeksema, and P.D. Klein
1991   Uniformly ^{13}C-labeled algal protein used to determine amino acid essentiality *in vivo*. Proc. Natl. Acad. Sci. USA 88:8091–8095.

Berthold, H.K., P.F. Crain, I. Gouni, P.J. Reeds, and P.D. Klein
1995   Evidence for incorporation of intact dietary pyrimidine (but not purine) nucleosides into hepatic RNA. Proc. Natl. Acad. Sci. USA 92(2):10123–10127.

Bier, D.M.
1987   The use of stable isotopes in metabolic investigation. Bailliere's Clin. Endocrinol. Metab. 1(4):817–836.

Boutton, T.W.
1991   Stable carbon isotope ratios of natural materials: I. Sample preparation and mass spectrometric analysis. Pp. 155–171 in Carbon Isotope Techniques, D.C. Coleman and D.M. Jones, eds. San Diego: Academic Press, Inc.

Cobelli, C., G. Toffolo, D.M. Bier, and R. Nosadini
1987   Models to interpret kinetic data in stable isotope tracer studies. Am. J. Physiol. 253:E551–E564.

Cobelli, C., G. Toffolo, and D.M. Foster
1992   Tracer-to-tracee ratio for analysis of stable isotope tracer data: Link with radioactive kinetic formalism. Am. J. Physiol. 262:E968–E975.

Des Rosiers, C., L. Di Donato, B. Comte, A. Laplante, C. Marcoux, F. David, C.A. Fernandez, and H. Brunengraber
1995   Isotopomer analysis of citric acid cycle and gluconeogenesis in rat liver. Reversibility of isocitrate dehydrogenase and involvement of ATP-citrate lyase in gluconeogenesis. J. Biol. Chem. 270:10027–10036.

Goodman, K.J., and J.T. Brenna
1992   High sensitivity tracer detection using high-precision gas chromatography-combustion isotope ratio mass spectrometry and highly enriched [U-^{13}C]-labeled precursors. Anal. Chem. 64:1088–1095.

Hellerstein, M.K., and R.A. Neese
1992   Mass isotopomer distribution analysis: A technique for measuring biosynthesis and turnover of polymers. Am. J. Physiol. 263:E998–E1001.

Hellerstein, M.K., J-M. Schwarz, and R. Neese
1996   Regulation of hepatic *de novo* lipogenesis in humans. Ann. Rev. Nutr. 16:523–527.

Hoyt, R.W., T.E. Jones, C.J. Baker-Fulco, D.A. Schoeller, R.B. Schoene, R.S. Schwartz, E.W. Askew, and A. Cymerman
  1994   Doubly labeled water measurement of human energy expenditure during exercise at high altitude. Am. J. Physiol. 266:R966–R971.
Katz, J., and W-NP. Lee
  1991   Application of mass isotopomer analysis for determination of pathways of glycogen synthesis. Am. J. Physiol. 261:E332–E336.
Landau, B.R., V. Chandramouli, W.C. Schumann, K. Ekberg, K. Kumaran, S.C. Kalhan, and J. Wahren
  1995   Estimates of Krebs cycle activity and contributions of gluconeogenesis to hepatic glucose production in fasting healthy subjects and IDDM patients. Diabetologia 38:831–838.
Leitch, C.A., and P.J.H. Jones
  1993   Measurement of human lipogenesis using deuterium incorporation. J. Lipid Res. 34:157–163.
Neese, R.A., J-M. Schwartz, D. Faix, S. Turner, A. Letscher, D. Vu, and M.K. Hellerstein
  1995   Gluconeogenesis and intrahepatic triose phosphate flux in response to fasting or substrate loads. Application of the mass isotopomer distribution analysis technique with testing of assumptions and potential problems. J. Biol. Chem. 270:14452–14463.
Segel, I.H.
  1968   Biochemical Calculations. How to Solve Mathematical Problems in General Biochemistry. New York: John Wiley & Sons.
Shipley, R.A., and R.E. Clark
  1972   Tracer Methods for *In Vivo* Kinetics. Theory and Applications. New York and London: Academic Press.
Yang, L-Y., A. Kuksis, J.J. Myher, and G. Steiner
  1996   Contributions of *de novo* fatty acid synthesis to very low density lipoprotein triacylglycerols: Evidence from mass isotopomer distribution analysis of fatty acids synthesized from [^{2}H$_6$]ethanol. J. Lipid Res. 37:262–274.
Yarasheski, K.E., K. Smith, M.J. Rennie, and D.M. Bier
  1992   Measurement of muscle protein fractional synthetic rate by capillary gas chromatography-combustion-isotope ratio mass spectrometry. Biol. Mass Spectrom. 21:486–490.

Emerging Technologies for Nutrition Research, 1997
Pp. 215–230. Washington, D.C.
National Academy Press

9

Measurement of Energy Substrate Metabolism Using Stable Isotopes

Robert R. Wolfe[1]

INTRODUCTION

Atoms that are chemically identical but differ slightly in weight are called isotopes. Mass differences of isotopes are due to different numbers of neutrons. A variety of atoms have naturally occurring stable isotopes. Conveniently, hydrogen (^{1}H and ^{2}H, or deuterium), carbon (^{12}C and ^{13}C), nitrogen (^{14}N and ^{15}N), and oxygen (^{16}O, ^{17}O, and ^{18}O) all have stable isotopes. In each of these cases, the most abundant is the one that is the lowest possible weight, and the heavier mass isotope is naturally present to a much smaller degree. Thus, the percent natural abundance of ^{2}H, ^{13}C, ^{15}N ,and ^{18}O is 0.015, 1.11, 0.37, and 0.20 percent, respectively. Atoms can be enriched so that a "mixture" is entirely a heavy stable isotope. These heavy stable isotopes can then be incorporated into molecules to create tracers.

[1] Robert R. Wolfe, Metabolism Unit, Shriners Burns Institute and University of Texas Medical Branch, Galveston, TX 77550
Supported by Shriners Hospital Grant 15849.

An ideal tracer is chemically identical to the compound of interest (the tracee) but distinct in some characteristic that enables its precise detection. In the case of tracers labeled with stable isotopes, the principal characteristic of distinction is their difference in mass from the naturally occurring form. Thus, mass spectrometry is the most precise means of detecting the abundance of tracers labeled with stable isotopes. Consequently, the focus of this chapter will be on techniques relying on mass spectrometry to quantify the abundance of stable isotopes of carbon and hydrogen in order to gain insight into the regulation of substrate metabolism.

Conventionally, the methodology involves the infusion of a compound labeled in a specific position of the molecule with a stable isotope (e.g., $[1\text{-}^{13}C]$-palmitic acid) in tracer doses. The infusion rate of the tracer, therefore, is trivial by comparison to the endogenous kinetics of the tracee. Blood, tissue, and/or breath samples are then obtained, and kinetic parameters are calculated using a mathematical model of varying complexity. The aim of this chapter will be to present examples of tracer methods to quantify both the plasma kinetics of glucose and free fatty acids (FFA) and also the relative contributions of the oxidation of intracellular glycogen and triglyceride to the total rate of oxidation of carbohydrate and fat, respectively. An exhaustive exposition on all possible methods of studying glucose and fat metabolism with stable isotopes is beyond the scope of this report. Because it is possible to make use of varying abundances of ^{13}C that occur naturally, a method also will be presented in this chapter that enables the quantitation of total carbohydrate and fat oxidation using the measurement of the rate of total carbon dioxide excretion ($\dot{V}CO_2$) and the natural abundance of ^{13}C in breath, and in the glucose, fat, and protein in the body. This method will be referred to as the "breath ratio method."

BREATH $^{13}C/^{12}C$ RATIO METHOD TO MEASURE SUBSTRATE OXIDATION

Description of Methodology

The method is based on the measurement of the absolute $^{13}C/^{12}C$ ratios in expired breath and in endogenous glucose, fat, and protein (Romijn et al., 1992). Because of a small amount of fractionation of ^{13}C in certain synthetic pathways such as photosynthesis, the natural abundance of ^{13}C in glucose, fat, and protein varies. Whereas the macronutrients may differ in enrichment, over time in one individual, the values should be reasonably constant if the diet is stable. The differences can be further amplified by the ingestion of ^{13}C-enriched cornstarch for a few days before the study.

The enrichment of the CO_2 in the breath (R_B) will be the sum of the proportional contribution of the oxidation of carbohydrate (x), fat (y), and protein (z) to produce CO_2, multiplied by the respective enrichments of each substrate (R_x, R_y, and R_z). Thus,

$$R_B = xR_x + yR_y + zR_z \qquad \text{(Equation 9-1)}$$

Only carbohydrate, fat, and protein oxidation contribute to the total CO_2 production. Consequently,

$$1 = x + y + z. \qquad \text{(Equation 9-2)}$$

R_x, R_y, and R_z can be determined (see below). Also, z can be calculated from urinary nitrogen excretion. Therefore, equations 9-1 and 9-2 can be solved for x and y (the proportion of CO_2 from carbohydrate and fat, respectively):

$$x = \frac{R_B - R_y(1-z) - zR_z}{R_x - R_y} \qquad \text{(Equation 9-3)}$$

and

$$y = 1 - x - z. \qquad \text{(Equation 9-4)}$$

Note that x and y can be determined without the use of indirect calorimetry. When compared to the values for proportional oxidation rates of carbohydrate and fat as determined by indirect calorimetry, a close agreement was observed (Romijn et al., 1992). It also may be of interest to quantify glucose and fat oxidation in terms of actual rates (in g/min) of oxidation, which can be accomplished with this methodology. However, the measurement of either oxygen consumption ($\dot{V}O_2$) or CO_2 production ($\dot{V}CO_2$) also is required. The situation in which only the $\dot{V}O_2$ is known will be considered first. It is first necessary to express total $\dot{V}CO_2$ as follows:

$$\dot{V}CO_2 \text{ (liters/min)} = 0.746c + 1.43f + 4.89n,$$

where c is the quantity of carbohydrate oxidized (in grams), f is the quantity of fat oxidized (in grams), and n is the quantity of urinary nitrogen excreted (in grams) per minute (keeping in mind that 1 g of nitrogen excretion represents the oxidation of approximately 6.25 g protein) (from Frayn, 1983). From equations 9-2 and 9-5, it can be seen that

$$x = \frac{0.746c}{0.746c + 1.43f + 4.89n}$$

$$y = \frac{1.43f}{0.746c + 1.43f + 4.89n}$$

$$z = \frac{4.89n}{0.746c + 1.43f + 4.89n}.$$

Therefore, substituting these values into Equation 9-1, R_B can be expressed as

$$R_B = \frac{0.746c \cdot R_x + 1.43f \cdot R_y + 4.89n \cdot R_z}{0.746c + 1.43f + 4.89n}. \qquad \text{(Equation 9-6)}$$

Solving for c,

$$c(g/min) = \frac{1.917f(R_y - R_B) + 6.555n(R_z - R_B)}{R_B - R_x}$$

(Equation 9-7)

to express in terms of $\dot{V}O_2$:

$$\dot{V}O_2 \text{ liters/min} = 0.746c + 2.03f + 6.04n.$$

(Equation 9-8)

Therefore,

$$c(g/min) = \frac{0.945\dot{V}O_2(R_y - R_B) + n[6.555(R_z - R_B)] - 5.7036n(R_y - R_B)}{R_B - R_x + 0.70354(R_y - R_B)}$$

(Equation 9-9)

$$f(g/min) = \frac{\dot{V}O_2 - 0.746c - 6.04n}{2.03}.$$

(Equation 9-10)

From these equations, both the proportion of carbohydrate and fat oxidation (Equations 9-3 and 9-4) and the total rate of each in g/min (Equations 9-7 and 9-10) can be calculated with knowledge of only the $\dot{V}CO_2$ or the $\dot{V}O_2$. The reliance on the isotope ratio of expired CO_2, rather than the total amount of CO_2 excretion, has significant benefits in two regards. First, the isotope ratio of CO_2 can be determined with much greater accuracy than can the total $\dot{V}CO_2$. Therefore, the precision of c and f, calculated from the isotope ratio method described above, can be much greater than when indirect calorimetry is used. Second, the isotope ratio method is not directly affected by ventilatory losses of CO_2 that are not directly due to substrate oxidation, such as occurs during high-intensity exercise. In this latter circumstance, measurement of $\dot{V}O_2$ represents much less of a problem than measurement of $\dot{V}CO_2$, since it does not change for reasons other than physiological changes in substrate oxidation.

Performance of Breath Ratio Method

In order to apply the breath ratio method, it is not necessary to administer tracers, although pretreatment with ingested ^{13}C-enriched cornstarch will amplify the differences among substrates and therefore improve accuracy. The enrichments of carbohydrates, fat, and protein can be obtained from a single blood sample. It has been shown that circulating lipids are a good reflection of peripheral fat stores, and, given a constant source of carbohydrate in the diet, blood glucose reflects muscle and liver tissue glycogen enrichment (Romijn et al., 1992). The procedure involves simple extraction, combustion, and isotope ratio mass spectrometry analysis. The breath ^{13}C/^{12}C ratio can be determined on a 15- to 20-ml sample collected through a mouthpiece and injected into a vacutainer for later analysis using an isotope ratio mass spectrometer (IRMS). $\dot{V}O_2$ must be determined if the relative contributions of fat and carbohydrate are to be converted into absolute rates. Conventionally, this is accomplished by indirect calorimetry, but portable devices are available that can accomplish this in the field. Alternatively, $\dot{V}CO_2$ can be used in the calculations. For field studies, $\dot{V}CO_2$ may be approximated by a stable isotope technique involving a bolus injection of $NaH^{13}CO_3$, and collection of multiple 15-ml samples of breath for subsequent IRMS analysis (Wolfe, 1992).

Current Research Using Breath Ratio Method

Application of this method has been limited to one study of endurance-trained cyclists at rest and during steady-state exercise at 80 percent of $\dot{V}O_2$max (Romijn et al., 1992). Figure 9-1 shows the change in breath $^{13}C/^{12}C$ ratio with exercise, and Table 9-1 shows the individual values compared with values obtained from the more conventional measurement of substrate oxidation using indirect calorimetry. The results show the breath ratio method to be a reliable alternative approach to quantify substrate oxidation, both at rest and during strenuous exercise.

Scientific Advantages and Disadvantages of the Breath Ratio Methodology

The major advantage of the breath ratio method to determine the relative contributions of carbohydrate and fat oxidation to overall energy expenditure is

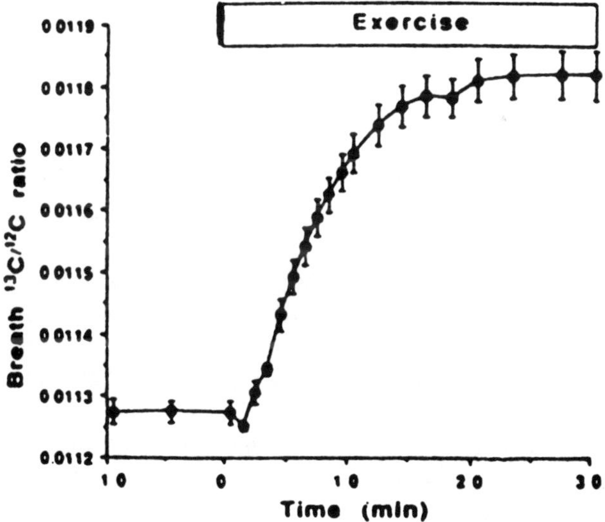

FIGURE 9-1 Absolute $^{13}C/^{12}C$ molar ratios in expired air at rest and during 30 minutes of exercise at 80 to 85 percent $\dot{V}O_2$max. Plateau value in $^{13}C/^{12}C$ enrichment is reached after 15 to 20 minutes. SOURCE: *American Journal of Physiology* (Romijn et al., 1992), used with permission.

TABLE 9-1 Substrate Oxidation Rates at Rest and During Exercise

	Carbohydrate		Fat	
Subject	Indirect Calorimetry	Ratio Method	Indirect Calorimetry	Ratio Method
		Rest		
1	1.81	1.58	1.50	1.58
2	0.59	1.00	1.80	1.65
3	0.00	0.26	2.25	2.12
4	0.27	0.65	1.86	1.72
5	2.27	2.38	1.48	1.44
6	0.93	0.80	1.72	1.77
Means ± SE	0.98 ± 0.36	1.11 ± 0.31	1.77 ± 0.12	1.71 ± 0.09
		Exercise		
1	60.48	59.41	2.92	3.37
2	36.83	29.89	5.78	8.62
3	33.98	32.99	8.38	8.80
4	37.00	38.02	9.74	9.34
5	22.49	30.44	11.25	8.03
6	45.71	59.38	5.77	3.22
Means ± SE	39.42 ± 5.20	41.69 ± 5.72	7.31 ± 1.25	6.90 ± 1.15

NOTE: Values are in $mg \cdot kg^{-1} \cdot min^{-1}$.

SOURCE: Adapted from Romijn et al. (1992).

the portability of the method, as no equipment is required. For quantifying rates of oxidation, however, there is less advantage because either $\dot{V}O_2$ or $\dot{V}CO_2$ must also be determined, and this is best accomplished with indirect calorimetry. While indirect calorimetry can be performed easily to determine either $\dot{V}O_2$ or $\dot{V}CO_2$, the conventional use of indirect calorimetry to determine the rate of substrate oxidation requires calculation of $\dot{V}CO_2 / \dot{V}O_2$, and thus both $\dot{V}CO_2$ and $\dot{V}O_2$ must be determined with great precision. This is a particular problem during intense exercise because loss of breath CO_2 occurs, not only as a result of metabolic production, but also in order to maintain acid-base balance. The resulting depletion of the bicarbonate pool invalidates indirect calorimetry as a tool to quantify substrate oxidation, yet this problem does not affect the validity of the breath ratio method because $\dot{V}O_2$ can still be determined accurately. The breath ratio method has an important advantage over traditional precursor-product tracer methods to measure substrate oxidation, in that isotopic exchange is not a problem. This is because no exogenous tracer is administered. Further, the true precursor enrichment for the formation of labeled CO_2 from an infused tracer is extremely difficult to determine accurately, since oxidation occurs intracellularly. In contrast, by utilizing the measured $^{13}C/^{12}C$ ratios in all compounds in the body (carbohydrate, fat, and protein), all possible precursor enrichments have been taken into account. Another advantage of the new ratio method, compared with the traditional tracer methods used to quantify substrate oxidation, is that changes in bicarbonate recovery that occur during exercise (Barstow et al., 1990) need not be considered. Alterations in bicarbonate recovery have no influence on the $^{13}C/^{12}C$ ratio in the expired air, since no exogenous tracer is infused. Thus, whatever pathways of CO_2 retention occur, these pathways cannot distinguish whether the CO_2 has been derived from carbohydrate or fat oxidation, and therefore the enrichment (in excreted CO_2) will not be affected by retention.

The only significant disadvantage is that the accuracy of the breath ratio method is highly dependent on the inherent differences in the ratio of $^{13}C/^{12}C$ in carbohydrate as compared to fat and protein. For this reason, it may be desirable to add ^{13}C-enriched carbohydrate to the diet. To use this method for an exercise study, however, it is necessary to use a glycogen-depleting exercise before starting the ^{13}C-glucose ingestion so that the muscle glycogen pool will be labeled (Romijn et al., 1992). Use of this protocol obviously limits the flexibility of the method.

Cost/Benefit of New Technology

The major cost incurred with this methodology is that of an IRMS, which is generally in the $200,000 to $230,000 range, with service being as much as $30,000 per year. Some less versatile units can be bought for closer to $100,000. If it is necessary to increase the enrichment of the body's carbohydrate stores, about 1 g of ^{13}C-glucose is required (Romijn et al., 1992), and this costs about $500. All other apparatus and supplies cost about $100. While the cost of the methodology may be exaggerated by these figures, it should be noted that an IRMS can be used for many other applications simultaneously.

How Practical is the Technology?

Operation of an IRMS requires a skilled technician and supervision by an experienced scientist. Training of a technician requires about 3 months. In the field, procedures are extremely simple, and all necessary procedures can be learned in about 1 hour. Data can be computed easily, as only algebraic equations are involved. However, due to extremely small differences in enrichment, an experienced investigator must be involved to ensure validity of data.

Can the Method Be Used in the Field?

One of the major advantages of this method is that it can be used easily in the field to determine the relative contributions of fat and carbohydrate oxidation to total energy production. However, field use would be limited by the requirement for quantitative oxidation rates, as indirect calorimetry would be needed.

TRACER INFUSION MEASUREMENT OF SUBSTRATE OXIDATION

When indirect calorimetry (or the breath ratio method) is used to quantify substrate oxidation, the additional use of stable isotopes to quantify substrate kinetics (i.e., the rate of release into blood and clearance from blood can provide valuable insight into the regulation of the processes involved. Substrate kinetics can only be accomplished at the whole-body level by the infusion of tracers. The basic idea of infusing a substrate such as glucose or a fatty acid such as palmitate that is labeled with ^{13}C to determine its rate of oxidation by the excretion of $^{13}CO_2$ is elegant for its simplicity. However, whereas the use of ^{13}C-labeled tracers to measure substrate oxidation is in fact feasible when proper correction factors are used to account for isotopic exchange, the methodology is far more complex than was thought in earlier years.

Description of Methodology

In this section, a specific application of tracers to quantify fatty acids and glucose kinetics in exercise will be discussed. With substrate oxidation quantified by indirect calorimetry, it is possible with tracers to distinguish the source (i.e., plasma vs. intracellular stores) of the substrate being oxidized and the regulation of the processes that make them available for oxidation. It should be kept in mind that the general approach to be presented is only representative of tracer methods and is by no means the only possible methodology using stable isotopes.

The rate of appearance of glucose in the plasma, and rate of tissue uptake, can be quantified by traditional tracer techniques using glucose with two deuterium atoms attached at the 6-carbon position (6, 6-D_2-glucose) (Wolfe, 1992). Although widely used in a variety of circumstances, this methodology has been used infrequently in exercise. One major problem has been the complications arising from the nonsteady-state kinetics induced by exercise. The limitations in calculating glucose kinetics in the nonsteady state have been well documented (e.g., Wolfe, 1992). The problems caused by rapid changes in plasma enrichment can be overcome to a great extent, however, by appropriate changes in tracer infusion rate

(Romijn et al., 1993). By first running a pilot study to determine the magnitude of change in enrichment caused by exercise, it is possible to adjust the tracer infusion rate appropriately to maintain a relatively steady state in isotopic enrichment during exercise, even when large changes in plasma glucose concentration occur (Romijn et al., 1993). This approach enables accurate calculation of glucose appearance and uptake, even in strenuous exercise.

From the total rate of carbohydrate oxidation, obtained by indirect calorimetry, and the rate of tissue glucose uptake (R_d), determined by means of the tracer, the minimum contribution of muscle glycogen stores to carbohydrate oxidation can be calculated, assuming that 100 percent of plasma glucose uptake is oxidized during exercise (Romijn et al., 1993). If less than 100 percent is oxidized, the calculated value for intramuscular glycogen oxidation will be underestimated. Therefore, the following equation provides the minimal rate of muscle glycogen oxidation:

$$\text{muscle glucogen oxidation} = \text{total carbohydrate oxidation} - \text{glucose } R_d.$$

Thus, by this method, any glycogen breakdown that leads to lactate production rather than complete oxidation will not be included in the calculation of rate of oxidation. Glycogen breakdown therefore exceeds the calculated rate of glycogen oxidation by a percentage amount equal to the percent of plasma glucose converted to lactate, since the metabolic pathways of glycogen and glucose converge at glucose 6-phosphate and are the same thereafter.

Fatty acids are the predominant energy substrate in almost all circumstances in the fasting state, except during extremely strenuous exercise. Understanding the factors controlling the release of fatty acids as a result of the breakdown of stored triglyceride (TG) (lipolysis) and the oxidation of fatty acids therefore is central to understanding the metabolic response in exercise. Recent advances in stable isotope methodology now allow the quantitative aspects of many components of fatty acid kinetics and oxidation to be determined.

Because the enzyme glycerol kinase is necessary for the first step in the metabolism of glycerol, and this enzyme is found only in the liver (Dixon and Webb, 1979, 842–843), glycerol can only be metabolized in the liver. Hence, lipolysis can be quantified by means of the determination of the rate of appearance of glycerol, as determined by a stable isotope tracer of glycerol such as $^2H_5$ or $2\text{-}^{13}C$-glycerol (Wolfe, 1992). Furthermore, since glycerol dissolves freely in water, there is no limitation to the amount of glycerol that can diffuse from the intracellular site of lipolysis into the plasma. Also, there is no endogenous metabolic production of glycerol (Wolfe and Peters, 1987). Finally, there is virtually no partial hydrolysis of triglyceride (Arner and Ostman, 1974), meaning that three fatty acids are released uniformly with every glycerol molecule that is released.

The fatty acids released into the intracellular space of the adipocyte have two potential fates—entry into the plasma or reesterification into triglycerides within the adipocyte. The process of reesterification involves the attachment of three fatty acids to α—glycerol phosphate derived from the metabolism of plasma glucose.

This may occur because of an abundance of α—glycerol phosphate, as occurs during hyperglycemia (Wolfe and Peters, 1987), or because of a low rate of blood flow through the fat. A decrease in blood flow is important because FFA are not soluble in water. They are carried in plasma bound to albumin, and availability of binding sites on albumin can be rate limiting for transport when blood flow is low.

Once released into the plasma, the fatty acids can be cleared, by tissues such as muscle, for oxidation, or they can be cleared by the liver and reesterified into TG and transported back to the periphery as very low density lipoprotein. Thus, in the general sense, TG-FFA cycling can be considered to involve the reesterification of fatty acids that have been initially released as a consequence of lipolysis.

The difference between the total release of fatty acids and the rate of appearance (Ra) of fatty acids in the plasma (FFA Ra) is equal to the rate of reesterification of fatty acids within the adipocyte. The FFA Ra can be determined by means of a labeled tracer of any individual FFA (e.g., [1-^{13}C]-palmitate), and then converted to total FFA turnover by dividing Ra palmitate by the fraction of the total FFA concentration represented by palmitate (determined by gas chromatography). As mentioned earlier, this calculation presumes that all fatty acids released by lipolysis either enter the plasma or are reesterified. It also is possible that fatty acids might be "directly" oxidized without entering the plasma. This would cause an overestimation of the intracellular recycling of FFA. However, it seems unlikely that this pathway of oxidation occurs to a great extent at rest. Data from a large number of experiments demonstrate the ratio of FFA Ra/Ra glycerol to be about 3/1 (e.g., Miyoshi et al., 1988; Wolfe et al., 1987). Since "direct" oxidation of FFA would involve the release of glycerol into the plasma, the ratio of FFA Ra/Ra glycerol would be significantly less than 3 if there was much of this type of oxidation. This is precisely the observation in strenuous exercise, as will be discussed below.

Given the rate of total lipolysis and total FFA release into (and uptake from) plasma and the rate of total fat oxidation, it is possible to distinguish quantitatively between lipolysis in adipose tissue (peripheral lipolysis) and intramuscular lipolysis. If all FFA taken up from the plasma during exercise can be assumed to be oxidized (Romijn et al., 1993), then the following equation provides a minimal rate of intramuscular fatty acid oxidation:

$$\text{intramuscular fatty acid oxidation } (\mu\text{mol·kg}^{-1}\text{·min}^{-1})$$
$$= \text{total fatty acid oxidation } (\mu\text{mol FFA·kg}^{-1}\text{·min}^{-1}) - \text{FFA R}_d,$$

where FFA R_d is the rate of tissue uptake of FFA. For every three fatty acids released from the intramuscular triglyceride pool, one glycerol will be released into plasma. Consequently, the minimum rate of release of glycerol from the intramuscular TG pool (intramuscular lipolysis) will be calculated as follows:

$$\text{intramuscular lipolysis } (\mu\text{mol·kg}^{-1}\text{·min}^{-1})$$
$$= \frac{\text{intramuscular fatty acid oxidation } (\mu\text{mol FFA·kg}^{-1}\text{·min}^{-1}).}{3 \ \mu\text{mol FFA}/\mu\text{mol glycerol}}$$

The total rate of glycerol release is equal to the glycerol released from peripheral adipocytes plus the glycerol released from the intramuscular pool. Consequently, it is possible to calculate the rate of adipocyte (peripheral) lipolysis as follows:

$$\text{peripheral lipolysis } (\mu\text{mol·kg}^{-1}\text{·min}^{-1})$$
$$= \text{total glycerol Ra} - \text{intramuscular lipolysis } (\mu\text{mol·kg}^{-1}\text{·min}^{-1}).$$

Review of Application of Methodology

Tracer infusion has been used to assess substrate metabolism in highly trained endurance cyclists at three different exercise intensities (25, 65, and 80% $\dot{V}\text{O}_2\text{max}$). The subjects were studied in the postabsorptive state on 3 consecutive days. On each day, a different exercise intensity was performed; the order of the intensities was randomized. On each occasion, stable isotopes were infused, and indirect calorimetry was used to determine substrate oxidation. The following tracers were infused: 6,6-D_2-glucose; $^2\text{H}_5$-glycerol; and $^2\text{H}_2$-palmitate. Changes in tracer infusion rates maintained plasma enrichments relatively constant.

The contribution to energy expenditure derived from glucose and FFA taken up from blood and from muscle glycogen and triglyceride are shown in Figure 9-2. The total amount of calories available from plasma does not change in relation to exercise intensity. At higher exercise intensities, muscle stores of glycogen and triglyceride become more important as energy substrates.

Scientific Advantages and Disadvantages

Alternative methodologies utilizing stable isotope tracers include the tissue or organ balance technique, biopsy analysis, and the use of radioactive tracers.

The balance technique, in which the arteriovenous difference of a substrate is multiplied by the rate of blood flow, can provide useful information about regional metabolism, but the balance approach cannot be used to quantify glucose production or the whole-body rate of lipolysis. The leg balance technique can give information about muscle, but strict interpretation of the data is made difficult by the inclusion of blood from skin and fat in the femoral vein. Finally, no information about the metabolism of the intramuscular stores of carbohydrate (i.e., glycogen) or TG can be obtained with the balance technique.

Considerable information about muscle glycogen metabolism has been obtained from biopsy data, but this approach has been far less successful in analyzing intramuscular TG metabolism. Limitations of the biopsy approach are its invasiveness and the unquantitative nature of the data as related to whole-body substrate metabolism.

The use of tracer methodology as described in this paper is relatively noninvasive, in that only peripheral venous catheters are required (for infusion of tracer and removal of samples). Further, a continuum of data can be obtained, as opposed

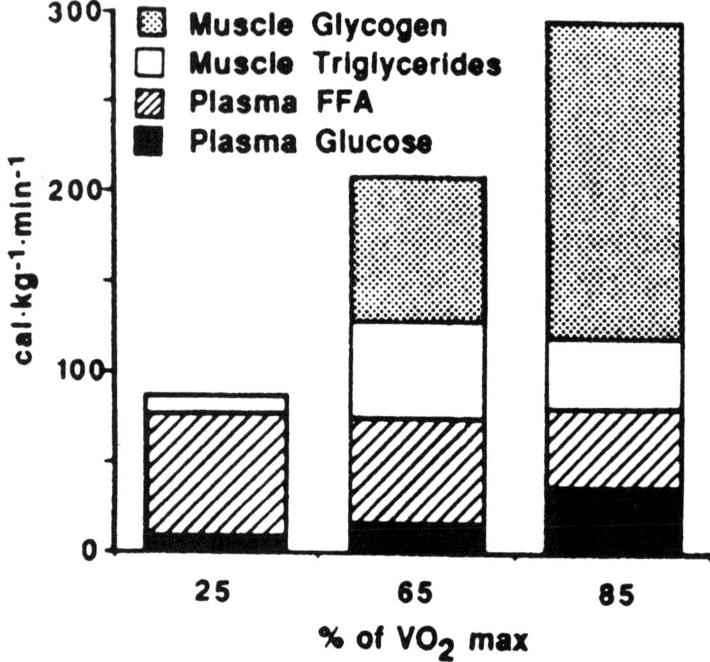

FIGURE 9-2 Maximal contribution to energy expenditure derived from glucose and free fatty acids (FFA) taken up from blood and minimal contribution of muscle triglyceride and glycogen stores after 30 minutes of exercise, expressed as function of exercise intensity. Total energy (cal) available from plasma does not change in relation to exercise intensity. SOURCE: *American Journal of Physiology* (Romijn et al., 1993), used with permission.

to the spot samples obtained by biopsy. Although assumptions are required to quantify intramuscular glycogen and TG metabolism, these assumptions are reasonable, and this is the only way to obtain such estimates, as well as the only method to quantify plasma fatty acid and glucose kinetics. In theory, the experiments described in this paper could be done with radioactive tracers. Advantages provided by stable isotopes are that they pose no health risk, and the isolation of compounds by gas chromatography prior to mass spectrometry not only provides a high degree of precision in analysis but also enables the concurrent use of multiple tracers. In the example provided in which glucose, glycerol, and FFA kinetics were determined during exercise, three different tracers labeled with ^{2}H were used. It would be extremely difficult (or impossible) with routine analytical procedures to use simultaneously three tracers labeled with the radioactive label ^{3}H and sort out the relative contributions of the three compounds to the observed radioactivity.

The only potential disadvantage of stable isotope methodology is that a larger amount of stable isotope tracer must be infused then when a radioactive tracer is used. This limits the experimental protocols so that the experimental procedure does not affect the endogenous kinetics of the substrate being traced.

AUTHOR'S CONCLUSIONS AND RECOMMENDATIONS

The use of tracers labeled with stable isotopes is the most effective means by which to quantify plasma substrate kinetics. The technology is readily available, and gas chromatography-mass spectrometers (GC-MS) are being produced at progressively lower prices as computers become available. An adequate GC-MS for the procedures described in this paper can be purchased for about $75,000. The cost of stable isotopes varies according to the tracer, but an individual experiment will cost about $200. The use of stable isotopes to quantify substrate oxidation is complicated by the need to make appropriate corrections for isotopic exchange, and in many circumstances, it can be more easily accomplished by classical indirect calorimetry. However, for specific applications, the use of tracers is valuable and can be accomplished with precision and accuracy.

Support of further development of the methodology is probably not required. The limitation of the methodology to field studies is significant because infusion pumps and intravenous infusions are required for optimal performance of the techniques. As currently used, this methodology is limited to a lab setting. Modifications to enable field studies are possible but not yet developed.

REFERENCES

Arner, P., and J. Ostman
  1974   Mono and di-acyl glycerols in human adipose tissue. Biochem. Biophys. Acta 369:209–221.
Barstow, T.J., D.M. Cooper, E.M. Sobel, E.M. Landau, and S. Epstein
  1990   Influence of increased metabolic rate on ^{13}C-bicarbonate washout kinetics. Am. J. Physiol. 259:R163–R171.
Dixon, M., and E.L. Webb
  1979   Enzymes. New York: Academic.
Frayn, K.N.
  1983   Calculation of substrate oxidation rates *in vivo* from gaseous exchange. J. Appl. Physiol. 55:628–634.
Miyoshi, H., G.I. Schulman, E.J. Peters, M.H. Wolfe, D. Elahi, and R.R. Wolfe
  1988   Hormonal control of substrate cycling in humans. J. Clin. Invest. 81:1545–1555.
Romijn, J.A., E.F. Coyle, J. Hibbert, and R.R. Wolfe
  1992   Comparison of indirect calorimetry and a new breath ^{13}C/^{12}C ratio method during strenuous exercise. Am. J. Physiol. 263(28):E64–E71.
Romijn, J.A., E.F. Coyle, L.S. Sidossis, A. Gastaldelli, J.F. Horowitz, E. Endert, and R.R. Wolfe
  1993   Regulation of endogenous fat and carbohydrate metabolism in relation to exercise intensity and duration. Am. J. Physiol. 265 (28):E380–E391.
Wolfe, R.R.
  1992   Radioactive and Stable Isotope Tracers In Biomedicine: Principles and Practice of Kinetic Analysis. New York: Wiley-Liss.

Wolfe, R.R., and E.J. Peters
  1987   Lipolytic response to glucose infusion in human subjects. Am. J. Physiol.
         252(15):E189–E196.
Wolfe, R.R., E.J. Peters, S. Klein, O.B. Holland, J. Rosenblatt, and H. Gary, Jr.
  1987   Effect of short-term fasting on the lipolytic responsiveness in normal and obese
         human subjects. Am. J. Physiol. 252:E189–E196.

DISCUSSION

VERNON YOUNG: Bob, would you just remind me what the protocol is with respect to the slide about three slides back where you brought the oxidative contribution of plasma and intracellular fats, what is the actual protocol?

ROBERT WOLFE: The subjects are infused with ^{13}C-oleate and ^{14}C-octanoate.

VERNON YOUNG: No, I do not mean the oleate, but the earlier one which you indicated was totally noninvasive.

ROBERT WOLFE: In that protocol, the subjects are infused with ^{13}C-palmitate and deuterated glucose. Then the substrate oxidation is measured by indirect calorimetry.

In the calculation of the data, the assumption was made that during exercise, 100 percent of plasma glucose uptake is oxidized, so the calculation gives you a minimal value for intramuscular glycogen.

Alternatively, if ^{13}C-glucose was infused, plasma glucose oxidation could be measured directly by collecting $^{13}CO_2$. However, previous data indicate that most glucose uptake is oxidized in exercise, and in any case, plasma glucose makes a small contribution to the total rate of oxidation. Therefore, the assumption is reasonable.

JOHANNA DWYER: Is that published somewhere?

ROBERT WOLFE: Yes, that experiment is in *The American Journal of Physiology* (Romijn et al., 1993) about a year or two ago.

WENDY KOHRT: Does your model take into account the possibility that fatty acids hydrolyzed from intramuscular triglycerides could be released into the plasma?

ROBERT WOLFE: I kind of skipped over some of the details. To the extent to which free fatty acids [FFA] are released into the plasma, then they become part of the plasma pool, so they are included in the measurement of the plasma FFA enrichment. The evidence would indicate that this process does not occur to any significant extent, and the reason is that in situations in which significant intramuscular triglyceride hydrolysis occurs, the rate of release of glycerol into blood increases dramatically in relation to free fatty acid release. There are three fatty acids relative to one glycerol normally released as a consequence of the hydrolysis of triglyceride, but the muscle has a very limited ability to use glycerol.

As the exercise intensity increases, the rate of whole-body glycerol/FFA Ra drops from approximately 3:1 to as low as 1:1, indicating almost all the fatty acid that is released from muscle triglyceride is directly oxidized in the muscle and the glycerol released into the plasma.

DONALD McCORMICK: It bothered me that this technique could not be made to do good kinetic work. You gave examples of releases of cellular drug in the plasma. Unless another very significant correction is made, every time one passes a membrane, one has the problem of diffusion. So every time you are going from wherever the site of origin is, whether oral or injected, to a series of membranes, mitochondria and otherwise, you are discriminating between ^{12}C and ^{13}C or ^{12}C and ^{14}C, and that is a multiple effect. You are not getting a reflection of the real kinetics of the predominant ^{13}C pool compound. The smaller the molecule, the greater the discrimination.

What I am really after is obviously the question of whether you can do a ^{13}C mass spectrometric analysis and a ^{14}C radiotracer and get at what the effects are of multiple membranes, say, in fatty acid oxidation, whether you can get the time factor. When you are doing steady state or whole body, it does not matter. But do you or others have those factors in the kinetic sense?

ROBERT WOLFE: The extent to which ^{13}C is discriminated as opposed to ^{12}C, I think, is of minimal concern, and the reason I say that is that if you look at the data on which we based the total oxidation of carbohydrate, protein, and fat, using the ^{13}C/^{12}C breath ratio method, the values come out almost exactly the same as with indirect calorimetry, which means the same rates are obtained without use of isotopes. Furthermore, kinetic studies with radio-labeled tracers and stable isotope tracers yield comparable data.

DONALD McCORMICK: Those are long lump times, though.

ROBERT WOLFE: I presented values derived almost entirely in steady state conditions. The kinetic modeling in nonsteady state with a stable isotope is more complex, but I would say it can be done. But I think that in terms of nutritional aspects and total substrate oxidation I would definitely recommend staying away from that. The problems, however, are more with modeling than isotope discrimination.

DENNIS BIER: With regard to the isotope effects, there are rather sizable isotope effects if you are talking about deuterium and tritium. If you look at the mass differences that are smaller, I mean, people have investigated ^{13}C and ^{12}C isotope effects on the molecular level, on the biochemical level, on the cellular level, and even with totally ^{13}C-labeled enzymes, for example, compared to their substrates, the differences are about 1 to 2 percent. I mean, they are small enough that we cannot measure them.

Now, we can tell those differences by isotope ratio mass spectrometry because that can measures parts per 100,000. That is exactly the basis of isotope fractionation in breath, the kind of thing Bob talked about with substrate oxidation, but it is below the limits of any detection that you can do.

DONALD McCORMICK: At steady state.

DENNIS BIER: Right. There is at least one set of experiments that I know of where people tried to look at transport in an organ with different isotope-labeled materials, specifically glucose, and that was done by Riccardo Bonnadonna, Ralph DeFronzo, Clyde Epidelli, myself, and others, where we gave ^{13}C with different labels and modeled the differences between those isotopes as they appeared inside the cell and they appeared in metabolites, et cetera, to discriminate transport, and in fact, we think we were successful.

Emerging Technologies for Nutrition Research, 1997
Pp. 231–257. Washington, D.C.
National Academy Press

10

Combined Stable Isotope-Positron Emission Tomography for *In Vivo* Assessment of Protein Metabolism

*V. R. Young,[1] Y-M. Yu, H. Hsu, J. W. Babich, N. Alpert,
R. G. Tompkins, and A. J. Fischman*

INTRODUCTION

The improved biochemical assessment of protein nutritional status and determination of quantitative dietary needs to maintain homeostasis and function in individuals, especially those who may be subjected to significant stress as in military combat situations, remain important research challenges for nutritional physiologists and biochemists. The advantages and limitations of approaches that have been taken so far to assess protein nutritional status have been discussed previously (Young et al., 1990). In that review it was proposed that an expanded application of stable isotope tracer techniques and of sophisticated

[1] V. R. Young, Laboratory of Human Nutrition, Massachusetts Institute of Technology, Cambridge, MA 02139; Shriners Burns Institute and Departments of Surgery and Radiology, Massachusetts General Hospital, Boston, MA 02114

The authors' studies were supported by grants from the Shriners Hospitals for Crippled Children and the National Institutes of Health (GM 21700, DK 15856, T 32-GM 07035, and T 32-CA 09362).

physicochemical measurements ought to offer an opportunity to make significant progress in nutritional evaluation. Therefore, this possibility has continued to be explored, and in this short review paper, particular attention will be given to presenting preliminary results from recent studies in this laboratory involving simultaneous use of stable isotope tracers and of imaging techniques involving positron emission tomography (PET).

To establish a reasonable framework for the discussion to follow, a general organization of body protein and amino acid metabolism is depicted in Figure 10-1; this includes some examples of the types of biochemical measures used to assess the status of the different metabolic-organ systems indicated. In the present context of a consideration of emerging technologies, however, the working hypothesis is that, by accumulating reliable data on the quantitative rates of protein anabolism and catabolism in various regions and organs of the body, practical new diagnostic tools can be developed for assessment of protein nutritional status in individuals under various pathophysiological states. Hence, the goal has been to refine, apply, and further develop noninvasive methods for determination of (1) protein turnover at the whole body and organ-tissue levels and (2) turnover of specific proteins *in vivo*. The principal analytical methods that have been exploited by this laboratory to date are those of isotope ratio and selected ion monitoring mass spectrometry and, more recently, positron emission tomography imaging.

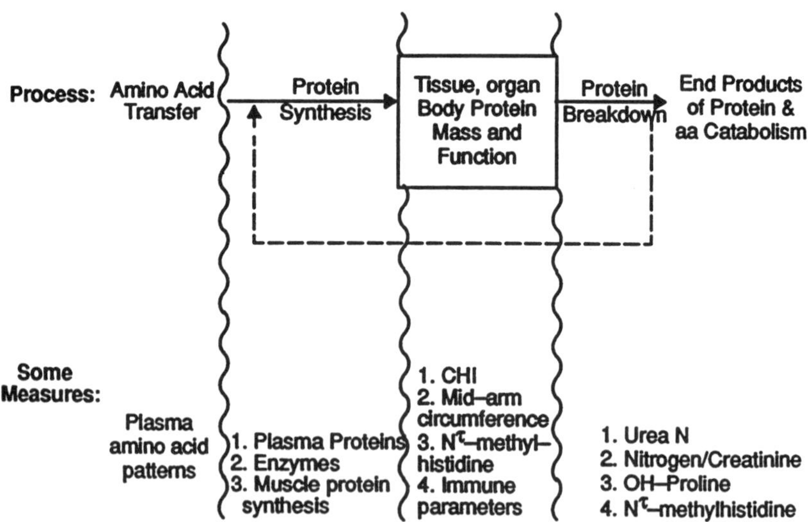

FIGURE 10-1 A simplified organization of protein and amino acid metabolism, with an indication of the major systems involved and measures used to assess the status of these systems. CHI, creatine height index; Urea N, urea nitrogen; OH-Proline, hydroxyproline. SOURCE: Young et al. (1990) © *J. Nutr.* (120:1496–1502), American Society for Nutritional Sciences. Figure is based on G. Arroyave.

Because there has been substantial discussion previously, as well as elsewhere in these workshop proceedings, on the use of stable isotope tracer techniques in protein nutritional metabolic research (Halliday and Rennie, 1982; Matthews and Bier, 1983; Waterlow et al., 1978; Young et al., 1991), the major focus of attention in this paper will be with respect to PET. This is a technique familiar to many concerned with clinical nuclear medicine, but it is the authors' position that emission computed tomography has not yet been embraced sufficiently or understood as an experimental tool for nutritional metabolic research. Hence, it will first be indicated why it is an exciting prospect to use PET, and then a general account will be presented of the physical principles involved in PET and methods used for imaging. For this purpose, summary tables and figures will be used to illustrate major points and then discussion will turn briefly to some actual or potential applications of these techniques in nutritional research before a summary and a series of conclusions are drawn.

ISOTOPE TRACER ESTIMATES OF PROTEIN AND AMINO ACID TURNOVER *IN VIVO*

Stable Isotope Techniques

The advantages and disadvantages of use of stable isotope tracers for nutritional metabolic studies have been discussed by Bier in these proceedings (see Chapter 8) and also elsewhere (Matthews and Bier, 1983). However from the present perspective, it is pertinent to emphasize that these tracers have been applied extensively in studies of whole body protein (nitrogen) and amino acid kinetics in human subjects. A widely used model for estimation of whole body rates of protein turnover is the "two-pool plasma precursor model" (Figure 10-2); this might involve, for example, use of $[1\text{-}^{13}C]$leucine as tracer, with the rates then being based on isotopic data obtained with blood and expired air samples, following intravenous and/or oral administration of amino acids labeled with ^{13}C or ^{15}N and/or ^{2}H (Garlick and McNurlan, 1994; Waterlow, 1995). In addition, ^{15}N-end product methods have been applied for determination of rates of whole body protein synthesis, most often by giving $[^{15}N]$glycine as tracer and then measuring the isotopic abundance of nitrogen in urinary urea and ammonia (Grove and Jackson 1995; Waterlow 1995). This latter approach is sufficiently safe and noninvasive to be applied in studies involving infants, pregnant women, and repeated measurements in other individuals or patients where blood sampling and/or venous puncture could not be justified or where it is not practical to do so. In both instances (precursor method and end-product method), whole body measurements of protein synthesis and breakdown rates are obtained. These parameters have been found to be quite valuable for enhancing understanding of human protein metabolism and nutrition, and it is clear that they represent a major investigative advance over information gained from the whole-body nitrogen balance method. However, they do not give any informa-

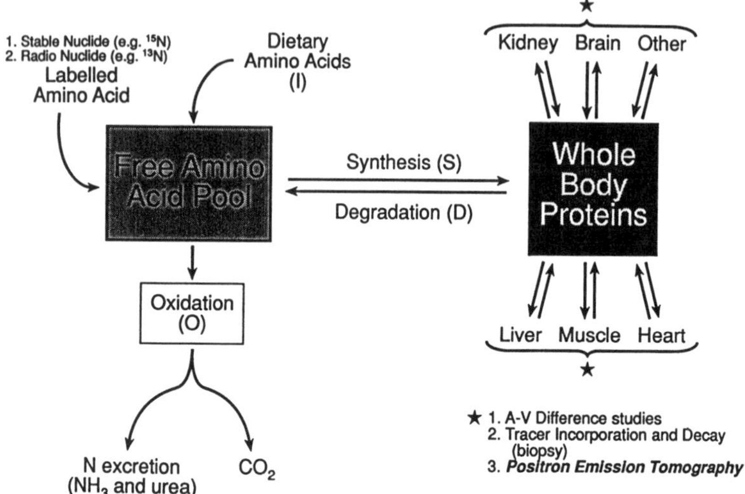

FIGURE 10-2 The two-pool model that is used widely to calculate rates of whole body protein synthesis and degradation (turnover) from data obtained with stable isotope (e.g., ^{15}N or ^{13}C) labeled amino acids. This diagram indicates that the turnover of whole body proteins is the sum of those occurring in the different organs and tissues. In separate or simultaneous studies, along with stable isotope tracers, rates in these specific regions might be determined from arteriovenous (A-V) difference studies, by measurement of incorporation of labeled tracers into and their loss from proteins and/or by positron emission tomography, using a short-lived radionuclide such as ^{13}N. SOURCE: Adapted from Garlick and McNurlan (1994).

tion about the quantitative contribution made by the major organs and tissues that collectively contribute to the status of whole-body protein balance and its integrity, nor do the parameters elucidate the changes occurring within those organs and tissues, possibly in different directions. Attempts are made to emphasize this point in Figure 10-2, which attempts to convey the need to dissect the kinetic parameters of whole body protein turnover into its major components, particularly by developing estimates of protein synthesis and breakdown in the principal protein-active organs such as liver, muscle, and the intestines.

Indeed, various approaches have been used to examine the dynamic status of protein and amino acid metabolism within individual tissues and organs, and these basically involve (1) arteriovenous (A-V) balance determinations across an organ (Tessari et al., 1995; Yu et al., 1990) or limb (Biolo et al., 1995; Cheng et al., 1985), while infusing a labeled amino acid such as ^{2}H-phenylalanine or [^{15}N, ^{13}C]leucine, or (2) a direct measurement of the incorporation of a labeled amino acid into tissue protein by taking a biopsy of the specific tissue (e.g., Essen et al., 1992; Nair et al. 1988, 1995; Welle et al., 1993; Yarasheski et al.,

1992, 1993). Although analytical developments now allow these types of studies to be conducted with much smaller tissue samples than were required previously (Calder et al., 1992), both of these major approaches are invasive, which limits their broad and convenient application in human nutritional-metabolic research.

Finally, in relation to an understanding of the integration of amino acid metabolism *in vivo* and how stressful conditions might compromise metabolism and homeostasis, it would be of considerable interest to develop a detailed picture of the quantitative metabolic fate of the individual amino acids within and among various organs. As illustrated in Figure 10-3, there is an organ specificity or orientation to the metabolism of the individual amino acids (e.g., Munro 1983; Young and El-Khoury, 1995), and the nutritional status of the individual will depend in part on how well the roles of the organs involved and their interactions with other organs are maintained. These could well be affected by dietary, hormonal, and other factors, including infection and physical and psychological stressors. Furthermore, the status of protein and amino acid metabolism within discrete areas of an organ, including the brain (Williams et al., 1994), also might be affected by such factors. It is within this metabolic framework that investigators in this laboratory have turned recently to an exploitation of PET for assisting in the inquiry into human protein metabolism under different conditions of health and disease. Therefore, the principles and some of the practical issues involved in PET and its application to nutritional research will now be

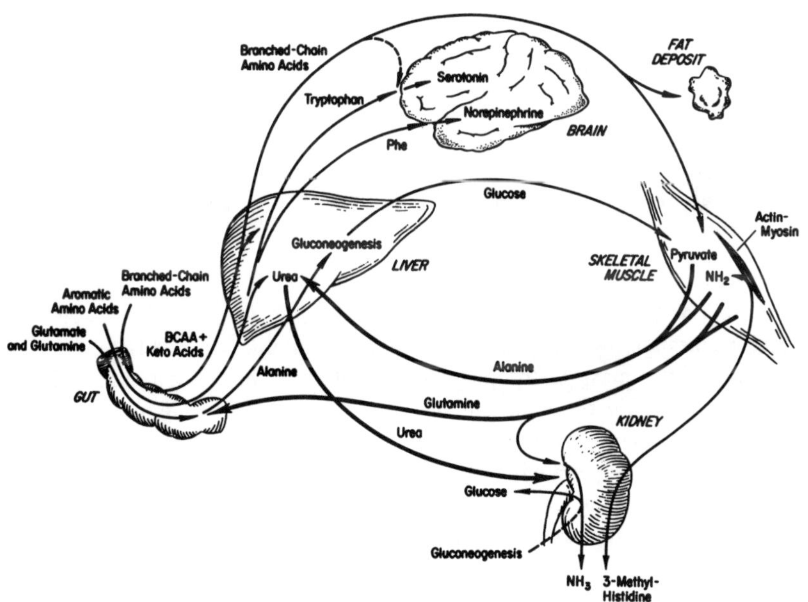

FIGURE 10-3 A simplified outline of the organ fate and origin of various amino acids. SOURCE: Adapted from Munro (1983).

considered in brief. This is done to help the informed reader, who may nevertheless be unfamiliar with PET, to perhaps better appreciate both its advantages and limitations. The discussion is, therefore, somewhat superficial, but consultation of the references will serve to elaborate upon the points made here.

Positron Emission Tomography

PET is a technique for measuring the concentration of a positron-emitting radio isotope, within a three-dimensional body, via external detection of the radiation emerging from the isotope. Positron-emitting radio nuclides of carbon, nitrogen, oxygen, and fluorine can be prepared readily, and because these elements are present in compounds that are relevant to the study of *in vivo* aspects of amino acid-protein metabolism, PET offers an opportunity to enhance current investigations of specific organ and tissue protein metabolism by the noninvasive means that will be discussed below. The basic principles of PET and measurement techniques are as follows, while the reader is referred to more extensive discussions for further detail (Christian, 1994; Daghighian et al., 1990; Fowler and Wolf, 1986; Hoffman and Phelps, 1986; Links, 1994; Ter-Pogossian et al., 1980).

Positron Decay and Coincidence Detection of Radiation Annihilation

Proton-rich nuclides decay to a more stable isotope by two possible decay processes: (1) by electron capture and (2) by positron decay, which is the particular emission of interest in this paper. In this latter process, a proton (p) is converted to a neutron (n), a positron (a positive electron, β^+), a neutrino (v), and energy, as follows:

$$p = n + \beta^+ + v + energy.$$

The emitted positron, after traveling a short distance, combines with an electron in the surroundings, resulting in an annihilation interaction.[2] This latter event converts all of the mass of the positron and electron into electromagnetic energy, which results in the emission of two 0.511-MeV photons (gamma rays) (Christian, 1994). These two gamma rays travel in very nearly opposite directions (Figure 10-4), penetrate the surrounding tissue, and are recorded outside of the subject by a circular array of detectors, which permit measurement of both the quantity and the location of the positron-emitting radio isotope (Daghighian et al., 1990; Links, 1994). Because the two annihilation photons are created si-

---

[2] In an annihilation interaction, the rest mass of the electron-positron pair disappears and is replaced by the two 511-KeV photons, in accord with conservation of energy and momentum.

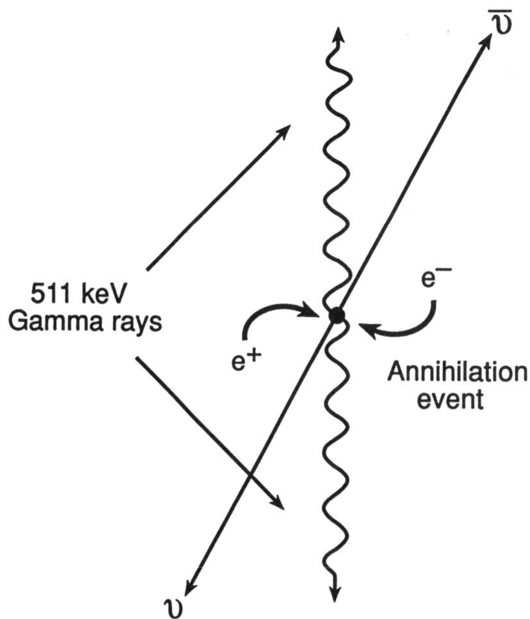

FIGURE 10-4 Annihilation of positron and electron produces two 0.511-MeV gamma photons. υ, neutrino; $\overline{\upsilon}$, antineutrino. SOURCE: P. E. Christian in *Nuclear Medicine, Technology and Techniques*, 3d ed., D. R. Bernier, P. E. Christian, and J. K. Langan, eds., St. Louis, 1994, Mosby.

multaneously, as well as being emitted at 180° angles to each other, the electronics of the detectors are arranged so as to count only coincident events in the opposite detectors (i.e., within a 5 billionth of a second). This, then, is the principle of annihilation coincidence detection (Figure 10-5) (Hoffman and Phelps, 1986). Gamma rays originating outside of the space between the two detectors interact with only one of the detectors per annihilation, and these rays are not counted, also as illustrated in Figure 10-5. It might be appreciated, therefore, that the accuracy of the tissue localization of activity and the detection efficiency depend on the size and cross-sectional geometry of the detectors and the detector materials used in their construction. These factors influence the cost of the equipment used in measurements, with scanners generally now costing over $2 million. Additional details concerning detector systems and image reconstruction are given elsewhere (Daghighian et al., 1990; Links, 1994), but it should be evident that PET can be used to image, in a quantitatively functional context, *in vivo* aspects of tissue metabolism, blood flow, and receptor occupancy, for example. However, PET cannot distinguish among different chemical (metabolic) species since it only measures radioactivity concentration. This is a major limitation of this technique, where, for example, specific meta-

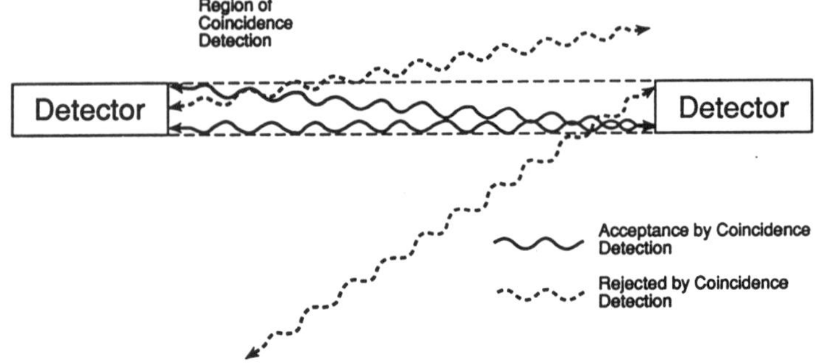

FIGURE 10-5 Schematic diagram of the principle of annihilation coincidence detection. SOURCE: Hoffman and Phelps, "Positron emission tomography: Principles and quantitation" in *Positron Emission Tomography and Autoradiography: Principles and Applications for the Brain*, 1986, pp. 237–286, reprinted with permission of Lippincott-Raven Publishers.

bolic interconversions are of particular interest in addition to where they are occurring within body tissues and organs.

Nuclide Production and Radiotracer Synthesis

While a large number of positron-emitting radionuclides exist, the physical properties of some positron (β^+)-emitters are summarized in Table 10-1. Additionally for comparison, information also is listed here about the more traditional radioisotopes, ^{14}C and ^3H. The half lives of the four positron emitters given in this table range from 2 minutes (^{15}O) to 110 minutes (^{18}F), and these physical properties offer some flexibility in tailoring the design of metabolic PET studies. For example, it is possible to use $H_2^{15}O$ to measure blood flow in a particular tissue or organ and then, after a short while, to give ^{18}F-deoxyglucose

TABLE 10-1 Physical Properties of ^{11}C, ^{15}O, ^{13}N, ^{18}F, ^3H, and ^{14}C

Nuclide	Half Life	Decay Mode
^{11}C	20.4 min	β+
^{15}O	2.07 min	β+
^{13}N	9.96 min	β+
^{18}F	109.7 min	β+
^3H	12.35 yr	β–
^{14}C	5,730 yr	β–

as a tracer to measure the glucose metabolic rate in the same organ. These nuclides are produced within a cyclotron whose design varies, and this determines cost and production capability (Fowler and Wolf, 1986). However, this aspect of PET-related technology will not be detailed further here.

With respect to carbon-11 (^{11}C), it is produced by ^{11}B (p,n)^{11}C and ^{14}N (p,α)^{11}C nuclear reactions (Table 10-2), with ^{11}C-labeled carbon monoxide (^{11}CO), carbon dioxide (^{11}CO$_2$), and cyanide (^{11}CN) being used as precursors for radiotracer synthesis (Table 10-3). ^{13}N is also cyclotron produced, generally via the ^{16}O (p,α)^{13}N nuclear reaction, which is performed using a water target to yield a [^{13}N]nitrate ion (Quaim et al., 1993). ^{13}N-ammonia can be produced directly by deuteron bombardment of methane and then, following purification, can be used for the synthesis of ^{13}N-labeled amino acids or other compounds using both biosynthetic and synthetic strategies (Fowler and Wolf, 1986). Some examples of the types of ^{11}C-, ^{13}N-, and ^{18}F-labeled compounds that can be made and could, perhaps, be used as probes of protein amino acid and substrate metabolism *in vivo* are listed in Table 10-3. This table was generated from data presented in the extensive review about positron-emitter tracers by Fowler and Wolf (1986).

APPLICATIONS OF PET

Although PET has not yet found extensive use in nutritional or metabolic research, its spatial resolution and quantitative features allow quantification of metabolic parameters in volumes of tissue as small as 1.0 cm^3. Thus, PET techniques have been validated for measurement of regional blood flow, blood volume, pH, and oxygen utilization (Huang et al., 1986) and applied in studies of glucose metabolism in the brain (Phelps et al., 1986), for measuring blood flow (Huang et al., 1983; Raichle et al., 1983), glucose metabolism and tricarboxylic acid cycle activity in the myocardium (Huang and Phelps, 1986; Schelbert and Schwaiger, 1986), and regional glucose uptake (leg, arm, and heart) (Nautila et al., 1993). Only limited studies using PET have been conducted on amino acid metabolism in peripheral tissues (e.g., Hawkins et al., 1989; Planas et al., 1992),

TABLE 10-2 Production of Positron-Emitting Radionuclides

Nuclide	Production
^{11}C	^{14}N(p,α)^{11}C
^{15}O	^{14}N(α,n)^{15}O
^{13}N	^{16}O(p,α)^{13}N
^{18}F	^{18}O(p,n)^{18}F

TABLE 10-3 Some Positron-Labeled Compounds that Have Been Synthesized for Biomedical Studies

Compound	Labeled Precursor
[^{11}C] Amino Acids	
L-[1-^{11}C]phenylalanine	H[^{11}C]N
L-[1-^{11}C]alanine	[^{11}C]O$_2$
L-[methyl-^{11}C]methionine	[^{11}C]O$_2$
L-[1-^{11}C]leucine	H[^{11}C]N
^{18}F-Labeled Compounds	
2-deoxyl-2[^{18}F]fluoro-D glucose	[^{18}F]F$_2$
3-deoxy-3-[^{18}F]fluoro-D glucose	H[^{18}F]anhydrous
^{13}N-Labeled Compounds	
L-[^{13}N]asparagine	[^{13}N]H$_3$
L-[^{13}N]leucine	[^{13}N]H$_3$
L-[^{13}N]methionine	[^{13}N]H$_3$

SOURCE: Adapted from Fowler and Wolf (1986).

although this technique is particularly attractive because in principle it is possible to make sequential, site-specific, time-dependent physiological and biochemical measurements within the same subject. More importantly, due to its relatively noninvasive nature, PET measurements can be made routine for application in experiments with human subjects.

L-methyl-[^{11}C]methionine (^{11}C-Met) has been found to be a useful tracer with PET for evaluation of amino acid kinetics *in vivo* (e.g., Stalnacke et al., 1982) and for detection of tumors (Bustany et al., 1986; Kubota et al., 1985; LaFrance et al., 1987; Mosskin et al., 1987). Therefore, and because it was possible to prepare ^{11}C-Met without a considerable synthetic or analytical research developmental effort (Figure 10-6), this laboratory has explored recently whether and how ^{11}C-Met might be used to estimate the rate of mixed protein synthesis in skeletal muscle. The major reasons for doing this and a summary of the initial results are given below.

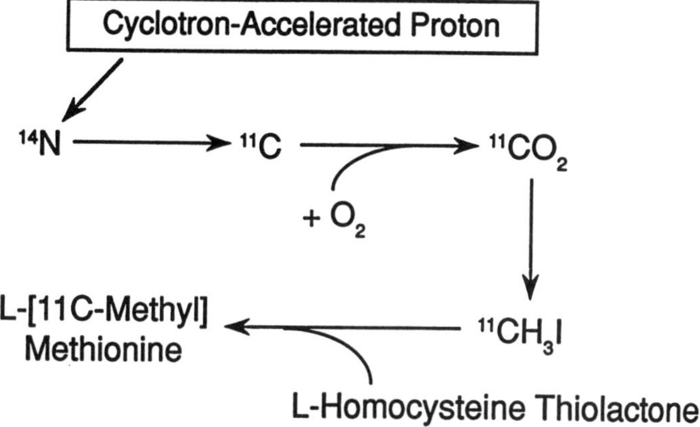

FIGURE 10-6 A general outline of one route of synthesis of L-[^{11}C-methyl]methionine. Further details given in Fowler and Wolf (1986) and Meyer et al. (1993).

Muscle Protein Synthesis as Measured with PET

Importance of Skeletal Muscle

The maintenance of lean body mass is critical for continued cell and organ function, whether this relates to the physical performance of the individual or the capacity to withstand a stressful condition, such as systemic infection. A major contributor to the total lean mass of the body is the skeletal musculature. This accounts for about 40 percent of body weight (Forbes, 1987, 171) and approximately 52 percent of the combined protein in the muscle and nonmuscle mass of the body (Cohn et al., 1980). Hence, it might be predicted that changes in the size and metabolic status of the skeletal musculature would have significance for the well-being and functional capacity of the individual. For example, in reference to energy metabolism, the skeletal musculature (1) is the principal site of facultative thermogenesis in response to excess carbohydrate (Astrup and Christensen, 1992), (2) acts as a buffer to maintain glucose homeostasis during postprandial energy-yielding substrate storage (Taylor et al., 1993), (3) is a major determinant of daily basal energy expenditure (Zurlo et al., 1990), and (4) accounts (Tzankoff and Norris, 1977) for a large proportion, if not all, of the decline in basal or resting energy expenditure during aging (McGandy et al., 1966; Vaughan et al., 1991; Young, 1992). Further, the skeletal musculature plays a key role in the regulation, maintenance, and integration of whole-body nitrogen homeostasis (Young, 1970). An example of this latter point is depicted in Figure 10-7, which shows that branched chain amino acids, glutamine, and arginine metabolism interact via the active participation of the skeletal musculature, intestines, kidney, and liver. The point to be emphasized here is that there are metabolically significant interactions and signaling among these major anatomic regions, in amino acid and protein metabolism. Hence, it is important to

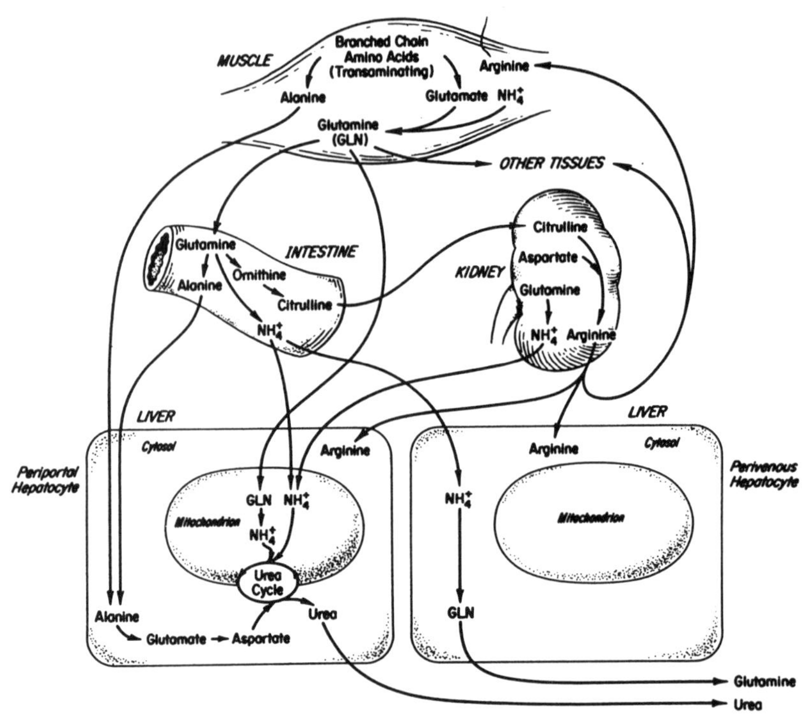

FIGURE 10-7 Outline of the metabolism of arginine, with reference to the cooperative involvement of the skeletal musculature intestines, kidney, and liver. SOURCE: Adapted from Brusilow and Horwich (1989).

learn how changes in the size, and possibly metabolic status, of the musculature under various physiological and stressful conditions affect the integrity of these metabolic interrelationships and, in consequence, the ability of the individual to cope with the environment.

Additionally, body protein wasting is a significant contributor to morbidity and death in a variety of catabolic disease states (Hill, 1992; Manning and Shenkin, 1995), with the major source of this loss being from skeletal muscle (Kinney, 1995; Kinney and Elwyn, 1983; Rennie, 1994). However, it should be pointed out that Muller et al. (1995) did not find that either the absolute level of muscle mass or the change in muscle mass during the advancing years in male subjects, who were participants in the Baltimore Longitudinal Study of Aging, was related to all-cause mortality. Perhaps, upon more detailed examination, muscle may be found to be more important in relation to morbidity and death due to infection and trauma while less so in relation to that associated with degenerative disease, including cardiovascular and arteriosclerotic disease and cancers at some organ sites.

For these various reasons a detailed, quantitative understanding of the *regional* distribution of protein and amino acid utilization and of the ways by which imbalances between protein synthesis and breakdown occur in the major organs will be required if more effective nutritional-pharmacological strategies for attenuating these losses and for improving upon the tools used for assessment of nutritional status are to be developed. Furthermore, a more complete and secure understanding of the metabolic etiology for changes in muscle mass under various conditions might begin with reliable *in vivo* estimates of the rates of myofibrillar and sarcoplasmic protein synthesis and breakdown under various pathophysiological conditions. For example, recent studies using ^{13}C-leucine as a tracer, followed by tissue biopsy, have shown that the fractional rate of mixed muscle or myofibrillar protein synthesis is significantly lower (about 30–40%) in elderly subjects (Welle et al., 1993; Yarasheski et al., 1993) as compared with younger adults. This age-related change in synthesis might represent an important mechanism that accounts for the diminished muscle mass in the elderly (Muller et al., 1995). However, a greater research effort needs to be focused on the *in vivo* regulation of muscle protein and amino acid metabolism, including determination of protein synthesis and breakdown rates, in adult human subjects under various pathophysiological conditions, such as those conditions experienced by military personnel in field operations. This is made more pertinent because measurements of protein synthesis may correlate with muscle strength, as suggested by the recent studies of Urban et al. (1995) concerning the effects of testosterone on muscle function and metabolism in elderly men. Of course, it also is equally important to determine whether and to what extent inflammatory mediators, such as interleukin-1 and tumor necrosis factor, determine the status of protein synthesis and breakdown (e.g., Goodman, 1991; Roubenoff and Rall, 1993; Zamir et al., 1992a, b) in skeletal muscle and to identify the multiple proteolytic pathways that might be involved (Goldberg and St. John, 1976; Sugden and Fuller, 1991; Thorne and Lockwood, 1993). These mediators are altered by infection as well as by vigorous exercise.

Initial Studies with PET

For the various reasons given above, as well as to establish a basis for the design and conduct of a series of studies in healthy adult control subjects and in preparation for later studies in different groups of hospitalized patients, an initial experiment was carried out with the aid of PET using ^{11}C-Met (Hsu et al., 1996) on the transport and metabolism of methionine in the skeletal muscle of anesthetized dogs. Data analyses were performed by fitting tissue- and metabolite-corrected, arterial blood-time-activity curves to a three-compartment model. The model structure included vascular space, tissue precursor, and protein compartments. The results of the PET measurements then were compared with data from simultaneous studies using A-V difference measurements during primed constant infusion of L-[1-^{13}C-methyl-^{2}H$_3$]methionine (^{13}C-^{2}H$_3$-Met). The A-V difference-stable isotope tracer approach has been applied by this laboratory and other investigators to quantify muscle protein metabolism within the limbs of human subjects (e.g., Biolo et al., 1995; Cheng et al., 1985; Tessari et al., 1991).

The details of this approach and the methods involved are presented in a recent publication (Hsu et al., 1996), but a few points might first be made before a summary of the results of this laboratory is presented below. First, the decision to conduct an initial study with ^{11}C-Met as a tracer was made, in part, because it has been shown that while isoenzymes of methionine adenosyltransferase, which catalyze synthesis of S-adenosylmethionine, are active in liver, kidney, and bone marrow, the specific activity of this enzyme is about 30-fold lower in heart and skeletal muscle (Finkelstein, 1990; Mudd et al., 1965). Therefore, it is reasonable to assume that most of the radioactivity that is retained in skeletal muscle following a dose of ^{11}C-Met would reflect its incorporation into proteins. Furthermore, in contrast to some other ^{11}C-labeled tracers, such as 1-^{11}C-leucine, analysis of PET studies with ^{11}C-Met, at least with reference to muscle, is not complicated by a contribution of ^{11}CO$_2$ to total blood radioactivity (Hawkins et al., 1989; Ishiwata et al., 1988). Nevertheless, much research remains to be carried out with respect to determination and evaluation of the choice and application of specific positron emitter-labeled amino acids for studies of regional aspects of body protein and specific amino acid metabolism in the human subject.

Second, for purposes of data analysis, the compartmental model that is illustrated in Figure 10-8 was applied. The rate constants K$_1$ (or K$_{2,1}$) and k$_2$ (or k$_{1,2}$) represent forward and reverse transport of methionine between plasma and tissue, and k$_3$ (or k$_{3,2}$) represents incorporation of the label into proteins, nucleic acids, creatine, and lipids. Due to the expected low level of transmethylation in

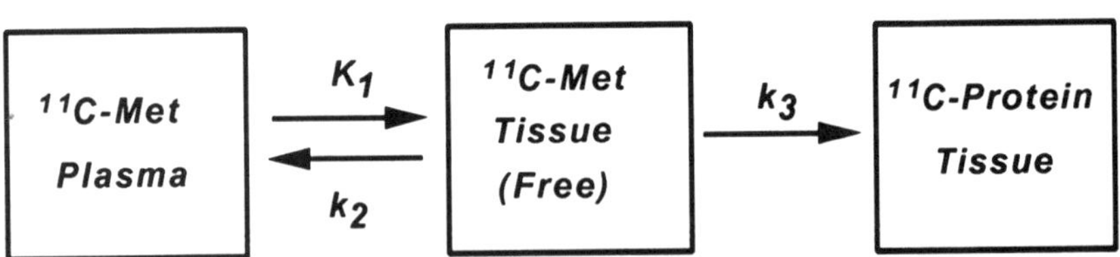

FIGURE 10-8 Kinetic model for ^{11}C-Met utilization by skeletal muscle. The model assumes that the rates of transamination and transmethylation of methionine in this tissue are low and it contains vascular space, tissue precursor, and protein compartments. The rate constants K$_1$ (K$_{2,1}$) and k$_2$ (k$_{1,2}$) represent forward and reverse transport of methionine between plasma and tissue, and k$_3$ (k$_{3,2}$) represents incorporation into proteins. SOURCE: Hsu et al. 1996. Measurement of muscle protein synthesis by positron emission tomography with L-[methyl^{11}C]methionine. Proc. Natl. Acad. Sci. USA 93:1841–1846. Copyright (1996) National Academy of Sciences, U.S.A.

muscle as already noted above, $k_{2,3}$ is taken to reflect the rate of total protein synthesis in this tissue (PSR = Protein Synthetic Rate). Radioactivity in the vascular compartment was represented by a blood volume fraction parameter; the model parameters were estimated by least squares fitting of the predicted tissue concentrations of methionine (based on measured whole blood ^{11}C radioactivity and the concentration of free labeled methionine plasma) to the tissue concentrations measured by PET (Hsu et al., 1996). Third, in the PET component of this PET-stable isotope tracer investigation, it was possible to assess the rate of muscle protein synthesis in two regions of the skeletal musculature: in the paraspinal muscles and in those in the hind leg. This was accomplished by first carrying out a 90-min ^{11}C-Met tracer study with the scanner oriented over the paraspinal muscle region. Then a second injection of ^{11}C-Met was given followed with a 90-min study and imaging over the hind leg region.

The Results and Their Interpretation

Estimated model parameters and values for PSR and $T_{\frac{1}{2}}$ (half life) of the tissue precursor (methionine) pool from PET for paraspinal and hind limb muscles are summarized in Table 10-4. No significant differences between hind limb and paraspinal muscles were detected for $K_{2,1}$; $k_{1,2}$; $k_{3,2}$; and PSR, and as shown in Figure 10-9, PSRs calculated for hind limb and paraspinal muscle were highly correlated.

PSR_{A-V} in the limb, as determined using a primed constant infusion of ^{13}C-^{2}H$_3$-Met together with A-V difference measurements of methionine isotopomer concentrations across the hind limb, was equivalent to 0.27 ± 0.05 nmol methionine $min^{-1} \cdot g^{-1}$. Hence, these results demonstrate that PSR_{A-V}, expressed in relation to the weight of limb tissue, is somewhat, but not greatly, higher than that based on the PET approach. Since the stable isotope procedure

TABLE 10-4 Kinetic Parameters for L-[Methyl-^{11}C]Methionine Metabolism in Paraspinal and Hind Limb Muscles

Muscle Region	$K_{2,1}$ (ml·min^{-1}·g^{-1})	$k_{1,2}$ (min^{-1})	$k_{3,2}$ (min^{-1})	PSR (nmol·min^{-1}·g^{-1})
Paraspinal	0.0154[*]	0.0266	0.0124	0.172
	± 0.0058	± 0.0094	± 0.0049	± 0.062
Hind Limb	0.0170	0.0304	0.0155	0.208
	± 0.0055	± 0.0100	± 0.0058	± 0.048

[*] Mean ± SEM.

SOURCE: Adapted from Hsu et al. (1996).

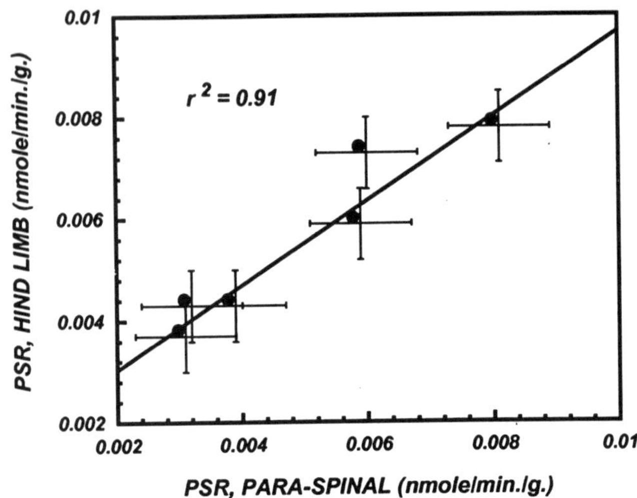

FIGURE 10-9 Relationship between the estimate of PSRs determined by PET for hind limb and paraspinal muscle. SOURCE: Hsu et al. 1996. Measurement of muscle protein synthesis by positron emission tomography with L-[methyl^{11}C]methionine. Proc. Natl. Acad. Sci. USA 93:1841–1846. Copyright (1996) National Academy of Sciences, U.S.A.

measures methionine utilization across the entire limb, whereas the PET-derived estimate is for muscle tissue specifically, some of the difference appears to be explained by bone marrow methionine metabolism and by the higher fractional rate of protein synthesis in the skin (Biolo et al., 1994).

Whole-body methionine kinetics also were measured in these dogs (Unpublished data, Y-M. Yu, Shriners Burns Institute, Boston, Mass., 1996), and so it was possible to estimate the relative contribution made by hind limb protein synthesis to the whole-body protein synthesis rate. A summary of these findings is presented in Table 10-5. According to these data, about 7 percent of the whole-body protein breakdown was accounted for by the breakdown of proteins in the left leg. This is a value that seems to be in reasonable line with the anticipated contribution by skeletal muscle to body protein metabolism if it can be compared with data for the adult human, where the entire skeletal musculature accounts for about 25 percent of total whole-body protein turnover. This latter value was arrived at by assuming (1) a whole-body protein breakdown rate of approximately 4 g·kg^{-1}·day^{-1} (Waterlow, 1995), (2) a muscle protein mass of 3.8 kg (Cohn et al., 1980), and (3) a muscle mixed protein fractional synthesis rate of about 1.95 percent per day (Garlick and McNurlan, 1994; Smith and Rennie, 1990).

TABLE 10-5 Rates of Protein Synthesis and Breakdown in the Whole Body and Hind Leg of Dogs Given a Constant Intravenous Infusion of L-[^{2}H$_3$-methyl-1-^{13}C]Methionine

Parameter	Value
Whole body (g·kg^{-1}·day^{-1})	
Protein synthesis	3.4 ± 0.5[*†]
Protein breakdown	4.5 ± 0.5
Hind limb as percentage of whole body	
Protein synthesis	7.3 ± 0.7
Protein breakdown	8.0 ± 0.5

[*] Mean ± SEM for seven dogs.

[†] The whole-body rate was based on the model of Storch et al. (1988) and the values for the hind leg based on the approach described by Yu et al. (1990) for leucine and as discussed in Hsu et al. (1996).

The Implications and Some Comments

A number of additional comments might be made in reference to this initial PET study. First, this investigation into the use of PET for purposes of quantifying protein metabolism *in vivo* has encouraged this laboratory to begin to plan a preliminary series of studies in human subjects, especially because the available estimates of amino acid metabolism in specific organs and tissues have been derived mostly from A-V difference or tissue biopsy studies, as mentioned earlier. However, the A-V difference technique has several limitations when applied in human studies: (1) measurements cannot be performed in tissues and organs that do not have a discrete venous drainage; (2) for organs with a single venous drainage (such as kidney), the catheterization required for measuring A-V differences may be unsuitable for routine application; (3) the measurements have limited anatomic resolution (i.e., A-V differences across the entire region alone cannot be used to determine the individual contributions made by muscle, bone marrow, fat, and skin to substrate utilization); and (4) relatively long tracer infusion times (~5 hours) are required for many of these studies.

However, PET provides a rapid, routine noninvasive, *in vivo* method for the quantitative analysis of some tissue-specific biochemical processes. Compared then with the A-V difference techniques, PET has several advantages: (1) the measurements require only a metabolite-corrected arterial input function and imaging, (2) the anatomic resolution of PET allows measurements to be performed on tissue volumes as small as 1.0 cm^3, and (3) due to the short half lives of the tracers, repetitive studies can be performed in the same subject. The limitations of the PET methodology include: (1) an exposure of the subject to ionizing radiation, (2) inability to make a direct estimate of the specific metabolic pathways followed by the tracer, and (3) in comparison with the A-V difference method, PET does not provide a measure of protein breakdown.

The second comment is that the potential importance of the influence of blood flow rate and substrate delivery on metabolism emerges from these data. Thus, from the present stable isotope and leg weight data, the rate of protein synthesis in the total hind limb of these experimental animals was found to be equivalent to 7.3 ± 1.7 (mean $\pm$ SD) g·day^{-1}. This compares with limited published values of about 3.2 g·day^{-1} (Barrett et al., 1987) and 8.6 to 11.5 g·day^{-1} (Biolo et al., 1992) for the hind limbs of dogs of comparable body weight. The authors believe that these differences might well be related to the blood flow rate across the limb during the study. In the study described here, PET measurements required that the leg of the dog be immobile. Hence, the dogs were heavily sedated and the hind limb restrained. These are procedures that could well have affected regional blood flow and the status of protein and amino acid metabolism in the limb. Recent reviews (Clark et al., 1995; Elia, 1995) emphasize the importance of blood flow on oxygen and substrate delivery in affecting metabolism in tissues and organs. In the present study, mean hind limb blood flow rate was 91 ml·min^{-1}, whereas it was about 228 to 240 ml·min^{-1} in studies by Biolo et al. (1992, 1994) and 33 ml·min^{-1} in that of Barrett et al. (1987). Thus, when differences in blood flow rates are taken into consideration, the rate of limb protein synthesis measured in the present study appears to be similar to these other published values.

Of further relevance to these workshop proceedings is the fact that cold exposure induces changes in blood flow to the skin and extremities, and high-altitude exposure can result in reduced blood flow in peripheral tissues (IOM, 1996). As noted above, blood flow can be accurately measured using oxygen-15 [^{15}O]water, and due to the short half life of ^{15}O, this tracer permits blood flow measurements to be made in conjunction with other metabolic studies involving positron emitter-labeled compounds in physiological studies. A major limitation, of course, is that such blood flow studies have to be carried out in the physical proximity of the cyclotron.

Third, in this study, high levels of ^{11}C-Met utilization by bone marrow also were noted (Hsu et al., 1996). This finding emphasizes the further potential value of PET in that it allows a simultaneous, discrete examination of the metabolic activity of different tissues within a particular organ.

Finally, in view of the authors' interest in the regulation of muscle protein mass and the metabolic basis that underlies changes in physical performance, it ought to be recognized that the PET approach described briefly above does not directly lead to an estimate of the rate of muscle protein breakdown. However, it would be entirely feasible to combine PET with one of the stable isotope protocols described elsewhere in this volume. The model that is proposed is the one described by Rathmacher et al. (1995), involving a bolus dose of L-3[^{2}H$_{3}$-

methyl]histidine given into the vein, followed by compartment modeling of the plasma tracer data. This is based on the principle that 3-methylhistidine, a component of actin and myosin, is a marker of muscle protein breakdown (Young and Munro, 1978). The model described by Rathmacher and coworkers (1995) is presented in Figure 10-10; for the present purpose it is shown to illustrate yet another example of the research value to be derived from a combined stable isotope-PET approach for *in vivo* assessment of protein metabolism in human subjects.

AUTHORS' SUMMARY AND CONCLUSIONS

This paper has attempted to illustrate the potential, as well as the limitations, of PET as an investigative technique in nutritional research. Within the past 10 years, major improvements in the production and handling of short-lived isotopes have occurred (Stocklin and Pike, 1993), and this has gone in step with advances in the design and use of instrumentation for radiation detection and tomography. Now, more than a hundred PET groups have been established worldwide. It might be anticipated, therefore, that there will be an expanded use of PET in nutritional-metabolic research. However, at the same time, it is recognized that PET is not likely to become widely available to the entire nutri-

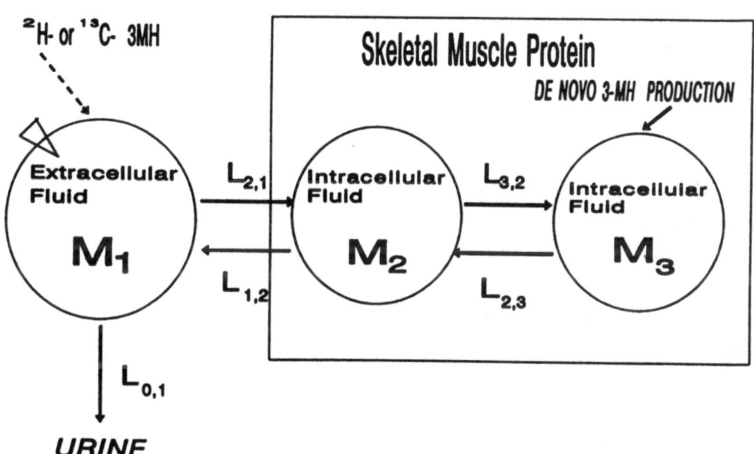

FIGURE 10-10 Schematic of a three-compartment model to analyze the kinetics of distribution, metabolism, and *de novo* production of 3-methylhistidine (3-MH) in human subjects. M_1, M_2, and M_3 represent the mass of 3-MH in compartments 1, 2, and 3, respectively. $L_{2,1}$, $L_{1,2}$, $L_{0,1}$, $L_{2,3}$, and $L_{3,2}$ are fractional transfer rate coefficients of 3-MH within the system. The tracer, 3-[^{2}H$_3$-methyl]-methylhistidine (D$_3$.3-MH), is injected into compartment 1. Sampling is performed from compartment 1(∇). *De novo* production of 3-MH occurs in compartment 3. SOURCE: Adapted from Rathmacher et al. (1995).

tional research community, even in the United States, and so it will probably remain a valuable technique at a limited number of academic research centers during the foreseeable future.

Finally, in preparing this paper the authors were asked to address a number of questions that relate to the technology discussed, and these, together with their brief answers, are presented in Table 10-6. As pointed out by Faulkner et al. (1991), the technology associated with positron imaging is extremely complex; a successful PET clinical research program requires a highly skilled team of scientists and technologists working in well-equipped, specialized laboratories and involves a significant annual financial expenditure. Nevertheless, the authors believe that it is entirely reasonable to suggest that, where the necessary mixture of technical expertise, collaborative interest and physical facilities exist, or where there is an obvious institutional commitment, PET must be considered among the exciting new and emerging technologies for nutritional and metabolic research.

TABLE 10-6 PET in Reference to Emerging Technologies: Some Questions and Answers

---

Will the technology be a significant improvement over current technologies?

    There is no alternative to a noninvasive "view" of the distribution of human amino acid metabolism *in vivo*.

How likely is the technology to mature sufficiently for practical use, and if so, how soon will it be available?

    It is available now but only in selected medical-academic centers.

Cost-benefit ratio?

    High cost: $2 million for camera, $2 million for cyclotron.

    Benefit: Probably also very high, but who knows?

What about Small Business Innovative Research?

    Certainly in the area of tracer development.

Practicality?

    It is demanding and complex but exciting! Multidisciplinary.

Field-testing scenarios?

    Not at all.

REFERENCES

Astrup, A., and N.J. Christensen
  1992 Role of the sympathetic nervous system in obese and post-obese subjects. Pp. 299–309 in Energy Metabolism: Tissue Determinants and Cellular Corollaries, J.M. Kinney and H.G. Tucker, eds. New York: Raven Press.

Barrett, E.J., J.H. Revkin, L.H. Young, B.L. Zavel, R. Jacob, and R.A. Gelfand
  1987 An isotopic method for measurement of muscle protein synthesis and degradation *in vivo*. Biochem. J. 245:223–228.

Biolo, G., D. Chinkes, X-J. Zhang, and R.R. Wolfe
  1992 A new model to determine *in vivo* the relationship between amino acid transmembrane transport and protein kinetics in muscle. J. Parenter. Enteral Nutr. 16:305–315.

Biolo, G., A. Gastaldelli, X-J. Zhang, and R.R. Wolfe
  1994 Protein synthesis and breakdown in skin and muscle: A leg model of amino acid kinetics. Am. J. Physiol. 267:E467–E474.

Biolo, G., R.Y.D. Fleming, and R.R. Wolfe
  1995 Physiologic hyperinsulinemia stimulates protein synthesis and enhances transport of selected amino acids in human skeletal muscle. J. Clin. Invest. 95:811–819.

Brusilow, S.W., and A.L. Horwich
  1989 Urea cycle enzymes. Pp. 629–663 in The Metabolic Basis of Inherited Disease, C.R. Scriver, A.L. Beaudet, W.S. Sly, and D. Valle, eds. New York: McGraw-Hill Info. Services Co., Health Professions Division.

Bustany, P., M. Chatel, J.M. Derlon, P. Sgouropoulos, F. Soussaline, and A. Syrota
  1986 Brain tumor protein synthesis and histological grades; a study by positron emission tomography (PET) with C-11-L-methionine. J. Neurooncol. 3:397–404.

Calder, A.G., S.E. Anderson, I. Grant, M.A. McNurlan, and P.J. Garlick
  1992 The determination of low d_5-phenylalanine enrichment (0.001–0.09 atoms percent excess), after conversion to phenylethylamine, in relation to protein turnover studies by gas chromatography/mass spectrometry. Rapid Commun. Mass Spectrom. 6:421–424.

Cheng, K.N., F. Dworzak, G.C. Ford, M.J. Rennie, and D. Halliday
  1985 Direct determination of leucine and protein metabolism in humans using L-[1-^{13}C,^{15}N]-leucine and the forearm model. Eur. J. Clin. Invest. 15:349–354.

Christian, P.E.
  1994 Physics of nuclear medicine. Pp. 35–52 in Nuclear Medicine. Technology and Techniques, 3rd ed., D.R. Bernier, P.E. Christian, and J.K. Langan, eds. St. Louis, Mo.: Mosby.

Clark, M.G., E.Q. Colquhoun, S. Rattigon, K.A. Dora, T.P.D. Eldershaw, J.L. Hall, and J. Ye
  1995 Vascular and endocrine control of muscle metabolism. Am. J. Physiol. 268:E797–E812.

Cohn, S.H., D. Vartsky, S. Yasamura, A. Sawitsky, I. Zoni, A. Vaswani, and K.J. Ellis
  1980 Compartmental body composition based on total-body nitrogen, potassium and calcium. Am. J. Physiol. 239:E524–E530.

Daghighian, F., R. Sumida, and M.E. Phelps
  1990 PET imaging: An overview and instrumentation. J. Nucl. Med. Technol. 18:5–15.

Elia, M.
  1995 General integration and regulation of metabolism at the organ level. Proc. Nutr. Soc. (London) 54:213–232.

Essen, P., M.A. McNurlan, J. Wernerman, E. Vinnars, and P.J. Garlick
  1992 Uncomplicated surgery, but not general anesthesia, decreases muscle protein synthesis. Am. J. Physiol. 262:E253–E260.

Faulkner, D.B., K.J. Kearfott, and R.G. Manning
 1991   Planning a clinical PET center. J. Nucl. Med. Technol. 19:5–19.
Finkelstein, J.D.
 1990   Methionine metabolism in mammals. J. Nutr. Biochem. 1:228–237.
Forbes, G.B.
 1987   Human Body Composition. Growth, Aging, Nutrition and Activity. New York: Springer-Verlag.
Fowler, J.S., and A.P. Wolf
 1986   Positron emitter-labeled compounds: Priorities and problems. Pp. 391–450 in Positron Emission Tomography and Autoradiography: Principles and Applications for the Brain, M.E. Phelps, T.C. Mazziotta, and H.R. Schelbert, eds. New York: Raven Press.
Garlick, P.J., and M.A. McNurlan
 1994   Isotopic methods for studying protein turnover. Pp. 29–47 in Protein Metabolism During Infancy, N.C.R. Räihä, ed. New York: Raven Press.
Goldberg, A.L., and A. St. John
 1976   Intracellular protein degradation in mammalian and bacterial cells. Annu. Rev. Biochem. 45:747–802.
Goodman, M.N.
 1991   Tumor necrosis factor induces skeletal muscle protein breakdown in rats. Am. J. Physiol. 260:E727–E730.
Grove, G., and A.A. Jackson
 1995   Measurement of protein turnover in normal man using the end-product method with oral [^{15}N]glycine: Comparison of single-dose and intermittent-dose regimens. Br. J. Nutr. 74:491–507.
Halliday, D., and M.J. Rennie
 1982   The use of stable isotopes for diagnosis and clinical research. Clin. Sci. 63:485–496.
Hawkins, R.A., S-C. Huang, J.R. Barrio, R.E. Keen, D. Feng, J.C. Mazziotta, and M.E. Phelps
 1989   Estimation of local cerebral protein synthesis rates with 1-[1-^{11}C]leucine and PET: Methods, model and results in animals and humans. J. Cereb. Blood Flow Metab. 9:446–460.
Hill, G.L.
 1992   Disorders in Nutrition and Metabolism in Clinical Surgery. Edinburgh: Churchill Livingstone.
Hoffman, E.J., and M.E. Phelps
 1986   Positron emission tomography: Principles and quantitation. Pp. 237–286 in Positron Emission Tomography and Autoradiography: Principles and Applications for the Brain, M.E. Phelps, J.S. Mazziotta, and H.R. Schelbert, eds. New York: Raven Press.
Hsu, H., Y-M. Yu, J.W. Babich, J.F. Burke, E. Livini, R.G. Tompkins, V.R. Young, N.M. Alpert, and A.J. Fischman
 1996   Measurement of muscle protein synthesis by positron emission tomography with L-[methyl^{11}C]methionine. Proc. Natl. Acad. Sci. USA 93:1841–1846.
Huang, S-C., and M.E. Phelps
 1986   Principles of tracer kinetic modeling in positron emission tomography and autoradiography. Pp. 287–346 in Positron Emission Tomography and Autoradiography: Principles and Applications for the Brain and Heart, M. Phelps, J. Mazziotta, and H. Schelbert, eds. New York: Raven Press.

Huang, S-C., R.E. Carson, E.J. Hoffman, J. Carson, N. MacDonald, J.R. Barrio, and M.E. Phelps
   1983   Quantitative measurement of local cerebral blood flow in humans by positron computed tomography and O-15 water. J. Cereb. Blood Flow Metab. 3:141–153.
Huang, S-C, D.G. Feng, and M.E. Phelps
   1986   Model dependency and estimation reliability in measurement of cerebral oxygen utilization rate with oxygen-15 and dynamic positron emission tomography. J. Cereb. Blood Flow Metab. 6:105–119.
IOM (Institute of Medicine)
   1996   Nutritional Needs in Cold and in High-Altitude Environments, Applications for Military Personnel in Field Operations, B.M. Marriott and S.J. Carlson, eds. A report of the Committee on Military Nutrition Research, Food and Nutrition Board. Washington, D.C.: National Academy Press.
Ishiwata, K., W. Vaalburg, P.H. Elsinga, A.M.J. Paana, and M.G. Waldreng
   1988   Comparison of L-[1-^{11}C]methionine and L-methyl-[^{11}C]methionine for measuring *in vitro* protein synthesis rates with PET. J. Nucl. Med. 29:1419–1427.
Kinney, J.M.
   1995   Metabolic responses of the critically ill patient. Crit. Care Clin. 11:569–585.
Kinney, J.M., and D.H. Elwyn
   1983   Protein metabolism and injury. Annu. Rev. Nutr. 3:433–466.
Kubota, K., T. Matsuzawa, M. Ito, K. Ito, T. Fujiwara, Y. Abe, S. Toshioka, H. Fukuda, J. Hatazawa, R. Iwata, S. Watanuki, and T. Ido
   1985   Lung tumor imaging by positron emission tomography using C-11-L-methionine. J. Nucl. Med. 26:37–42.
LaFrance, N.D., L. O'Tauma, V. Villemagne, J. Williams, K. Douglas, R.F. Dannals, H. Ravert, A. Wilson, H. Drew, J. Links, D. Wong, B. Carson, H. Brem, L. Strauss, and H.N. Wagner
   1987   Quantitative imaging and follow-up experience of C-11-L-methionine accumulation in brain tumors with positron emission tomography. J. Nucl. Med. 26:37–42.
Links, J.M.
   1994   Instrumentation. Pp. 53–85 in Nuclear Medicine Technology, D.R. Bernier, P.E. Christian, and J.K. Langan, eds. St. Louis, Mo.: Mosby.
Manning, E.M.C., and A. Shenkin
   1995   Nutritional assessment in the critically ill. Crit. Care Clin. 11:603–634.
Matthews, D.E., and D.M. Bier
   1983   Stable isotopes for nutritional investigation. Annu. Rev. Nutr. 3:309–339.
McGandy, R.B., C.H. Barrows, Jr., A. Spanias, A. Meredith, J.L. Stone, and A.H. Morris
   1966   Nutrient intakes and energy expenditure in men of different ages. J. Gerontol. 21:581–587.
Meyer G-J., H.H. Coenen, S.L. Waters, B. Langstrom, R. Contineau, K. Strijckmans, W. Vaalburg, C. Hallidin, C. Crouzel, B. Maziére, and A. Luxen
   1993   Quality assurance and quality control of short-lived radiopharmaceuticals for PET. Pp. 91–150 in Radiopharmaceuticals for Positron Emission Tomography, G. Stocklin and V.W. Pike, eds. Dordrecht, The Netherlands: Kluwer Academic Publishers.
Mosskin, M., H. von Holst, M. Bergstrom, V.P. Collins, L. Ericksson, P. Johnstrom, and G. Norén
   1987   Positron emission tomography with ^{11}C-methionine and computed tomography of intracranial tumors compared with histopathologic examination of multiple biopsies. Acta Radiol. 28:673–681.

Mudd, S.H., J.D. Finkelstein, F. Irreverre, and L. Laster
  1965 Transsulfuration in mammals. Microassays and tissue distributions of three enzymes of the pathway. J. Biol. Chem. 240:4382–4392.
Muller, D.C., D. Elahi, J.D. Sorkin, and R. Andres
  1995 Muscle mass: Its measurement and influence on aging. The Baltimore Longitudinal Study of Aging. Pp. 60–62 in Nutritional Assessment of Elderly Populations: Measure and Function, I.H. Rosenberg, ed. New York: Raven Press.
Munro, H.N.
  1983 Metabolic basis of nutritional care in liver and kidney disease. Pp. 93–105 in Nutritional Support of the Seriously Ill Patient, R.W. Winters and H.L. Green, eds. New York: Academic Press, Inc.
Nair, K.S., D. Halliday, and R.C. Creggs
  1988 Leucine incorporation into mixed skeletal muscle protein in humans. Am. J. Physiol. 254:E208–E213.
Nair, K.S., G.C. Ford, K. Ekberg, E. Fernqvist-Forbes, and J. Wahren
  1995 Protein dynamics in whole body and leg tissues in type I diabetic patients. J. Clin. Invest. 95:2926–2937.
Nautila, P., J. Knuuti, U. Ruotsalainen, V.A. Koivisto, E. Eronen, M. Teräs, J. Bergman, M. Haaparanta, L-M. Voipio-Pulkki, J. Viikari, T. Rönnemaa, U. Wegelius, and H. Yki-Järvomem
  1993 Insulin resistance is localized to skeletal but not heart muscle in type I diabetes. Am. J. Physiol. 264:E756–E762.
Phelps, M.E., J.C. Mazziotta, and H.R. Schelbert, eds.
  1986 Positron Emission Tomography and Autoradiography: Principles and Applications for the Brain and Heart. New York: Raven Press.
Planas, A.M., C. Prenant, B.M. Mazoyer, D. Comar, and L. DiGiamberardino
  1992 Regional cerebral L-[^{14}C-*Methyl*]methionine incorporation into proteins: Evidence for methionine recycling in the rat brain. J. Cereb. Blood Flow Metab. 12:603–612.
Quaim, S.M., J.C. Clark, C. Crouzel, M. Guillaume, H.J. Helmeke, B. Nebeling, V.W. Pike, and G. Stocklin
  1993 PET radionuclide production. Pp. 1–43 in Radiopharmaceuticals for Positron Emission Tomography, G. Stocklin and W.V. Pike, eds. Dordrecht, The Netherlands: Kluwer Academic Publishers.
Raichle, M.E., W.R.W. Martin, P. Herscovitch, M.A. Mintum, and J. Markham
  1983 Brain blood flow measured with intravenous H$_2$^{15}O. II. Implementation and validation. J. Nucl. Med. 24:790–798.
Rathmacher, J.A., P.J. Flakoll, and S.L. Nissen
  1995 A compartmental model of 3-methylhistidine metabolism in humans. Am. J. Physiol. 269:E193–E198.
Rennie, M.J.
  1994 Human skeletal and cardiac muscle proteolysis: Evolving concepts and practical applications. Pp. 23–48 in Organ Metabolism and Nutrition: Ideas for Future Critical Care, J.M. Kinney and H.N. Tucker, eds. New York: Raven Press.
Roubenhoff, R., and R.C. Rall
  1993 Humoral mediation of changing body composition during aging and chronic inflammation. Nutr. Rev. 51:1–11.
Schelbert, R.R., and M. Schwaiger
  1986 PET studies of the heart. Pp. 581–661 in Positron Emission Tomography and Autoradiography: Principles and Applications for the Brain and Heart, M. Phelps, J. Mazziotta, and H. Schelbert, eds. New York: Raven Press.

Smith, K., and M.J. Rennie
  1990   Protein turnover and amino acid metabolism in skeletal muscle. Ballière's Clin.
         Endocrinol. Metab. 4:461–498.
Stalnacke, C-G., B. Jones, B. Langstron, H. Lundquist, P. Malmborg, S. Sjoberg, and B.
         Larsson
  1982   Short-lived radionuclides in nutritional physiology. A model study with L-[Me-
         ^{11}C]methionine in the pig. Br. J. Nutr. 47:537–545.
Stocklin, G., and V.W. Pike, eds.
  1993   Radiopharmaceuticals for Positron Emission Tomography. Methodological As-
         pects. Dordrecht, The Netherlands: Kluwer Academic Publishers.
Storch, K.J., D.A. Wagner, J.F. Burke, and V.R. Young
  1988   Quantitative study, *in vivo*, of methionine cycle in humans using [methyl-^{2}H$_3$] and
         [1-^{13}C]methionine. Am. J. Physiol. 255:E322–E231.
Sugden, P.H., and S.J. Fuller
  1991   Regulation of protein turnover in skeletal and cardiac muscle. Biochem. J. 273:21–
         27.
Taylor, R., T.B. Price, L.D. Katz, R.G. Shulman, and G.I. Shulman
  1993   Direct measurement of change in muscle glycogen concentration after a mixed
         meal in normal subjects. Am. J. Physiol. 265:E224–E229.
Ter-Pogossian, M.M., M.E. Raichle, and B.E. Sobel
  1980   Positron-emission tomography. Sci. Am. 243:171–181.
Tessari, P., S. Inchiostro, B. Biolo, E. Vincent, and L. Sabadin
  1991   Effects of acute systemic hyperinsulinemia on forearm muscle proteolysis in
         healthy man. J. Clin. Invest. 88:27–33.
Tessari, P., S. Inchiostro, M. Zanett, and R. Barazzoni
  1995   A model of skeletal muscle kinetics measured across the human forearm. Am. J.
         Physiol. 269:E127–E136.
Thorne, D.P., and T.D. Lockwood
  1993   Four proteolytic processes of myocardium, one sensitive to thiol reactive agents
         and thiol protease inhibitor. Am. J. Physiol. 265:E10–E19.
Tzankoff, S.P., and A.H. Norris
  1977   Effect of muscle mass on age-related BMR changes. J. Appl. Physiol. 43:1001–
         1006.
Urban, R.J., Y.H. Bodenburg, C. Gilkison, J. Foxworth, A.R. Coggan, R.R. Wolfe, and A.
         Ferrando
  1995   Testosterone administration to elderly men increases skeletal muscle strength and
         protein synthesis. Am. J. Physiol. 269:E820–E826.
Vaughan, L., F. Zurlo, and E. Ravussin
  1991   Age and energy expenditure. Am. J. Clin. Nutr. 53:821–825.
Waterlow, J.C.
  1995   Whole-body protein turnover in humans—past, present and future. Annu. Rev.
         Nutr. 15:57–92.
Waterlow, J.C., P.J. Garlick, and D.J. Millward
  1978   Protein Turnover in Mammalian Tissues and in the Whole Body. Amsterdam:
         North-Holland Publishers.
Welle, S., C. Thornton, R. Jozefowicz, and M. Statt
  1993   Myofibrillar protein synthesis in young and old men. Am. J. Physiol. 264:E693–
         E698.
Williams, L.M., P.E. Ballmer, L.T. Hannah, I. Grant, and P.J. Garlick
  1994   Changes in regional protein synthesis in rat brain and pituitary after systemic inter-
         leukin 1-ß administration. Am. J. Physiol. 267:E915–E920.

Yarasheski, K.E., J.A. Campbell, K. Smith, M.J. Rennie, J.O. Halloszy, and D.M. Bier
1992   Effect of growth hormone and resistance exercise on muscle growth in young men. Am. J. Physiol. 262:E261–E267.

Yarasheski, K.E., J.J. Zachwieja, and D.M. Bier
1993   Acute effects of resistance exercise on muscle protein synthesis rate in young and elderly men and women. Am. J. Physiol. 265:E210–E214.

Young, V.R.
1970   The role of skeletal and cardiac muscle in the regulation of protein metabolism. Pp. 585–674 in Mammalian Protein Metabolism, H.N. Munro, ed. New York: Academic Press.
1992   Macronutrient needs in the elderly. Nutr. Rev. 50:454–462.

Young, V.R., and A.E. El-Khoury
1995   The notion of the essentiality of amino acids, revisited, with a note on the indispensable amino acid requirements of adults. Pp. 191–232 in Amino Acid Metabolism and Therapy in Health and Nutritional Disease, LC. Cynober, ed. Boca Raton, Fla.: CRC Press.

Young, V.R., and H.N. Munro
1978 N^τ-methylhistidine (3-methylhistidine) and muscle protein turnover: An overview. Fed. Proc. 37:2291–2300.

Young, V.R., J.S. Marchini, and J. Cortiella
1990   Assessment of protein nutritional status. J. Nutr. 120:1496–1502.

Young, V.R., Y-M. Yu, and M. Krempf
1991   Protein and amino acid turnover using the stable isotopes 15N, ^{13}C and ^{2}H as probes. Pp. 17–72 in New Techniques in Nutritional Research, R.G. Whitehead and A. Prentice, eds. San Diego: Academic Press.

Yu, Y-M., D.A. Wagner, E.E. Tredgett, J.A. Walaszewski, J.F. Burke, and V.R. Young
1990   Quantitative role of splanchnic region in leucine metabolism: L-[1-^{13}C,^{15}N]leucine and substrate balance studies. Am. J. Physiol. 259:E36–E50.

Zamir, O., P-O. Hasselgren, W. O'Brien, R.C. Thompson, and J.E. Fischer
1992a   Muscle protein breakdown during endotoxemia in rata and after treatment with interleukin-1 receptor antagonist (IL-Ira). Ann. Surg. 216:381–385.

Zamir, O., P-O. Hasselgren, S.L. Kunkel, J. Frederick, T. Higashiguchi, and J.E. Fischer
1992b   Evidence that tumor necrosis factor participates in the regulation of muscle proteolysis during sepsis. Arch. Surg. 127:170–174.

Zurlo, F., K. Larsen, C. Bogardus, and E. Ravussin
1990   Skeletal muscle metabolism is a major determinant of resting energy expenditure. J. Clin. Invest. 86:1423–1427.

DISCUSSION

DONALD McCORMICK: A couple of questions. One is that 30 mCi of labeled methionine did not sound like a heck of a lot, Vernon. How much methionine is delivered?

VERNON YOUNG: About 30 nmol methionine.

DONALD McCORMICK: In the case of a molecule where you label with an isotope like 11C, the decay is to nitrogen, is it not?

VERNON YOUNG: Yes, in that case.

DONALD McCORMICK: I am thinking of cases where you have a carbon and a nitrogen, and you generate an azide that is very toxic.

VERNON YOUNG: Oh, but the actual amount is so small. I thought what you were going to do was to ask me what the radiation load was, which I think is a very fair question. Well, I will tell you, since you did not ask. (Laughter)
 I understand that in studies of this kind the radiation dose is roughly somewhere between a CAT scan and a barium enema. It is certainly in that range.

ARTHUR ANDERSON: I am intrigued by the bone marrow observations that you made. Have you gotten any preliminary evidence now about whether the protein synthesis is related to cell division versus antibody production?

VERNON YOUNG: Oh, no. That is a darned good question. What this [PET] actually does is that it gives you rates of biochemical processes, but it does not tell you what that process is. So this particular approach does have significant limitations, but I think the combination of approaches is extremely powerful.

DENNIS BIER: I do not want to ask a question, but earlier Vernon said he only had one regret, that he was getting on a plane. He was too embarrassed to tell you that, really, his other real regret is that as a young person and a British citizen, he was not a member of the United States military. (Laughter)

VERNON YOUNG: Nor was I member of the British military. (Laughter)

Emerging Technologies for Nutrition Research, 1997
Pp. 259–272. Washington, D.C.
National Academy Press

11

Nuclear Magnetic Resonance Studies of Liver and Muscle Glycogen Metabolism in Humans

Gerald I. Shulman[1]

INTRODUCTION

This paper describes some of this laboratory's recent studies in which nuclear magnetic resonance (NMR) spectroscopy has been used to gain new insights into the regulation of liver and muscle glycogen synthesis in normal humans as well as into the pathogenesis of noninsulin-dependent diabetes mellitus (NIDDM) or Type II diabetes mellitus. This chapter will focus on the application of the technique to examine the regulation of peripheral glucose uptake and hepatic glucose output—the two major processes affected by insulin resistance. It provides an overview of the principles of NMR spectroscopy and introduces some of the different nuclei that can be studied using the technique. The use of carbon-13 (^{13}C) NMR spectroscopy on muscle to assess the rate of muscle glycogen synthesis in normal and diabetic humans is described, as is the use of phosphorus-31 (^{31}P) NMR spectroscopy to investigate the rate-limiting steps in

[1] Gerald I. Shulman, Department of Internal Medicine, Yale University School of Medicine, New Haven, CT 06520-8020

muscle glycogen synthesis. Finally, this paper will discuss the utilization of ^{13}C NMR spectroscopy in the noninvasive measurement of hepatic glycogen content for direct quantification of hepatic glycogenolysis and indirect quantification of gluconeogenesis in normal subjects and subjects with Type II diabetes mellitus.

BRIEF OVERVIEW OF THE BASIC PRINCIPLES OF NMR SPECTROSCOPY

This paper will provide only a brief overview of the basic principles of NMR spectroscopy, which are reviewed in detail elsewhere (Gadian, 1982; Jardetzky and Roberts, 1981). The technique of NMR spectroscopy relies on the spin properties of certain atomic nuclei, which make them behave like tiny bar magnets. Within molecules, these nuclei are usually oriented randomly in space. One might expect then that, when placed in a magnetic field, these nuclei will behave like a compass needle and line up with the field. However, as a result of the laws of quantum mechanics, these nuclei do not behave like conventional bar magnets but instead they tend to line up either with or against the field with the two different orientations having slightly different energies (Gadian, 1982; Jardetzky and Roberts, 1981). When subjected to an oscillating magnetic field, the nuclei can be made to move between these transition states. Under the applied magnetic field, the nuclei will precess (resonate) at a particular frequency. The higher the magnetic field, the faster the frequency of precession and the greater the difference between the two energy states. The electromagnetic frequency at which precession occurs depends on the particular nucleus being analyzed and its molecular environment (Gadian, 1982; Jardetzky and Roberts, 1981). Table 11-1 shows some of the nuclei that can be studied using NMR spectroscopy. Hydrogen nuclei, in the form of protons (^{1}H), when placed in a magnetic field of 2.1 Tesla (T) (the unit of magnetic field intensity) will precess at 89.5 megahertz (MHz). Overall, ^{1}H NMR spectroscopy is the most sensitive

TABLE 11-1 Properties of Nuclei that Can Be Studied Using Nuclear Magnetic Resonance Spectroscopy

Nucleus	Resonance at 2.1T (MHz)	Natural abundance (%)	Relative sensitivity (%)
^{1}H	89.5	99.98	100
^{31}P	36.2	100	6.6
^{13}C	22.5	1.1	0.016

NOTE: T, Tesla; MHz, megahertz.

nucleus to examine using NMR spectroscopy. It is the signals from protons in the body that are analyzed when whole-body magnetic resonance imaging (MRI) is performed. Since most of the protons in the body are associated with water and fat, it is the ^{1}H signals from these substances that are detected and constructed into a three-dimensional image by a computer.

In contrast to getting NMR signals from protons in the body to obtain images, this paper will focus on the application of phosphorus (^{31}P) and carbon (^{13}C) NMR spectroscopy in humans to measure intracellular metabolite concentrations for the study of metabolism. ^{31}P NMR spectroscopy takes advantage of the fact that ^{31}P is the only naturally occurring form of phosphorus, and it therefore represents approximately 100 percent of the phosphorus in all phosphate-containing compounds (Table 11-1). As will be shown, ^{31}P NMR spectroscopy can be used to quantify high-energy phosphate intermediates, such as adenosine triphosphate (ATP) and phosphocreatine in muscle. It also can be used to measure glucose-6-phosphate (G-6-P) concentrations in muscle, thus allowing the rate-limiting step of muscle glycogen synthesis to be analyzed. In contrast with ^{1}H and ^{31}P nuclei, only 1.1 percent of carbon nuclei occur naturally as the ^{13}C form; the rest occur as ^{12}C, which is NMR-invisible. Consequently, ^{13}C NMR spectroscopy of naturally occurring substances in the body is a relatively insensitive technique, having an overall relative sensitivity that is approximately 10,000 times less than that of ^{1}H NMR spectroscopy. However, as will be shown, it is possible to use ^{13}C NMR spectroscopy to measure natural abundance ^{13}C glucose in liver and muscle glycogen, which typically occurs in concentrations of greater than 50 mmol/liter. Furthermore, the sensitivity of this technique can be improved by up to almost 100-fold by using ^{13}C-enriched isotopes.[2]

NMR Spectrometer

In simple terms, an NMR spectrometer consists of a magnet, a probe, a radio-frequency generator, and a computer. In the studies described in this paper, the probe is placed under the gastrocnemius muscle or over the liver and acts like an antenna, both transmitting and receiving electromagnetic energy from the adjacent tissue. The radio-frequency generator sends electromagnetic pulses to the probe at the frequency at which the nuclei being investigated are oscillating. The nuclei in the tissue absorb some of the energy and in turn move to a higher energy state. When they return to their lower energy states, they give off energy that is then picked up by the probe, and a receiver picks up the signal bounced off the tissue. This signal is then passed to a computer, where it is transformed into a spectrum that yields chemical information. This ability to

---

[2] Natural abundance ^{13}C glucose represents 1.1 percent of the total glucose in liver and muscle glycogen. The use of ^{13}C-enriched isotopes can increase this up to 99 percent.

measure tissue metabolite concentration noninvasively makes NMR spectroscopy a very powerful technique for clinical investigation.

Applications of NMR Spectroscopy

NMR spectroscopy is a useful tool that has contributed to the better understanding of some of the basic pathophysiologic events that occur in Type II diabetes. It has provided a more accessible method of measuring muscle glycogen than the previously employed biopsy method. It also has been used to examine the extent to which the defect in insulin action in subjects with Type II diabetes can be attributed to impairment of muscle glycogen synthesis (Shulman et al., 1990).

In one study, five Type II diabetic subjects and six age- and weight-matched control subjects were subjected to a hyperglycemic-hyperinsulinemic clamp,[3] using somatostatin to inhibit endogenous insulin release in order to measure rates of muscle glycogen synthesis under similar concentrations of plasma glucose and insulin (Shulman et al., 1990). The target plasma glucose and insulin concentrations were approximately 190 mg/dl and approximately 70 μU/ml, respectively, simulating postprandial conditions. The infusate in the clamp was 20 percent enriched with 1-^{13}C glucose, to produce a 20-fold increase in the sensitivity of the ^{13}C NMR technique. The rate of incorporation of intravenously-infused 1-^{13}C glucose into muscle glycogen was measured directly in the gastrocnemius muscle using a 2.1T NMR spectrometer, allowing rates of muscle glycogen synthesis to be quantified.

When the incremental change in muscle glycogen concentration was measured over time in the diabetic subjects, the rate of muscle glycogen synthesis (as reflected by the slope of the plot) was approximately half that of the control subjects ($p < 0.05$) (Figure 11-1). Therefore, under similar concentrations of plasma glucose and insulin, there was a profound defect in muscle glycogen synthesis in the Type II diabetic subjects. When extrapolated to whole-body glucose metabolism, it was found that virtually all of the nonoxidative glucose disposal in the normal control subjects could be accounted for by muscle glycogen synthesis. Rates of whole-body glucose disposal were approximately 50 percent lower in the diabetic subjects than the control subjects under similar conditions of glucose and insulin, reflecting a profound impairment in insulin-stimulated glucose disposal (Figure 11-2). This decreased rate of glucose disposal could be attributed largely to decreased rates of nonoxidative glucose disposal. Similar to the normal control subjects, muscle glycogen synthesis accounted for virtually all of the nonoxidative glucose disposal in the diabetic subjects. This implies that a defect in the insulin-stimulated muscle glycogen

---

[3] A technique by which plasma glucose concentration is kept constant by a variable infusion of glucose.

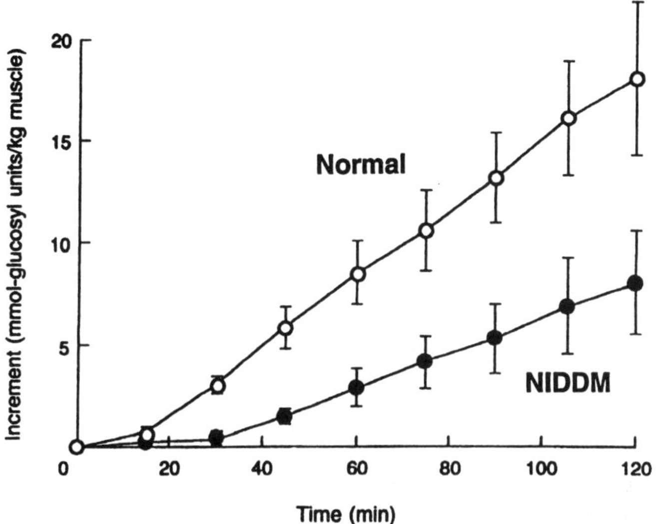

FIGURE 11-1 Incremental change in muscle glycogen concentration in both Type II diabetic subjects (NIDDM) and age- and weight-matched control subjects during a hyperglycemic-hyperinsulinemic clamp. (Error bars represent SEM.) SOURCE: Shulman et al., "Quantitation of muscle glycogen synthesis in normal subjects and subjects with non-insulin-dependent diabetes by ^{13}C nuclear magnetic resonance spectroscopy," *New England Journal of Medicine* 322:223–228. Copyright 1990 Massachusetts Medical Society. All rights reserved.

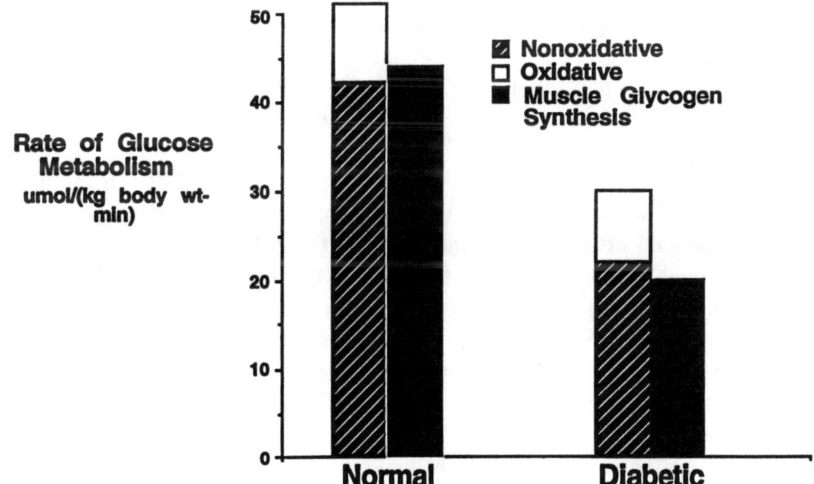

FIGURE 11-2 Rates of oxidative, nonoxidative glucose metabolism, and muscle glycogen synthesis in both Type II diabetic subjects and age- and weight-matched control subjects during a hyperglycemic-hyperinsulinemic clamp.

synthetic pathway is largely responsible for the slower rates of glucose disposal in patients with Type II diabetes mellitus.

GLUCOSE TRANSPORT-PHOSPHORYLATION: THE RATE-LIMITING STEP IN MUSCLE GLYCOGEN SYNTHESIS

In order to identify and understand the defect in the conversion of glucose to muscle glycogen in Type II diabetes, it is necessary to consider the two well-recognized steps in muscle glycogen synthesis that are insulin regulated and might be affected in patients with Type II diabetes mellitus. The first step involves the glucose transporter GLUT 4 (which is the primary protein involved in insulin-stimulated transport), whose response to insulin is known to cause its translocation from the intracellular membrane pools to the plasma membrane, allowing glucose to be transported into the cell in a facilitated manner (Denton and Tavaré, 1992). The other well-known, insulin-regulated step involves glycogen synthase, the enzyme that performs the final step of converting G-6-P to glycogen in muscle glycogen synthesis (Denton and Tavaré, 1992).

If glycogen synthase is defective in Type II diabetes, then it should be possible to see an increase in the concentration of G-6-P, as conversion of G-6-P into glycogen would be impaired in patients with Type II diabetes. However, if glucose transport or phosphorylation (hexokinase) is defective, then there should be no change or possibly a decrease in intracellular G-6-P concentration under insulin-stimulated conditions. ^{31}P NMR spectroscopy was therefore used to measure the concentration of G-6-P in the muscle in order to distinguish between these two possibilities (Rothman et al., 1992). Six Type II diabetic subjects and six age- and weight-matched controls were studied using a hyperglycemic-hyperinsulinemic clamp, with similar steady state plasma concentrations of insulin (approximately 70 µU/ml) and glucose (approximately 180 mg/dl) achieved in both groups. The concentration of G-6-P in the gastrocnemius muscle was measured using ^{31}P NMR spectroscopy. In the control subjects, there was an increase of approximately 0.1 mmol in G-6-P concentration in the muscle of normal subjects 30 minutes into the clamp study, compared with that measured at the start of the clamp (Figure 11-3). This increase was sustained throughout the study. In contrast, the diabetic subjects had approximately the same starting level of G-6-P but experienced virtually no change in the concentration of G-6-P in the muscle over the time span of the study (Figure 11-3). On average, the concentration of G-6-P measured in normal subjects was 0.24 ± 0.02 mmol/kg ($\pm$ SEM) muscle compared with 0.17 ± 0.02 mmol/kg ($\pm$ SEM) muscle in Type II diabetic subjects ($p < 0.01$). These data suggest that glucose transport or phosphorylation is defective in patients with Type II diabetes mellitus and that it is responsible for reduced rates of insulin-stimulated muscle glycogen synthesis. However, it is possible that, as the diabetic subjects have been hyperglycemic for some years and as chronic hyperglycemia itself is known to cause insulin resistance, the lack of effect observed on concentrations

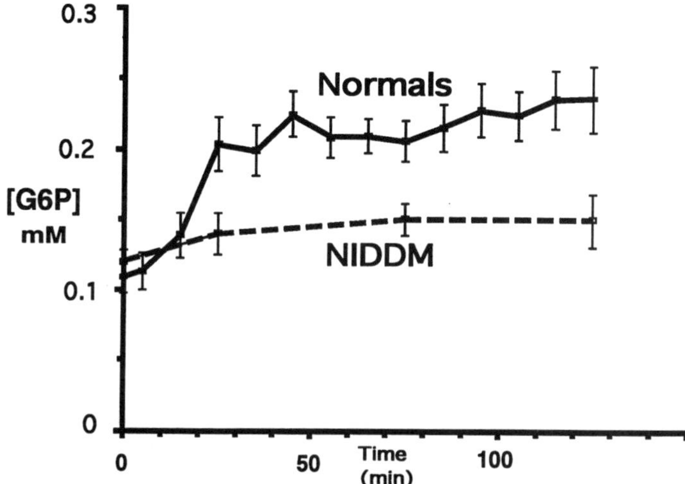

FIGURE 11-3 Glucose-6-phosphate (G-6-P) concentration during the hyperglycemic-hyperinsulinemic clamp study in both Type II diabetic subjects (NIDDM) and age- and weight-matched control subjects during a hyperglycemic-hyperinsulinemic clamp. (Error bars represent SEM.) SOURCE: Rothman et al. (1992). Reproduced from *The Journal of Clinical Investigation* (89:1069–1075) by copyright permission of The American Society for Clinical Investigation.

of G-6-P could be the result of glucose toxicity. In order to examine whether this observed defect in glucose transport-phosphorylation is a primary or an acquired defect in the pathogenesis of NIDDM, this laboratory recently measured muscle glycogen synthesis rate and muscle G-6-P concentration using ^{13}C and ^{31}P NMR spectroscopy as well as oxidative and nonoxidative glucose metabolism in six lean, normoglycemic offspring of parents with NIDDM and seven age- and weight-matched control subjects. These subjects were studied under hyperglycemic (~11 mM)-hyperinsulinemic (~480 pM) clamp conditions (Rothman et al., 1995). Offspring of NIDDM parents had a 50-percent reduction in total glucose metabolism, primarily due to a decrease in the nonoxidative component. The rate of muscle glycogen synthesis was reduced by 70 percent ($p < 0.005$), and the accumulation of muscle G-6-P was reduced by 40 percent ($p < 0.003$) in the offspring of NIDDM parents, which suggests impaired muscle glucose transport-hexokinase activity. These changes were similar to those previously observed in subjects with fully developed NIDDM as well as in control subjects under euglycemic-hyperinsulinemic conditions with matched rates of muscle glycogen synthesis. These data demonstrate that insulin resistant offspring of NIDDM parents have reduced rates of nonoxidative glucose metabolism and muscle glycogen synthesis, secondary to a defect in muscle glucose transport-hexokinase activity prior to the onset of overt hyperglycemia. The presence of this defect in these subjects suggests that it may be a primary factor in the pathogenesis of NIDDM.

NMR SPECTROSCOPIC STUDIES OF LIVER
GLYCOGEN METABOLISM

The application of NMR spectroscopy to the measurement of liver glycogen also has resulted in many significant new observations, as liver tissue is even more inaccessible than muscle tissue for biopsy. In one study that made use of the naturally occurring ^{13}C in liver glycogen, ^{13}C NMR spectroscopy was used to measure the net rate of hepatic glycogenolysis during a 68-h fast in seven young healthy subjects (Rothman et al., 1991). As the fast progressed, the decrease in hepatic glycogen content was measured every 3 to 6 hours. A relatively linear decrease in hepatic glycogen content was observed up to 40 hours after the start of the fast, after which there was no further significant decrease (Figure 11-4). By combining these measurements with liver volume measurements obtained from MRI, it was possible to calculate the net rate of hepatic glycogenolysis. Furthermore, by subtracting the net rate of hepatic glycogenolysis from the rate of glucose production in the whole body (determined by deuterated or tritiated glucose turnover techniques), the rate of gluconeogenesis was calculated. When this calculation was performed in young healthy subjects, gluconeogenesis accounted for 64 ± 5 percent (mean ± SEM) of the total glucose production during the first 22 hours (Figure 11-5). From 22 to 46 hours, gluconeogenesis comprised 82 ± 5 percent of glucose production, and during the

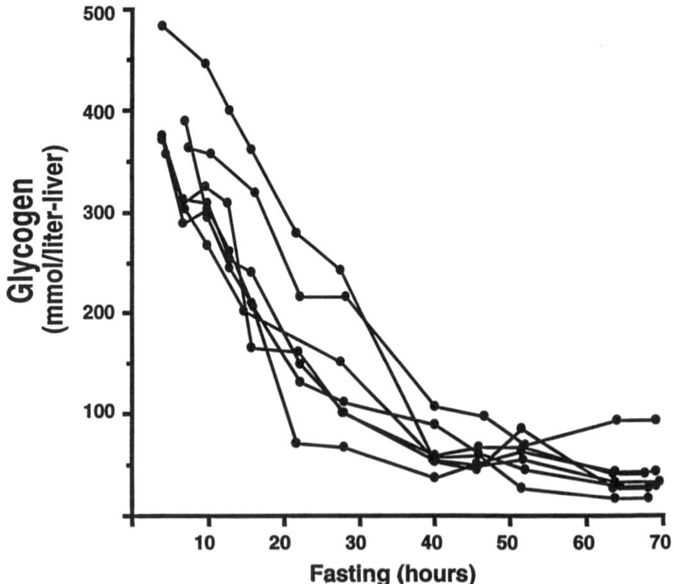

FIGURE 11-4 Hepatic glycogen concentration time course during a 68-h fast in seven normal subjects. SOURCE: Reprinted with permission from Rothman et al., "Quantitation of hepatic glycogenolysis and gluconeogenesis in fasting humans with 13C NMR," *Science* 254:573–576. Copyright 1991 American Association for the Advancement of Science.

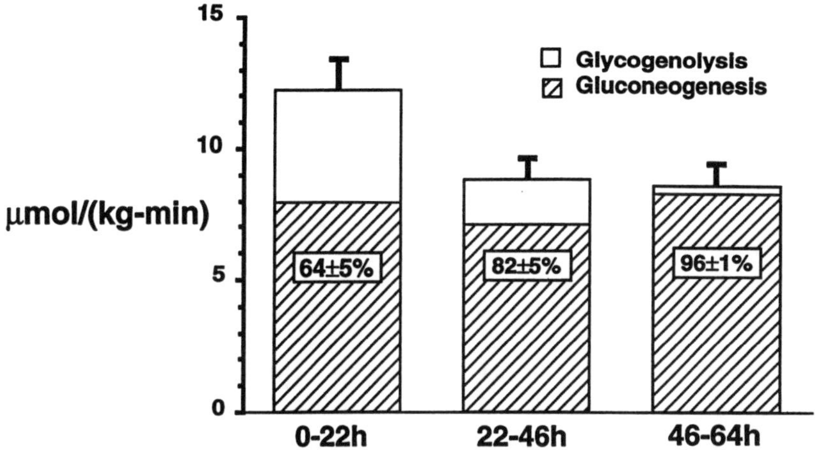

FIGURE 11-5 Mean rates of whole-body glucose production, net hepatic glycogenolysis, and gluconeogenesis in young normal subjects for three intervals (0 to 22 hours, 22 to 46 hours, and 46 to 64 hours) during a 68-h fast.

last 20 hours of the fast, virtually 100 percent of glucose production was due to gluconeogenesis. Therefore, even early on in a fast, gluconeogenesis appears to account for a larger proportion of total glucose production than previously was thought.

Subsequently, a study was performed to investigate whether the higher rates of hepatic glucose production that are known to occur in patients with poorly controlled Type II diabetes mellitus (DeFronzo et al., 1992) are due to increased rates of hepatic glycogenolysis, increase rates of gluconeogenesis, or a combination of both processes (Magnusson et al., 1992). In order to examine this question, seven Type II diabetic subjects were fed a diet identical to that of five age- and weight-matched control subjects for 3 days and then subjected to an overnight fast. Liver glycogen concentration, measured after 4 hours of fasting in Type II diabetic subjects, was approximately half that found in normal subjects ($p < 0.05$). The rate of hepatic glycogenolysis, as reflected by the slope of the plot, was also significantly less than in the normal control subjects ($p < 0.05$) (Figure 11-6). After performing the same kind of calculations as previously described, it was found that net hepatic glycogenolysis contributed approximately one-third and gluconeogenesis contributed two-thirds to rates of whole-body glucose production in the age- and weight-matched control subjects (Figure 11-7). In contrast, diabetic subjects had a rate of hepatic glucose production that was approximately 20 percent greater than that of the control subjects ($p < 0.01$). Since net rates of hepatic glycogenolysis in Type II diabetics

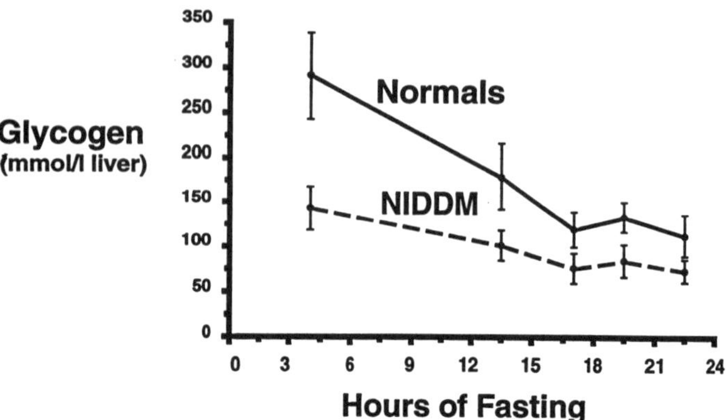

FIGURE 11-6 Hepatic glycogen concentration time course in both Type II diabetic subjects (NIDDM) and age- and weight-matched control subjects following an overnight fast. SOURCE: Magnusson et al. (1992). Reproduced from *The Journal of Clinical Investigation* (90:1323–1327) by copyright permission of The American Society for Clinical Investigation.

were lower than in the control subjects, virtually all of the increase in hepatic glucose production observed in the diabetic subjects could be attributed to increased rates of gluconeogenesis.

RELATIVE ADVANTAGES AND DISADVANTAGES OF NMR SPECTROSCOPY COMPARED TO OTHER TECHNIQUES

There are several unique aspects of the NMR technique that make it superior to other existing methods. First of all, in contrast to the biopsy method, which has been the traditional method to measure the concentration of intracellular metabolites, the NMR method is noninvasive, which allows the performance of multiple repeated measurements of a given metabolite in any organ in the body. This is especially useful when rates of a metabolic process need to be assessed, such as liver or muscle glycogen synthesis. Furthermore the interpretation of the results of enzyme activities or metabolite concentrations obtained from biopsy material is obscured by several limitations: (1) because of the invasiveness of the technique, muscle biopsies are typically limited to a few time points, (2) enzyme activities do not necessarily reflect *in vivo* substrate flux, and (3) the concentrations of certain metabolites in the biopsy sample change greatly following excision (for example, G-6-P concentrations in human muscle biopsies are typically artifactually high due to glycogen breakdown between sample excision and freezing).

Safety is another important advantage that NMR has over comparable techniques. No ionizing radiation is involved either in acquiring the spectra-image or in the isotopes utilized as compared to positron emission tomography

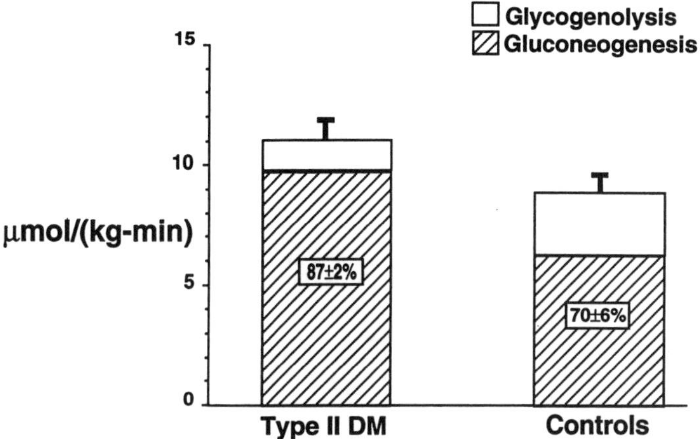

FIGURE 11-7 Mean rates of whole-body glucose production, net hepatic glycogenolysis and gluconeogenesis in both Type II diabetic subjects and age- and weight-matched control subjects following an overnight fast.

(PET) scanning, where radioactive isotopes are required for all studies, or computed axial tomography scanning, where ionizing radiation is used to obtain images. Since all ^{13}C and ^{31}P NMR studies involve stable nuclei, an additional advantage of this technique over PET is that these studies can be performed over relatively long periods of time without having to worry about the restrictions imposed by using radioactive isotopes, which typically have very short half-lives. Finally, the NMR technique yields chemical information. As discussed, ^{31}P NMR spectroscopy can be used to measure intracellular concentrations of high energy phosphate intermediates (e.g., ATP and phosphocreatine), inorganic phosphate, and intracellular pH, as well as some glycolytic intermediates. Furthermore, when ^{13}C-labeled isotopes are used in conjunction with ^{13}C NMR spectroscopy, an investigator can actually trace the metabolic fate of the ^{13}C label. For example, an investigator can measure the rate of label transfer from the C1 position of glucose to the C3 position of lactate into the C4 position of glutamate. Such information is very useful for estimating rates of metabolic fluxes *in vivo* (e.g., rates of glycolysis and glucose oxidation). In contrast, the PET method cannot directly assess the metabolic fate of an administered radio-labeled compound (e.g., distinguishing ^{11}C-labeled lactate from ^{11}C-labeled glutamate or which carbon in either metabolite is labeled).

The main disadvantage of the NMR technique is its relative insensitivity. At conventional magnetic field strengths (1–2T) an investigator typically is limited to measuring metabolites that exist in millimolar concentrations with either ^{13}C or ^{31}P NMR spectroscopy. However, with the advent of new editing techniques for ^{1}H NMR, which, as discussed, is the most sensitive nucleus for NMR studies as well as the development of magnets with higher field strengths, it likely will be possible to improve considerably on the overall sensitivity of this technique in the near future.

AUTHOR'S SUMMARY

In summary, NMR spectroscopy has become a useful tool for investigating the physiologic regulation of liver and muscle glycogen metabolism in normal humans as well as defining the metabolic defects that occur in patients with Type II diabetes mellitus. By applying NMR spectroscopy to the muscle, it was possible to demonstrate that muscle glycogen synthesis is the principal pathway of glucose disposal in both normal and Type II diabetic subjects. Furthermore, defects in muscle glycogen synthesis play a predominant role in insulin resistance that occurs in patients with Type II diabetes mellitus. From the ^{31}P NMR studies it was possible to show that this defect in muscle glycogen synthesis is secondary to a defect in glucose transport or phosphorylation. Furthermore, this same defect was observed in young, healthy, lean, normoglycemic, insulin-resistant offspring of Type II diabetic parents, suggesting that this defect in glucose transport or phosphorylation may have a primary role in the pathogenesis of Type II diabetes mellitus.

When applied to the liver, ^{13}C NMR spectroscopy can be used to assess the rate of net hepatic glycogenolysis and to quantify rates of gluconeogenesis noninvasively. Contrary to prevailing thought, gluconeogenesis was found to account for over half of the glucose production during the first 22 hours of a fast in young healthy subjects. In Type II diabetic subjects, rates of net hepatic glycogenolysis were decreased and rates of gluconeogenesis were increased following an overnight fast. Furthermore, this accelerated rate of gluconeogenesis can account for the higher rate of hepatic glucose production observed in these subjects, which is known to be an important contributing factor to fasting hyperglycemia.

Given the great potential of the NMR technique to measure metabolite concentrations and metabolic fluxes in any organ of the body noninvasively, it is likely that this technique will continue to provide new insights into the regulation of substrate metabolism in normal humans as well as into the pathogenesis of various metabolic diseases such as diabetes mellitus.

REFERENCES

DeFronzo, R.A., R.C. Bonadonna, and E. Ferrannini
  1992   Pathogenesis of NIDDM: A precarious balance between insulin action and insulin secretion. Pp. 569–663 in International Textbook of Diabetes Mellitus, vol. 1, K.G.M.M. Alberti, R.A. DeFronzo, H. Keen, and P. Zimmet, eds. Chichester: John Wiley and Sons.

Denton, R.M., and J.M. Tavaré
  1992 Action of insulin on intracellular processes. Pp. 385–408 in International Textbook of Diabetes Mellitus, vol. 1, K.G.M.M. Alberti, R.A. DeFronzo, H. Keen, and P. Zimmet, eds. Chichester: John Wiley and Sons.

Gadian, D.G.
  1982 Nuclear Magnetic Resonance and Its Application to Living Systems. New York: Oxford University Press.

Jardetzky, O., and G.C.K. Roberts
  1981 NMR in Molecular Biology. New York: Academic Press.

Magnusson I., D.L. Rothman, L.D. Katz, R.G. Shulman, and G.I. Shulman
  1992 Increased rate of gluconeogenesis in Type II diabetes mellitus. A ^{13}C nuclear magnetic resonance study. J. Clin. Invest. 90:1323–1327.

Rothman, D.L., I. Magnusson, L.D. Katz, R.G. Shulman, and G.I. Shulman
  1991 Quantitation of hepatic glycogenolysis and gluconeogenesis in fasting humans with ^{13}C NMR. Science 254:573–576.

Rothman, D.L., R.G. Shulman, and G.I. Shulman
  1992 ^{31}P nuclear magnetic resonance measurements of muscle glucose-6-phosphate. Evidence for reduced insulin-dependent muscle glucose transport or phosphorylation activity in non-insulin-dependent diabetes mellitus. J. Clin. Invest. 89:1069–1075.

Rothman, D.L., I. Magnusson, G. Cline, D. Gerard, C.R. Kahn, R.G. Shulman, and G.I. Shulman
  1995 Decreased muscle glucose transport/phosphorylation is an early defect in the pathogenesis of non-insulin-dependent diabetes mellitus. Proc. Natl. Acad. Sci. (USA) 92:983–987.

Shulman, G.I., B.L. Rothman, T. Jue, P. Stein, R.A. DeFronzo, and R.G. Shulman
  1990 Quantitation of muscle glycogen synthesis in normal subjects and subjects with non-insulin-dependent diabetes by ^{13}C nuclear magnetic resonance spectroscopy. N. Engl. J. Med. 322:223–228.

DISCUSSION

WENDY KOHRT: Do you envision this method being used to assess visceral lipolytic activity?

GERALD SHULMAN: We are very interested in that specific question in that increased visceral lipolytic activity has been proposed to be an important factor in the pathogenesis of insulin resistance in noninsulin-dependent diabetes mellitus. I think it may be possible in the future.

WM. CAMERON CHUMLEA: Can you do spectroscopy on a region of interest or is the coil just draped over?

GERALD SHULMAN: Yes, it is possible to do localized spectroscopy and obtain spectra from a specific voxel inside a tissue bed.

ROBERT NESHEIM: Thank you very much, that was very interesting. I cannot help but be struck by the fact that 50 years ago when I was in the Army, I do not recall that we were talking about any of these subjects.

(Laughter)

Forty-five years ago, when I was in graduate school, I do not remember the vocabulary that we are talking about here, even any reference to it. My, times have changed.

Emerging Technologies for Nutrition Research, 1997
Pp. 273–277. Washington, D.C.
National Academy Press

IV

Discussion

IRWIN TAUB: It is clear that, in any issue involving endurance when fatigue comes on and in other issues regarding the ability of people to function under stressful conditions, several of the techniques we have heard today certainly are applicable. In particular, what Gerald Shulman pointed out is very relevant.

In fact, the issue, as Jim Vogel brought up, is how performance is influenced by the intake of food, what you eat, in what form that food is, how quickly or how often you eat, and so on, which raises, then, the question that I have for Dr. Shulman. You demonstrated previously, and it is in some of your papers, that for an individual functioning at 30 percent $\dot{V}O_2max$, you can get a steady state between the depletion of the glycogen and the synthesis of the glycogen, by the slow infusion of glucose.

What do you expect would happen if one were to work harder and to counteract it by more rapid ingestion and digestion of the food? Do you still think there should be this equilibrium or, I should say, this steady state, which means greater endurance, or do you think there are some other issues, like insulin and so on, that might compromise the situation?

GERALD SHULMAN: I believe you are referring to our work on glycogen turnover in muscle, which I did not discuss today. We are now in the process of examining other factors that might impact on muscle glycogen turnover.

GILBERT LEVEILLE: In measuring glycogen, can you use the technique to look at glycogen disappearance during exercise?

GERALD SHULMAN: Yes.

GILBERT LEVEILLE: How long is your measurement period?

GERALD SHULMAN: We can get down to about 8 minutes per measurement, with reasonable signal to noise.

G. RICHARD JANSEN: Have you separated out the effects of glucose and insulin by giving a glucose load and, say, giving diazoxide, which inhibits insulin secretion?

GERALD SHULMAN: We just finished a study in humans, in which we looked at the role of glucose and insulin in the regulation of hepatic glycogen synthesis.[1] In the absence of insulin, hyperglycemia *per se* will not cause any ^{13}C label incorporation into glycogen. Only after portal vein insulin concentration rises to greater than 150 pµ does significant hepatic glycogen synthesis occur.

REED HOYT: I was curious about the ^{13}C-glucose costs for a given field strength and decoupling power, and how to balance it.

GERALD SHULMAN: When we first started these studies 10 years ago, it was $450.00 a gram, and we use about 20 grams per study. But now, when you buy in large quantities, you can get the cost down to about $45.00 to $50.00 a gram.

DENNIS BIER: I have probably been buying isotope longer than anybody in this room. Twenty-five years ago, it cost several thousand dollars for a few hun-

---

[1] M. Roden, G. Perseghin, K. F. Petersen, J. H. Hwang, G. W. Cline, K. Gerow, D. L. Rothman, and G. I. Shulman. 1996. The roles of insulin and glucagon in the regulation of hepatic glycogen synthesis and turnover in humans. J. Clin. Invest. 97:642–648.

dred milligrams for anything we tried to do. The first experiments we did cost several thousand dollars apiece.

Today you can buy the same material, like leucine, glucose, and various amino acids, in the order of $60.00 or $70.00 a gram. In fact, they often are cheaper than the corresponding radiotracers. So there is a whole host of things you can do at rates that are realistically $50.00 to $100.00 per subject, at the most, and some of them are $20.00 to $30.00.

I wanted to make a comment about the cost because this was something that used to be a problem with the first stable isotope experiments. You can do one $100,000 experiment and get the right answer or ten $10,000 experiments and get the wrong answer. Now, which would you rather do (which is what we are addressing here)? I mean, is it worth putting the money up front to get the answers that are correct and move the field ahead or is it worth continuing to do the wrong ones because they are cheaper? I know which route I would take.

(Laughter)

DAVID SCHNAKENBERG: Perhaps you said it, and forgive me if I missed it, but your methodology would allow you to follow glycogen repletion in muscle as well as depletion, right?

GERALD SHULMAN: That is right.

DAVID SCHNAKENBERG: Because I think in many instances, for military application, in terms of guidance to a commander or to a soldier it could very well be written on the label which foods inside that ration pack should be consumed to replete muscle stores most rapidly, when the soldier has just been through an exhausting, physically enduring event.

GERALD SHULMAN: We are now looking at optimal feeding and exercise regimens to achieve and maintain glycogen supercompensation.

DAVID SCHNAKENBERG: In some instances in the military situation, elements of a relatively small increase in the rate of recovery or the rate of (speed of) a response time (for example, if one guy happens to shoot one second before the other person) can have more than a 10-percent impact.

(Laughter)

So even a 10-percent increase in the rate of recovery may be militarily important.

DOUGLAS WILMORE: Can you see changes in muscle swelling?

GERALD SHULMAN: We are now combining these measurements with MRI to assess muscle volume and swelling.

HAL GOFORTH: Along the lines of the discussion earlier, with the optimum repletion you would have the opportunity to look at the effect of fructose versus glucose as a recommended food source for liver glycogen, which may be more important for cognitive performance than for, say, just leg muscles.

GERALD SHULMAN: Yes, it also is possible to use the same methods to assess optimal regimens for liver glycogen repletion.

REED HOYT: For Dr. Wolfe, what you presented was remarkable. I wanted to have you clarify whether we could apply your techniques concerning ^{13}C-^{12}C ratios in urea, for example, to some of these field studies where we do have reasonable estimates of energy expenditure and food intakes and so forth, to get at just what they are combusting for fuel or whether you would need other tracers in addition?

ROBERT WOLFE: The accuracy of that method depends on the different ratios (of ^{13}C to ^{12}C) in carbohydrate, fat, and protein. We performed the quantitation of substrate validation by the ratio technique in two ways. In one case, no tracer was given. In the other, carbohydrate containing some ^{13}C was given to stabilize the glycogen stores at a higher enrichment. The precision is improved with the additional ^{13}C-glucose, but the method nonetheless can be used without any modification of the diet at all. It actually just requires a breath sample. A urine sample could be used, however, and the carbon enrichment of urea analyzed since that is derived from the bicarbonate pool.

With a breath sample, if you have any independent means of measuring total oxygen consumption, then you can quantify oxidation in absolute terms. So I think it is optimal if you have some extra ^{13}C added to carbohydrate, but it is certainly not necessary.

HARRIS LIEBERMAN: To follow up on that, what sort of accuracies are you talking about in either case?

ROBERT WOLFE: It depends on exactly how you define accuracy in terms of the coefficient of variation. The determination in one person from day to day...

HARRIS LIEBERMAN: In a population sample of, say, eight people rather than an individual.

ROBERT WOLFE: I am just trying to recall the data. It depends on how you express it, because you are quantifying carbohydrate and fat oxidation, and if you have very low carbohydrate oxidation, then you will have a high percent error in that and a low percent error in the fat oxidation. Roughly, the error is about 5 or 10 percent, but the percent error depends on whether you are predominantly oxidizing fat or carbohydrate. The percentage error will be greater on the substrate that is the minimally oxidized substrate.

HARRIS LIEBERMAN: So 5 to 10 percent for individual variation?

ROBERT WOLFE: Right.

V

Ambulatory Techniques for Measurement of Energy Expenditure

MEASURING ENERGY EXPENDITURE AND fuel utilization during field (ambulatory) operations is critical to the military mission. Chapters 12 through 14 present techniques currently in use in the field, while Chapter 15 explores a laboratory-based technique.

The doubly labeled water method, the subject of Chapter 12, estimates energy expenditure and total body water by measuring production of singly labeled carbon dioxide and water after administration of water doubly labeled with stable isotopes of hydrogen and oxygen. After subjects digest the labeled water, samples of urine or saliva are taken and the respiratory quotient (carbon dioxide produced/oxygen consumed) is determined, which allows for a noninvasive, accurate estimate of energy expenditure in the field. Care must be taken to ensure the accuracy of analysis, and in longer field studies, consideration must be given to the variances in the natural abundance of the stable isotope of water due to geography.

In Chapter 13, three portable systems for determining minute ventilation and oxygen uptake are profiled. All have been validated in the laboratory, but only one has been validated in the field. The systems are costly and require trained personnel, but it is easy to learn the technique and analyze the data.

As a tool for the immediate assessment of physical activity and determination of energy needs, the ambulatory foot contact monitor is used to estimate the metabolic cost of locomotion, as described in Chapter 14. Estimations are based on the ratio of total body weight to foot contact time during each stride through an electronic device implanted in a shoe. While the technology is simple, easy to use, and inexpensive, it is unable as yet to determine total energy expenditure, needs to incorporate body weight, and does not account for up- and downhill movement.

The author of Chapter 15 details the use of near-infrared spectrometry as a method for the measurement of a single constituent within a complex organic mixture both *in vitro* and *in vivo*. After scanning a mixture over a range of wavelengths, the peaks in the resultant absorption patterns are analyzed using Beer's law or regression analysis to determine the concentration for the constituent of interest. One of the main uses of this technique is for monitoring blood metabolites noninvasively, but improvements in technology need to be made before its potential in the field can be tested.

Emerging Technologies for Nutrition Research, 1997
Pp. 281–296. Washington, D.C.
National Academy Press

12

Doubly Labeled Water for Energy Expenditure

James P. DeLany[1]

INTRODUCTION

The doubly labeled water (DLW) technique was developed as a method for measurement of free-living energy expenditure in animals (Lifson and McClintock, 1966). The method has since been validated in many animal species (for summary see Roberts, 1989; Schoeller, 1988). Twenty years after the initial report of the DLW method (Lifson et al., 1955), the economic feasibility of using the method in humans was considered (Lifson et al., 1975). The obstacle to applying the method to humans was the cost of the large quantities of oxygen-18 labeled water ($H_2^{18}O$) needed to attain an adequate isotopic enrichment for calculation of valid elimination rates. This obstacle was overcome by improvements in gas isotope ratio mass spectrometers and a decrease in the cost of $H_2^{18}O$. Another 7 years passed before the DLW method eventually was validated against the intake balance (I/B) method in humans (Schoeller and van Santen, 1982). The method has since been validated against indirect calorimetry

---

[1] James P. DeLany, Pennington Biomedical Research Center, Baton Rouge, LA 70808

and I/B in many different subject populations by several laboratories, with a demonstrated precision (coefficient of variation) of 2 to 8 percent (Schoeller, 1988).

THEORY OF DOUBLY LABELED WATER

The DLW method is based on the premise that after a dose of doubly labeled water, $^2H_2^{18}O$, the two isotopes equilibrate with total body water (TBW) and then are eliminated differentially from the body (Figure 12-1). Deuterium (^2H) leaves the body as water, while ^{18}O leaves as water (H_2O) and carbon dioxide (CO_2). Therefore, CO_2 production can be calculated by subtracting ^2H elimination from ^{18}O elimination. The DLW method is an ideal method for military nutrition studies because it is an accurate field technique for determination of free-living energy expenditure. There are no requirements for subject compliance (except giving urine and/or saliva samples) such as filling out logs; there is no fear of equipment breakage; and it can be used to validate other field techniques. The initial validations of DLW were conducted under sedentary conditions, while military studies generally have involved soldiers undergoing strenuous activity. In a study of subjects under sedentary conditions (1.4 × sleeping metabolic rate) and in subjects undergoing heavy bicycle ergometer workouts (2.6 × metabolic rate), the DLW method was shown to be accurate compared to indirect calorimetry (Westerterp et al., 1988). The method

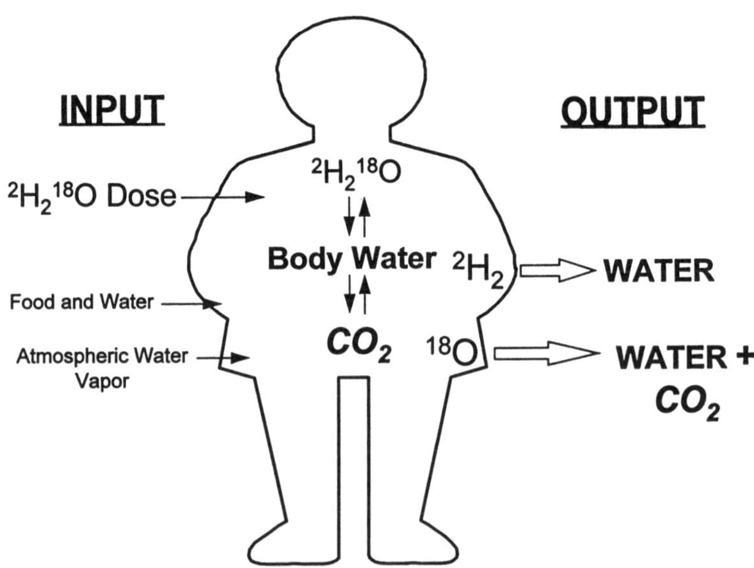

^{18}O elimination (water + CO_2) - $^2H_2$ elimination (water) = CO_2 Production

FIGURE 12-1 Theory of doubly labeled water method.

has since been validated in soldiers under various conditions (DeLany et al., 1989; Forbes-Ewan et al., 1989; Hoyt et al., 1991, 1994).

In addition to providing measurement of integrated energy expenditure, the DLW method provides simultaneous measures of TBW (from which body composition can be calculated) and water turnover, key measurements for many military nutrition studies. Hydration status is perhaps more critical to the sustained performance of soldiers than energy balance, and water requirements have been studied during many field studies. Use of ^{2}H elimination for measurement of water turnover was initially validated in animal studies (Lifson and McClintock, 1966). It was pointed out that water intake can be overestimated unless corrections are made for water turnover in the lungs (Figure 12-1) and fractionation (preferential loss of one isotope due to different physical properties) of ^{2}H. Water intake by ^{2}H elimination also was investigated in the first validation of DLW in humans (Schoeller and van Santen, 1982). The isotope method was within 1.3 ± 6.7 percent (coefficient of variation) of the measured water intake, although the range was from –6.3 percent to +8.0 percent. Data compiled from analysis of 77 male soldiers in a variety of field settings were used to compare water intake measured by deuterium oxide (^{2}H$_2$O) elimination with logbook self-reports with canteens as a unit of consumption (Jones et al., 1993). Water intake by the ^{2}H$_2$O elimination method agreed very well with that obtained by the logbook method ($3,750 \pm 1,120$ vs. $3,810 \pm 1,450$ g/d).

Doubly Labeled Water Protocol

A typical DLW protocol is depicted in Figure 12-2. The study begins with the collection of baseline urine and/or saliva samples, followed by oral administration of the ^{2}H$_2$^{18}O dose. Saliva samples are obtained 2 to 4 hours after the dose for calculation of dilution spaces (Schoeller et al., 1980). A urine sample is collected the following morning for measurement of initial enrichment. Urine samples then are collected at the end of the period for measurement of final isotopic enrichment. The length of time a DLW study can be carried out depends

FIGURE 12-2 Typical doubly labeled water protocol. TBW, total body water.

on the turnover of the two isotopes, which is dependent on H_2O and CO_2 output. For studies in typical adults, the optimal metabolic period is 4 to 21 days (Schoeller, 1988), with military nutrition studies generally limited to the shorter time periods. If TBW is expected to change over the metabolic period, deuterium oxide will need to be readministered at the end of the study for a final TBW measurement.

Since the DLW dose and the analyses are so expensive, it is imperative that enough specimens are obtained to have backup samples at the beginning and end of the period of interest. Problems with specimens, such as inability to obtain a specimen, loss of a specimen, or contamination of a specimen, can occur in the field or in the lab. The protocol depicted in Figure 12-2 illustrates the minimum number of specimens to be collected for a DLW study. This protocol provides backup samples for the initial and final time points. If there is a problem with the 24-h urine, the 4-h saliva specimen can be used as the initial time point. If the final sample is bad, the urine from the previous day can be used as the final enrichment for elimination rate calculations. The ^{18}O isotope abundances are measured on a gas-inlet isotope ratio mass spectrometer with a CO_2-water equilibration device (DeLany et al., 1989). Briefly, urine and saliva samples are equilibrated with CO_2 at a constant temperature in a shaking water bath for at least 12 hours. The CO_2 then is purified cryogenically under vacuum before introduction into the mass spectrometer. The hydrogen isotope abundances usually are measured on a gas-inlet isotope ratio mass spectrometer, after microdistillation and zinc (or uranium) reduction (DeLany et al., 1989).

The ^2H and ^{18}O isotope elimination rates (k_H and k_O) can be calculated by the two-point method using the initial (i) isotopic enrichment and the final (f) enrichments: $k = (\ln \text{enrichment}_f - \ln \text{enrichment}_i)/\Delta t$, where ln is the natural log, enrichment is the enrichment above baseline, and Δt is the number of days between the initial and final sample. CO_2 production has been calculated according to Schoeller (1988):

$$rCO_2 = (N/2.078)(1.01k_O - 1.04k_H) - 0.0246rH_2O_f \qquad \text{(Equation 12-1)}$$

where N is the TBW calculated from the ^{18}O enrichment in the 4-h saliva (or average of initial and final 4-h saliva samples if TBW is expected to change), and rH_2O_f is the rate of fractionated evaporative water loss, which is estimated to be $1.05N(1.01k_O - 1.04k_H)$.

Two-Point versus Multipoint Sampling

There has been some debate about the number of time points needed to obtain accurate measures of isotope elimination rates. As originally developed for experiments in animals and in the first human validations, elimination rates were calculated from an initial and a final time point, which has become known as the two-point method (although more than two points are often collected). For the multipoint DLW protocol, samples are obtained throughout the period, and elimination rates are calculated by regression analyses. The rationale of the multiple-point method is that by using more time points to calculate elimination rates, sample-to-sample variation (analytical error) is averaged out, and a more precise measure of energy expenditure might be obtained. Although multiple samples may provide an advantage with regard to increased precision, there are several disadvantages to this method. The obvious problems with obtaining multiple samples are that it intrudes more into the subject's daily routine, may interfere with the habitual daily energy expenditure, and increases the laboratory work load. The less obvious and major concern with the multiple-sample method is that it does not give an exact average over the metabolic period if there are systematic variations in the water (Lifson et al., 1955; Nagy and Costa, 1980) or CO_2 flux (Lifson et al., 1955; Speakman and Racey, 1986). However, in contrast to earlier comments by other investigators (Coward, 1988; James et al., 1988), the two-point method gives the arithmetically correct energy expenditure. This is because the two-point method gives an exact average of elimination rates over time even in the face of systematic variations, while the regression models do not (Coward, 1990; Nagy and Costa, 1980; Schoeller and Coward, 1990; Speakman and Racey, 1986; Welle, 1990). Variations in energy expenditure and water turnover often occur during military nutrition studies, either due to the nature of a field training exercise or due to environmental factors.

Two U.S. Army Research Institute of Environmental Medicine studies demonstrate the advantage of the two-point method over the multiple-point method in military studies. A multipoint sampling strategy was employed that would incorporate the best aspects of the two-point with those of the multipoint protocol. Samples were analyzed from the first 2 and the last 3 days of the metabolic period for calculation of elimination rates by linear regression. This is similar to the optimal sampling design suggested to minimize error (Cole and Coward, 1992). Results were compared with those obtained by the two-point method using isotope enrichments measured on samples from the first and last days. In a high-altitude study (Edwards et al., 1991) in which energy expenditure and water turnover were relatively constant throughout the study, energy expenditure by the two-point method (3,550 ± 610 kcal/d) was nearly identical to that obtained using the multipoint method (3,565 ± 675 kcal/d). This study demonstrated that energy expenditure could be measured accurately with only two time points, eliminating the need for extra sample collection and laboratory analyses. A summary of the available data on repeat DLW measures of energy expenditure also showed that there was no improvement in accuracy or precision for the multipoint method over the two-point method (Cole and Coward, 1992). The variance of repeat measures in two studies using the two-point method (7.4% and 7.3%) was similar to that observed in two studies using the multipoint method (7.4% and 6.7%).

A second study demonstrated the major potential disadvantage of the multipoint methods. During a cold-weather study, there was a significant change in energy expenditure and water turnover towards the end of the metabolic period due to environmental extremes (DeLany et al., 1991). During the second to the last day of the metabolic period, the soldiers moved and set up a defensive position, underwent live-fire exercises, and moved back to camp (February 12–13). During the previous day and the day following the live-fire exercises, the soldiers "stood down" (remained inactive) the entire day because of helicopter support and extreme cold weather. Therefore, H_2O and CO_2 elimination were very different over these 3 days. Deviations from a linear isotope elimination were apparent from a close examination of a plot of the log of ^2H enrichment (^{18}O data were similar) versus time (Figure 12-3). Examination of regression coefficients that were 0.99 or better suggested a linear response. However, this physiologic variation (as opposed to analytical error) introduced an error in calculation of isotope elimination by the regression method, giving an energy expenditure that was significantly ($p < 0.01$) lower than that obtained using the two-point method ($5,015 \pm 510$ vs. $5,140 \pm 630$ kcal/d). Therefore, as has been described previously, the two-point and regression methods are both accurate when there are no deviations in energy expenditure and water turnover during the measurement period (assuming isotope enrichments are measured accurately). However, when there are systematic variations during the period, the multipoint methods using simple linear regression do not give true measures of elimination rates.

The Importance of Isotope Dilution Space Ratios

Another recent debate has centered on the relationship between the two isotope dilution spaces and TBW. When the original equation for humans was developed (Equation 12-1 above), there were few available data on the relation-

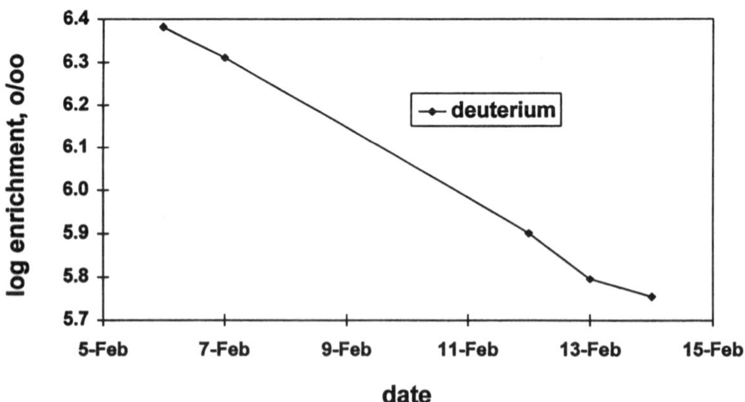

FIGURE 12-3 Deviation in isotope elimination due to physiologic variation. o\oo, per mille derivations in heavy isotope ratio relative to standard mean ocean water (smow).

ship between the two isotope dilution spaces. The ratio between the ^{2}H and ^{18}O dilution spaces (N_D/N_O) in 23 subjects was 1.033, which was rounded to three significant digits to give a ratio of 1.03 (Schoeller et al., 1986). The ratio between N_O and TBW based on available animal data, and the theoretical estimate of the nonaqueous exchangeable oxygen pool was estimated to be 1.007, which was rounded to 1.01 (Schoeller et al., 1980). This gave a ratio of 1.04 for N_D/TBW. In a recent review of available data, a new ratio of 1.0427 was recommended (Speakman et al., 1993). The following year, two independent investigators reviewed the available literature and came to a different conclusion (Coward et al., 1994; Racette et al., 1994). These investigators noted that differences in dilution space ratios reported in the literature appeared to be method dependent. Labs using the method of direct addition of biological fluid (urine or saliva) to the zinc reagent for reduction to hydrogen gas obtained a higher N_D/N_O ratio than those using uranium reduction or zinc reduction after distillation of the sample. A study of the effect of sample matrix (i.e., compounds in urine) in biological fluids demonstrated inaccuracies in the measurement of ^{2}H enrichment with the direct addition technique (Ritz et al., 1994). For a urine sample with an average solids concentration of 40 g/kg, the ^{2}H enrichment was underestimated by 2.4 percent, causing an overestimation in the calculated dilution space (Ritz et al., 1994). Based on these observations, the new recommended N_D/N_O ratio is 1.034 (Coward et al., 1994; Racette et al., 1994), and individual factors for N_D/TBW and N_O/TBW are 1.041 and 1.007. These modifications are made in Equation 12-1 to give Equation 12-2 below:

$$rCO_2 = (N/2.078)(1.007k_O - 1.041k_H) - 0.0246rH_2O_f \qquad \text{(Equation 12-2)}$$

The details are the same as for Equation 12-1 above, except the new factors also are used in the calculation of rH_2O_f to give $1.05N(1.007k_O - 1.041k_H)$.

This may seem like a small modification to Equation 12-1, but small differences in dilution space ratios introduce significant changes in the calculation of rCO_2. A 1 percent difference in the N_D/N_O ratio (e.g., 1.04 vs. 1.03) can introduce a 4 percent error in the calculation of CO_2 production and energy expenditure during a typical DLW study in soldiers. Errors would be even higher in studies where energy expenditure is lower. When the modified equation (Equation 12-2) was used to recalculate existing validation data, the accuracy of the DLW method improved from an overestimate of 3.3 ± 8.9 percent (when using the original Equation 12-1) to an energy expenditure that agreed within 1.2 ± 8.5 percent of that obtained by indirect calorimetry. However, when the higher proposed ratio was used, energy expenditure was underestimated by 3.1 ± 9.9 percent (Racette et al., 1994).

PARTICULAR CONCERNS FOR MILITARY NUTRITION DLW STUDIES

Additional concerns when applying the DLW method to military nutrition studies are changes in baseline isotope during the study, the possible need for a higher dose of isotope and the need for administration of multiple doses of DLW to obtain energy expenditure during a long training study. For typical DLW studies, the baseline isotope abundance is measured before administration of the DLW and is assumed to remain constant throughout the study. The problem of baseline isotope shifts occurs in military studies because the soldiers often are transported to a different geographical location to carry out a field-training study. This poses a problem because ^2H and ^{18}O are naturally occurring isotopes, and variations in the isotopic enrichment of water occur based on geographical location (Dansgaard, 1964). When the soldiers move to the location of a field-training study, drinking water with a different isotopic abundance will mix with TBW (Figure 12-1) and appear as a change in elimination rates, leading to errors in the measurement of energy expenditure. This phenomenon has been observed in patients receiving parenteral nutrition, in infants changing parenteral formulas or switching to oral formula, and in soldiers during field-training studies (DeLany et al., 1989; Hoyt et al., 1991, 1994; Jones et al., 1988; Schoeller et al., 1986). Therefore, in military nutrition studies employing DLW, a control group not receiving isotope must also be studied to correct for background shifts in isotope.

Another concern in military nutrition studies is the possible requirement for higher DLW dose due to high water turnover and high energy expenditure that occur during field-training exercises. For example, during one phase of a Ranger training course (Moore et al., 1992), water turnover during the first 3 days was over 9 liters/d, while energy expenditure was $5,350 \pm 770$ kcal/d. The high water turnover and energy expenditure combined to flush out the isotope, with over half of the administered dose eliminated in the first 4 days (Figure 12-4). This posed a problem because there also was interest in ascertaining energy expenditure over the next 11 days. However, there was only enough isotope remaining to measure energy expenditure with any degree of accuracy over the next 6 days. A high water turnover had been anticipated, and a higher dose than usual was given. However, with such high turnover rates (even higher than anticipated), giving a higher DLW dose is not very effective. The only way to obtain DLW data for this entire period of interest would be to administer a second dose of $^2H_2^{18}O$ on day 10, or perhaps even on day 4 (Figure 12-4).

A multiple-dosing (administration of a dose of DLW) strategy was used in an earlier study to obtain data on energy expenditure during a 28-d field-training exercise (DeLany et al., 1989). Multiple doses have also been used in Ranger training studies to obtain energy expenditure during much of the 63-d course (Moore et al., 1992). In the Ranger studies, multiple dosings have been administered and samples have been collected at various times throughout a dosing pe-

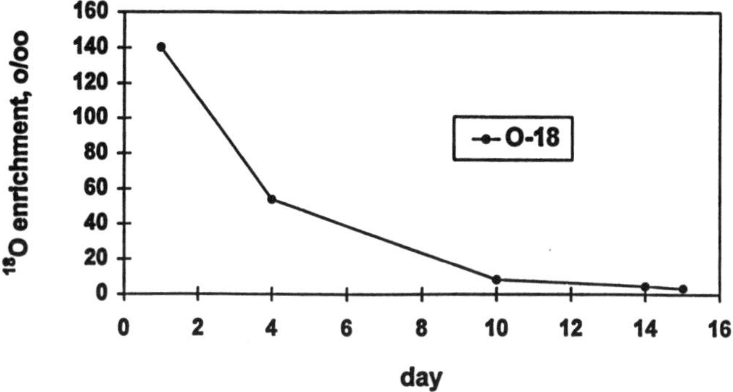

FIGURE 12-4 Washout of isotope due to high water turnover. o/oo, ratio per mille derivations in heavy isotope ratio relative to standard mean ocean water (smow).

riod to obtain data from multiple phases within a period (Figure 12-5). The days
between the arrows indicate the training phases covered by four separate DLW
dosings, and the points indicate the energy expenditure for a typical subject for
each period. Note that in the first and third period, two measurements of energy
expenditure were obtained, corresponding to two separate portions of that phase
of the training course. This was accomplished by obtaining a specimen in the
middle of the period as well as at the end of the period. The data presented in
Figure 12-4 correspond to Period 3 in Figure 12-5. The day 4 sample (Figure
12-4) served as the final time point for the first 3 days of the study, as well as
the initial time point for measurement of energy expenditure over the next 6
days. Using this strategy, it was possible to calculate energy expenditure during
two distinct portions of the training program.

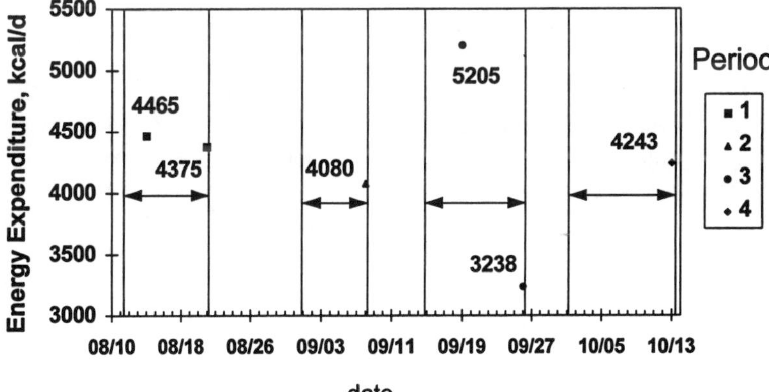

FIGURE 12-5 Multiple administrations of doubly labeled water doses to obtain energy
expenditure during much of a Ranger training course.

Drawbacks of the DLW Method

The major drawbacks of the DLW method are cost of the ^{18}O-labeled water and the cost and technical difficulties associated with the isotope analyses. The need for an expensive isotope ratio mass spectrometer and sample preparation systems limits the number of laboratories that can carry out the method on-site. In addition, the technical difficulties of measuring the isotope enrichments with the required accuracy are formidable. High accuracy in isotope measurements is required because energy expenditure is calculated based on a small difference between the two isotope elimination rates. The primary difficulties arise from fractionation of the isotopes during sample preparation and measurement due to the different physical characteristics of the heavy isotopes compared with the major isotope. Furthermore, sample matrix can interfere with isotope measurements (as discussed above). However, there are several labs throughout the world that have considerable experience with the method and have overcome the analytical difficulties.

Price and availability of the ^{18}O-labeled water have been drawbacks of the DLW method. In early 1990, the price of a gram of $H_2{}^{18}O$ (10 g of a 10% solution) had risen to $36, with a dosing for a typical 70-kg man costing $400. Due to increased demand and production problems over the next couple of years, the price of $H_2{}^{18}O$ rose to over $63/g, with delivery times often exceeding 12 months. This price increase brought the cost of dosing a single subject to at least $700. By early 1995, the shortage was overcome, with the price dropping to $35/g and delivery within a few weeks, bringing the cost of dosing a typical 70-kg subject down to $385. The increased availability of $H_2{}^{18}O$ at a lower price will allow more widespread use of the DLW method. In addition, it will allow an entire training course to be covered with DLW measurements, with no gaps, as has been done in the past (see Figure 12-5).

AUTHOR'S CONCLUSIONS AND RECOMMENDATIONS

The doubly labeled water method is an ideal tool for military nutrition research. It is a true field technique for accurate measurement of free-living energy expenditure of soldiers undergoing training exercises. The only intrusion into the soldier's daily routine is collection of urine and saliva samples at the beginning and end of the study. The method also provides simultaneous measures of TBW, body composition, and water turnover. When applying the DLW method to military nutrition research, the following recommendations are made:

- The two-point method should be utilized to calculate elimination rates, with backup specimens collected for the initial and final time points.
- A control group should be included to correct for baseline isotope shifts due to changes in food and water supply.

- Careful planning is required so that the optimum dosing and specimen collection protocol are utilized based on (1) estimated water turnover and energy expenditure, and (2) maximization of information gained from study.
- When calculating energy expenditure, use Equation 12-2, which incorporates new dilution space factors based on the latest available data.
- Multiple DLW dosings can be used to obtain data on energy expenditure for long training exercises.
- The decrease in cost of the $H_2^{18}O$ dose should allow for adequate dosings to cover an entire training study, with no gaps in energy expenditure data.

REFERENCES

Cole, T.J., and W.A. Coward
  1992   Precision and accuracy of doubly labeled water energy expenditure by multipoint and two-point methods. Am. J. Physiol. 263 (26):E965–E973.
Coward, A.
  1990   The doubly labeled water method for measuring energy expenditure. Technical recommendations for use in humans. Calculation of pool sizes and flux rates. Pp. 48–68 in NAHRES-4, A Consensus Report by the IDECG Working Group, A.M. Prentice, ed. Vienna: IAEA.
Coward, W.A.
  1988   The doubly labeled water ($^2H_2^{18}O$) method: Principles and practice. Proc. Nutr. Soc. 47:209–218.
Coward ,W.A., P. Ritz, and T.J. Cole
  1994   Revision of calculations in the doubly labeled water method for measurement of energy expenditure in humans. Am. J. Physiol. 267 (30):E805–E807.
Dansgaard, W.
  1964   Stable isotopes in precipitation. Tellus 16:436–468.
DeLany, J.P., D.A. Schoeller, R.W. Hoyt, E.W. Askew, and M.A. Sharp
  1989   Field use of $D_2^{18}O$ to measure energy expenditure of soldiers at different energy intakes. J. Appl. Physiol. 67(5):1922–1929.
DeLany, J.P., R.J. Moore, and R.W. Hoyt
  1991   Use of doubly labeled water for measurement of energy of soldiers during training exercises in a cold environment and at high altitude [abstract]. Int. J. Obes. 15:48.
Edwards, J.S.A., E.W. Askew, N. King, C.S. Fulco, R.W. Hoyt, and J.P. DeLany
  1991   An assessment of the nutritional intake and energy expenditure of unacclimatized U.S. Army soldiers living and working at high altitude. Technical Report No. T10-91. Natick, Mass.: U.S. Army Research Institute of Environmental Medicine.
Forbes-Ewan, C.H., B.L.L. Morrissey, G.C. Gregg, and D.R. Waters
  1989   Use of doubly labeled water technique in soldiers training for jungle warfare. J. Appl. Physiol. 67(1):14–18.
Hoyt, R.W., T.E. Jones, T.P. Stein, G.W. McAninch, H.R. Lieberman, E.W. Askew, and A. Cymerman
  1991   Doubly labeled water measurement of human energy expenditure during strenuous exercise. J. Appl. Physiol. 71(1):16–22.
Hoyt, R.W., T.E. Jones, C.J. Baker-Fulco, D.A. Schoeller, R.B. Schoene, R.S. Schwartz, E.W. Askew, and A. Cymerman
  1994   Doubly labeled water measurement of human energy expenditure during exercise at high altitude. Am. J. Physiol. 266:R966–R971.

James, W.P.T., J.P. Haggarty, and B.A. McGaw
  1988   Recent progress in studies on energy expenditure: Are the new methods providing answers to old questions? Proc. Nutr. Soc. 47:195–208.
Jones, P.J.H., A. Winthrop, D.A. Schoeller, R.M. Filler, P.R. Swyer, J.Smith, and T. Heim
  1988   Evaluation of doubly labeled water for measuring energy expenditure during changing nutrition. Am. J. Clin. Nutr. 47:799–804.
Jones, T.E., R.W. Hoyt, J.P. DeLany, R.L Hesslink, and E.W. Askew
  1993   A comparison of two methods of measuring water intake of soldiers in the field [abstract]. FASEB J. 7:A610.
Lifson, N., and R. McClintock
  1966   Theory of use of turnover rates of body water for measuring energy and material balance. J. Theor. Biol. 12:46–74.
Lifson, N., G.B. Gordon, and R. McClintock
  1955   Measurement of total carbon dioxide production by means of D_2O^{18}. J. Appl. Physiol. 7:705–710.
Lifson, N., W.S. Little, D.G. Levitt, and R.M. Henderson
  1975 $D_2^{18}O$ method for CO_2 output in small mammals and economic feasibility in man. J. Appl. Physiol. 39(4):657–664.
Moore, R.J., K.E. Friedl, T.R. Kramer, L.E. Martinez-Lopez, R.W. Hoyt, R.E. Tulley, J.P. DeLany, E.W. Askew, and J.A. Vogel
  1992   Changes in soldier nutritional status and immune function during the Ranger training course. Technical Report No. T13-92. Natick, Mass.: U.S. Army Research Institute of Environmental Medicine.
Nagy, K.A., and D.P. Costa
  1980   Water flux in animals: Analysis of potential errors in the tritiated water method. Am. J. Physiol. 238:R454–R465.
Racette, S.B., D.A. Schoeller, A.H. Luke, K. Shay, J. Hnilicka, and R.F. Kushner
  1994   Relative dilution spaces of ^2H- and ^{18}O-labeled water in humans. Am. J. Physiol. 267 (30):E585–E590.
Ritz, P., P.G. Johnson, and W.A. Coward
  1994   Measurements of ^2H and ^{18}O in body water: Analytical considerations and physiological implications. Br. J. Nutr. 72:3–12.
Roberts, S.B.
  1989   Use of doubly labeled water method for measurement of energy expenditure, total body water, water intake, and metabolizable energy intake in humans and small animals. Can. J. Physiol. Pharmacol. 67:1190–1198.
Schoeller, D.A.
  1988   Measurement of energy expenditure in free-living humans by using doubly labeled water. J. Nutr. 188:1278–1289.
Schoeller, D.A., and A. Coward
  1990   The doubly-labeled water method for measuring energy expenditure. Technical recommendations for use in humans. Practical consequences of deviations from the isotope elimination model. Pp. 166–190 in NAHRES-4, A Consensus Report by the IDECG Working Group, A.M. Prentice, ed. Vienna: IAEA.
Schoeller, D.A., and E. van Santen
  1982   Measurement of energy expenditure in humans by doubly labeled water method. J. Appl. Physiol. 53(4):955–959.
Schoeller, D.A., E. van Santen, D.W. Peterson, W. Dietz, J. Jaspan, and P.D. Klein
  1980   Total body water measurement in humans with ^{18}O and ^2H labeled water. Am. J. Clin. Nutr. 33:2686–2693.

Schoeller, D.A., R.F. Kushner, and P.J.H. Jones
  1986   Validation of doubly labeled water for measuring energy expenditure during parenteral nutrition. Am. J. Clin. Nutr. 44:291–298.
Speakman, J.R., and P.A. Racey
  1986   Measurement of CO_2 production by the doubly labeled water technique. J. Appl. Physiol. 61:1200–1202.
Speakman, J.R., K.S. Nair, and M.I. Goran
  1993   Revised equations for calculating CO_2 production from doubly labeled water in humans. Am. J. Physiol. 264 (27):E912–E917.
Welle, S.
  1990   Two-point vs. multipoint sample collection for the analysis of energy expenditure by use of the doubly labeled water method. Am J. Clin. Nutr. 52:1134–1138.
Westerterp, K.R., F. Brounds, W.H.M. Saris, and F.T. Hoor
  1988   Comparison of doubly labeled water with respirometry at low- and high-acitivity levels. J. Appl. Physiol. 65(1):53–56.

DISCUSSION

JOHANNA DWYER: How long is long term with multiple doses?

JAMES DeLANY: We attempted to cover a 2-mo time period. We did not quite make it. We would have needed at least six to eight dosings, maybe seven, to cover the whole Ranger training study.

JOHANNA DWYER: But it is within the realm of possibility?

JAMES DeLANY: Yes. But that was all the isotope Reed Hoyt had.

DENNIS BIER: I, like most of the other people in the room, I would guess, are enamored with this method for its advantages, but I still have a problem with the two-dose approach. You showed us several lines which clearly were not linear; I mean, they had breakpoints. In one case, it was because the subjects had eaten more, as I remember. With the last line, you had the last two points 1 day apart, and there was a change in the slope of the curve.

JAMES DeLANY: That was actually from the same study.

DENNIS BIER: Two points will always define a straight line, so you are okay there, but then when you have these other lines, there may be breakpoints because there is a change in energy expenditure. If that is the case, if they break in short periods of time, then you no longer have the steady state circumstance you need to make the calculation because you are not far enough into the decay period of the water. Or depending on what point you have, if you are taking only two of them, you can change the slope of that line, depending on where you are. You showed us lines at several points.

Finally, I want to comment on just the simple matter of when people collect samples. I can imagine a situation in the field where a guy is supposed to collect a sample at noon. But then noon passes and next it's "Oh, 12:20 or 1:00, I forgot," and he puts it in the noon bottle. That happens to us all the time. It may not happen to you.

JAMES DeLANY: Oh, I am sure it does. Okay, let us start with your first point.

DENNIS BIER: Could you just go back to one slide for an example, just about the second or the third from the end?

(Slide)

Depending on which one of those last three points you pick, or the last two points . . .

JAMES DeLANY: The last two points, right.

This is the same study that I showed you where on this day, the subjects were on a 12-mi march, and on this day they were stuck in the tent. The advantage of the two-point method is it gives the true cumulative elimination. If this was appropriately modeled with a modeling technique, you would get the correct answer, but no one does that.

This is actually a lower-energy expenditure day. Doubly labeled water does not give you a day-by-day breakdown; it is integrated, so you measure it over 7 to 10 days and then divide by 7, and you get an average. But that does not mean that the energy expenditure was 6,000 calories a day every day during this study.

For instance, on this day I am sure it was 2,500 or less; they were stuck in the tent sleeping all day. The two-point method, though, will give you the true elimination over that time period.

DENNIS BIER: Which two points did you pick?

JAMES DeLANY: The beginning and end. Between this day and this day, the average energy expenditure would be 100 kcals more than this final day. I do not know, I am just pulling a number out of the hat. But we were interested in the whole time period.

ROBERT WOLFE: Since you made the case so strongly for the two-point method, the other thing I would add that there is a potential advantage to collecting multiple points. It is that you use the jackknife technique to examine bad data points. For example, if you have seven data points, you calculate energy expenditure using all of the data points. Then you recalculate energy expenditure, sequentially eliminating each data point. You end up with a series of values that can be used to calculate a standard deviation of the energy expenditure determination in that individual.

That has some practical advantages in two senses. One, if you get an outlier that is way off, you can preset the standard deviation beyond which you will not accept a value. Where we found that to be particularly useful was when we were studying the energy expenditure of the U.S. swimmers prior to the Olympics. It turned out they were using much more energy than we had anticipated.

So by doing that, you can work backwards. In other words, if we had used the original whole period, that enrichment was so low and the variability was so much that the standard deviation for each individual was very large. We just kept removing the last time points from regression analysis until we reached the point where we had an acceptable standard deviation when we did this technique of dropping one point and using the remainder.

It is kind of a different issue than Denny and you were just arguing, but it gives you at least some sort of a statistical basis to decide whether an outlier is one that should be discarded and, also, the point at which you would say, again, in an objective way, whether the rest of the data points are giving us more variability than information.

DAVID SCHNAKENBERG: In the first study you did for us up in the mountains of Vermont, we were interested in water consumption, and you used this methodology to do water flux and estimate of water consumption over that entire period. You did not mention that. Is that at all feasible to do?

JAMES DeLANY: In fact, in many of the studies, particularly when the ^{18}O was a problem, we did a lot of studies with turnover of total body water. In some of the altitude studies, we were interested just in water. I meant to bring that up, but you are right, we do measure water flux and have done some studies with canteen measurement of water intake versus the isotope and got very good agreement.

DAVID SCHNAKENBERG: What do you feel the reliability of that method is for estimating actual fluid consumption over extended periods?

JAMES DeLANY: It does not appear to be as good as energy expenditure, but some of the data that Tanya Jones has been compiling, some of the data that we have collected regarding the use of isotope versus the canteen measurements, look really good, with a correlation of maybe 0.85 between the measured intake and the isotope measurement of water turnover.

JOAN CONWAY: Do you need doubly labeled water to do the water flux?

JAMES DeLANY: No, just deuterium.

DAVID SCHNAKENBERG: It [water flux] is a by-product of going through all the calculations of the DLW method.

JAMES DeLANY: Yes, you get it because you calculate water turnover in the DLW method, yes.

Emerging Technologies for Nutrition Research, 1997
Pp. 297–314. Washington, D.C.
National Academy Press

13

Measurement of Oxygen Uptake with Portable Equipment

John F. Patton[1]

INTRODUCTION

The energy balance of an organism is a function of energy intake and energy expenditure. Energy intake, the amount of food consumed in a given period, is theoretically easy to assess through careful quantification of food intake. In contrast, the measurement of energy expenditure under free-living conditions has been one of the more elusive goals of research scientists. Energy expenditure is an important measurement in many nutritional, epidemiological, and ergonomic studies, whether it be in determining daily energy requirements, calculating energy balance, measuring habitual physical activity, or quantifying energy cost of physical task performance.

Generally, two approaches have been used to assess energy expenditure: indirect estimates and direct measurement of oxygen uptake. Indirect methods include such procedures as activity questionnaires (Montoye, 1971),

[1] John F. Patton, Military Performance Division, U.S. Army Research Institute of Environmental Medicine, Natick, MA 01760-5007

heart-rate recording (Spurr et al., 1988), pedometers and accelerometers (Kashiwazaki et al., 1986; Montoye, et al., 1983), and doubly labeled water (Stager et al., 1995). In general, many of these suffer from various practical and/or theoretical limitations, and some have not been evaluated to determine their reliability or validity.

The validity of the direct measurement of oxygen uptake as a basis for measuring energy expenditure, however, has been well established and has been used to determine the energy cost of a great variety of human activities. In field studies, the classical method has been to collect expired air in Douglas bags (DB) carried by the subject or the experimenter. While this technique has been widely used, it is cumbersome, limited to fairly short collection periods, and requires timed collections of expired gas and subsequent analysis of expired oxygen and carbon dioxide concentrations using conventional laboratory techniques.

The modified Kofranyi-Michaelis (KM) respirometer (Consolazio, 1971), which also has been used extensively for energy exchange studies in a field environment, represents an early portable system to measure expired volume. The KM meter is a simple, compact, lightweight unit consisting of a dry gas meter for measuring the total volume and temperature of the expired air. An aliquoting device continuously removes a small percentage of each breath into a bag that is then analyzed for oxygen and carbon dioxide concentrations in the laboratory.

A truly portable system, however, is one that not only is capable of measuring the volume of the expired or inspired air for determination of minute ventilation ($\dot{V}E$ or $\dot{V}I$), but also is capable of measuring gas concentrations so that oxygen uptake ($\dot{V}O_2$) can be calculated by the instrument. In addition, such a system must be light enough to be easily transported and must be battery operated, and the analysis of both gas volume and concentration must be rapid and integrated with a high-speed microprocessor. Currently, there are three systems available that possess these technological advancements and allow for the measurement of $\dot{V}O_2$ in humans under free-living conditions. This paper will describe the specifications of each of these and present data on their validity, reliability, and operability in the laboratory and, where applicable, in a field environment.

PORTABLE SYSTEMS FOR MEASURING OXYGEN UPTAKE

The three portable systems capable of providing a continuous measurement of $\dot{V}O_2$ and ventilation for long periods are (1) the Total Energy Expenditure Measurement system (TEEM 100, AeroSport, Ann Arbor, Mich.), (2) the COSMED K2 (Vacumed, Ventura, Calif.), and (3) the Oxylog (P. K. Morgan, Andover, Mass.). Each of these has unique features but contains the basic technological advances previously mentioned to allow for the rapid measurement and integration of ventilation and gas concentrations and, thus, the calculation of oxygen uptake.

TEEM 100

Specifications

The TEEM 100 is the newest of the portable systems and has been available commercially for approximately 4 years (TEEM 100 Operator's Manual, 1993). The principal features of this instrument are depicted in Table 13-1.

Briefly, the TEEM 100 uses an open-circuit continuous sampling system for the measurement of oxygen uptake ($\dot{V}O_2$) and carbon dioxide production ($\dot{V}CO_2$). A simple orifice plate pneumotachometer located in the face mask measures expired flow. A high-frequency pulse-modulated valve extracts proportional samples of expired gas over the flow wave form. These samples are introduced into a closed-loop mixing chamber and then passed into a gas analysis chamber, both of which are located in the base unit. An electronic variable sampling system provides a constant flow of gas independent of the expired flow rate. This means equilibration time is constant over a wide range of $\dot{V}E$. The oxygen and carbon dioxide percentages are measured using an absolute oxygen (O_2) sensor (galvanic fuel cell) and a nondispersive, infrared CO_2 detector, respectively. The microprocessor integrates $\dot{V}E$ with expired O_2 and CO_2 percentages to calculate $\dot{V}O_2$, $\dot{V}CO_2$, $\dot{V}E$, and respiratory exchange ratio

TABLE 13-1 TEEM 100 Specifications

Weight: 3.3 kg

$\dot{V}E$: Pneumotachometer in facemask (range: 2–200 liters $\cdot$ min^{-1})

FeO$_2$: Galvanic fuel cell (range: 0–25%)

FeCO$_2$: Nondispersible infrared (range: 0–10%)

Power: 12-volt rechargeable battery (timed use/charge: 2 hours)

Output: Parallel and serial ports
Digital panel meter

Variables: $\dot{V}E$, FeO$_2$, FeCO$_2$, $\dot{V}O_2$, $\dot{V}CO_2$, RER,

NOTE: TEEM, Total Energy Expenditure Measurement system; $\dot{V}E$, expired minute ventilation; FeO$_2$, fractional concentration of oxygen in expired air; FeCO$_2$, fractional concentration of carbon dioxide in expired air; $\dot{V}O_2$, oxygen uptake; $\dot{V}CO_2$, carbon dioxide production; RER, respiratory exchange ratio.

SOURCE: Adapted from TEEM 100 Operator's Manual (1993).

(RER). The measurement of CO_2 and calculation of the RER are unique features of the TEEM 100 and represent important variables in many nutrition studies.

Validity-Reliability Data

Available data evaluating the TEEM 100 for the measurement of $\dot{V}O_2$ are limited. Segal et al. (1994) compared the TEEM 100 to the Sensormedics 2900 (S2900) Metabolic Analysis System during low-intensity cycle ergometer exercise (0, 25, and 50 W) and found no significant differences in either $\dot{V}O_2$ or $\dot{V}E$ at any intensity. Also, correlations between the two systems ranged from $r = 0.85$ to $r = 0.96$ ($p < 0.001$), with no significant differences between the regression line and the line of identity. The authors concluded that the findings support the validity of the TEEM 100 for low-intensity exercise and suggest that it is an acceptable alternative to the more cumbersome, expensive systems for gas exchange and metabolic measurements in the laboratory.

In a study to evaluate the TEEM 100 at higher exercise intensities, Clure et al. (1995) compared it to the S2900 during maximum exercise testing of well-conditioned athletes. At peak $\dot{V}O_2$, $\dot{V}E$ (liters $\cdot$ min^{-1}) was significantly lower with the TEEM 100 compared to the S2900 (146 $\pm$ 15 vs. 135 $\pm$ 16, $p < 0.05$) but no difference was seen in $\dot{V}O_2$ (60.7 $\pm$ 6.2 vs. 58.0 $\pm$ 6.5 ml $\cdot$ kg^{-1} $\cdot$ min^{-1}). The correlation between the two systems for $\dot{V}O_2$ at all levels of exercise was 0.71, suggesting that while the TEEM 100 appears to provide valid data for maximum performance testing, considerable individual variability may occur.

Because of its portability, apparent ease of use, and validity at low-exercise intensities compared to the SensorMedics 2900 system, it can be concluded that the TEEM 100 has potential for use in the areas of exercise science, nutrition, and rehabilitation and athletic medicine. Certainly more validity studies need to be performed using different exercise protocols and under conditions where the instrument is worn by the subject to establish its robustness. Also its suitability for use in environments other than the laboratory must be determined.

COSMED K2

Specifications

The COSMED K2 is a relatively new, integrated, portable, telemetric oxygen uptake system (K2 Operator's Manual, 1991). Its attractiveness lies in its capability to obtain $\dot{V}O_2$ and $\dot{V}E$ from individuals performing work in the field or in conditions such as space flight where large, more cumbersome equipment would be unmanageable. The basic features of this system are depicted in Table 13-2.

TABLE 13-2 COSMED K2 Specifications

Weight: 0.85 kg (transmitter + battery pack)

$\dot{V}_E$: Turbine flowmeter in facemask (range: 2 to > 300 liters $\cdot$ min^{-1})

FeO_2: Polarographic (range: 9–23%)

Power: NiCd rechargeable batteries (timed use/charge: 2–4 hours)

Output: Receiver unit (range: 600 m [1,967 ft])

Variables: $\dot{V}_E$, FeO_2, $\dot{V}_{O_2}$, R_f

NOTE: $\dot{V}_E$, expired minute ventilation; FeO_2, fractional concentration of oxygen in expired air; NiCd, nickel-cadmium; $\dot{V}_{O_2}$, oxygen uptake; R_f, respiratory rate.

SOURCE: Adapted from K2 Operator's Manual (1991).

The COSMED K2 consists of a specially designed facemask that contains a photoelectric turbine-type flowmeter (response range over 300 liters $\cdot$ min^{-1}) and a capillary tube for sampling expired air. An extra valve located at the bottom of the face mask reduces inspiratory resistance and helps eliminate condensation for the comfort of the subject.

The system is equipped with an FM radio transmitter that broadcasts signals to a receiver unit. The receiver includes a microcomputer that processes, archives, and displays calculated data (on screen and in print) in real time. The receiver is equipped with an interface for downloading to a computer. The range of the transmitter in an open field is 600 m (1,967 ft), using the small antenna supplied.

The transmitter is composed of two subunits carried by the subject in a specially designed harness, with the front unit containing the gas-sampling and transmitter apparatus on the subject's chest and the rear unit containing the battery pack on the subject's back. Both the receiver and transmitter are powered by rechargeable nickel-cadmium (NiCd) batteries.

As ambient air passes through the facemask, it is sampled by the capillary tube at a rate proportional to the ventilatory rate by way of a dynamic sampling pump. It then passes through a desiccant and into a miniature mixing chamber located inside the transmitter, which also contains the oxygen polarographic electrode.

The transmitter sends data for $\dot{V}_{O_2}$ and $\dot{V}_E$ to the receiver, which displays and prints the $\dot{V}_{O_2}$, $\dot{V}_E$, respiratory rate (R_f), tidal volume, and fractional concentration of oxygen in expired air (FeO_2). Because the COSMED K2 does not analyze CO_2 in the expired air, it is not able to determine the RER. It assumes that RER equals 1.00 for every value of $\dot{V}_{O_2}$. The equation used to calculate $\dot{V}_{O_2}$ at standard temperature and pressure, dry gas (STPD) is:

$$\dot{V}_{O_2} = \dot{V}_E \times (F_IO_2 - FeO_2), \qquad\qquad \text{(Equation 13-1)}$$

where fractional concentration of oxygen in inspired air (F_IO_2) is assumed to be 20.93 percent.

Validity-Reliability Data

The COSMED K2 has been evaluated by a number of researchers over the past few years (Crandall et al., 1994; Kawakami et al., 1992; Lucia et al., 1993). Kawakami et al. (1992) compared the COSMED to the DB method during continuous cycle ergometry exercise of gradually increasing loads and found, with a few exceptions, little difference between systems over ranges of 0.5 to 2.5 liters $\cdot$ min^{-1} for $\dot{V}_{O_2}$ and 10 to 90 liters $\cdot$ min^{-1} for $\dot{V}_E$. These authors also used the COSMED during such sporting events as rowing and soccer and found it to be useful in assessing training.

Crandall et al. (1994) compared the COSMED to a breath-by-breath (BBB, the criterion method) metabolic measurement system during a maximal graded exercise test (GXT) using the Bruce protocol (treadmill exercise test) (Bruce et al., 1973). As expected with a system that lacks the capacity to measure CO_2, at the lower exercise intensities the COSMED tended to underestimate the $\dot{V}_{O_2}$ measured by the BBB system and at higher intensities tended to overestimate the BBB $\dot{V}_{O_2}$. However, there were no significant differences between systems at any stage of the GXT. COSMED ventilation volumes, however, were significantly higher than those measured with the BBB system, but this did not have any apparent effect on the validity of the $\dot{V}_{O_2}$ data.

In the most comprehensive evaluation of the COSMED, Lucia and coworkers (1993) compared it to the DB technique during submaximal progressive treadmill exercise consisting of six stages of 3 minutes each after which a maximal test was performed following a rest period. In addition, a comparison also was made between two different COSMED systems. Tables 13-3, 13-4, and 13-5 present average values for $\dot{V}_E$, FeO_2, and $\dot{V}_{O_2}$, respectively, for three of the exercise stages and at maximal exercise.

All comparisons between mean values of $\dot{V}_E$ (Table 13-3) measured by the two COSMEDs or DB indicated no significant differences and, indeed, were remarkably close at all stages with the exception of maximal exercise. At this latter intensity, the difference was less than 6 percent. Correlation coefficients among the three systems were significant ($p < 0.01$) and above 0.90 for all intensities.

Comparisons among mean values of FeO_2 measured by COSMED1, COSMED2, and the DB showed significant differences for the submaximal stages (Table 13-4). Correlation coefficients among testing sessions were significant ($p < 0.01$) but relatively low for most exercise intensities, consistently below 0.80.

TABLE 13-3 Average Values of Minute Ventilation (liters $\cdot$ min^{-1}, BTPS)

Intensity	COSMED1	COSMED2	DB
Stage 2	79 ± 19	79 ± 19	78 ± 19
Stage 4	99 ± 24	98 ± 26	97 ± 25
Stage 6	121 ± 33	119 ± 32	122 ± 33
Maximal	151 ± 35	151 ± 32	159 ± 40

NOTE: BTPS, body temperature and pressure, saturated gas; DB, Douglas bag.

SOURCE: Adapted from Lucia et al. (1993).

TABLE 13-4 Average Values of Fractional Concentration of Oxygen in Expired Air (%)

Intensity	COSMED1	COSMED2	DB
Stage 2	16.3 ± 0.5	16.3 ± 0.4	16.0 ± 0.5
Stage 4	16.7 ± 0.5	16.6 ± 0.4	16.4 ± 0.5
Stage 6	16.9 ± 0.6	16.8 ± 0.5	16.7 ± 0.5
Maximal	17.2 ± 0.4	17.3 ± 0.4	17.1 ± 0.5

NOTE: DB, Douglas bag.

SOURCE: Adapted from Lucia et al. (1993).

TABLE 13-5 Average Values of Oxygen Uptake (liters $\cdot$ min^{-1}, STPD)

Intensity	COSMED1	COSMED2	DB
Stage 2	2.32 ± 0.46	2.35 ± 0.51	2.43 ± 0.51
Stage 4	2.70 ± 0.53	2.70 ± 0.55	2.80 ± 0.58
Stage 6	3.09 ± 0.65	3.09 ± 0.60	3.22 ± 0.68
Maximal	3.57 ± 0.76	3.51 ± 0.70	3.69 ± 0.76

NOTE: STPD, standard temperature and pressure, dry gas; DB, Douglas bag.

SOURCE: Adapted from Lucia et al. (1993).

Mean values of $\dot{V}O_2$ among systems showed significant differences only at Stage 6 of the submaximal exercise test (Table 13-5). The percent variation among mean $\dot{V}O_2$ levels over the three testing sessions was consistently below 5 percent across all exercise intensities. Correlation coefficients among COSMED1, COSMED2, and the DB were significant at all intensities ($p < 0.01$) and relatively high, always above 0.86.

Because the COSMED K2 does not measure CO_2, it is predisposed to an inherent error in calculating $\dot{V}O_2$. However, Lucia et al. (1993) found that if the average RER obtained from the DB technique is used to correct the $\dot{V}O_2$ measured by the COSMED, this value does not differ significantly from that of the actual value obtained across all exercise intensities. Thus, the results indicate that the COSMED K2 is a reliable and valid instrument for the measurement of $\dot{V}O_2$ during laboratory exercise testing at submaximal and maximal intensities. Also the assumption made by the COSMED of a constant respiratory gas exchange ratio of 1.00 did not have a significant influence on $\dot{V}O_2$ measurements.

Oxylog

The Oxylog, initially reported on by Humphrey and Wolff (1977), was the first of the portable systems able to provide a continuous, direct measure of $\dot{V}O_2$ and $\dot{V}E$ for long periods.

Specifications

The specifications for the Oxylog are presented in Table 13-6. In 1994, the instrument was completely updated with respect to its electronics, data acquisition, and storage capability and the method used to measure O_2 concentration in inspired and expired gases (Oxylog Operator's Manual, 1994).

The instrument is equipped with an oronasal mask that is held against the face by an elastic head harness. On the inspired side of the mask, a turbine flowmeter is attached for measurement of inspiratory volume, a unique feature of this instrument. Expired air passes through flexible respiratory tubing connected to the Oxylog. The older model measured the inspired ventilation over a range of only 6 to 80 liters $\cdot$ min^{-1}, which, due to the limitations of the system, limited the measurement of $\dot{V}O_2$ to 3.0 liters $\cdot$ min^{-1}. The new model, with a larger flowmeter and greater ventilatory range, can measure $\dot{V}O_2$ up to 10 liters $\cdot$ min^{-1}.

The O_2 fraction of the inspired air is measured separately from that of the expired air by using two fuel cells (the older model used polarographic electrodes) in samples dried by passing through a desiccant. The use of two fuel

TABLE 13-6 Oxylog Specifications

Weight: < 2 kg
$\dot{V}$I: Turbine flowmeter in facemask (range: 2–150 liters · min^{-1})
F_1O_2 and FeO_2: Figaro fuel cell (range: 0–25%)
Power: NiCd rechargeable battery (timed use/charge: 12 hours)
Output: Panel display meter
Serial port
Variables: $\dot{V}$I, F_1O_2, FeO_2, $\dot{V}O_2$

NOTE: $\dot{V}$I, inspired minute ventilation; F_1O_2, fractional concentration of oxygen in inspired air; FeO_2, fractional concentration of oxygen in expired air; NiCd, nickel-cadmium; $\dot{V}O_2$, oxygen uptake.

SOURCE: Adapted from Oxylog Operator's Manual (1994).

cells to determine the difference in O_2 concentrations (between inspired air vs. expired air) is also a unique feature among portable systems. The TEEM 100 and COSMED K2 both assumed an inspired O_2 concentration of 20.93 percent.

The Oxylog uses the same formula as the COSMED K2 for calculating $\dot{V}O_2$ and is, therefore, subject to the same error when RER is other than 1.00. At RERs of 0.8 and 0.9, this underestimation is approximately 3.5 percent and 1.8 percent, respectively (Harrison et al., 1982).

The Oxylog is powered by NiCd batteries that provide a timed use per charge of up to 12 hours. This represents a major advantage over the previous systems. $\dot{V}O_2$ and $\dot{V}E$ data are stored internally each minute during use and may be retrieved by serial link when connected to an IBM-compatible computer. The total inclusive storage time is over 2,000 minutes.

Validity-Reliability Data

Over the past few years, several authors have evaluated the accuracy of the Oxylog for use in both the laboratory and the field environment for measurement of $\dot{V}O_2$ (Ballal and MacDonald, 1982; Harrison et al., 1982; Louhevaara and Ilmarinen, 1985).

Harrison et al. (1982) compared steady-state values of minute ventilation and $\dot{V}O_2$ measured by the Oxylog and a standard laboratory system comprising a dry gas meter and mass spectrometer during cycle ergometer exercise at intensities ranging from 75 to 150 W. They found that mean differences between $\dot{V}$I (Oxylog) and $\dot{V}E$ (standard) were significant ($p < 0.05$) only at the highest intensity (4.9% lower for Oxylog), while Oxylog values for $\dot{V}O_2$ were 4.4 percent lower ($p < 0.01$) than standard values for all intensities.

In the study by Louhevaara and Ilmarinen (1985), similar results were found in a comparison between the Oxylog and the DB technique during both dynamic exercise (walking) and combined static (lifting) and dynamic exercise at various intensities. While the correlation coefficients between these two systems were 0.99 and 0.91 for walking and lifting, respectively, the Oxylog underestimated the $\dot{V}O_2$ by an average of 4.1 percent for walking and 6.4 percent for lifting.

The Oxylog also was evaluated in this laboratory (Unpublished data, J. F. Patton, M. M. Murphy, R. P. Mello, T. Bidwell, and M. Harp, U.S. Army Research Institute of Environmental Medicine, Natick, Mass., 1992) by comparing it to the DB method in 12 men during steady-state treadmill walking at 3.5 mph at grades of 0 percent, 5 percent, and 10 percent. The data for inspired ventilation and $\dot{V}O_2$ are presented in Tables 13-7 and 13-8, respectively.

As seen, these data agree quite closely with previous reports that found the Oxylog to underestimate $\dot{V}O_2$ by 4 to 5 percent. Again, if the correction factor for RER is applied (1.8% for an RER of 0.9; 3.5% for 0.8), the underestimation is reduced to approximately 2 to 3 percent since the RER at the above intensities was between 0.83 and 0.90.

The correlation coefficient for $\dot{V}O_2$ between the DB technique and the Oxylog was 0.98 ($p < 0.001$), indicating a very good relationship over the range of exercise intensities studied.

Other Studies Using the Oxylog

In a report by the World Health Organization (WHO) on energy and protein requirements (1985), emphasis was placed on the importance of relying on

TABLE 13-7 Ventilation, liters · min^{-1} (mean ± SE)

Grade (%)	Oxylog	DB	% Difference
0	30.5 ± 0.8	29.5 ± 1.0	−3.3
5	42.3 ± 1.1	40.6 ± 1.0	−4.0
10	59.3 ± 1.8	56.5 ± 1.3	−4.7

NOTE: SE, standard error; DB, Douglas bag.

SOURCE: Adapted from J. F. Patton, M. M. Murphy, R. P. Mello, T. Bidwell, and M. Harp (Unpublished data, U.S. Army Research Institute of Environmental Medicine, Natick, Mass., 1992).

TABLE 13-8 Oxygen uptake, liters $\cdot$ min^{-1} (mean $\pm$ SE)

Grade (%)	Oxylog	DB	% Difference
0	1.22 ± 0.03	1.17 ± 0.04	–4.1
5	1.71 ± 0.04	1.64 ± 0.04	–4.1
10	2.31 ± 0.05	2.21 ± 0.05	–4.3

NOTE: SE, standard error; DB, Douglas bag.

SOURCE: Adapted from J. F. Patton, M. M. Murphy, R. P. Mello, T. Bidwell, and M. Harp (Unpublished data, U.S. Army Research Institute of Environmental Medicine, Natick, Mass., 1992).

measures of energy expenditure rather than energy intake as a basis for arriving at possible estimates of energy requirements of various individuals and populations. As a result, a number of investigators have reported on the use of the Oxylog for the direct measurement of metabolic rate to validate daily energy expenditure estimates and to standardize methodology.

In a study by Chiplonkar et al. (1992), the Oxylog was used to measure resting metabolic rate (RMR) in both men and women to validate the FAO/WHO/UNU (Food and Agriculture Organization/World Health Organization/United Nations University) equation for RMR which, in turn, was applied using FAO/WHO/UNU factors for energy cost of physical activities as multiples of RMR to calculate daily energy expenditure estimates.

Soares et al. (1989) measured the basal metabolic rates (BMRs) of 34 healthy individuals with the Oxylog and compared these values to other procedures, such as the Hartmann and Braun Metabolator, ventilated tent and hood, and whole-body indirect calorimeter, and found no significant differences among instruments. This comparison was made because it is important to know whether errors in methodology could account for differences in BMR when collating worldwide measurements.

McNeill et al. (1987), in another metabolic study, modified the Oxylog turbine flowmeter to operate at low flow rates and then compared its use to the DB method for the measurement of RMR. They reported a correlation coefficient of 0.94 between systems, with an underestimation of $\dot{V}O_2$ of 4 to 5 percent by the Oxylog, similar to that previously seen during exercise, and concluded that it was sufficiently accurate for field studies of energy expenditure.

In other applications of the Oxylog, Ikegami et al. (1988) described the development of a telemetry system for the Oxylog and then applied it to the measurement of $\dot{V}O_2$ during a doubles tennis game lasting 80 minutes. This probably represented the first reported successful continuous measurement of $\dot{V}O_2$ during actual sports activity.

Patton et al. (1995) also used the Oxylog to quantify the increase in energy cost for both men and women of performing physical tasks (such as load carriage, lifting, lift and carry, and obstacle course navigation) in chemical protective clothing. These tasks were conducted in both laboratory and field conditions. It was concluded that the Oxylog provided a very accurate measure of $\dot{V}O_2$ and represented the only practical way such information could be obtained.

Finally, Riley et al. (1992) have employed the Oxylog to assess the functional capacity of patients with chronic cardiac failure during corridor walk testing.

It is evident from these reports that the Oxylog has proven to be an acceptable instrument for the measurement of $\dot{V}O_2$ in nutritional, physiological, and physical rehabilitation type studies.

AUTHOR'S CONCLUSIONS AND RECOMMENDATIONS

The portable systems described herein feature state-of-the-art technology and represent considerable improvements to previously available systems for the direct measurement of $\dot{V}O_2$.

Available data suggest that all three systems are valid and reliable for the measurement of ventilation and oxygen uptake under laboratory conditions. However, only the Oxylog has been thoroughly tested under a variety of field scenarios and been found sufficiently accurate for reliable determinations of $\dot{V}O_2$.

The technology in these systems has matured sufficiently for practical use and is being used in numerous laboratories throughout the world. Further advances in technology will undoubtedly continue, but it is not expected that any significant changes will be made in these instruments in the immediate future since all have been recently developed or updated.

The major drawback to the wide-scale use of these portable systems is their cost (the Oxylog and TEEM 100 are approximately $8,000 and the COSMED K2 is approximately $35,000). This limits the use of these systems to relatively few subjects. This cost, however, should be weighed against that of techniques that estimate only energy expenditure, that is, a cost/benefit (accuracy) analysis must be considered.

The use of Department of Defense funds for further technological developments of portable systems does not seem warranted since these systems encompass the latest in available technology.

The technology utilized in these systems is very practical and requires trained personnel to operate the equipment, but it is not inordinately complex or exotic. The techniques can be learned readily, and the data provided are easily analyzed and interpreted.

REFERENCES

Ballal, M.A., and I.A. MacDonald
1982   An evaluation of the Oxylog as a portable device with which to measure oxygen consumption. Clin. Phys. Physiol. Meas. 3:57–65.

Bruce, R.A., F. Kusumi, and D. Hosmer
1973   Maximal oxygen intake and nomographic assessment of functional aerobic impairment in cardiovascular disease. Am. Heart J. 85:546–562.

Chiplonkar, S.A., V.V. Agte, M.K. Gokhale, V.V. Kulkarni, and S.T. Mane
1992   Energy intake and resting metabolic rate of young Indian men and women. Indian J. Med. Res. 96:250–254.

Clure, C., P.B. Watts, P. Gallagher, R. Hill, S. Humphreys, and B. Wilkins
1995   Accuracy of the TEEM 100 metabolic analyzer during maximum oxygen uptake testing of Nordic skiers [abstract]. Med. Sci. Sports Exerc. 27:S86.

Consolazio, C.F.
1971   Energy expenditure studies in military populations using Kofranyi-Michaelis respirometers. Am. J. Clin. Nutr. 24:1431–1437.

Crandall, C.G., S.L. Taylor, and P.B. Raven
1994   Evaluation of the COSMED K2 portable telemetric oxygen uptake analyzer. Med. Sci. Sports Exerc. 26:108–111.

Harrison, M.H., G.A. Brown, and A.J. Belyavin
1982   The "Oxylog": An evaluation. Ergonomics 25:809–820.

Humphrey, S.J.E., and H.S. Wolff
1977   The Oxylog. J. Physiol. 267:12P.

Ikegami, Y., S. Hiruta, H. Ikegami, and M. Miyamura
1988   Development of a telemetry system for measuring oxygen uptake during sports activities. Eur. J. Appl. Physiol. 57:622–626.

K2 Operator's Manual
1991   Operator's Manual for the K2. Ventura, Calif.: Vacumetrics, Inc., Vacumed Division.

Kashiwazaki, H., T. Inaoka, T. Suzuki, and Y. Kondo
1986   Correlations of pedometer readings with energy expenditure in workers during free-living daily activities. Eur. J. Appl. Physiol. 54:585–590.

Kawakami, Y. D. Nozake, A. Matsuo, and T. Fukunaga
1992   Reliability of measurement of oxygen uptake by a portable telemetric system. Eur. J. Appl. Physiol. 65:409–414.

Louhevaara, V., and J. Ilmarinen
1985   Comparison of three field methods for measuring oxygen consumption. Ergonomics 28:463–470.

Lucia, A., S.J. Fleck, R.W. Gotshall, and J.T. Kearney
1993   Validity and reliability of the COSMED K2 instrument. Int. J. Sports Med. 14:380–386.

McNeill, G. M.D. Cox, and J.P.W. Rivers
1987   The Oxylog oxygen consumption meter: A portable device for measurement of energy expenditure. Am. J. Clin. Nutr. 45:1415–1419.

Montoye, H.J.
1971   Estimation of habitual physical activity by questionnaire and interview. Am. J. Clin. Nutr. 24:1113–1118.

Montoye, H.J., R. Washburn, S. Servais, A. Ertl, J.G. Webster, and F.J. Nagle
1983   Estimation of energy expenditure by a portable accelerometer. Med. Sci. Sports Exerc. 15:403–407.

Oxylog Operator's Manual
   1994   Operator's Manual. Oxylog 2. Andover, Mass.: P.K. Morgan Instruments, Inc.
Patton, J.F., M. Murphy, T. Bidwell, R. Mello, and M. Harp
   1995   Metabolic cost of military physical tasks in MOPP 0 and MOPP 4. Technical
           Report T95-9, AD A294059. Natick, Mass.: U.S. Army Research Institute of Envi-
           ronmental Medicine.
Riley, M., J. McFarland, C.F. Stanford, and D.P. Nicholls
   1992   Oxygen consumption during corridor walk testing in chronic cardiac failure. Eur.
           Heart J. 13:789–793.
Segal, K.R., B. Chatr-Aryamontri, and D. Guvakov
   1994   Validation of a new portable metabolic measurement system [abstract]. Med. Sci.
           Sports Exerc. 26(5):S54.
Soares, M.J., M.L. Sheela, A.V. Kurpad, R.N. Kulkarni, and P.S. Shetty
   1989   The influence of different methods on basal metabolic rate measurements in human
           subjects. Am. J. Clin. Nutr. 50:731–736.
Spurr, G.B., A.M. Prentice, P.R. Murgatroyd, G.R. Goldberg, J.C. Reina, and N.T. Christman
   1988   Energy expenditure from minute-by-minute heart-rate recording: Comparison with
           indirect calorimetry. Am. J. Clin. Nutr. 48:552–559.
Stager, J.M., A. Lindeman, and J. Edwards
   1995   The use of doubly labeled water in quantifying energy expenditure during
           prolonged activity. Sports Med. 19:166–172.
TEEM 100 Operator's Manual
   1993   Operator's Manual. AeroSport TEEM 100 Total Energy Expenditure Measurement
           Manual. Ann Arbor, Mich.: AeroSport, Inc.
WHO (World Health Organization)
   1985   Energy and protein requirements. Report of a joint FAO/WHO/UNU Expert
           Committee. WHO Technical Report Series 724. Geneva, Switzerland: World
           Health Organization.

DISCUSSION

KARL FRIEDL: Are those underestimations something that can be fixed with just a screw or something?

(Laughter)

JOHN PATTON: The only way you can really fix them is to know what your respiratory exchange ratio is at that level of exercise. If you knew that, and you never do when you are using these systems, you could correct it, because there are correction factors for that.

For example, if the RER of exercise is 0.9, then the Oxylog and the COS-MED will underestimate oxygen uptake about 1.8 percent, so if your underestimation is 4 percent, about half of that is due to the fact that you are not measuring carbon dioxide and using that in the equation to calculate oxygen uptake. That is a problem.

JOHANNA DWYER: John, I did not see a clear advantage, and I saw a big cost of the COSMED versus the Oxylog. Did I miss something?

JOHN PATTON: Advantage between them?

JOHANNA DWYER: Yes, for the COSMED.

JOHN PATTON: The cost difference is the big factor, I think.

DOUGLAS WILMORE: Why? That one was out of line with the other two.

JOHN PATTON: It is telemetry.

JOHANNA DWYER: I just wondered what the advantage was in terms of . . .

JAMES DeLANY: But it is not lighter.

JOHN PATTON: Oh, yes, it is. The COSMED K2 is very light.

JOHANNA DWYER: Then that is what it is. Sorry. It is lots lighter.

JOHN PATTON: The data you get out of all these systems appear to be very similar in terms of the underestimation. I kind of am wedded to the Oxylog. I have used it, I know it, I feel comfortable with it. I am not that knowledgeable with the other systems, but that is not to say that the other systems are not good, too.

WENDY KOHRT: What about calibration procedures, and how long is the calibration stable?

JOHN PATTON: The Oxylog is very stable. I cannot really comment on the other two systems, I really do not know. We calibrate the Oxylog at the beginning of the experiment, and it usually holds its calibration for at least an hour or two without any problem—you might want to check it. You can usually tell. You start seeing a little drop-off in the oxygen uptake, but it is pretty stable for 3 or 4 hours.

WENDY KOHRT: And you just calibrate it to room oxygen?

JOHN PATTON: Yes, and barometric pressure. That is all you are going to need. Well, we can also run gases through it to calibrate the fuel cell. You can do that, too. And volume, you can put volume through it, too, sure. But it is fairly stable.

DOUGLAS WILMORE: John, what do you do with these data? Do you convert them to energy equivalencies? What do you do with them?

JOHN PATTON: As far as oxygen uptake, we do not really, at least in my lab, convert it very frequently to kilocalories. You can calculate the data in terms of oxygen uptake consumed per kilogram body weight per minute.

DOUGLAS WILMORE: So you use it in a relative way, basically?

JOHN PATTON: Right.

DOUGLAS WILMORE: In other words, you say, here [at this time point] they are at rest, and here [at another time point] they are doing a task.

JOHN PATTON: Yes, just to quantify the level of intensity of the activity or whatever they are doing.

DOUGLAS WILMORE: Have you ever used just heart rate or something like that?

JOHN PATTON: Oh, sure.

DOUGLAS WILMORE: Does that get you to the same place?

JOHN PATTON: Sure, you can do a heart rate-oxygen uptake relationship. Is that what you mean? You can do that on the treadmill. But when you go out to the field, I do not think that heart rate remains reliable. If you did a load carriage study on the treadmill and got a heart rate-oxygen uptake relationship, and then you were to go out in the field and do load carriage, you could see some relationship there between heart rate and oxygen uptake, but very seldom do soldiers go out and do just one type of exercise.

DOUGLAS WILMORE: So thermal loads and things [affect the results]?

JOHN PATTON: That is another thing that will affect it, certainly, the length of activity; all kinds of variables will affect the heart rate. I just do not think heart rate has been too reliable as a measure of energy expenditure.

KARL FRIEDL: John, as an example of the application that we used this for, didn't you do a big MOPP [Military Oriented Protective Posture] study? Did you talk about that?

JOHN PATTON: No, I did not, really.

KARL FRIEDL: That is a beautiful example. I think that is what he is asking. How do you use this?

JOHN PATTON: I did not present any of those data. Certainly one thing that we used it for is to look at the difference in energy cost between performance of physical tasks in the MOPP-4 condition[2] compared with a MOPP-0 condition,[3] looking at changes and at the effect of the MOPP gear itself on physical task performance, and this entailed all kinds of things, from load carriage to lifting and carrying to litter carrying to obstacle course and all kinds of militarily relevant tasks, so we could get quantification of the MOPP gear per se.

Yes, thank you, Karl, that is one way in which we have used it.

ARTHUR ANDERSON: I have a question from the perspective of a scuba diver concerned about oxygen utilization while diving. Apropos of the MOPP gear comment, I felt it was important to ask the question of whether or not you tested this equipment in a MOPP gear environment in Riyadh during Operation Desert Storm, when the extreme emotional stress of having false alarms go off caused people to put their MOPP gear on. Would the hyperventilation associated with stress interfere with the benefit of the data that you get out of that oxygen utilization versus breathing in a nonstressful laboratory?

JOHN PATTON: You mean in a masked condition? I do not think it is going to change the oxygen uptake too much. Sure, your ventilation will change, and the amount of oxygen that actually is extracted is going to change. But when you

---

[2] Condition where soldier is clothed in full protective uniform over battle dress uniform (BDU). This includes protective mask, battle dress overgarment, boots, and gloves.

[3] Condition where soldier is clothed only in BDU.

apply it to the equation for oxygen uptake, there is going to be little change, little effect on oxygen uptake per se. I mean with just the masked condition itself, you tend to hypoventilate a little bit, but you extract more oxygen, so when you make the calculation for oxygen uptake there is little change.

ARTHUR ANDERSON: Hyperventilation, where you are inefficiently ventilating and blowing off air and not necessarily . . .

JOHN PATTON: Okay, then, your extractions would be much less, so when you calculate oxygen uptake, you are quite likely to get similar values.

JOHN VANDERVEEN: Did they have any evaluation of how well the carbon dioxide analyzer works in the TEEM 100?

JOHN PATTON: I have not seen any data on that, no. All I presented were the data on ventilation and the oxygen uptake. That is a good question. I know that is being looked at right now, as a matter of fact, both the oxygen and the carbon dioxide.

Emerging Technologies for Nutrition Research, 1997
Pp. 315–343. Washington, D.C.
National Academy Press

14

Advances in Ambulatory Monitoring: Using Foot Contact Time to Estimate the Metabolic Cost of Locomotion

Reed W. Hoyt[1] and Peter G. Weyand

INTRODUCTION

Physical activity plays a pivotal role in maintaining the physical fitness, trim appearance, and health of members of both the public and the U.S. military (AR 600-9, 1986; Byers, 1995; U.S. Department of the Army, 1992). However, a shortage of valid and reliable instrumentation to assess the physical activity and physical fitness of free-living humans has hampered understanding of this complex subject (Montoye and Taylor, 1984; Powell and Paffenbarger, 1985; Taube, 1995). The ambulatory foot contact monitor (FCM), which accurately estimates the metabolic cost of locomotion, is a new addition to the existing array of methods used to assess physical activity (Hoyt et al., 1994; LaPorte et al., 1985; Saris, 1986). This technology offers new opportunities to study the

[1] Reed W. Hoyt, Altitude Physiology and Medicine Division, U.S. Army Research Institute of Environmental Medicine, Natick, MA 01760

dose-response relationships of walking and running to macronutrient requirements, weight control, physical fitness, and the incidence of disease and injury.

The first of the following sections describes FCM technology and some potential applications. Next, the fundamental research linking the energetics and mechanics of human locomotion is reviewed. Finally, advantages and disadvantages of the FCM technology and suggestions for future research are discussed.

DESCRIPTION OF FOOT CONTACT MONITOR TECHNOLOGY

The ambulatory FCM accurately estimates the metabolic cost of locomotion ($\dot{M}_{loco}$ = total rate of energy expenditure – estimated rate of resting energy expenditure) from the ratio of total body weight to the time during each stride that a single foot is in contact with the ground (Hoyt et al., 1994). As discussed below, laboratory research has shown that the $\dot{M}_{loco}$ is determined primarily by the rate of force generation needed to support total body weight (Kram and Taylor, 1990). The rate of force generation can be estimated from the ratio of total body weight to foot contact time. At a given total body weight, increases in the speed of locomotion are associated with decreases in foot contact time, increases in the rate of force generation, and increases in the $\dot{M}_{loco}$.

The FCM is a relatively simple electronic device that measures the time the foot is in contact with the ground, and the time the foot is in the air, during each stride (see Figure 14-1). This is accomplished by a sensor circuit, an analog-to-

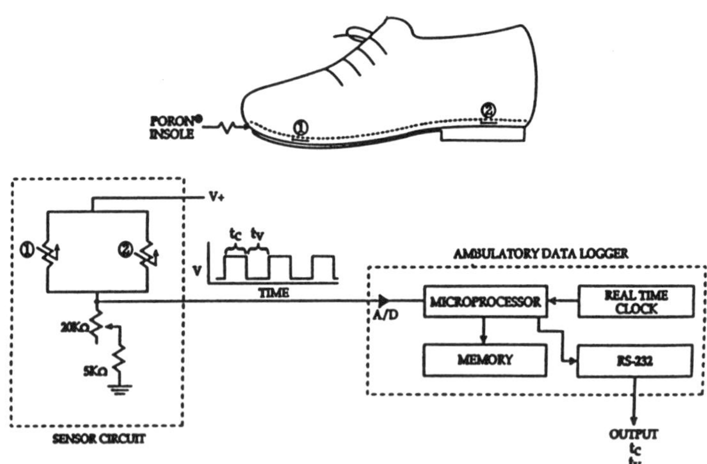

FIGURE 14-1 Schematic diagram of ambulatory electronic foot contact monitor. Force-sensing resistors (1,2) were placed under the ball and heel of one foot. A/D, analog to digital converter; t_c, time of foot contact for each stride; t_v, time foot is in the air for each stride; V, voltage; Ω, ohm (the unit of electric resistance equal to the resistance of a circuit in which a potential difference of 1 volt produces a current of 1 ampere). SOURCE: *Journal of Applied Physiology* (Hoyt et al., 1994), used with permission.

digital converter, and a microcontroller (microprocessor, memory, real time clock, and interface). The sensor circuit consists of two force sensors (consisting of either switches or force-sensitive resistors) located in the insole of a shoe or boot, one sensor under the ball and the other under the heel of the foot. These force sensors, which form part of a voltage divider circuit,[2] simply indicate whether or not the foot is in contact with the ground. During foot contact, the sensor circuit resistance decreases dramatically, and the voltage output becomes more positive. When the foot is elevated, sensor circuit resistance increases, and the voltage output becomes less positive. An analog-to-digital converter converts the output of the voltage divider sensor circuit into a digital signal that is processed and stored by a low cost microcontroller. The duration of each foot contact and noncontact period is recorded, and minute-to-minute averages of the $\dot{M}_{loco}$ are calculated and displayed and/or stored.

The FCM was used in a laboratory study to derive and cross-validate an equation for estimating $\dot{M}_{loco}$ from body weight (W_b) and foot contact time (t_c) (Hoyt et al., 1994). Indirect calorimetry was the criterion method used to measure the total rate of energy expenditure. Specifically, the rate of energy expenditure at each speed during treadmill exercise was calculated from oxygen consumption ($\dot{V}O_2$) and carbon dioxide production ($\dot{V}CO_2$) using conventional indirect calorimetric relationships (Lusk, 1928, 61–74). Each subject was tested at three walking speeds and three running speeds. Resting energy expenditure was estimated from height, weight, and age by the Harris-Benedict equation (Harris and Benedict, 1919). $\dot{M}_{loco}$ was calculated by subtracting resting energy expenditure from total energy expenditure. Twelve young males were tested during horizontal treadmill walking and running. The equation to estimate $\dot{M}_{loco}$ was derived in six randomly selected subjects:

$$\dot{M}_{loco} = 3.702(W_b/t_c) - 149.6(r^2 - 0.93).$$

Cross-validation in the remaining six subjects showed that *estimated* and *measured* $\dot{M}_{loco}$ were highly correlated ($r^2 = 0.97$) (Figure 14-2). The average individual error between estimated and measured $\dot{M}_{loco}$ was 0 percent (range = –22 to 29%). A simple ambulatory FCM, calibrated only for the individual's body weight, apparently can be used to estimate the $\dot{M}_{loco}$ (kcal/min, watts) accurately over a full range of walking and running intensities.

APPLICATIONS OF FCM TECHNOLOGY

The FCM can be used to estimate the $\dot{M}_{loco}$ of individuals in their natural environment without complex equipment. Minute-to-minute or day-to-day pat-

---

[2] A voltage divider circuit is a series of resistors connected across a voltage source from which various lesser values of voltage may be obtained.

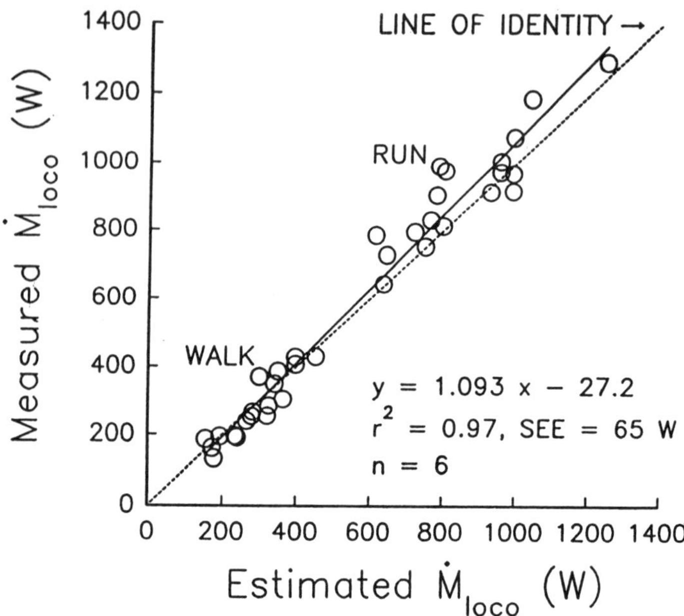

FIGURE 14-2 Relationship of measured metabolic cost of locomotion and the estimated metabolic cost of locomotion. Estimated $\dot{M}_{loco}$ was calculated using the equation $\dot{M}_{loco} = 3.702(W_b/t_c) - 149.6$ derived in a separate group of six young men. The 36 data points represent 6 subjects tested at 6 speeds (3 walking speeds and 3 running speeds). W, watts. SOURCE: *Journal of Applied Physiology* (Hoyt et al., 1994), used with permission.

terns of energy expended in walking and/or running can be determined. In addition, FCMs can be used to monitor changes in absolute or relative aerobic fitness.

The FCM could be used to address a variety of basic questions regarding physical activity patterns and physical fitness in free-living humans, particularly in relationship to the incidence of obesity, disease, and injury (Blair, 1993; Blair et al., 1992). Assessing low-level activity such as walking is of particular interest, given its apparent importance in maintaining health and energy balance and avoiding obesity (Hovell et al., 1992). Furthermore, FCMs with alphanumeric displays could provide the user with an immediate source of information about energy expenditure and physical fitness. This type of feedback could be beneficial in weight management, aerobic conditioning, and rehabilitation programs (Dausch, 1992).

Detailed information on the energetic costs of locomotion could also be useful in (1) determining the macronutrient and water requirements of soldiers in the field, (2) defining the metabolic cost of the numerous military tasks that involve movement by foot and load bearing (Patton et al., 1991), (3) improving heat strain prediction models (Kraning, 1991), and (4) clarifying the relationship of walking and running with the incidence of training injuries.

Macronutrient Requirements of Soldiers in the Field

A recurrent theme of meetings of the Committee on Military Nutrition Research is the need for more accurate and detailed estimates of the intensity, duration, and frequency of exercise performed by soldiers. This type of information, which FCM technology could help obtain, is needed to calculate actual macronutrient requirements and design better operational rations. In addition, quantitative data on the energy expenditure of soldiers are necessary in calculating water requirements (Hoyt and Honig, 1996; Kraning, 1991).

Weight Management

Obesity and lack of physical fitness are common in the United States (Russell et al., 1995) and often go hand in hand. This is reflected in the primary goal of Army Regulation 600-9 (1986), "The Army Weight Control Program," which "is to insure that all personnel—(1) Are able to meet the physical demands of their duties under combat conditions. (2) Present a trim military appearance at all times."

In a behavioral treatment program for obesity, an experimental group that used an interactive computer program to monitor energy balance was more successful at losing weight and maintaining a lower body weight than was a control group (Burnett et al., 1985). Analogously, an FCM displaying cumulative and real time estimates of the energy cost of locomotion, and even estimated speed and distance traveled, may encourage walking and running. More effective monitoring of personal physical activity patterns also may improve the typically poor adherence to exercise routines (Hakala, 1994; King et al., 1992).

Another way to promote regular physical activity may be to encourage an increase in the level of routine activities (Brownell et al., 1980). Walking and running, two major components of normal physical activity (Perrier Study of Fitness in America, 1979), could be fostered through the use of FCM technology. The FCM method is unique among ambulatory monitoring technologies in its ability to estimate the energy cost of walking. While walking is often very low in intensity, it is more effective than higher intensity exercise in promoting body fat combustion (Zierath and Wallberg-Henriksson, 1992).

Physical Fitness

The FCM technology could be used to help athletes and soldiers meet physical fitness goals (U.S. Department of the Army, 1992) in two ways. First, the FCM method can be used to monitor the frequency, duration, and absolute intensity of walking or running exercise. Second, the relationship of heart rate to the $\dot{M}_{loco}$ estimated by the FCM method can be used to improve the effectiveness of aerobic training programs. Total energy expenditure can be estimated from heart rate if the relationship of heart rate to oxygen consumption and energy expenditure is established for each individual. The $\dot{M}_{loco}$ also can be calculated as the difference between total energy expenditure and resting energy expenditure. The heart rate method provides useful estimates of energy expenditure at moderate-to-high work rates but is inaccurate at low activity levels (Ceesay et al., 1989; Christensen et al., 1983; Meijer et al., 1989; Spurr et al., 1988).

Although it is easy to set guidelines for exercise duration and frequency, it is much more difficult to specify the exercise intensity needed for an aerobic training effect since it varies widely both among and within individuals as a function of fitness (Åstrand and Rodahl, 1986; Pollock, 1973; Shephard, 1968). Classically, the effects of aerobic training on cardiorespiratory fitness are assessed by measuring maximal oxygen uptake during exercise to exhaustion (Clausen, 1977).

A simpler approach is to use FCM estimates of $\dot{M}_{loco}$ to monitor aerobic fitness. When an accurate comparison of different individuals is needed, absolute aerobic fitness can be estimated from measurements of the maximal $\dot{M}_{loco}$. However, a submaximal test can be used to assess relative changes in individual aerobic conditioning reliably during the course of an exercise program.

Specifically, the efficacy of aerobic fitness programs can be assessed by following changes in the linear relationship of heart rate to $\dot{M}_{loco}$ in response to training. A relative increase in an individual's aerobic fitness will be reflected in decreases in heart rate at specific work loads, and vice versa (Kappagoda et al., 1979). The feedback provided by periodic determination of heart rate at various standardized submaximal $\dot{M}_{loco}$ solves the central problem of defining the intensity required for an individual to increase aerobic fitness.

Unfit or obese individuals, or those with metabolic disorders, may benefit from a progressive approach to exercise training (Young, 1995). Additionally, the individually tailored aerobic training programs made possible by FCM technology should help reduce high attrition rates often associated with training programs involving high-intensity physical activity (Westerterp et al., 1992).

Epidemiology and Patient Rehabilitation

Although the impact of physical activity on long-term and short-term health is significant (Blair et al., 1992; Byers, 1995; Paffenbarger et al., 1986; Siscovick et al., 1985), the dose-response relationships have been difficult to quantify in free-living humans (LaPorte et al., 1985). The FCM could help solve this problem by facilitating the collection of detailed information on the intensity, frequency, and duration of walking and running. This type of information also is needed in studies of the etiology of running injuries (van Mechelen, 1992). The FCM technology could also facilitate the monitoring and management of patients involved in orthopedic and cardiorespiratory rehabilitation (Ettinger and Afable, 1994; Todd et al., 1992).

FOOT CONTACT TIMES AND METABOLIC RATES DURING LOCOMOTION: A CENTURY OF EXPERIMENTATION LINKING ENERGETICS AND MECHANICS

The relationship between energetics and mechanics during exercise was considered by Nobel Laureate A. V. Hill and his coworkers early in this century. While performing isolated muscle experiments that established the fundamental mechanical properties of skeletal muscle, Hill's group also was interested in understanding how muscles are used during exercise. Hill's original ideas were both intuitive and reasonable, but they proved to be incorrect. Today's answers, based in part on his isolated muscle experiments, are less intuitive, but nonetheless simple. A century of experimentation has led to a general theory of how muscles are used during locomotion and how their use is related to the metabolic costs that are incurred. The theory is based on the invariant properties of the muscles, bones, and tendons used for support and movement. It incorporates functional principles from molecular, cellular, and tissue levels to explain how muscles function in the multijointed lever systems of whole animals. It provides simple quantitative relationships that account for the energy cost of running, virtually over the entire continuum of animal sizes and running speeds. Although it was developed to explain the metabolic cost of locomotion, the general nature of the theory suggests that it also will apply to other forms of exercise.

One practical outcome of the progress in scientific understanding of the energetics and mechanics of locomotion is the potential for accurate determination of energy expenditure without the collection of expired gases. The development of the less cumbersome technology will allow metabolic rate to be quantified more accurately in many settings. What follows is the experimental evolution of our understanding of the energetics and mechanics of terrestrial locomotion that provided the background for the development of this technology.

Fundamentals of Terrestrial Locomotion

The first measurements of the energetic requirements of locomotion were made by the German scientist Zuntz (1897) at the end of the nineteenth century. He measured the rates of oxygen consumption to determine the metabolic energy expended by humans and dogs walking and running on a treadmill at different speeds over various inclines. He found that metabolic rate increased linearly with speed for both humans and dogs during both level and inclined running. Subsequent measures showed that this relationship is linear for nearly all terrestrial animals that run (Figure 14-3) and established the linear increase in metabolic rate with running speed as the first fundamental principle of the energetics of terrestrial locomotion (Taylor et al., 1970, 1982).

One consequence of the linear increase of oxygen consumption with speed is that the same amount of energy is expended to run a mile (calculated as the slope of the oxygen consumption vs. running speed) regardless of running velocity. This cost is generally expressed in body mass-specific terms (J/nm) and is referred to as the cost of transport. The measurements taken on animals of different sizes since Zuntz's initial experiments have shown that oxygen consumption increases more rapidly with speed in smaller animals. The systematic nature of these differences established the second fundamental principle of the energetics of terrestrial locomotion: the cost of transport decreases in a regular manner with increases in body size, scaling with body mass to the −0.30 power (Taylor et al., 1980) (Figure 14-4). Thus, if size extremes in nature are considered, the 10-g shrew expends 100 times more energy per unit body mass than the 2,000-kg elephant to run a given distance.

Hill (1950) attributed both the linear increase in metabolic cost with running speed and the lower transport costs of larger animals to differences in the rate at which muscles performed the mechanical work of running. This explanation later proved to be incorrect due to Hill's assumptions about the relationship

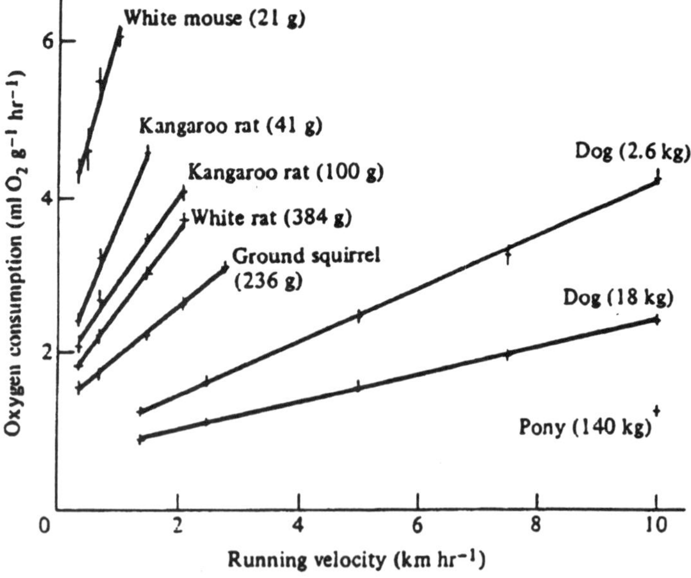

FIGURE 14-3 Oxygen consumption increases linearly with running speed in terrestrial animals. SOURCE: *American Journal of Physiology* (Taylor et al., 1970), used with permission.

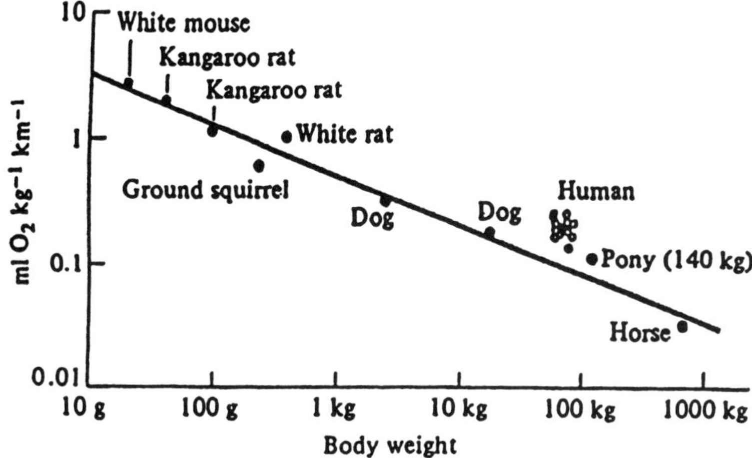

FIGURE 14-4 The cost of transport (the slope of the relationship between oxygen consumption and running speed) is higher in small animals than in large, scaling with body mass to the -0.30 power. SOURCE: *American Journal of Physiology* (Taylor et al., 1970), used with permission.

between metabolic cost and the work of running. It would require decades of experimentation before it would become clear which of the mechanical tasks performed during running required metabolic energy.

What Sets Cost?

The Mechanical Work of Running and Metabolic Cost

The movements of an animal or a human running steadily at a brisk pace must be finely coordinated in time and space. Airborne and grounded periods alternate regularly. Limbs oscillate in relation to one another and the torso. The center of mass rises and falls, and it accelerates and decelerates during the period of support. These movements involve fluctuations in both the kinetic and gravitational potential energy of the animal's center of mass and limbs, and it is logical to hypothesize that muscles perform the work necessary to effect these energy changes as efficiently as possible. Indeed, the scientists who first considered the question started with this hypothesis.

Cavagna and Margaria were among the first to attempt to determine muscular efficiency (mechanical work of running/metabolic energy expended) during locomotion (Cavagna et al., 1964). They expected to find that the mechanical work of running would be performed at the maximal efficiency (20–25%) that Hill had measured for isolated muscle. Using a force platform and video analysis to measure the work of running, their measurements produced a surprising result. The efficiency of running exceeded the maximal efficiency of isolated muscle. In fact, at high speeds, the efficiency reached 70 percent, roughly three times the maximal value for isolated muscle. How could such a result be explained? They concluded that muscles did not perform all of the positive work done during each running stride. The cyclical positive and negative oscillations of the kinetic and gravitational potential energy that corresponded to the changes in the speed and height of the body apparently allowed much of the work to be performed conservatively by springs. Because the fluctuations that they measured in the kinetic and gravitational potential energy of the body's center of mass were in phase, they concluded that muscles and tendons stored potential energy elastically during one portion of the stride and released it during another, in a manner analogous to a spring or bouncing ball. Clearly, not all of the work of running required metabolic energy.

Perhaps the energy saved by "running springs" was related to the linear increase in oxygen consumption with running speed and to the higher transport costs of smaller animals. Subsequent investigations upheld this possibility. Models of the mechanics of running, which treated humans and animals as "linear springs" with masses concentrated above their support limbs, predicted almost perfectly the changes in stride lengths, frequencies, landing, and takeoff angles that occurred during actual running (Blickhan, 1989; McMahon and Cheng, 1990). Mechanical tests on tendons, conducted by Alexander and colleagues (1981), indicated that in running humans, 50 percent of the mechanical work required could be stored and released by the springs in the Achilles tendon and the arch of the foot alone (Ker et al., 1987). Furthermore, Cavagna's force platform and video technique indicated that there might be important differences in how well springs worked in different-sized animals (Cavagna et al., 1964). The efficiencies of large, fast animals, such as ponies, reached values as high as 150 percent, while those of small animals, such as rats and mice, reached only 6 percent at their top aerobic speeds (Heglund et al., 1982). Did the better springs of larger animals explain their lower transport costs?

This question was difficult to resolve because the relationship of the efficiencies of whole animals indicated little about the efficiencies of their running muscles. This was true for several reasons. It was not possible to partition the total mechanical work into that performed by the muscles and that conserved by springs and pendulums. Neither the energy stored elastically in springs nor the energy transferred among body segments and the torso could be quantified directly. This made it impossible to know how much of the total work the muscles actually were doing. Also, these work measurements included only the positive work done during each stride. The running muscles were certainly active while they were being lengthened by gravity. The forces they generated during lengthening incurred a metabolic cost, but this was not included in this analysis. Therefore, determining how much of the chemical energy released by the running muscles was converted into mechanical work (as in Hill's isolated muscle experiments) was simply not possible with this technique. More evidence was needed before the mechanical tasks performed by the running muscles that required metabolic energy could be identified.

Generating Force to Support the Weight of the Body

The lack of definitive answers from measurements of the mechanical work of running and further consideration of running mechanics prompted C. R. Taylor and colleagues to adopt a different approach. These scientists recognized that doing work is not the only requirement of an animal running on level ground at a constant speed. Because the height of the body's center of mass does not change over time and the amount of work required to overcome wind resistance is generally small, the net work done by the body on the environment is very close to zero. However, even if the conservation of the mechanical energy required for running at a constant speed were perfect (i.e., 100%, so that the muscles need not perform any work), the active muscles would still be required to generate a time-averaged ground force equal to the weight of the body. With these thoughts in mind, Taylor and colleagues undertook a number of experiments to test the relationship between supporting body weight and metabolic cost.

One of their first experiments involved having animals ranging in size from mice to horses run on treadmills while carrying loads weighing between 5 and 30 percent of their body masses (Taylor et al., 1980). They found that at the same speeds, animals ran with the same stride lengths and stride frequencies in the weighted and unweighted conditions. This finding was fortuitous because it meant that the forces generated by the running muscles to support the weight of the body increased in direct proportion to the load on the animal. The results showed that metabolic cost increased in direct proportion to the weight carried by the animal; that is, a 10 percent increase with a load equal to 10 percent of body weight, a 20 percent increase with a load equal to 20 percent of body weight, and so on. This was an important result. It suggested that generating force to support the weight of the body during running was directly related to metabolic cost.

Equivalent experiments were conducted in simulated reduced gravity, which allowed the vertical force that was generated to be reduced by different amounts (Farley and McMahon, 1992). In these experiments, the metabolic cost of running decreased in direct proportion to the amount of force required to support the weight of the body under the different conditions. In both the weighting and the reduced gravity experiments, there was a 1:1 relationship between the force generated to support the weight of the body and the metabolic cost of running.

The weighting and reduced gravity experiments indirectly supported the related conclusion that the metabolic importance of swinging limbs was small. If the kinetic energy required to swing limbs was responsible for a significant portion of the metabolic energy expended by the animal, loading or unloading a person or animal by a percentage of its body weight ought to alter the metabolic cost by some lesser factor. However, this was not the case under any of the conditions. This conclusion reinforced one reached previously through a different experimental approach (Taylor et al., 1974). These researchers selected animals of the same weights (goats, cheetahs, and gazelles) but different distributions of that weight between the limbs and torso. They found that the energetic cost of treadmill running in the three species was identical. This was true despite vast differences in the amount of work necessary to swing the slight limbs of the gazelle in comparison to the sturdy limbs of the cheetah. If the work of swinging limbs demanded metabolic energy, the cheetah should have higher metabolic costs, but this was not the case.

The view that emerged from the weighting, reduced gravity, and limb inertia experiments differed but did not contradict that provided by the mechanical work experiments. Measurements of the mechanical work of running and its relationship to metabolic cost (i.e., efficiency) were not meaningful if much or all of the mechanical work being performed was conserved by springs and pendulums. The direct relationship between metabolic cost and the forces generated by the active muscles to support the weight of the body raised what seemed to be an unlikely possibility: springs and pendulums performed all of the work of running regardless of animal size and running speed.

Linking Force Generation to Energetic Fundamentals

Even though the results of the mechanical work, reduced gravity, and weighting experiments were consistent and suggested a direct relationship between vertical force and metabolic cost, these experiments were indirect and not completely conclusive. The results did not provide an explanation for the linear increase in metabolic rate with running speed, nor for the lower transport costs of larger animals. Explaining the basic energetic principles of locomotion required linking the mechanical and metabolic properties of muscles to force generation during locomotion in whole animals.

The mechanics of running, like the energetics of running, appeared to conform to general patterns. For example, the mechanics of running at different speeds and in different-sized animals appeared to be achieved through equivalent movements that took place at different rates. In both humans and animals, the mechanics of what the muscles and tendons did during the support phase, and when the critical vertical forces were generated, were virtually the same across the range of running speeds. This was true of the angles of individual joints during support (Biewener et al., 1981; McMahon and Cheng, 1990), the stiffness of leg springs (force/leg displacement) (Farley et al., 1993; McMahon and Cheng, 1990), and step lengths (defined as the horizontal distance moved by the center of mass while the foot is in contact with the ground) (Taylor et al., 1980) (see Figure 14-5). However, at faster running speeds, and in smaller animals, these movements took place more rapidly.

STEP LENGTH

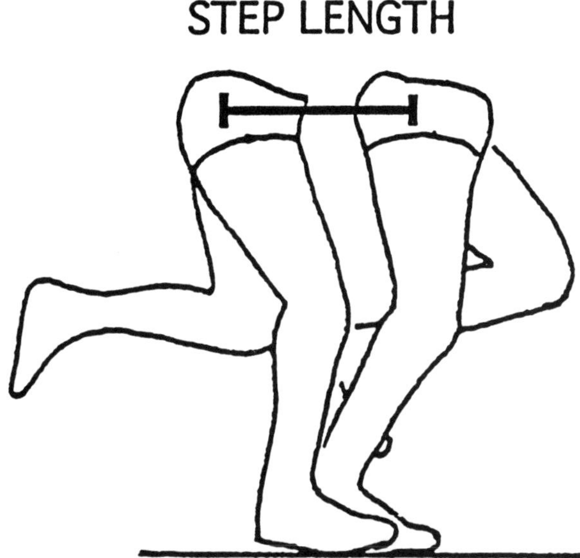

FIGURE 14-5 Step length is the horizontal distance moved by the center of mass while a single foot is in contact with the ground. SOURCE: Wright (1995), used with permission.

There also was evidence from different-sized animals that the differences in mechanical activity were directly related to the differences in metabolic cost (Heglund and Taylor, 1988). Smaller animals had higher metabolic costs and ran with higher stride frequencies. With increases in running speed, the metabolic cost per stride increased in all animals. However, when metabolic cost was expressed on a per stride basis at equivalent speeds, such as the trot-gallop transition, it was the same for all animals. The fact that at equivalent speeds, different-sized animals had the same ratio of support time/total time indicated that the size differences in metabolic cost were proportional to the periods of ground contact (tc) in large and small animals and suggested a link to the time available for force development (Rome, 1992).

If the time course of foot contact was a determinant of metabolic cost, as previous results suggested it might be, changing this variable ought to change cost. This easily could be achieved by having humans change their natural stride frequencies and support periods by running in time to a metronome. When humans either increased or decreased their freely chosen step lengths, the metabolic cost of running was greater than that at their naturally chosen frequency (Cavanaugh and Williams, 1982; Farley and Gonzalez, 1996). Clearly, the freely chosen step lengths and corresponding contact times minimized metabolic cost.

Insights from Changing Contact Times

What then dictated the lengths of the steps and contact times that were naturally selected at any running speed? Again, the answer was provided by human experiments in which the naturally chosen frequencies during running and hopping were altered (Farley and Gonzalez, 1996; Farley et al., 1991). During both running and hopping, the body behaved as a spring; that is, force had the same relationship to displacement during both the yield and rebound stages of the support phase. When stride or hopping frequency was decreased and the ground contact period increased, the body no longer behaved this way. The higher forces during the rebound phase and the increased metabolic rate suggested that additional mechanical work from the muscles had to be supplied to replace the work not being performed by the body's springs (Figure 14-6). Slowing the rate of force generation disrupted the body's springs and made the muscles do more work.

Metabolic rate also increased when humans ran at higher-than-preferred stride frequencies, which decreased the period of ground contact at any running or hopping speed. Force displacement curves indicated that the running springs worked nearly perfectly under this condition, as they did at the preferred frequency, which suggested that muscular work did not change, but that the mus-

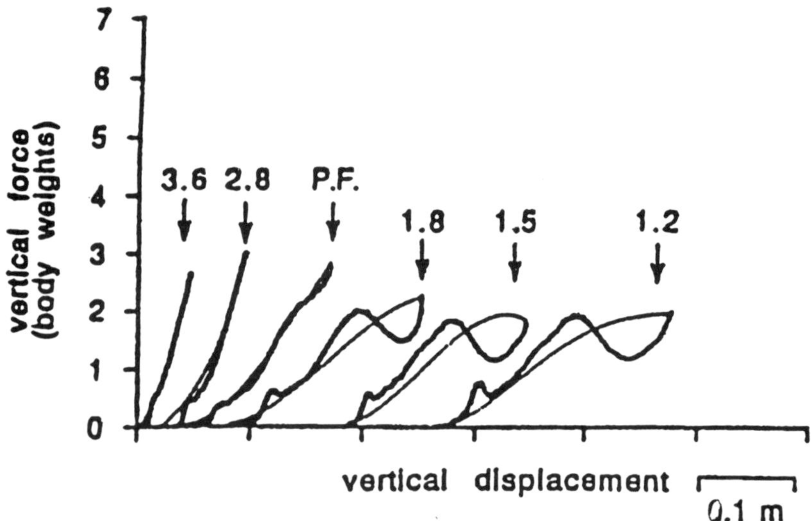

FIGURE 14-6 During human hopping (and also running) at natural frequencies (PF) and above, forces when the body moves toward (thick lines) and away (thin lines) from the earth during the support phase are the same at any displacement of the center of mass; that is, the body behaves as a spring. At lower frequencies, the higher forces during the rebound phase indicate the body no longer behaves this way. SOURCE: *Journal of Applied Physiology* (Farley et al., 1991), used with permission.

cles had to support the weight of the body in a shorter period of time. The increase in metabolic cost when humans ran at higher-than-preferred frequencies was directly related to the decreased period of contact during which the muscles developed vertical force (Farley and Gonzalez, 1996). The stride length experiments added further evidence that the rate of vertical force development was a fundamental determinant of the metabolic cost of running. Specifically, they indicated that chosen step lengths and periods of force generation minimized metabolic cost by allowing force to be developed at the slowest rates that still allowed the body to behave as a natural spring.

Equally interesting was the finding that the step lengths that dictated ground contact times were nearly unchanged across running speeds. This suggested an optimal mechanical solution for minimizing the muscular forces and the cost of generating vertical force against the ground. A consequence of the near constancy of step lengths was a regular decrease in the period of time the foot was in contact with the ground, with increases in running speed. This was true regardless of whether the increases in running speed were brought about by increases in stride frequency or stride length. Thus, the generation of a time-averaged ground force equal to body weight takes place in progressively shorter periods of time as running speed is increased (Figure 14-7). Taylor and colleagues recognized that the period of ground contact must set the rate at which force is developed to support the weight of the body. This prompted them to examine the relationship between the metabolic cost of running and the period of ground contact in different-sized animals across their range of aerobic running speeds where cost could be measured (Kram and Taylor, 1990). Using the inverse of ground contact times to estimate the rates of muscular force generation needed to support the weight of the body, they found a constant relationship between metabolic rate and the inverse of the ground contact (1/tc) period across a 10-fold range of running speeds and a 4,500-fold range of body masses in both quadrupeds and bipedal hoppers.

Why Do Contact Times Set Metabolic Rates?

The implications of this intriguing result brought Taylor and colleagues back to the experiments and questions of Hill almost 70 years earlier and provided an attractive link between the classic responses of muscle in *in vitro* and *in situ* preparations and their operation in living animals. The explanation for the constant relationship between the rate of force generation and metabolic rate was simple. The inverse of the time of foot-ground contact and corresponding rates of force generation dictated the speed of the muscle fibers recruited to generate the required force. As running speed increased, the time available for force generation (tc) decreased, and the rate at which force was developed (1/tc) increased. The proposed links among running speed, rates of force generation, and fiber speed was consistent with what was known about the metabolic cost of force generation in isolated muscle (Rome et al., 1990; Woledge et al., 1985)

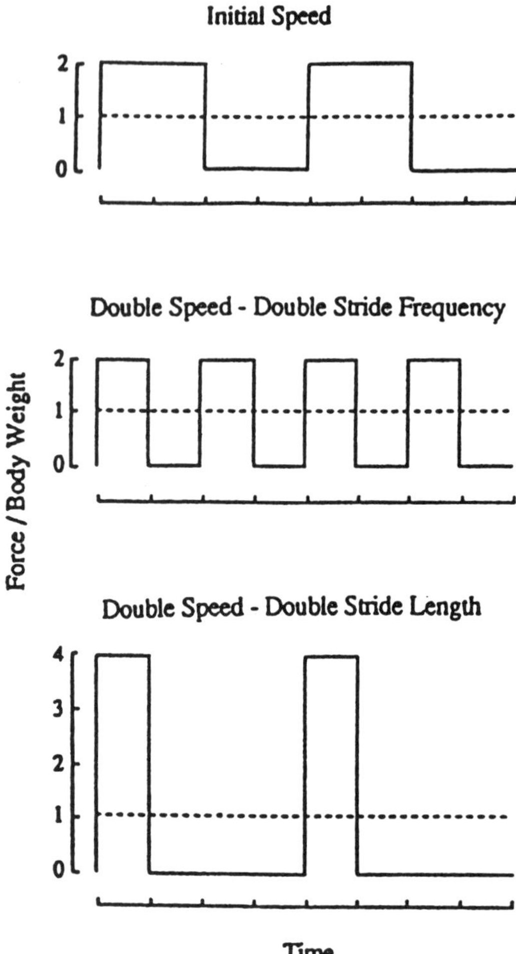

FIGURE 14-7 Whether running speed is increased by increasing stride length (period of zero force) or stride frequency (frequency of force pulses), the time of foot-ground contact (force pulse width) decreases as speed increases if step lengths are nearly constant. Shorter contact times require greater rates of force generation to support the weight of the body. The dashed line, equal to one body weight, is the time-averaged force exerted against the ground. SOURCE: Reprinted from Taylor (1992) by courtesy of Marcel Dekker, Inc.

and fiber recruitment patterns in whole animals (Armstrong and Laughlin, 1985; Henneman et al., 1965; Walmsley et al., 1978). The explanation also was supported by the close agreement between the ranges of 1/tc and those of the maximal shortening velocities of the muscles reported for both individual and different-sized animals (Rome et al., 1990). Furthermore, the constant rate-normalized cost indicated that the muscular activity at different running speeds was equivalent. If running faster was achieved through shortening the muscles faster, as Hill had suggested, the metabolic cost of force generation also should increase as it did in isolated muscle, but this was not the case. This explanation also was consistent with the relative constancy of the mechanics of support across running speed. The simple relationship between rates of force generation and fiber speed provided a compelling explanation for how the mechanical properties of muscle on molecular, cellular, and tissue levels operate within the lever systems of animals to satisfy the mechanical requirements of running.

Why is the Metabolic Cost of Generating Force the Same in Large and Small Animals?

The truly remarkable finding was that rates of force generation could explain completely the metabolic cost of force generation in running animals, not only across running speeds but also across the entire spectrum of animal sizes. It indicated that both the activities and the volumes of muscle recruited by different-sized animals were the same. This was curious given the identical need of large and small animals to support their body weights and the more crouched posture of small animals. These postural differences required higher muscle forces in small animals to generate the same ground reaction force. Biewener (1989) defined this ratio (ground force/muscle force) as the effective mechanical advantage (EMA) and quantified it by measuring muscle moment arms (r, the distance from the muscle-tendon insertion point on the bone to the joint axis of rotation) and the perpendicular distances from the ground reaction force vectors during running to the joint axis of rotation (R) (Figure 14-8). He found that EMA scaled with body mass to the 0.80 power. How then could small animals generate higher muscle forces, which required greater muscle cross-sectional areas, with the same muscle volumes? The only possibility was for the smaller animals to generate this force with shorter muscle fibers. Indeed, nature had provided this solution. Alexander and colleagues (1981) had shown that muscle fiber length changes with body size, scaled with body mass to the 0.20 power, exactly offsetting the size differences in EMA and muscle forces to result in the same muscle volumes being recruited by large and small animals to generate force against the ground (Biewener, 1989).

Summary

In conclusion, nearly a century of experimentation produced considerable progress in the understanding of the relationship between the energetics and mechanics of exercise. The work of running was not related to metabolic cost, as Hill and others had initially hypothesized, because the muscles of animals running on level ground performed very little work. Rather, metabolic cost was set by the forces generated by the muscles to support the weight of the body.

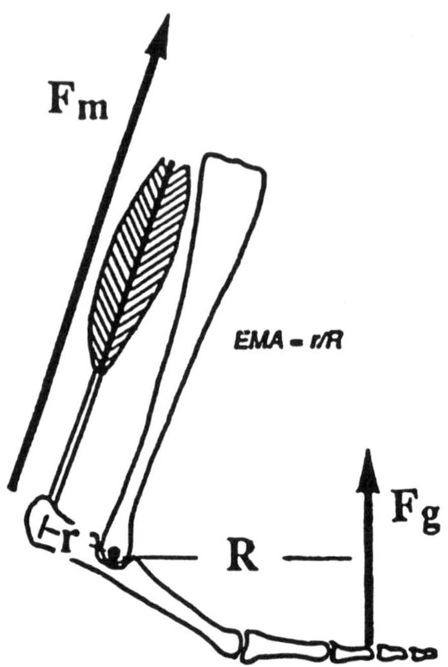

FIGURE 14-8 The effective mechanical advantage (EMA), the ratio of ground reaction force to muscle force, is determined by the ratio of the muscle moment arm (r) to the perpendicular distance at the force vector from the joint axis of rotation (R). F_m, muscle force; F_g, ground force. SOURCE: Reprinted with permission from Biewener, "Scaling body support in mammals: Limb posture and muscle mechanics," *Science* 245:45–48. Copyright 1989 American Association for the Advancement of Science.

The rates at which these forces were generated resolved the mechanism underlying the fundamental energetic principles of locomotion. Both the linear increase in metabolic rate with running speed and the lower running costs of larger animals were directly accounted for by the rates at which muscular forces were generated. The establishment of this remarkable relationship accompanies the experimental evolution of a general model of how muscles are used during exercise that also may explain the metabolic costs of other activities.

ADVANTAGES AND DISADVANTAGES OF FCM TECHNOLOGY

The FCM appears to have a number of advantages compared to other techniques used to estimate $\dot{M}_{loco}$ in the field:

• It provides accurate estimates of the metabolic cost of both walking and running. The ability to estimate accurately the metabolic cost of both high-intensity running and low-intensity walking is unique among ambulatory monitors. This method offers new opportunities to study activity patterns in aged, handicapped, and sedentary humans.

- Output is in standard energy units. The linear relationship between body weight, foot contact time, and the metabolic cost of locomotion allows easy and direct calculation of the $\dot{M}_{loco}$ in standard units (e.g., joules, kcal, watts, kcal/min).
- FCM requires no individual calibration beyond a determination of body weight. If confirmed, this FCM characteristic should make it easier to study large groups of people.
- FCM provides a simple means of monitoring aerobic fitness. The FCM can be used alone to estimate an individual's maximal $\dot{M}_{loco}$ and work capacity. It also can be used in conjunction with determinations of heart rate to assess changes in relative aerobic fitness.
- FCM is simple enough to be useful in epidemiologic studies. The FCM is simple, inexpensive, compact, lightweight, and has a low power requirement. The FCM method requires less subject cooperation than diaries and is potentially less time consuming and expensive than other techniques involving observation, diaries, activity questionnaires, and interviews (Montoye and Taylor, 1984).

Current disadvantages of the FCM are as follows:

- The FCM does not account for energy costs of other concurrent activities such as upper body work. Humans engage in many types of physical activity. Combining the FCM with activity monitors, heart rate monitors, or questionnaires may help identify energy costs for physical activities other than walking and running (Haskell et al., 1993; Montoye and Taylor, 1984).
- Body weight must be determined and may change over time. Total body weight is probably relatively stable over the course of a day in the general population. However, total weight can fluctuate in soldiers as equipment is donned and doffed. It is technologically possible to monitor both total weight and foot contact time.
- Current FCM algorithms do not account for uphill or downhill movement. Research in progress suggests uphill and downhill movement can be accounted for through the changing relationship of the time the foot contacts the ground to the time the foot is in the air. As an individual moves uphill, the time of contact remains constant, but the length of time the foot is raised is reduced. The converse occurs during downhill movement.
- Further research is needed. Studies with larger and more heterogeneous subject populations that include women, children, and the elderly are needed to establish the general validity of this method. In addition, studies are needed (1) to confirm that measurements of $\dot{M}_{loco}$ can be made by the FCM method without complex individual calibration, (2) to quantify the effects of grade on $\dot{M}_{loco}$,

and (3) to compare $\dot{M}_{loco}$ estimates by the FCM method with those measured by heart rate, doubly labeled water, and other methods.

AUTHORS' CONCLUSIONS AND RECOMMENDATIONS

The ability of ambulatory monitors such as the FCM to assess physiologic function in free-living humans is rapidly improving, in parallel to the marked progress in electronic sensors, microprocessors, data storage, and telemetry. These new personal status monitors will be used to answer practical scientific questions, help meet the medical needs of soldiers injured in remote locations, and provide field commanders with the data they need to prevent environmental injuries among their troops.

The FCM technology is practical, simple to use, and represents a significant addition to existing technologies. This technology should help meet the research need for detailed information on energy expenditure patterns and physical fitness of free-living humans. The cost-benefit ratio of this technology seems favorable. Each FCM should be inexpensive enough (about $50 to $100) to be useful in large-scale epidemiologic studies. Support for continued FCM technology development is needed to expedite the production and testing of FCMs.

REFERENCES

Alexander, R. McN., A.S. Jayes, G.M.O. Maloiy, and E.M. Wathuta
   1981   Allometry of the leg muscles of mammals. J. Zool. (Lond.) 194:539–552.
AR 600-9 (Army Regulation 600-9)
   1986   *See* U.S. Department of the Army.
Armstrong, R.B., and M.H. Laughlin
   1985   Metabolic indicators of fibre recruitment in mammalian muscles during locomotion. J. Exp. Biol. 115:201–213.
Ästrand, P.O., and K. Rodahl
   1986   Textbook of Work Physiology, Physiological Bases of Exercise, 3d ed. New York: McGraw-Hill Book Co.
Biewener, A.A
   1989   Scaling body support in mammals: Limb posture and muscle mechanics. Science 245:45–48.
Biewener, A., R.M. Alexander, and N.C. Heglund
   1981   Elastic energy storage in the hopping of kangaroo rats (*Dipodomys spectabilis*). J. Zool. (Lond.) 195:369–383.
Blair, S.N.
   1993   Evidence for success of exercise in weight loss and control. Ann. Intern. Med. 119:702–706.
Blair, S.N., H.W. Kohl, N.F. Gordon, and R.S. Paffenbarger, Jr.
   1992   How much physical activity is good for health? Annu. Rev. Public Health 13:99–126.
Blickhan, R.
   1989   The spring-mass model for running and hopping. J. Biomech. 22:1217–1227.

Brownell, K.D., A.A. Stunkard, and J.M. Albaun
  1980   Evaluation and modification of exercise patterns in the natural environment. Am. J. Psychiatry 137:1540–1545.
Burnett, K.R., C.B. Taylor, and W.S. Agras
  1985   Ambulatory computer-assisted therapy for obesity: A new frontier for behavior therapy. J. Consult. Clin. Psychol. 53:698–703.
Byers, T.
  1995   Body weight and mortality [editorial]. New Engl. J. Med. 333:723–724.
Cavagna, G.A., F.P. Sabiene, and R. Margaria
  1964   Mechanical work in running. J. Appl. Physiol. 19:249–256.
Cavanaugh, P.R., and K.R. Williams
  1982   The effect of stride length variation on oxygen uptake during distance running. Med. Sci. Sports Exerc. 14:30–35.
Ceesay, S.M., A.M. Prentice, K.C. Day, P.R. Murgatroyd, G.R. Goldberg, and W. Scott
  1989   The use of heart rate monitoring in the estimation of energy expenditure: A validation study using indirect whole-body calorimetry. Br. J. Nutr. 61:175–186.
Christensen, C.C., H.M.M. Frey, E. Foenstelien, E. Aadland, and H.E. Refsum
  1983   A critical evaluation of energy expenditure estimates based on individual O_2 consumption/heart rate curves and average daily heart rate. Am. J. Clin. Nutr. 37:468–472.
Clausen, J.P
  1977   Effects of physical training on cardiovascular adjustments to exercise in man. Physiol. Rev. 57:779–816.
Dausch, J.G.
  1992   The problem of obesity: Fundamental concepts of energy metabolism gone awry. Crit. Rev. Food Sci. Nutr. 31:271–298.
Ettinger, W.H., Jr., and R.F. Afable
  1994   Physical disability from knee osteoarthritis: The role of exercise as an intervention. Med. Sci. Sports Exerc. 26:1435–1440.
Farley, C.T., and O. Gonzalez
  1996   Leg stiffness and stride frequency in human running. J. Biomech. 29(2):181–186.
Farley, C.T., and T.A. McMahon
  1992   Energetics of walking and running: Insights from reduced gravity. J. Appl. Physiol. 73:2709–2712.
Farley, C.T., R. Blickhan, J. Saito, and C.R. Taylor
  1991   Hopping frequency in humans: A test of how springs set stride frequency in bouncing gaits. J. Appl. Physiol. 71:2127–2132.
Farley, C.T., J. Glasheen, and T.A. McMahon
  1993   Running springs: Speed and animal size. J. Exp. Biol. 185:71–87.
Hakala, P.
  1994   Weight reduction programmes at a rehabilitation centre and a health centre based on group counselling and individual support: Short- and long-term follow-up study. Int. J. Obes. 18:483–489.
Harris, J.A., and F.G. Benedict
  1919   A biometric study of basal metabolism in man. Publication no. 279. Washington, D.C.: Carnegie Institute of Washington.
Haskell, W.L., M.C. Yee, A. Evans, and P.J. Irby
  1993   Simultaneous measurement of heart rate and body motion to quantitate physical activity. Med. Sci. Sports Exerc. 25:109–115.
Heglund, N.C., and C.R. Taylor
  1988   Speed, stride frequency, and energy cost per stride: How do they change with body size and gait? J. Exp. Biol. 108:429–439.

Heglund, N.C., M.A. Fedak, C.R. Taylor, and G.A. Cavagna
    1982   Energetics and mechanics of terrestrial locomotion. IV. Total mechanical energy
            changes as a function of speed and body size in birds and mammals. J. Exp. Biol.
            97:57–66.
Henneman, E., G. Somjen, and D.C. Carpenter
    1965   Functional significance of cell size in spinal motoneurons. J. Neurophysiol.
            28:581–598.
Hill, A.V.
    1950   The dimensions of animals and their muscular dynamics. Sci. Prog. 38:209–230.
Hovell, M.F., C.R. Hofstetter, J.F. Sallis, M.J.D. Rauh, and E. Barrington
    1992   Correlates of change in walking for exercise: An exploratory analysis. Res. Q.
            Exerc. Sport 63:425–434.
Hoyt, R.W., and A. Honig
    1996   Environmental influences on body fluid balance during exercise: Altitude. Pp.
            187–200 in Body Fluid Balance in Exercise and Sport, E.R. Buskirk and S.M.
            Puhl, eds. Boca Raton, Fla.: CRC Press, Inc.
Hoyt, R.W., J.J. Knapik, J.F. Lanza, B.H. Jones, and J.S. Staab
    1994   Ambulatory foot contact monitor to estimate the metabolic cost of human locomo-
            tion. J. Appl. Physiol. 76:1818–1822.
Kappagoda, C.T., R.J. Linden, and J.P. Newell
    1979   Effect of the Canadian Air Force training programme on a submaximal exercise
            test. Q. J. Exp. Physiol. 64:185–204.
Ker, R.F., M.B. Bennett, S.R. Bibby, R.C. Kester, and R.M. Alexander
    1987   The spring in the arch of the human foot. Nature 325:147–149.
King, A.C., S.N. Blair, D.E. Bild, R.K. Dishman, P.M. Dubbert, R.H. Marcus, N.B. Oldridge,
            R.S. Paffenbarger, Jr., K.E. Powell, and K.K. Yeager
    1992   Determinants of physical activity and interventions in adults. Med. Sci. Sports
            Exerc. 24:S221–S236.
Kram, R., and C.R. Taylor
    1990   Energetics of running: A new perspective. Nature 346(6281):265–267.
Kraning, K.K., II
    1991   A computer simulation for predicting the time course of thermal and cardiovascu-
            lar responses to various combinations of heat stress, clothing and exercise. Techni-
            cal Report T13-91. Natick, Mass.: U.S. Army Research Institute of Environmental
            Medicine.
LaPorte, R.E., H.J. Montoye, and C.J. Casperson
    1985   Assessment of physical activity in epidemiologic research: Problems and pros-
            pects. Public Health Rep. 100:131–146.
Lusk, G.
    1928   The Elements of the Science of Nutrition, 4th ed. New York: Academic Press.
            Reprint: New York: Johnson Reprint Corp., 1976.
McMahon, T.A., and G.C. Cheng
    1990   The mechanics of running: How does stiffness couple with speed? J. Biomech.
            23:65–78.
Meijer, G.A., K.R. Westerterp, H. Koper, and F. Ten Hoor
    1989   Assessment of energy expenditure by recording heart rate and body acceleration.
            Med. Sci. Sports Exerc. 21:343–347.
Montoye, H.J., and H.L. Taylor
    1984   Measurement of physical activity in population studies: A review. Hum. Biol.
            56:195–216.

Paffenbarger, R.S., R.T. Hyde, A.L. Wing, and C. Hsieh
   1986   Physical activity, all-cause mortality, and longevity of college alumni. N. Engl. J. Med. 314:605–613.
Patton, J.F., M. Murphy, T. Bidwell, R. Mello, and M. Harp
   1991   Metabolic cost of military physical tasks in MOPP 0 and MOPP 4. Technical Report T95-9. Natick, Mass.: U.S. Army Research Institute of Environmental Medicine.
Perrier Study of Fitness in America
   1979   Study No. S2813. New York: Louis Harris and Associates Inc.
Pollock, M.L.
   1973   The quantification of endurance training programs. Exerc. Sport Sci. Rev. 1:155–188.
Powell, K.E., and R.S. Paffenbarger
   1985   Workshop on epidemiologic and public health aspects of physical activity and exercise: A summary. Public Health Rep. 100:118–126.
Rome, L.C.
   1992   Scaling of muscle fibers and locomotion. J. Exp. Biol. 168:243–252.
Rome, L.C., A.A. Sosnicki, and D.O. Goble
   1990   Maximum velocity of shortening of three fiber types from the horse soleus: Implications for scaling with body size. J. Physiol. (Lond.) 431:173–185.
Russell, C.M., D.F. Williamson, and T. Byers
   1995   Can the Year 2000 objective for reducing overweight in the United States be reached?: A simulation study of the required changes in body weight. Int. J. Obes. 19:149–153.
Saris, W.H.M.
   1986   Habitual physical activity in children: Methodology and findings in health and disease. Med. Sci. Sports Exerc. 18:253–263.
Shephard, R.J.
   1968   Intensity, duration and frequency of exercise as determinants of the response to a training regimen. Int. Z. Angew Physiol. 28:272–278.
Siscovick, D.S., R.E. LaPorte, and J.M. Newman
   1985   The disease-specific benefits and risks of physical activity and exercise. Public Health Rep. 100:180–188.
Spurr, G.B., A.M. Prentice, P.R. Murgatroyd, G.R. Goldberg, J.C. Reina, and N.T. Christman
   1988   Energy expenditure from minute-by-minute heart-rate recording: Comparison with indirect calorimetry. Am. J. Clin. Nutr. 48:552–559.
Taube, G.
   1995   Epidemiology faces its limits. Science 269:164–169.
Taylor, C.R.
   1992   Cost of running springs. In Physiological Adaptations in Vertebrates: Respiration, Circulation, and Metabolism, S. Wood, R. Weber, A. Hargens, and R. Millard, eds. New York: Dekker.
Taylor, C.R., K. Schmidt-Neilsen, and J.L. Raab
   1970   Scaling of the energetic cost of running to body size in mammals. Am. J. Physiol. 219:1104–1107.
Taylor, C.R., A. Shkolnik, R. Dmi'el, D. Bahrav, and A. Borut
   1974   Running in cheetahs, gazelles, and goats: Energy cost and limb configuration. Am. J. Physiol. 227:848–850.
Taylor, C.R., N.C. Heglund, T.A. McMahon, and T.R. Looney
   1980   Energetic cost of generating muscular force during running: A comparison of large and small animals. J. Exp. Biol. 86:9–18.

Taylor, C.R., N.C. Heglund, and G.M.O. Maloiy
  1982   Energetics and mechanics of terrestrial locomotion. I. Metabolic energy consumption as a function of speed and body size in birds and mammals. J. Exp. Biol. 97:1–21.
Todd, I.C., D. Wosornu, I. Stewart, and T. Wild
  1992   Cardiac rehabilitation following myocardial infarction. Sports Med. 14:243–259.
U.S. Department of the Army
  1986   Army Regulation 600-9. "The Army Weight Control Program." September 15. Washington, D.C.
  1992   U.S. Army field manual FM 21-20. "Physical Fitness Training." September 30. Washington, D.C.
van Mechelen, W.
  1992   Running injuries. A review of the epidemiological literature. Sports Med. 14:320–335.
Walmsley, B., J.A. Hodgson, and R.E. Burke
  1978   Forces produced by the medial gastrocnemius and soleus muscles during locomotion in freely moving cats. J. Neurophysiol. 41:1203–1216.
Westerterp, K.R., G.A.L. Meijer, E.M.E. Janssen, W.H.M. Saris, and F. ten Hoor
  1992   Long-term effect of physical activity on energy balance and body composition. Br. J. Nutr. 68:21–30.
Woledge, R.C., N.A. Curtin, and E. Homsher
  1985   Energetic Aspects of Muscle Contraction. London: Academic Press.
Wright, S.
  1995   Turning the other cheeks: Insights into the cost of locomotion from running backwards. Undergraduate thesis, Harvard University, Cambridge, Mass.
Young, J.C.
  1995   Exercise prescription for individuals with metabolic disorders. Practical considerations. Sports Med. 19:43–54.
Zierath, J.R., and H. Wallberg-Henriksson
  1992   Exercise training in obese diabetic patients. Sports Med. 14:171–189.
Zuntz, N.
  1897   Über den Stoffverbauch des Hundes bei Muskelarbeit. Arch. Gesamte Physiol Menschen Tiere 68:191–211.

DISCUSSION

BERNADETTE MARRIOTT: What about arm swing in relation to motion?

REED HOYT: It is basically unaccounted for. The calibration group swung their arms, and the experimental group swung their arms as well. If they are carrying a load in their hands, the total load would be accounted for in terms of total body weight. The extra energy needed to swing that load would not be accounted for.

JOAN CONWAY: What do these devices look like?

REED HOYT: I will pass one around. The one that is coming around is just standard type technology. Under that insole, you can see the four sensitive resistors. The surface-mount technology probably could be fitted into the heel of a shoe fairly easily and, as MIT suggests, perhaps the force of walking could be used to generate some electricity with some piezoelectric stuff to get rid of the batteries.

(Laughter)

GILBERT LEVEILLE: Have you looked at telemetry of the data so that you could be manipulating [it] during the course of the experiment?

REED HOYT: The device is compatible with telemetry. In other words, there is a data output port. The way the device is configured right now, you gather the data, plug it into your computer, and download it. It is set up electronically so that you could hook a display on to it, so there could be a display on the shoe, or you could telemeter it with the appropriate telemetry feed—you would have to feed to a telemetry unit—so it is possible.

JOHN VANDERVEEN: What information does the sensor actually give you, other than the contact?

REED HOYT: That is strictly it.

JOHN VANDERVEEN: So if they are going uphill, you cannot tell versus . . .

REED HOYT: The uphill-downhill work is an issue. The Concord field station is working on it. The initial suggestion is that contact time does not change; the time spent with the foot in the air does change. So clearly, as you go uphill, you have a mass gravity change and an increase in potential energy, and depending on the grade, you will be more or less efficient in that movement. I think we have a shot at sorting that out as well.

DOUGLAS WILMORE: Reed, this comes out of some discussions several of us had at lunch, and it seems to me that the future is going to be to develop a set of microelectric monitors and detectors for people to tell not only supervisors when someone is in trouble or what they need, but maybe even to sense to the individual when homeostatic mechanisms may break down, for example, hydration status, energy status, and things of that sort.

Tell us how you see this evolving. Give us your thoughts about the next 10 or 15 years of development, because clearly the electronics are available and a lot of other stuff is available, too.

REED HOYT: Things are changing very quickly in terms of the electronics. The engine, the data logger, that is on this device was $500 a year and a half ago, and it is $15 now. I think in certain instances there will be a need to monitor people.

In chemical protective suit gear, the soldiers are at risk of cooking themselves. In Ranger school, they are perhaps at risk of hypothermia or hyperthermia. I see a cascade of monitoring from a personal monitor, where it will tell you when you start to become hyperthermic and give you a yellow light or a red light to drop out of whatever activity you are engaged in. That kind of monitoring could include heat production from this device as part of the puzzle.

There is keen interest, as I mentioned, within the command and even wider, to pour some money into personal monitoring. I think that as problems arise, there may be a need to then bring that to the next stage, where the team leader might be informed or the medic might be informed. Or with somebody having a problem, they could plug in by telemedicine to Walter Reed, or wherever the experienced clinicians are, to help the medic through a problem.

I think there is a lot of interest in refining that whole process, and there will be many little pieces of the puzzle, body temperature pills, foot contact monitors, canteen drinkometers, and on and on.

ROBERT NESHEIM: One of the things that occurs to me is that this technique could be used, knowing the weight of the individual and knowing the kind of work that he is going to do, to tell that individual how many calories he had to consume at that particular time during that task in order to be able to keep himself in balance.

One issue that this committee has addressed, of course, is that soldiers tend to underconsume. Maybe this might be a way of helping to get them to think about what they are eating.

REED HOYT: That is true. You can say you have so much body fat and so much body carbohydrate stores and you are going in a hole, so you need to keep pace. It has been a dilemma for us for a while.

JOHN VANDERVEEN: I was just curious. How are these systems relative to marching in water and things of that sort? Will you get them so that you can do that?

REED HOYT: Well, I think it is easy enough to make them waterproof. There has been a variety of work done on effects of substrate on energy requirements, and postholing through the snow or walking around on loose sand or walking in water up to your knees certainly is going to have an energy cost associated with it that will not necessarily be dealt with by this device. You need to know independently what the substrate conditions were like. That would be another sensor.

DOUGLAS WILMORE: But you could code that in, too. That would be a variable that you could code in.

REED HOYT: That is right, you would have a water sensor out there.

DAVID SCHNAKENBERG: I do not know if everyone in the room is aware of it, but I think that at least a year and a half ago when I left, the Army was looking at soldier modernization, soldiers of the twenty-first century.

You now are looking at a combat soldier or infantryman carrying a sophisticated data-acquisition system and a data-processing system and necessary uplinks to a satellite computer that would involve geopositioning, where he is specifically on the battlefield, sensing something about the environment, certainly detecting an infrared target and feeding that back into microoptics that he would be wearing on his helmet, to where you could have a variety of information that could be provided either automatically or on demand.

Initially it was to provide information about the environment and perhaps about his equipment and about the enemy. We always were trying to convince those that were involved in this process that it was a great opportunity to feed the soldier some information about himself.

The question comes back to: what is the short list of biosensors that we can put noninvasively on a human, preferably, that could be used to provide information with an on board algorithm to convert it into a useful tool, the red light and the green light?

REED HOYT: From the Rangers' point of view they had two problems. One was "Where am I?" So that requires a global positioning system solution, perhaps. And the other was "How do you tell the difference between an exhausted, sleep-deprived Ranger and one who is hypothermic?" So there you need some measure of body temperature in a situation where they are at risk.

DAVID DINGES: I was going to add a comment along that line. I think you have to distinguish between the technical feasibility, which, frankly, I consider to be trivial at this point—the only reason that these miniaturized devices are not right now in systems is because the companies who have the ability to make them do not do so until they see a market for them.

The real issues are, what do you measure physiologically that is scientifically valid, and what are the countermeasures? How do you feed that information back, or what do you tell a soldier to do when he or she is imperiled? Those are the substantive scientific issues, from my perspective.

The others are engineering issues and I think Dr. Wilmore said we have the potential right now to monitor almost anything with a miniaturized capacity with technology. The substantive issues are what, on whom, with what kind of feedback to prevent what?

KARL FRIEDL: You are exactly right. We do not want to feed individual soldiers a lot of medical or physiological information, giving them heart rate, blood pressure, and core temperature, and all that, which is really meaningless and it confuses them and it turns into something they will use for contests.

(Laughter)

We are talking about piggybacking onto a system that is going into effect with global positioning and all that. That is part of the twenty-first century land warrior system. And it finally allows the medical people to say, okay, you can put some stuff on here, now what do you want on this? And nobody really knows. We have not figured out exactly how we are going to interpret that and that is the big question. You hit it right on the head.

JAMES VOGEL: Just in follow-up, I might mention something you might be interested in, that the Ranger training regimen has agreed to be a test bed for these personal monitors, if this is interesting. Probably the very first version that will be tried this coming year will include the positioning monitoring, probably heart rate and temperature, though the other day we argued for hours about what temperature to record.

The technology is available; it is a question of where you record it from and, of course, what you do with it. Of course, these personal monitors will be monitored not by the individual, probably, to begin with, but by physician assistants or the command structure, at least in the Ranger training situation.

ARTHUR ANDERSON: Will the frequencies of these signals be in a form that cannot be monitored by the adversary? I mean, would it help them to know you are afraid?

REED HOYT: They are very sensitive about being identified by electronic emanation. Certainly the radio-temperature pill, which is one way to get a core body temperature, has a signal that goes approximately a yard and they are concerned, so with these more powerful systems you have that as a general concern.

G. RICHARD JANSEN: I guess what I am thinking is that if something can be done, it will be done, and I am thinking about information overload. I think this is what we are seeing with computers. What we see with computers is that the more the program has to do, the slower it does it, until you need to upgrade the computer. So there are limits. I think it really comes down to what is needed, because the soldier can only process, in a minute amount of time, the most important information, and there is going to be a lot of noise transmitted as we are talking here.

ROBERT NESHEIM: As Jim Vogel was pointing out, where this information goes and who is going to have the responsibility for acting on it is one of the key issues. I do not think you can have 100 individual soldiers in a platoon reacting to their own individual data. There has to be some command structure that is going to be able to control that or we are going to have chaos out there.

REED HOYT: These systems that they are setting up now are really for command and control. The early versions of the personal status monitors are probably going to be casualty assessment tools, to know who is still out there and what level of function they are at.

DOUGLAS WILMORE: . . . given that the physician assistant will then have a computer that information will dump into, or he can use algorithms or something like that.

Emerging Technologies for Nutrition Research, 1997
Pp. 345–358. Washington, D.C.
National Academy Press

15

Noninvasive Measurement of Plasma Metabolites Using Near-Infrared Spectroscopy

Donald Bodenner[1]

INTRODUCTION

The rapid, noninvasive measurement of organic analytes (substances) in blood or tissue would be tremendously useful in the treatment of battlefield injuries. Monitoring of hemoglobin, renal function, and liver metabolites would allow early detection of circulatory compromise and other conditions. Peacetime applications would include screening, diagnosis, and monitoring of diseases such as diabetes, liver dysfunction, renal disease, and abnormalities of lipid metabolism. Military training exercises could be enhanced by in-field monitoring of lactate and other biological markers of extreme physical exertion. A noninvasive instrument for accomplishing these tasks must meet several criteria. It should be accurate and precise over a clinically useful range of values for a particular analyte. The instrument should be small enough to be transported easily and able to operate for long periods of time without recharging the power

---

[1] Donald Bodenner, University of Rochester School of Medicine and Dentistry, Rochester, NY 14642

source. The device also must be rugged enough to withstand harsh conditions and must be reliable over time.

Modalities that satisfy these criteria are currently in very early stages of development. Of these, near-infrared (NIR) spectrophotometry appears to have the most potential at the present time for meeting these rigorous demands. NIR spectrophotometry requires no reagents and is very rapid and safe. Moreover, the sample can consist of complex organic mixtures (blood) and is not consumed by analysis.

This chapter focuses on NIR as a modality showing great promise as a noninvasive method of measuring multiple organic compounds in humans. A discussion of the theoretical basis for NIR biomedical applications will be followed by examples of the use of NIR *in vitro* and *in vivo*.

BACKGROUND

All organic compounds, by definition, consist of various combinations of carbon and hydrogen in combination with other atoms such as oxygen, nitrogen, and sulfur. The bonds joining these atoms undergo molecular vibrations when exposed to NIR light, whose wavelength extends from the end of the visible spectrum (approximately 700 nm) to the beginning of the infrared spectrum (2,500 nm). The NIR absorptions of these bonds usually consist of diverse combinations and overtone bands. Most organic compounds, therefore, will produce unique spectra (absorption patterns) when scanned over the range of NIR wavelengths. For example, NIR is capable of differentiating between the six hexose sugar isomers. NIR has been widely used for the identification and characterization of pure compounds, but the complexity of the spectra has in the past precluded the use of NIR to measure individual compounds within complex mixtures encountered in blood or tissue. Recent advances in methods of NIR spectral analysis (discussed below) have made possible the identification of spectral perturbations induced by concentration changes of a single compound despite changing concentrations of other organic metabolites in the sample.

CHEMOMETRIC METHODS

The first step in the analysis of NIR data is the evaluation of the spectra that are obtained by scanning over the range of NIR wavelengths. The absorbance spectrum obtained for a pure compound exhibits multiple peaks and troughs corresponding to maximum and minimum absorbance over a range of wavelengths. The dependence of peak height on analyte concentration is then used to measure the substance of interest. However, the identification of peaks, particularly in complex mixtures, is often very difficult. Calculation of the first or second derivative of the absorbance with respect to wavelength allows for more accurate identification of a peak and the measurement of peak heights for a particular compound. This is usually accomplished by plotting the difference in absorbance at two different wavelengths. The advantages of such a derivative analysis of an NIR spectrum is illustrated in Figure 15-1, which depicts a hypothetical spectrum with a peak at point B. The change in absorbance (log 1/transmittance) is constant and positive from point A to point B. The first derivative from point B to C also is constant but negative. The peak at point B is sharply defined at the point where the slope of the line changes. The second derivative of the spectrum measures the differences in the slope, measuring the change in the optical curve just prior to and after a point in the spectrum. The second derivative of the simple curve will be 0 when the slope is constant (Figure 15-1c) but will change suddenly when a peak is encountered with a sud-

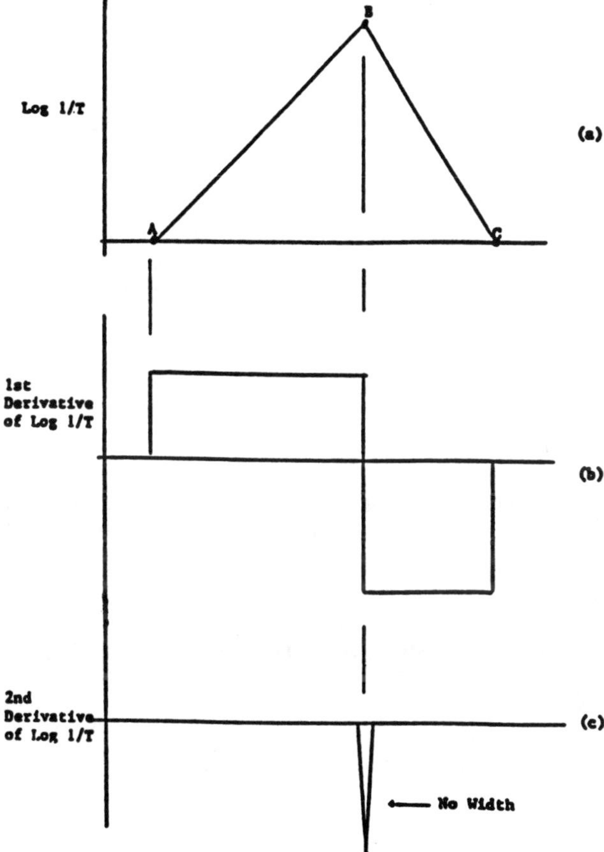

FIGURE 15-1 Model spectrum illustrating derivative analysis. (a) Absorbance increasing from point A to a peak at point B and then decreasing to point C. (b) First derivative of the model spectrum identifying the peak at point B by a deflection from positive to negative. (c) Second derivative of the model spectrum identifying the peak at point B by a sharply negative deflection.

den deflection in the slope. An added benefit is that derivative analysis, measuring changes in absorbance spectra, compensates for baseline drifts. Derivative analysis is not unique to NIR spectroscopy but has been used in other spectroscopic methods to enhance spectral resolution.

The second step in the analysis of NIR data is the construction of a standard curve or calibration. Traditional calibration techniques using standard solutions of purified compounds are not applicable to complex biological mixtures. Peaks from other constituents in the mixture routinely overlap with the peak of interest. Moreover, hydrogen bonding and other variations in the chemical composition make direct comparison of NIR absorbance of biological samples with that of solution standards impractical. Instead, calibration must be made using standard samples that accurately reflect the environment actually present during sampling. For instance, the construction of a NIR calibration to measure glucose in whole blood should involve patient-derived whole blood samples containing various concentrations of glucose measured by an independent, established method of glucose determination. Ideally the variations in glucose concentrations within these samples should be diet induced, because interfering substances will be affected concurrently with changes in glucose concentrations. Simply spiking a blood sample with glucose would not reflect these subtle changes in the calibration mixture. Calibration of NIR absorbance data from complex mixtures, therefore, often requires more refined methods of data analysis such as least-squares and multiple linear regression algorithms (Haaland, 1990, 1992; Honigs et al., 1983; Martens and Naes, 1989; Thomas and Haaland, 1990).

Univariate Least Squares

Converting absorbance data to concentration measurements is accomplished through the application of Beer's Law (Equation 15-1), which states that the light absorbance of a particular analyte at a specific wavelength is proportional to the concentration:

$$\text{Absorbance} = \text{molecular absorptivity} \times \text{path length} \times \text{concentration} \qquad \text{(Equation 15-1)}$$
$$A = elc,$$

where e is molecular absorptivity, l is path length, and c is concentration. Beer's Law is derived for pure compounds without overlapping absorptions. For practical purposes, a constant incorporating the molecular absorptivity, path length, and contribution from interfering substances is substituted for the l term in Equation 15-1 and rearranged in the form of a linear equation (Equation 15-2).

$$c = K + J \cdot A(ln) \qquad \text{(Equation 15-2)}$$

This univariate least-squares regression equation is used by simultaneously measuring concentration of the analyte in question and the absorbance A at wavelength ln. This process is repeated for several concentrations of analyte. The correlation between the concentration and absorbance, or linearity of the fit, is reflected in the slope J. The y-intercept is the constant K. This process is repeated for all wavelengths in the NIR light spectrum. Criteria for choosing wavelengths applicable to practical measurement of the analyte are a linear correlation between absorbance and concentration (high correlation coefficient) and robust absorbance at that wavelength. These criteria are met by plotting correlations obtained at each wavelength and absorbance at each wavelength. Potentially useful wavelengths can be identified by inspection. The clinical utility of the regression can be determined by calculating the standard error of calibration (SEC), representing the deviation of data points from the regression line. This term is expressed in concentration units employed for the calibration and can be compared to SECs obtained using standard laboratory methods.

The final step in the process of NIR data analysis is to use the regression equation identified by the calibration procedure to predict the concentration of unknown samples of the analyte in question. Again, it is important to have a wide range of concentrations of the compound in question to test all regions of the regression generated. Moreover, it is vital that the unknown samples tested be derived from the identical, or nearly identical, source. The absorbance at the best-fit wavelength is measured for the unknown samples and the concentration predicted using Equation 15-2 containing the empirically determined constants K and J. The predicted concentrations are plotted versus the measured concentrations. The correlation coefficient obtained is indicative of the ability of the regression equation to measure the analyte in the sample. An example of this type of calibration is illustrated in Figure 15-2 for NIR-predicted albumin in human plasma. Standard laboratory determination of albumin using a Kodak Ektachem analyzer is plotted along the x-axis and the NIR-predicted albumin concentration along the y-axis. A perfect calibration would result in all the data points falling on a straight line through the origin with a correlation of 1.0. The correlation obtained in this particular study using univariate least-squares analysis was 0.96 with a standard error of calibration of 1.8 g/liter (Hall and Pollard, 1992).

In practice, univariate least squares rarely can predict adequately the concentration of an analyte in a complex mixture such as blood or plasma over the full range of clinically useful analyte concentrations. Errors may be distributed evenly over the entire concentration measured, or the regression may break down at extremes of the sample set. These errors are caused by scattering differences or absorbance contributions at the chosen wavelength by interfering substances. Advanced chemometric techniques utilizing multivariate regression recently have been developed to address these problems (for review, see Beebe and Kowalske, 1987).

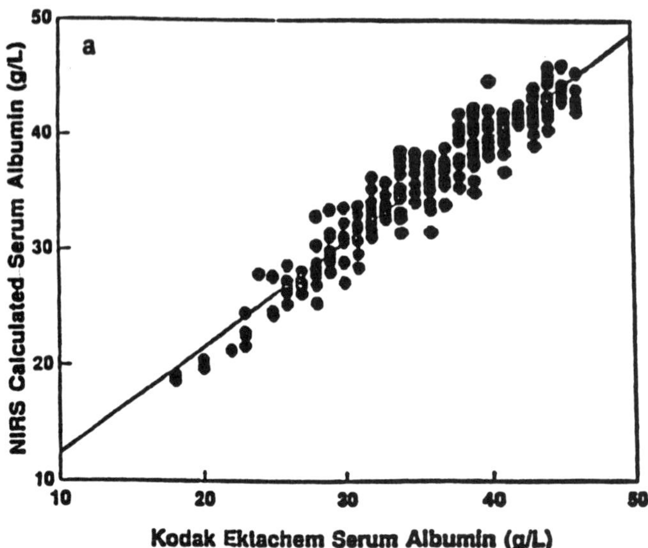

FIGURE 15-2 Testing of a near-infrared (NIR) calibration to standard laboratory analysis. NIR absorbance data and a least-squares calibration model were used to calculate serum albumin (y-axis) and then compared with albumin measured using a Kodak Ektachem (x-axis). Correlation of the best fit line was 0.96 with standard error of calibration of 1.8 g/liter. SOURCE: Hall and Pollard (1992), used with permission.

Multivariate Regression

As mentioned above, substances other than the one of interest in a complex mixture may absorb NIR light at the wavelength used to generate a univariate least-squares calibration equation, invalidating the subsequent prediction of analyte concentration. The fact that changes in all absorbance peaks of a particular compound are directly related to changes in concentration of that analyte can be used to correct for absorbance contributions from interfering substances. A wavelength is identified that ideally is absorbed only by the interfering substance. Absorbance changes at this wavelength secondary to changes in the concentration of the interfering substance will be directly related to interfering absorbance contributions to the principal wavelength used to measure the analyte of interest. Additional terms can thus be added to the univariate Equation 15-2 to correct for interfering substances (Equation 15-3), where c is the predicted analyte concentration, K is the y-intercept, and the constants J(1) through J(n) are slope terms.

$$c = K + J(1) \cdot A(l1) + J(2) \cdot A(l2) + \ldots + J(n) \cdot A(ln) \qquad \text{(Equation 15-3)}$$

The calibration method for this simple multivariate equation is similar to that outlined for the univariate regression described above. Samples are analyzed representing a broad range of concentrations of the analyte of interest measured by reference laboratory methods. The constants $J(n)$ are derived using standard algorithms for solving such multiple regression equations. One of the advantages of this method of regression analysis is that the identity of the interfering substance is not necessary for calibration. An equation that correlates best with analyte concentration can be derived empirically by measuring absorbance at multiple wavelengths, in addition to that of the analyte, over a range of analyte samples. Although time consuming, empirically solving for the constants J(n), which best relate optical data to analyte concentration, can then be carried out.

Principal component regression (PCR) and partial least squares (PLS) are chemometric tools that extend many of the basic principles inherent within classical least-squares and multivariate least-squares approaches. A detailed discussion of these methods is beyond the scope of this article (for review, see Beebe and Kowalske, 1987; Haaland, 1990, 1992). Particular strengths of these algorithms include maximization of signal-to-noise ratios by taking advantage of the entire NIR spectra, more efficient measurement of low-concentration analytes in complex mixtures, and resistance to the effects of instrument noise. There are advantages and disadvantages to each of the chemometric methods available for measurement of organic analytes. The superiority of one over the other is dependent upon the sample composition and information desired.

APPLICATIONS

In Vitro Analysis

NIR has been widely used in the agricultural industries since the 1970s (Watson, 1977) to measure protein in wheat flour (Hruschka and Norris, 1982), and sugar content of breakfast cereals (Baker and Norris, 1985). Biomedical applications of NIR have been explored only recently. Early NIR reflectance experiments using standard multiple linear regression techniques predicted human serum cholesterol concentration with a correlation of 0.985 (Peuchant et al., 1987). Similar techniques also were used by the same investigators to measure fecal fat (Peuchant et al., 1988). NIR measurement of fat and conjugated bilirubin in feces can be used to screen infants for biliary atresia (Akiyama and Yamauchi, 1994).

Recent advances in chemometric methods of NIR analysis discussed above have made possible the measurement of a variety of biological substances in complex mixtures. Fourier transform analysis of near-infrared was used to model glucose levels in aqueous solutions with a R^2 correlation of 99.4 percent (Arnold and Small, 1990). Reflectance NIR spectroscopy and linear regression were used to predict glucose in blood with a correlation of 0.969 (Mendelson et al., 1990). NIR analysis using a two-wavelength multiple linear least-squares method predicted serum albumin with a correlation of 0.98 compared with standard laboratory methods (Hall and Pollard, 1993). Partial least-squares analysis of human serum triglycerides produced a correlation of 0.98 with reference measurement techniques (Hall and Pollard, 1993).

In Vivo Analysis

The primary noninvasive application of NIR spectroscopy has been the measurement and monitoring of tissue oxygenation. The ratio of the absorbance peak of deoxyhemoglobin at 760 nm and total hemoglobin (measured by the absorbance at the isosbestic point of oxyhemoglobin and deoxyhemoglobin, that is, where the extinction coefficients are identical) represents an accurate index of tissue oxygenation (Jobsis, 1977; Yoshiya et al., 1980). This observation has led to a number of clinical applications of NIR to the measurement of hemoglobin saturation in the liver (Kitai et al., 1993), noninvasive measurement of blood flow and oxygen consumption in the forearm (De Blasi et al., 1994), estimation of circulating blood volume (Christensen et al., 1993), fetal monitoring (Faris et al., 1994), and noninvasive methods of measuring cerebral blood flow and oxygenation (Carney et al., 1993; Skov et al., 1991; Williams et al., 1994; Wyatt, 1993).

Because a ratio of NIR absorbances is being measured in many of these clinical applications, an internal control is present that corrects for differences in finger size, skin pigmentation, and other possible confounding variables among patients. Such and internal control is not present in the measurement of other biological compounds of clinical interest such as glucose, lipids, and hepatic enzymes, where a more complex chemometric analysis is necessary for these blood analytes. Moreover, the analysis is complicated further by the dynamic nature of the *in vivo* setting. As opposed to measurement of analytes in an *in vitro* setting, the composition of blood and tissue is in a constant state of flux.

Very few reports of studies have appeared that have overcome these formidable obstacles. Transcutaneous measurement of blood glucose by NIR light through the finger was achieved in three patients with Type I diabetes who had been fed a mixed meal consisting of carbohydrate, fat, and protein that generated a blood glucose range of between 2.5 and 27 mmol/liter (45–486 mg/dl) (Robinson et al., 1992). NIR spectral data were obtained using three spectrometer configurations and either PLS or PCR chemometric methods of data analysis. The results show some inconsistencies among spectrophotometer configurations and among the chemometric methods used. A Fourier transform spectrophotometer and PLS data analysis yielded the best correlation, with an average absolute error of 1.1 mmol/liter (19.8 mg/dl) (Figure 15-3). The absolute error of predicted glucose concentration was similar using a grated monochrometer, producing light at 1 nm increments, and the PLS algorithm with (2.1 mmol/liter [37.8 mg/dl]) and without (1.6 mmol/liter [28.8 mg/dl]) fiberoptics. This study demonstrated the feasibility of measuring blood glucose noninvasively over a wide range of blood glucose concentrations. The absolute errors of prediction

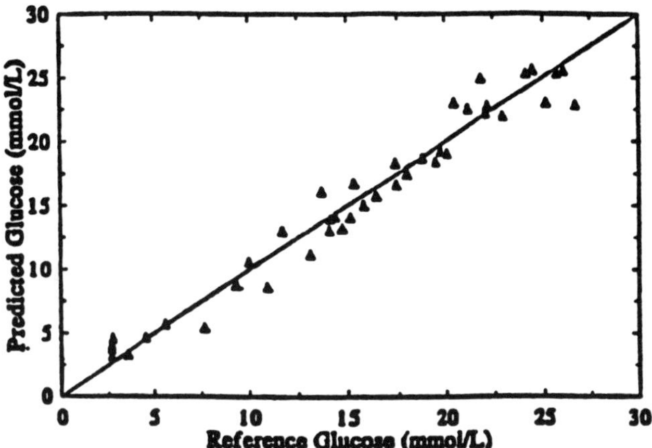

FIGURE 15-3 Transcutaneous measurement of blood glucose using near-infrared (NIR) light transmitted through the finger. Correlation between NIR-predicted blood glucose using a partial least-squares calibration model and measurement of glucose by reference techniques. Average error of prediction 1.1 mmol (19.8 mg/dl). SOURCE: Robinson et al. (1992), used with permission.

approach clinical usefulness, approximating the range encountered with current lancet-based glucose meters (Meehan et al., 1992; Vallera et al., 1991). The predictions were unique for each patient, however, and did not represent a calibration equation that could be generalized to diabetic patients as a group. Moreover, the effect on the calibration of changes in concentration of other organic analytes in high concentration in the bloodstream, such as hemoglobin, fat, and urea, is unknown.

A different approach to noninvasive measurement of blood glucose recently has been reported, using reflectance NIR spectroscopy rather than NIR light transmitted through tissue (Heise et al., 1994). Several glucose excursions with values ranging from 30 to 600 mg/dl were induced on different days in a single diabetic patient through the administration of glucose and insulin. NIR reflectance was measured on the inner lip, and PLS was used to correlate blood glucose to NIR-predicted glucose. The mean-square prediction error for 132 spectra obtained from single-day glucose excursions was 45.6 mg/dl (2.54 mmol/liter). The error was improved slightly when a time-delay filter, or constant accounting for venous to tissue equilibration of glucose, was added. Random blood glucose values also were predicted in the same patient on subsequent days (Figure 15-4). Of 216 random spectra, the error was 51.9 mg/dl (2.88 mmol/liter) (Heise et al., 1994). Glucose was also predicted from a grouped analysis of spectra obtained from inner-lip reflectance data measured in 133 diabetic patients. The glucose values in the study group ranged between 35 and 417 mg/dl. Again using PLS algorithms, the mean-square prediction error was 57.9 mg/dl (3.2 mmol/liter).

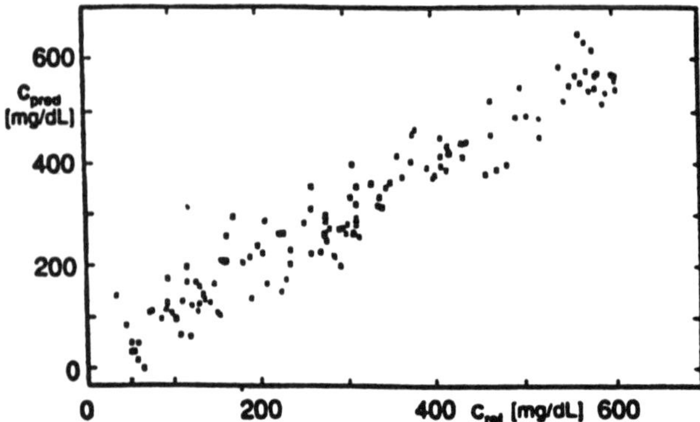

FIGURE 15-4 Blood glucose measurement using reflected near-infrared (NIR) light from the inner lip. Scatter plot of 216 random NIR glucose measurements from a single individual using a partial least-squares calibration model versus reference glucose values (mean-square glucose prediction error of 51.9 mg/dl.) SOURCE: Heise et al. (1994), used with permission.

The errors encountered are significantly greater than those observed using the transcutaneous approach, exceeding acceptable standards based upon lancet-based glucose meters. It is unclear whether this is secondary to sampling error or inherent within the reflectance approach. The results do show, however, that a single regression equation is capable of predicting blood glucose among individuals, implying that a general calibration applicable to large populations may be feasible.

AUTHOR'S CONCLUSIONS AND RECOMMENDATIONS

NIR spectroscopy is an emerging technology with numerous potential applications for the rapid and noninvasive monitoring of organic blood analytes. New methods of data analysis have demonstrated the feasibility of measuring single constituents within a complex organic matrix both *in vitro* and *in vivo*. Direct military applications would include biochemical evaluation of wounded soldiers in the field, monitoring metabolites during training, and the routine screening and health maintenance of military personnel. Difficult issues remain unresolved before an instrument will be available to meet these goals. Preliminary studies suggest, however, that these problems are now primarily technical in nature. Thus, significant advances in the development of noninvasive methods of organic analyte measurement are expected. The great potential inherent in this evolving technology suggests that continued research efforts are warranted.

REFERENCES

Akiyama, T., and Y. Yamauchi
  1994   Use of near infrared reflectance spectroscopy in the screening for biliary atresia. J. Pediatr. Surg. 29(5):645–647.
Arnold, M.A., and G.W. Small
  1990   Determination of physiological levels of glucose in an aqueous matrix with digitally filtered Fourier transform near-infrared spectra. Anal. Chem. 62:1457–1464.
Baker, D., and K.H. Norris
  1985   Near-infrared reflectance measurement of total sugar content of breakfast cereals. Appl. Spec. 39(4):618–621.
Beebe, K.R., and B.R. Kowalske
  1987   An introduction to multivariate calibration and analysis. Anal. Chem. 59:1007a–1017a.
Carney, J.M., W. Landrum, L. Mayes, Y. Zou, and R.A. Lodder
  1993   Near-infrared spectrophotometric monitoring of stroke-related changes in the protein and lipid composition of whole gerbil brains. Anal. Chem. 65(10):1305–1313.
Christensen, P., B. Eriksen, and S.W. Henneberg
  1993   Precision of a new bedside method for estimation of the circulating blood volume. Acta Anaesthesiol. Scand. 37(6):622–627.
De Blasi, R.A., M. Ferrari, A. Natali, G. Conti, A. Mega, and A. Gasparetto
  1994   Noninvasive measurement of forearm blood flow and oxygen consumption by near-infrared spectroscopy. J. Appl. Physiol. 76(3):1388–1393.
Faris, F., M. Doyle, Y. Wickramasinghe, R. Houston, P. Rolfe, and S. O'Brien
  1994   A non-invasive optical technique for intrapartum fetal monitoring: Preliminary clinical studies. Med. Eng. Phys. 16(4):287–291.
Haaland, D.M.
  1990   Multivariate calibration methods applied to quantitative FT-IR analyses. Pp. 395–468 in Practical Fourier Transform Infrared Spectroscopy, J.R. Ferraro and K. Krishnan, eds. New York: Academic Press.
  1992   Multivariate calibration methods applied to the quantitative analysis of infrared spectra. Pp. 1–30 in Computer-Enhanced Analytical Spectroscopy, vol. 3, P.C. Jurs, ed. New York: Plenum Press.
Hall, J.W., and A. Pollard
  1992   Near-infrared spectrophotometry: A new dimension in clinical chemistry. Clin. Chem. 38(9):1623–1631.
  1993   Near-infrared spectroscopic determination of serum total proteins, albumin, globulins, and urea. Clin. Biochem. 26(6):483–490.
Heise, H.M., R. Marbach, T. Koschinsky, and F.A. Gries
  1994   Noninvasive blood glucose sensors based on near-infrared spectroscopy. Artif. Organs 18(6):439–447.
Honigs, D.E., J.M. Freelin, G.M. Hieftje, and T.B. Hirschfeld
  1983   Near-infrared reflectance analysis by Gauss-Jordan linear algebra. Appl. Spec. 37(6):491–497.
Hruschka, W.R., and K.H. Norris
  1982   Least-squares curve fitting of near-infrared spectra predicts protein and moisture content of ground wheat. Appl. Spec. 36(3):261–264.
Jobsis, F.F.
  1977   Noninvasive, infrared monitoring of cerebral and myocardial oxygen sufficiency and circulatory parameters. Science 198:1264–1267.

Kitai, T., A. Tanaka, A. Tokuka, K. Tanaka, Y. Yamaoka, K. Ozawa, and K. Hirao
   1993   Quantitative detection of hemoglobin saturation in the liver with near-infrared spectroscopy. Hepatology 18(4):926–936.
Martens, H., and T. Naes
   1989   Multivariate Calibration. New York: John Wiley and Sons.
Meehan, C.D., L.A. Bove, and A.S. Jennings
   1992   Comparison of first-generation and second-generation blood glucose meters for use in a hospital setting. Diabetes Educ. 18(3):228–231.
Mendelson, Y., A.C. Clermont, R.A. Peura, and B.C. Lin
   1990   Blood glucose measurement by multiple attenuated total reflection and infrared absorption spectroscopy. IEEE Trans. Biomed. Eng. 37(5):458–465.
Peuchant, E., C. Salles, and R. Jensen
   1987   Determination of serum cholesterol by near-infrared reflectance spectrometry. Anal. Chem. 59(14):1816–1819.
   1988   Value of a spectroscopic "fecalogram" in determining the etiology of steatorrhea. Clin. Chem. 34(1):5–8.
Robinson, M.R., R.P. Eaton, D.M. Haaland, G.W. Koepp, E.V. Thomas, B.R. Stallard, and P.L. Robinson
   1992   Noninvasive glucose monitoring in diabetic patients: A preliminary evaluation. Clin. Chem. 38(9):1618–1622.
Skov, L., O. Pryds, and G. Greisen
   1991   Estimating cerebral blood flow in newborn infants: Comparison of near infrared spectroscopy and 133-Xe clearance. Pediatr. Res. 30(6):570–573.
Thomas, E.V., and D.M. Haaland
   1990   Comparison of multivariate calibration methods for quantitative spectral analysis. Anal. Chem. 62:1091–1099.
Vallera, D.A., M.G. Bissell, and W. Barron
   1991   Accuracy of portable blood glucose monitoring. Effect of glucose level and prandial state. Am. J. Clin. Pathol. 95(2):247–252.
Watson, C.A.
   1977   Near infrared reflectance spectrophotometric analysis of agricultural products. Anal. Chem. 49:835a–840a.
Williams, I.M., A.J. Picton, S.C. Hardy, A.J. Mortimer, and C.N. McCollum
   1994   Cerebral hypoxia detected by near infrared spectroscopy. Anaesthesia 49(9):762–766.
Wyatt, J.S.
   1993   Near-infrared spectroscopy in asphyxial brain injury. Clin. Perinatol. 20(2):369–378.
Yoshiya, I., Y. Shimada, and K. Tanaka
   1980   Spectrophotometric monitoring of arterial oxygen saturation in the finger tip. Med. Biol. Eng. Comp. 18:27–32.

DISCUSSION

GAIL BUTTERFIELD: How did you chose the finger rather than the ear lobe [as the site of measurement]?

DONALD BODENNER: The finger was chosen after some initial study showed that the ear lobe, surprisingly, is too squishy. It is very deformable, and in the initial studies, anyway, if you want to have a set path length for any particular patient, the ear lobe would not qualify.

JOHN VANDERVEEN: I would imagine that virtual blood flow changes would affect your reading, would they not?

DONALD BODENNER: That has not been studied. We have indirect evidence that that is probably not true, because many patients for the population study said in the patient history that they had serious peripheral vascular disease from their diabetes. In other words, they already had preexisting blood flow problems, but that was not measured directly. That is one of the variables we do have to test.

JOHN VANDERVEEN: Even temperature would have an impact on blood flow.

DONALD BODENNER: To examine temperature as a variable, a temperature sensor for both the finger tip and the proximal finger was used. Surprisingly, temperature differences introduced only a minor error in the determinations.

JOHANNA DWYER: If two things are changing simultaneously, for instance blood glucose and urea or something else, what happens? Can you get a useful measurement?

DONALD BODENNER: The answer is yes, the reason being—and that is why I wanted to spend some time on basic principles—is that everything according to Beer's Law is directly proportional. So if the absorption of BUN [blood urea nitrogen] is increasing and if it is overlapping on your area of interest, this overlapping contribution will be proportional to the direct contribution at a wavelength outside of your area of interest.

Thus, using this reasoning, you can correct for a variety of different substances in a complex mixture.

JOAN CONWAY: I have a comment. I was the one who used NIR for body composition, and what I found was that every population that I used needed a new calibration, and I also found that true for anything that you tried to use this for. It is very similar to our problem in body composition studies, where if you use BIA [bioelectrical impedance analysis], or almost any method, each time you want a study population you have a different calibration. I just raise it as a problem that I never saw until I started doing that research.

DONALD BODENNER: It was a very big consideration, and it still remains one. The idea, I should stress, is between an individual calibration, which is what you are discussing, where every time you do one of these analyses on individual patients you have to do a new individual calibration, versus a general calibration that you can apply to the entire population, off-the-shelf technology. That was a main concern that we had as well, and we still do.

JOAN CONWAY: The other comment I have is I know that this is being used to measure oxygen concentration in blood.

DONALD BODENNER: In a variety of places.

DONALD McCORMICK: Isn't it true that you have to fingerprint based on absorptions . . . My point is, is it not quite severely limited by the number of metabolites that you can reliably know you are looking at?

It is going back to Johanna Dwyer's question, because I do not think you can select a large number of things and filter them out.

DONALD BODENNER: Once again, getting back to how the equations are made, if you can find an overtone or any kind of a band in the NIR region that absorbs adequately that is representative of interfering substances, then their contribution to the glucose absorbance can be accounted for.

ROBERT WOLFE: Yes, but the question is how many do you need for a generalizable calibration equation?

DONALD BODENNER: We found that you can get by with about 200 in terms of glucose measurement, but we have not looked at a lot of the different potential contributors, especially in diabetics, or people in dialysis. What, for instance, happens when the BUN, which is a measure of renal failure, is 150? Or when patients are profoundly anemic? There are a large number of pathophysiolgic states where it is unclear whether this type of analysis will hold true.

Emerging Technologies for Nutrition Research, 1997
P. 359. Washington, D.C.
National Academy Press

V

Discussion

GILBERT LEVEILLE: This is just a reaction. I thought it was a very exciting day. For those of us who have been away from the bench for a long time, it is exciting to see what is happening. The intriguing things to me are how the technology is evolving, and the tremendous number of things we can do with much greater efficiency than we could ever do them before.

Still, the issue that remains is the basic fundamental question that one poses to be answered with the new technology. It is interesting to look at the basic biochemistry that we are now able to explore in noninvasive ways, or at least with minimal invasion. But we still are playing the same tracer games when we chase a few carbons around a metabolic cycle, this is still fun, but I think it still leads us back to what questions we really want to ask.

Someone raised the question of whether what we really need to look at is what is happening at the membrane level and what impact that is having at the total organism level. Clearly that is an important question that we have not addressed, and we need to get to it.

VI

Molecular and Cellular Approaches to Nutrition

IN PART VI, CHAPTERS 16 AND 17 FOCUS on molecular approaches to nutrition research, while Chapters 18 and 19 concentrate on cellular approaches.

In Chapter 16, metal-regulated gene expression is reviewed. Trace metals can play a role in gene expression in three ways: structural, catalytic, or regulatory. The regulation of gene expression by trace metals is more specific and interactive than the other two levels of interaction. Iron and zinc provide the best examples of metals involved in gene regulation, with the role of zinc being the best understood of any of the metals. The chapter discusses the zinc-finger motif of some proteins that are involved in DNA binding, as well as the role of zinc as an activator of trans-acting factors for regulating specific gene expression.

Chapter 17 provides an overview of the processes that contribute to gene expression and describes techniques used to study the regulation of gene expression associated with nutrient metabolism. While protein synthesis can be regulated at the level of transcription, translation, or posttranslational modification, particular emphasis in this chapter is given to the process of gene transcription and its control, and several model systems are described that show how changes in transcription of specific genes occur in response to nutritional factors.

Chapters 16 and 17 describe molecular techniques that may permit the identification of stress-responsive genes whose expression would be beneficial to control, and the authors indicate that in the future it may be possible to combine nutritional therapy with gene modification. However, the use of techniques to study gene expression is still limited in its application to nutritional problems.

The use of isolated cell techniques to study the cellular uptake and metabolism of naturally occurring glucosides of water-soluble vitamins is the subject of Chapter 18. While micronutrients are clearly essential to performance capability, a number of questions remain to be answered regarding their exact roles. Much work has been done to elucidate the cellular import of water-soluble vitamins, their metabolism, and their bioavailability.

Finally, Chapter 19 examines cellular dysfunction during physiologic stress by discussing the use of isolated cell systems to study the impact of hypoxia and oxidative stress on cellular function. Cellular responses to these stimuli are dependent on the cell type, the nature of the stress, and the environment (cellular, exocrine, and endocrine) of the cells. It is emphasized that if the purpose of using an isolated cell system is to model a more complex *in vivo* counterpart, the choice of cell system becomes critical. As a general rule, to maximize the utility of a particular cell model, the cell type chosen must display a pattern of response and sensitivity to the stimulus similar to the tissue or system of interest.

These two chapters show how isolated cell systems can be used to examine the effects of stimuli at the organelle or cellular level. Caution is warranted in that care must be taken to choose cell culture models that are as similar in response as possible to the entire organism and situation in question, and like the molecular approaches to nutritional problems, application is still limited.

Emerging Technologies for Nutrition Research, 1997
Pp. 363–373. Washington, D.C.
National Academy Press

16

The Role of Metals in Gene Expression

Raymond K. Blanchard and Robert J. Cousins[1]

The concept that metals are able to influence gene expression has been understood in general terms for decades. Growth responses associated with the addition of trace elements to the nutrient supply of both plants and animals supported such a role. Subsequent to this, the demonstration that enzymes associated with nucleic acid biochemistry were metalloenzymes more firmly established the metal-gene expression relationship.

All living organisms require metals to sustain various cellular processes. These metals include the macrominerals, for example calcium, which is not believed to directly influence gene expression, but may do so indirectly through secondary messenger roles. Trace metals (elements) required in the diet include copper, iron, manganese, nickel, selenium, and zinc. In humans, these trace elements are required in microgram to milligram amounts per day. Cellular mechanisms control the transport of trace metals into and out of cells so that the

---

[1] Robert J. Cousins, Center for Nutritional Sciences and Food Science and Human Nutrition Department, University of Florida, Gainesville, FL 32611

influences of natural abundance and thermodynamic properties do not determine the cellular content and function of a specific metal (da Silva and Williams, 1991). Nevertheless, these mechanisms can be overwhelmed by very high intakes of a trace metal.

INVOLVEMENT OF METALS IN GENE EXPRESSION

There are three ways trace metals can be involved in gene expression. One is structural, where metals facilitate interaction among various binding groups to provide the altered conformation necessary for interactions such as between specific proteins and DNA (Cousins, 1995). The second type of involvement is catalytic, where the metal is required for the activity of an enzyme associated with gene expression. The third class involves specific regulation, where metal occupancy of a transacting protein modulates transcription of a specific gene. This type of involvement is different from the first in that it is much more specific, being more interactive than structural in function. Since the catalytic role appears to be relatively unalterable in humans except, perhaps, in extreme deficiency situations during development, this chapter will concentrate on the structural and regulatory aspects of metals in gene expression.

The best examples of the regulation of gene expression by metals are iron and zinc. In the case of iron, metal occupancy decreases the binding of a metal-regulatory binding protein to ferritin mRNA, allowing the translation of ferritin mRNA to increase while simultaneously increasing binding to transferrin receptor mRNA, which increases the degradation of mRNA (O'Halloran, 1993). Because iron exhibits oxidation-reduction (redox) chemistry, rapid control of ferritin synthesis at the level of translation is necessary to provide rapid control of free iron levels within cells.

Far more is known about the involvement of zinc in gene expression than that of other elements. The intracellular binding affinity is greater for zinc than for virtually all other metals found in cells, with the exception of copper. However, unlike iron, zinc does not exhibit redox chemistry but has the properties of a Lewis acid and exhibits fast ligand exchange, which is important for its catalytic role (da Silva and Williams, 1991). A principal example of this catalytic role in gene expression is exhibited by the family of RNA nucleotidyl transferases (RNA polymerases I, II, and III). Zinc also plays a structural role in the zinc-finger motif of proteins that are involved in DNA binding, as is discussed below. Finally, as an activator of trans-acting factors,[2] zinc is responsible for regulating the expression of specific genes. The latter is discussed below.

---

[2] Proteins that bind to a gene (usually in the promoter region) to help regulate transcription of the gene.

ZINC FINGERS

Zinc ions serve an important structural function by tetrahedrally coordinating to cysteine or histidine residues of certain proteins to stabilize the structure of a small functional domain. The most prominent role of proteins with zinc-finger motifs is sequence-specific binding to DNA during transcription, and this is one of the most common eukaryotic DNA-binding motifs (Klug and Schwabe, 1995). Transcription factors that use zinc fingers as DNA-binding domains range from basal transcription components such as Sp1, to tissue type-specific factors such as GATA-1, to inducible factors such as glucocorticoid receptors (Lewin, 1994). In addition, some zinc fingers have been shown to mediate protein-protein interactions. The degree of influence of the level of dietary zinc on zinc interaction with finger proteins is not known.

Four major but distinct families of zinc-finger motifs have been identified. The first type is the original or classic zinc finger, as exemplified in transcription factor TFIIIA (Klug and Schwabe, 1995). A single, independent motif contains 1 zinc ion coordinated to 2 cysteine and 2 histidine residues, with a loop or finger of 12 amino acids between the 2 pairs of coordinating residues. This DNA-binding structure often functions as a multimer in which the finger motif is repeated in tandem one to nine times, with the spacing between the coordinating residues being highly conserved. This primary structure has served as the starting point for identifying other zinc-finger motifs based on DNA- and amino acid-sequence homology.

The second family of zinc-finger proteins contains a "zinc twist" (Vallee et al., 1991). This motif consists of two tandem zinc fingers with only cysteines as the zinc coordinating residues. Unlike the classic zinc finger, these two fingers twist around each other to form a single functional unit with two faces. The zinc-twist motif is characteristic of the DNA-binding domain of the steroid hormone receptor super family. These receptors frequently function as dimers (Lewin, 1994).

The third zinc-finger type motif to be recognized is referred to as a "zinc cluster." In this structure, just six conserved cysteines[3] coordinate two zinc ions in a single cluster, and the first and third cysteines are shared between both zinc ions. This motif is responsible for sequencing specific DNA binding of proteins, such as in the transcription factor GAL4.

The LIM domain is the fourth type of zinc-finger motif. It is composed of two tandem finger-like zinc-binding sites (Dawid et al., 1995). The first zinc is coordinated by three cysteines and a histidine, while the second zinc is coordinated by four cysteines. The LIM domain occurring in some proteins is followed by a homeodomain,[4] which may mediate DNA binding. In contrast, for

---

[3] Cysteines that appear in the same relative position within the molecule throughout the entire family of this type of protein.

[4] An amino acid motif that is similar or identical to a sequence originally identified in some *Drosophila* transcription factors (homeodomain proteins) as the site that binds to a

LIM-only proteins, there is mounting evidence that the LIM motif is involved in protein-protein interactions (Schmeichel and Beckerle, 1994).

With such a wide distribution among proteins involved in different cellular processes, zinc fingers are an important focus of research for therapeutic applications. For example, with their high sequence specificity, they are being evaluated as alternatives to anti-sense DNA approaches to modulating gene expression, and new DNA specificities for zinc fingers are being developed by mutagenesis and phage display library screening (Rebar and Pabo, 1994; Wu et al., 1995). In this way, engineered zinc-finger proteins could be selected based on their ability to bind a specific sequence of interest in order to target specific genes or points of regulation.

METAL-RESPONSIVE GENE REGULATION

The mechanisms of transcriptional regulation operate through protein interactions with specific sequences of DNA known as response elements. These response elements provide the specificity for protein factors to interact with each other on the promoter and ultimately result in the unique regulation of different genes. One widely studied eukaryotic response element that confers increased transcription by metals was first identified in the promoter of the metallothionein I gene (Stuart et al., 1984). This metal response element, or MRE, is a 15-base pair (bp) consensus sequence found in multiple copies that potentiates a large increase in gene expression when zinc or cadmium is present (Cousins, 1994). MRE consensus sequences are generally found in the first several hundred base pairs of the promoter and are often near or overlapping with response elements for other transcriptional factors, such as AP1 (Lewin, 1994). In addition, MREs are orientation independent and confer metal responsiveness when placed in heterologous promoters.

Recently a protein factor that binds to MREs, and is essential for metal responsiveness, has been cloned and characterized from the mouse and human sources. This MRE-binding transcription factor (MTF-1) has a DNA-binding domain consisting of six classical zinc fingers and a separate transcriptional activation domain (Brugnera et al., 1994). It is not yet clear, however, whether MTF-1 binds or interacts directly with zinc or cadmium to activate transcription or whether another metalloregulatory protein binds zinc or cadmium and then interacts with MTF-1.

The fact that MRE elements function independently of other regulatory elements makes them valuable in the construction of chimeric genes for transgenic animals (Palmiter et al., 1982). One or several MREs can be incorporated into the promoter of a chimeric gene and allow the expression of the gene to be controlled *in vivo*. In this way, dietary zinc acting through MREs

---

class of genes known as homeotic or homeobox genes. This motif is found throughout eukaryotes.

might eventually be coupled to gene therapy to provide some degree of control for therapeutic gene expression, as discussed below.

mRNA DIFFERENTIAL DISPLAY

As international genome mapping projects progress, it has become an increasing priority in biology to identify the genes contained in these vast sequences in order to characterize the function of each gene product. Consequently, detection of genes regulated by nutritional status or altered physiological situations has become increasingly important. Most of the techniques for analyzing regulation by nutrition and other factors, however, require information about the gene as a prerequisite, and it is estimated that current international databases have only identified approximately 30 percent of the total genes in the human genome (Orr et al., 1994). A recently developed polymerase chain reaction (PCR) technique, mRNA differential display, can detect genes that are regulated under different physiological states with no prior information about the gene (Liang et al., 1993). This method is currently being used to detect genes regulated by dietary micronutrients such as zinc and selenium (Blanchard and Cousins, 1996; Kendall and Christensen, 1995).

The technique of mRNA differential display begins with the isolation of RNA from animals, tissues, or cells exposed to different physiological conditions. The RNA is reverse transcribed using an oligo d(T) primer that has an additional two non-T bases at its 3' end in order to anchor the start of the cDNA synthesis to the junction of the 3' untranslated region and the poly A tail. A total of four anchor primers are needed. The resulting cDNAs are then subjected to the polymerase chain reaction using the oligo d(T) primer and a decanucleotide primer of arbitrary sequence that will only amplify cDNAs representing a small subset of mRNAs from the original sample and incorporate a radioactive label. Gel electrophoresis and autoradiography are used to display the resulting PCR products. Any mRNA that contains the arbitrary decanucleotide sequence within approximately 400 bp of poly A tail will have that portion of its 3' end amplified by the primers in the PCR reaction, and this will produce a band of a specific size on the autoradiograph. In order to screen the entire population of mRNA in a given sample effectively, it is necessary to use a battery of at least 26 different arbitrary decamers, as well as the 4 oligo d(T) primers for all possible combinations at the 3' end. The intensity of the autoradiographic image is proportional to the amount of a particular mRNA in the samples. Therefore, cDNA bands of the same size that vary in intensity between experimental conditions represent an mRNA that is differentially expressed under those conditions. In addition, since the samples are displayed adjacent to each other on a gel with many lanes, more than two physiological conditions can be evaluated at the same time, which increases the versatility of this technique.

The cDNA for each differentially expressed mRNA is recovered from the electrophoresis gel and cloned into a plasmid to maintain a stable copy of cDNA for further analysis. The cDNA is first used as a probe for a Northern blot analysis of the original RNA samples to confirm the differential expression in the actual RNA and to quantify the levels of expression. Northern blot confirmation of mRNA differential display is important to eliminate false positives from further evaluation.

DNA sequencing is the next step in analyzing the cDNA clone. The sequence generally contains the 3' untranslated region of the mRNA and a small portion of the carboxyl terminal of the protein coding region. This incomplete sequence of an expressed mRNA is referred to as a 3' expressed sequence tag (EST) (Okubo et al., 1992). The sequence of the EST is used to search DNA sequence databases to determine if the mRNA has been previously identified and characterized. The novel aspect of 3' ESTs from mRNA differential display is that some information is already known about the expression of the gene. This information will greatly assist in selecting which newly identified genes should receive priority for further characterization in different metabolic processes.

USES OF METALS IN GENE REGULATION

There are two general areas in which metals introduced in the diet could regulate genes of interest to the support of military troops in the field. The first would relate to regulation of chimeric genes introduced through genetic manipulation. The field of molecular medicine has shown that it is possible to target specific genes, introduce them into human subjects, and observe expression (Morrow and Kucherlapati, 1995). This area is clearly at the forefront of molecular biology, but practical applications and resolution of ethical ramifications of these applications are at least decades away.

The regulation of transgenes by zinc is feasible because: metal response elements have been characterized, it is possible to produce multiple MREs in a single promoter, low basal-level expression of MRE-regulated genes usually occurs, there is a potential for a high level of expression, and duration of the elevated expression is directly correlated to the duration of increased zinc intake. The approach envisioned would be similar to that of the technology demonstrated earlier through use of a metal-responsive promoter (metallothionein promoter) linked to the growth hormone genes (Palmiter et al., 1982). Specifically, in mice and farm animals, transgenes were activated by increasing the level of zinc in the diet. The metal binds to the MRE-binding protein, which in turn initiates increased transcription of the growth hormone gene. This technology could be applied to virtually any gene of interest to military or public health situations.

The second area where metals could contribute to applications of interest to the military is that of gene expression associated with stress. It has been demonstrated repeatedly that zinc in high levels provides protection against cellular damage caused by ionizing radiation and various chemical toxins (Willson, 1989). The mechanism of this protection is believed to be through prevention of free radical formation, although this mechanism has yet to be firmly established. Since many genes are activated by zinc, it is likely that a spectrum of zinc-responsive genes are activated during a distinct supplementation period that provides the observed cellular protection. Providing supplemental zinc via the diet at high levels during periods of stress may well be advantageous to allow military troops the ability to better withstand stressful situations. Zinc is a relatively nontoxic metal and could easily be introduced through dietary means that would provide a programmed duration of response.

AUTHORS' CONCLUSIONS AND RECOMMENDATIONS

This brief review has tried to demonstrate how some aspects of metal-regulated gene expression could be put to use in applications related to military activities. Molecular biology has clearly evolved to the point where it is providing tools, such as differential display, that will allow identification of genes that are beneficial to control during stressful situations. It should then be possible through newly evolving techniques to use that information in a way that will allow altering the diet through various combinations of dietary components that activate genes to select specific types of responses. The key task for the immediate future is to identify the genes most likely to be of benefit when regulated by nutritional means. As technology advances, the application of this information will unfold.

REFERENCES

Blanchard, R.K., and R.J. Cousins
  1996   Differential display of intestinal mRNAs regulated by dietary zinc. Proc. Natl. Acad. Sci. USA 93:6863–6868.
Brugnera, E., O. Georgiev, F. Radtke, R. Heuchel, E. Baker, G.R. Sutherland, and W. Schaffner
  1994   Cloning, chromosomal mapping and characterization of the human metal-regulatory transcription factor MTF-1. Nucleic Acids Res. 22:3167–3173.
Cousins, R.J.
  1994   Metal elements and gene expression. Annu. Rev. Nutr. 14:449–469.
  1995   Trace element micronutrients. Pp. 898–901 in Molecular Biology and Biotechnology: A Comprehensive Desk Reference, R.A. Meyers, ed. New York: VCH Publishers.
da Silva, J.J.R., and R.J.P. Williams, eds.
  1991   The Biological Chemistry of the Elements: The Inorganic Chemistry of Life. Oxford: Clarendon Press.
Dawid, I.B., R. Toyama, and M. Taira
  1995   LIM domain proteins. C. R. Acad. Sci. Paris 318:295–306.

Kendall, S.D., and M.J. Christensen
1995　Modified differential display identifies genes in rat liver differentially regulated by selenium [abstract]. FASEB J. 9:A158.

Klug, A., and J.W.R. Schwabe
1995　Zinc fingers. FASEB J. 9:597–604.

Lewin, B.
1994　Genes V. Oxford: Oxford University Press.

Liang, P., L. Averboukh, and A.B. Pardee
1993　Distribution and cloning of eukaryotic mRNAs by means of differential display: Refinements and optimization. Nucleic Acids Res. 21:3269–3275.

Morrow, B.E., and R. Kucherlapati
1995　Molecular genetic medicine. Pp. 556–561 in Molecular Biology and Biotechnology: A Comprehensive Desk Reference, R.A. Meyers, ed. New York: VCH Publishers.

O'Halloran, T.V.
1993　Transition metals in control of gene expression. Science 261:712–725.

Okubo, K., N. Hori, R. Matoba, T. Niiyama, A. Fukushima, Y. Kojima, and K. Matsubara
1992　Large-scale cDNA sequencing for analysis of quantitative and qualitative aspects of gene expression. Nature Genetics 2:173–179.

Orr, S., T.P. Hughes, C.L. Sawyers, R.M. Kato, S.G. Quan, S.P. Williams, O.N. Witte, and L. Hood
1994　Isolation of unknown genes from human bone marrow by differential screening and single-pass cDNA sequence determination. Proc. Natl. Acad. Sci. USA 91:11869–11873.

Palmiter, R.D., R.L. Brinster, R.E. Hammer, M.E. Trumbauer, M.G. Rosenfeld, N.C. Birnberg, and R.M. Evans
1982　Dramatic growth of mice that develop from eggs microinjected with metallothionein-growth hormone fusion genes. Nature 300:611–615.

Rebar, E.J., and C.O. Pabo
1994　Zinc finger phage: Affinity selection of fingers with new DNA-binding specificities. Science 263:671–673.

Schmeichel, K.L., and M.C. Beckerle
1994　The LIM domain is a modular protein-binding interface. Cell 79:211–219.

Stuart, G.W., P.F. Searle, H.Y. Chen, R.L. Brinster, and R.D. Palmiter
1984　A 12-base-pair DNA motif that is repeated several times in metallothionein gene promoters confers metal regulation to a heterologous gene. Proc. Natl. Acad. Sci. USA 81:7318–7322.

Vallee, B.L., J.E. Coleman, and D.S. Auld
1991　Zinc fingers, zinc clusters, and zinc twists in DNA-binding protein domains. Proc. Natl. Acad. Sci. USA 88:999–1003.

Willson, R.L.
1989　Zinc and iron in free radical pathology and cellular control. Pp. 147–172 in Zinc in Human Biology, C.F. Mills, ed. New York: Springer-Verlag.

Wu, H., W-P.Yang, and C.F. Barbas, III
1995　Building zinc fingers by selection: Toward a therapeutic application. Proc. Natl. Acad Sci. USA 92:344–348.

DISCUSSION

HARRIS LIEBERMAN: How widely used is the technique, the differential display of RNA, and how practical is it?

ROBERT COUSINS: It was developed in late 1992. There was a very significant modification in 1993. Since then there have been a number of papers out on it. The first use with intact animals, I think, will be coming out fairly shortly. It is a technique that has some limitations, but nonetheless, it is, in my view, the most powerful screening method that one has available to look at what genes are turned on and turned off in a given physiologic state or a given nutritional state. I think the sequence information that is available in data banks, which this has to be drawn against, is the limiting factor.

G. RICHARD JANSEN: What is the physiological significance of the enhanced expression of metallothionein beyond the requirement level?

ROBERT COUSINS: That is another very active area of investigation, but it appears now that with cells that are transfected with this gene, the cells are protected from various types of radiation damage. Transgenic animals that are now commercially available are being studied. Animals that have overexpression of the gene are being studied to determine what physiologic changes they have in response to having more copies of that gene and more of the protein produced. I think it is a host defense type of mechanism that we are looking at.

WILLIAM BEISEL: This is a fascinating presentation, and it surely brings things up to date. Originally we had discovered the sequestration of zinc, the movement of zinc into the cells during the acute-phase response, and we were always wondering what it meant, why did the body do this? We were thinking years ago that it was probably to get more zinc into enzymes, because it was present in so many enzymes, but these studies of the gene expression certainly . . .

ROBERT COUSINS: You are right. Your work showed that the plasma zinc decreases right after exposure to endotoxin and other things. The plasma zinc goes into the liver and other tissues that produce metallothionein, as it turns out, because, kinetically, you can actually show where the metal goes. That has some function, but whether the function is related to controlling zinc fingers or signaling mechanisms has yet to be looked at.

ROBERT NESHEIM: Orville, I am sure you have some comment, particularly with your recent article in *Nature* discussing the role of selenium in this area.

ORVILLE LEVANDER: There is quite a bit of work going on with selenium right now in differential display as well. What I was wondering about, Bob, is, on your differential display analysis, that was rat intestine and you had a lot of sequences up there, but is anything happening with metallothionein under those conditions? I did not see it on the slides.

ROBERT COUSINS: No. In the one slide I showed where we wanted to prove that the technique was working, we actually used kidney RNA as the source material because in a dietary study, where zinc is provided over a long period of time, the kidney metallothionein RNA is a very nice titrator of intake. So we just wanted to show that the technique under nutritional conditions, feeding rats for two weeks, would show a difference in MRE [metal-responsive element]-regulated genes, so that is why we used the kidney for that purpose.

But in the intestine, where metallothionein also is produced, you should see that response, and we have not as yet picked it up. It is kind of interesting. I do not know what the reason is—we do not select for any given size—it just probably has not come up yet. We have gone through roughly half the combinations that are possible.

EDWARD HIRSCH: What was the time course of the response to the dietary supplement?

ROBERT COUSINS: Very quickly. We see changes within hours.

GABRIEL VIRELLA: Have any of the components of the immune system, for example cytokines or complement, been tested in this system?

ROBERT COUSINS: Yes, again, using a metallothionein system as the prototype, there has been a lot of research done on that.

GABRIEL VIRELLA: I mean in working with cytokines.

ROBERT COUSINS: Oh, working with the cytokines in differential displays and so on? Not to my knowledge, no. I think it is a technology that up until now has been limited primarily to differences in transformed versus nontransformed cells, and looking for what genes are differentially expressed. I do not think the physiologists and immunologists have caught on to it quite yet, but they will, certainly.

JOHN FERNSTROM: I am ignorant in this area. Is zinc something for which there is a regulated storage pool, such that one can think about the responsiveness from dietary changes as needing to be short responses or long responses?

ROBERT COUSINS: Yes. I did not have time to go into that aspect of things. There are at least two pools. One is the vast majority of zinc that is tied up in zinc-finger proteins and in enzymes and so on in cells, which are turning over, of course, at varying rates, and then there is a shorter response, a very small pool, that is yet to be defined. Some of that may well be bound to metallothionein.

There is something in the literature called a rapidly exchanging pool. The nature of that, outside of the fact that it occurs and can be shown kinetically to occur, is not known. But metallothionein could well serve part of that function because it expands and contracts, depending upon the amount of zinc available.

JOHN FERNSTROM: For a known zinc function, how fast does the deficiency become expressed in terms of loss of a particular function?

ROBERT COUSINS: It is believed to occur very quickly. Good examples of that are really hard to come by, but it is a Type II deficiency [tissue levels are maintained], where, as soon as you get to a certain point, things crash in a hurry. You will see reductions in growth and changes in various other things. In the case of zinc you see skin problems and so on. Immune problems occur very quickly.

WILLIAM BEISEL: I was just going to comment on the still very unexplored aspect of the cytokines because the proinflammatory cytokines do turn on this sequestration of zinc. Cytokines are the trigger. Within 15 minutes you see the increase in metallothionein generation, so it is a fantastically rapid response system and needs a lot more exploration.

ROBERT COUSINS: That is why I mentioned that zinc is in some ways an ideal entity if someone wanted to use a technology such as introduction of transgenes into human subjects by various means. You could then regulate those genes very quickly and with somewhat nontoxic conditions.

ROBERT NESHEIM: Thank you very much, Bob. In addition to the discussion of zinc, I learned that there is another MRE to explain.

Emerging Technologies for Nutrition Research, 1997
Pp. 375–387. Washington, D.C.
National Academy Press

17

Metabolic Regulation of Gene Expression

Howard C. Towle[1]

INTRODUCTION

Nutritional factors can influence virtually every aspect of the functioning of the human organism. This influence extends to the realm of gene expression. By influencing gene expression in specific tissues of the organism, nutritional factors help to adapt the organism to changes in the environment. This review will describe the technologies that have emerged for analyzing the effects of nutrition on gene expression, with particular emphasis on the process of gene transcription and its control. Several model systems then will be described in which changes in specific gene expression in response to nutritional factors have been elucidated and efforts to understand the molecular basis of these changes have been made. While this field is still in its infancy, the pace of change suggests that great strides will soon be forthcoming in understanding these important mechanisms and how they may relate to human health and disease.

---

[1] Howard C. Towle, Department of Biochemistry, University of Minnesota Medical School, Minneapolis, MN 55455

Gene expression refers to those processes by which the genetic information stored in the DNA is converted into proteins (including enzymes) within the cell. This is a multistep process that involves gene transcription, mRNA processing (capping, splicing, and polyadenylation), and mRNA transport and translation. Each of these processes in turn involves a complex series of biochemical events. Consequently, control of gene expression can be exerted at many different sites in the cell, and in fact, examples of regulation occurring at each step of this pathway have been elucidated. Such complexity of control is undoubtedly critical to the fine tuning of cellular function within the context of the overall organism. Despite this richness in terms of potential sites of control, it is clear that transcriptional regulation and, more specifically, control of transcriptional initiation provide the most commonly employed site for regulation. Given the importance of transcriptional regulation, much attention has been focused on this process in the past decade and much has been learned. Hence, this chapter will focus primarily on regulation occurring at the level of gene transcription.

TRANSCRIPTION AND ITS REGULATION

Transcription of protein-coding genes in all eucaryotes is performed by the enzyme RNA polymerase II. However, this enzyme lacks the inherent ability to recognize the proper site in DNA for initiation of transcription. Rather, RNA polymerase II functions together with a battery of general "transcription factors" to perform these processes (for review, see Zawel and Reinberg, 1993). To date, six factors essential to the process of promoter selection and initiation have been identified. These factors, together with RNA polymerase II, recognize specific sequences in the DNA helix at the initiation site that are frequently termed the basal promoter site. The most commonly recognized of these signals is the TATA box, a 7 base pair (bp)-conserved sequence occurring approximately 30 bp upstream from (to the 5' end of) the site of initiation in many genes. Other less-conserved signals at the site of initiation also play a role in the site selection. These sequences are recognized by general transcription factors to initiate assembly of the RNA transcription complex.

Although RNA polymerase II in combination with the general transcription factors is competent to recognize and initiate transcription from the basal promoter, the rate of this process is very low. To achieve effective production of mRNA, other transcription factors need to be brought into play. Because these transcription factors only function on a limited set of genes, they are termed specific transcription factors. There are in excess of 100 such factors present in any particular cell. These specific transcription factors function by binding to specific DNA sequences in the vicinity of the basal promoter site. Many times these sites are located immediately upstream of the basal promoter, within 100 to 200 bp of the initiation site. Other times these factors can function by binding at sites that can be several thousand base pairs removed from the initiation site in regions known as enhancers. These sites serve to localize the specific transcription factors in proximity to the basal transcriptional machinery. The factors in turn influence the rate of initiation, presumably by making protein-protein contacts with RNA polymerase II or its associated factors (Choy and Green, 1993). These contacts are thought to alter the stability or kinetics of initiation-complex formation to stimulate transcription. Thus, the rate of initiation from any specific promoter in any particular cell is determined in large part by the qualitative and quantitative nature of the binding sites for specific transcription factors present on the gene and the concentration and activity of the corresponding transcription factors present in the cell. Regulation can occur by controlling the activity of these specific transcription factors. Thus, understanding the control of transcriptional initiation requires the elucidation of the regulatory sequences present for binding specific transcription factors and the elucidation of the nature of the factors that bind to these sites. Technologies for unraveling these components have developed in the past decade and are essential tools in the arsenal of the molecular biologist.

TECHNOLOGIES FOR STUDYING GENE TRANSCRIPTION

The first issue that generally needs to be tackled when analyzing the control of specific gene transcription is the localization of DNA regulatory sequences. These sequences represent the binding sites for specific transcription factors and can be used as tools to help identify these factors. The fundamental assay that has been developed for addressing this question is the transfection assay. To perform a transfection assay, there are several prerequisites. First, one needs a cultured cell that is capable of responding to the nutrient or metabolite of interest. Second, one needs cloned DNA sequences from a gene that is transcriptionally regulated in response to the effector. Third, one needs a means of introducing the cloned DNA into the cultured cell. Finally, one needs an assay to assess promoter activity. This latter need is most often fulfilled by linking the gene of interest to a "reporter gene," which contains the coding sequences for an easily assayed enzyme activity. The most commonly employed reporter genes are chloramphenicol acetyl transferase, β-galactosidase, and luciferase. In the transfection assay, DNA sequences from the gene of interest containing the potential regulatory regions and basal promoter, as well as a reporter gene, are introduced into a cultured cell. These sequences are then transcribed by the endogenous machinery of the cell. By culturing the transfected cell in the presence of varying concentrations of a specific nutrient or metabolite, the presence of regulatory sequences can be detected by assessing changes in reporter gene activity. In combination with techniques that allow specific mutagenesis of the cloned DNA, the location of the regulatory sequences can be pinpointed. This is generally accomplished first by using deletion mutations to define the boundaries of the region of interest and then by making finer point mutations to locate the critical bases for control.

Once the regulatory sequences of a particular gene have been identified, they can be used to search for a particular transcription factor that binds to this site. A variety of assays are available for examining specific protein-DNA interactions, but of these the electrophoretic mobility shift ("band shift") assay has proven the most useful (Fried and Crothers, 1981). In this assay, a short DNA oligonucleotide is radiolabeled with ^{32}P. This radiolabeled oligonucleotide is mixed with nuclear extracts from the cell or tissue of interest in the presence of excess, unlabeled DNA. The latter serves to react with all nonsequence-specific binding proteins, so that only proteins with high affinity will bind to the radiolabeled probe. The presence of a bound protein is then detected by electrophoresis in a nondenaturing polyacrylamide gel. Under these conditions, the migration of the radiolabeled oligonucleotide will be retarded if bound to a specific protein. In this manner, the presence of a specific transcription factor can often be detected even when it is present in low abundance and purity.

Purification of specific transcription factors can be a technical challenge, given the small quantities of material often present and the very low relative abundance of these proteins. Great strides have been made in this process due to the development of DNA-affinity purification technology (Kadonaga and Tjian, 1986). In this case, a specific oligonucleotide containing the binding site for the transcription factor of interest is coupled to an inert support such as cellulose. Nuclear extracts are incubated with the DNA affinity columns. Again, excess nonspecific DNA is generally added to compete for nonspecific binding of other nuclear proteins with lower affinity. After binding, the transcription factor of interest is eluted by increasing ionic strength. DNA affinity can lead to purifications on the orders of several thousand-fold in a single pass and may make it feasible to recover sufficient quantities of specific transcription factors for biochemical analysis, such as protein sequencing. Alternatively, the genes encoding specific transcription factors can be directly cloned by screening cDNA expression libraries with radiolabeled probes containing the relevant binding site (Singh et al., 1988).

REGULATION OF GENE EXPRESSION BY CHOLESTEROL

All cells require cholesterol for membrane biosynthesis. Cholesterol can be derived from the diet or synthesized by cells. In order to achieve a balance in their cholesterol needs, cells have developed mechanisms to control these two sources (for review see Goldstein and Brown, 1990). Cholesterol uptake is mediated by the low-density lipoprotein receptor (LDL receptor). When cholesterol levels are low, the production of this receptor is induced to provide for more uptake, and when cholesterol levels are high, receptor production is repressed. The rate-limiting enzymes for cholesterol biosynthesis in the cells are HMG-CoA synthase and HMG-CoA reductase. These enzymes are regulated in terms of both their enzymatic activity and production. Cholesterol limitation leads to induction of the synthesis of these two enzymes, while excess cholesterol leads to repression. In this manner, the cell strives to ensure that adequate supplies of cholesterol are available for membrane biosynthesis and that excess levels that can lead to deleterious cell effects do not accumulate.

Efforts to understand the transcriptional regulation of the genes encoding LDL receptor, HMG-CoA synthase, and HMG-CoA reductase were conducted in the laboratories of Goldstein and Brown (1990). First, using transfection assays, the critical DNA regulatory sequences necessary for control by cholesterol were mapped. The 5'-flanking regions of each of these genes were linked to reporter genes and introduced into Chinese hamster ovary fibroblast cells. Cells were maintained in the absence of cholesterol or in the presence of exogenous cholesterol. After 48 hours, cells maintained in the absence of cholesterol were found to have markedly higher levels of reporter gene activity than cells maintained in the presence of cholesterol. This result implied that the regulatory sequences were present in the cloned 5'-flanking regions of each gene. By mutational analysis, the regulatory sequences of each gene were mapped and compared. A specific DNA motif with the sequence (5')CACCCCAC was found to be present in the regulatory sequences of each of the cholesterol metabolizing genes. Goldstein and Brown (1990) proposed that this motif, which they designated the SRE-1 for sterol response element, served as the binding site for a specific transcription factor involved in the coordinate control of these three genes. This factor presumably would be activated under conditions of low cholesterol to stimulate transcription of the corresponding genes.

To further analyze this system, the specific transcription factor recognizing the SRE-1 from the LDL receptor gene was purified to homogeneity (Wang et al., 1993). This purification took advantage of DNA affinity chromatography using the SRE-1 containing oligonucleotide. The purified factor was designated SREBP-1 for SRE-binding protein. A highly homologous gene, designated SREBP-2, was subsequently identified (Hua et al., 1993). Several properties suggest that these genes are critical for mediating the cholesterol regulatory pathway. First, binding of SREBP to SRE-1 oligonucleotides containing mutations of the binding site correlated with functional activity of the mutant binding sites (Briggs et al., 1993). Mutations that interfered with activity in the transfection assay blocked SREBP-1 binding *in vitro*, whereas mutations that did not interfere with activity did not block binding. Second, introducing a plasmid into a cultured cell, which led to overexpression of SREBP, led to increased promoter activity from cotransfected DNA containing the SRE-1 element (Sato et al., 1994). Third, a sterol-resistant mutant cell line was found to have a defect in the gene encoding SREBP-2 (Yang et al., 1994).

Identification of the specific transcription factor and its DNA binding site led to efforts to understand how the activity of this factor is regulated by cellular cholesterol levels (Wang et al., 1994). Cloning of the gene for SREBP-1 revealed that it encoded a protein of 125 kilodaltons (kDa), significantly larger than the 68 kDa SREBP-1 isolated by DNA affinity chromatography. Using specific antibodies to the SREBP-1, the 125-kDa form was found to be localized in the endoplasmic reticulum of the cell as an integral membrane-bound protein. The 68-kDa nuclear form represented the amino (N)-terminal segment of this larger precursor form. Control by cholesterol involved the cleavage of the 68-kDa N-terminal fragment from its endoplasmic reticulum precursor and subsequent nuclear localization of the active fragment. While it is unclear how cholesterol regulates this process, it is tempting to speculate that cholesterol as a normal membrane substituent may influence the properties of the protease involved in cleavage of the SREBP-precursor. In this manner, the levels of intracellular cholesterol can be directly linked to formation of the transcription factor involved in controlling intracellular cholesterol levels.

Many questions remain to be answered but are now experimentally tractable given the progress in this area. Is cholesterol itself a direct mediator of the control pathway, or does it need to be metabolized to an active metabolite? In cells, the oxysterol 25-hydroxycholesterol is more potent than cholesterol, suggesting that a metabolite of cholesterol may be the mediator. What is the nature of the protease involved in cleavage of the SREBP-1 precursor, and how is its activity regulated? Are other genes that are regulated by cholesterol controlled through the same pathway? Preliminary evidence indicates that the answer to this last question may be "no" and that other regulatory pathways may be important (Osborne, 1991; Spear et al., 1994). It also is known that expression of the genes involved in cholesterol metabolism may be regulated at steps other than transcription, and these pathways are largely unexplored. Clearly, there is much to learn, but given the progress of the past few years, the prognosis for answering these questions is excellent.

REGULATION OF HEPATIC GENE EXPRESSION BY CARBOHYDRATE

A second example of gene transcription that is regulated in response to nutritional factors involves the liver and enzymes involved in triglyceride formation. When mammals are fed a diet high in simple carbohydrates and low in fats, a significant portion of the excess carbohydrate is taken up by the liver and converted to triglycerides. Feeding of such a diet induces a response in the liver that involves both rapid changes in the enzymatic activity of the key rate-limiting enzymes in this pathway and a longer-term induction of the cellular concentration of these enzymes (for review, see Hillgartner et al., 1995). The latter is presumably an adaptive response of the organism and is the focus of this discussion. Enzymes that have been shown to be induced by carbohydrate feeding include enzymes of glycolysis, such as pyruvate kinase; enzymes of fatty acid synthesis, such as acetyl CoA carboxylase and malic enzyme; and enzymes of triglyceride formation, such as glycerol-3-phosphate acyltransferase. In all cases, the induction in enzyme production is due to increased mRNA levels. In several cases, but not all, transcription represents the key step in this regulation (Hillgartner et al., 1995).

The actual intracellular pathway leading to increased transcription in response to carbohydrate feeding is poorly understood. Feeding of a high-carbohydrate diet causes increased glucose metabolism in the liver, as well as increased insulin secretion and decreased glucagon secretion. All of these factors play a role in the induction. Using cultured primary hepatocytes as a model system, an important role of carbohydrate metabolism has been implicated. Comparing hepatocytes cultured in low (5.5 mM) or high (27.5 mM) concentrations of glucose, most of the enzymes that are induced in whole animals fed a high-carbohydrate diet also are induced in the hepatocytes cultured in the presence of high concentrations of glucose. This occurs in the presence of a constant concentration of insulin. Other carbohydrates that can feed into the glycolytic pathway at or above the level of pyruvate also are able to induce enzyme production (Mariash and Oppenheimer, 1983). This has led to the hypothesis that increased carbohydrate metabolism is responsible for initiating an intracellular signaling pathway that coordinately regulates this set of genes. The role of insulin appears to be to facilitate effective carbohydrate metabolism in the cell. In particular, the glucokinase step of glucose metabolism is highly insulin-sensitive in the hepatocyte (Lefrancois-Martinez et al., 1994).

To explore this signaling pathway, Towle and coworkers have attempted first to elucidate the DNA regulatory sequences and specific transcription factors responsible for transcriptional regulation. Two genes have been chosen to compare for this purpose: the liver-type pyruvate kinase (PK) and S_{14} genes. The latter encodes a polypeptide of unknown physiological function that is expressed in the liver, adipose tissue, and lactating mammary gland, all sites of active fatty acid metabolism (Oppenheimer et al., 1987). S_{14} mRNA is induced rapidly in the rat ($\leq$ 30 minutes) after feeding a high-carbohydrate meal, and this response is due to changes in gene transcription (Jump et al., 1990). By comparing the induction of the PK and S_{14} genes, the scientists in this laboratory hoped to identify common components that might be involved in coordinate regulation of this family.

Using transfection assays in primary hepatocytes, it was shown that the 5'-flanking region of either the PK or S_{14} genes were capable of supporting increased promoter activity in cells maintained in high glucose compared to cells in low glucose (Jacoby et al., 1989; Thompson and Towle, 1991). The regulatory sequences responsible for this effect were mapped by mutagenesis: for the S_{14} gene, critical sequences were found between −1457 and −1422 upstream from the promoter site (Shih and Towle, 1992, 1994). For the PK gene, the critical regulatory sequences mapped to a region between −172 and −144 (Bergot et al., 1992; Liu et al., 1993). Comparing the two regulatory sequences to each other revealed some significant similarities. In both cases, the binding motif (5')CACGTG is found within the regulatory site in two copies. In both cases, the spacing between the two motifs is 5 bp, and this spacing is critical to control by carbohydrate (Shih et al., 1995). The CACGTG motif is recognized as the core binding site for a family of transcription factors known as the *c-myc* family. All members of this family possess a similar DNA binding motif composed of a basic region that contacts the DNA and adjacent helix-loop-helix and leucine zippers motifs involved in dimerization (Kadesch, 1993). Based on this information, it was hypothesized that a member of the *c-myc* family expressed in liver binds to each of two similar sites oriented on the same side of the DNA helix. These proteins may interact with each other directly or form a contact site for a third component. These factors serve as the end of the signaling cascade that is activated by increased carbohydrate metabolism in the rat. The identity of the factor binding to the regulatory sequences of these two genes is currently unknown and is the target of future investigation.

METABOLITES AS DIRECT EFFECTORS OF TRANSCRIPTION FACTORS

Recent work has established a direct pathway by which nutrients and metabolites can influence gene transcription. This work comes from studies of a large family of genes known as the steroid receptor family. This family includes receptors for a wide variety of hormones that directly enter the cell to elicit their biological activity: steroid hormones, thyroid hormones, retinoic acids, and vitamin D_3. In this family, the receptor itself serves as a transcription factor for which the activity is regulated by binding of its ligand (for review see Evans, 1988).

During the cloning of the steroid receptors, a large group of related gene products of unknown physiological function were discovered. These gene products contained sequence homology with the steroid receptors, particularly in the DNA-binding domain, and hence were postulated to function as transcription factors as well. However, no ligand was known for activating these factors. This led to their designation as "orphan receptors" (O'Malley and Conneely, 1992). The hypothesis was proposed that these family members would be activated by yet unidentified ligands. Recently, activators have been found for several of the orphan receptors, and the nature of these activators suggests that intracellular nutrients or metabolites may be the natural ligands.

The peroxisome proliferator-activated receptors (PPARs) represent the best characterization of the orphan receptors. These receptors were first shown to be activated in response to a diverse group of xenobiotic substances known to induce a massive accumulation of peroxisomes in rodent hepatocytes (Issemann and Green, 1990). In addition to peroxisome proliferation, these agents also induce enzymes of the peroxisomal and microsomal fatty acid oxidation systems. This induction has been shown to be due to direct interaction of the PPARs with regulatory sequences in the genes encoding these enzymes, such as acyl-CoA oxidase (Dreyer et al., 1992; Tugwood et al., 1992). Although peroxisome proliferators were first shown to be activators of PPARs, the question arose as to what the natural ligands for these receptors might be. Recent work has shown that natural fatty acids activate PPARs (Keller et al., 1993). This finding is consistent with observations that high dietary fat intake induces the peroxisomal β-oxidation system. A preference for polyunsaturated fatty acids over monounsaturated or saturated fatty acids was found. With polyunsaturated fatty acids, activation was observed with concentrations of 50 μM, which is within the range found in blood. To date, the mechanism by which fatty acids activate PPARs is unknown. No direct binding of fatty acids to the PPARs has been demonstrated. It is reasonable to speculate that a product formed by metabolism of fatty acids may be the actual ligand for these receptors. It also is conceivable that fatty acids could act by release of an unknown second messenger. PPARs represent the first group of mammalian transcription factors that are activated by nutrients.

A second group of orphan receptors from the steroid receptor family that appears to be activated in response to a nutrient has been recently identified. In this case, the orphan receptor was found by pharmacologic screening to be activated by farnesol and certain of its metabolites (Forman et al., 1995). Again, activation occurred within the micromolar range for the most active agents, which is thought to be physiological for these compounds. Similar to the PPARs, direct binding of farnesol to the receptor has not been demonstrated, which suggests that a farnesoid-induced metabolite may serve as an authentic ligand for the receptor. The farnesol derivative, farnesyl pyrophosphate, is a key metabolic intermediate as the last common precursor in the mevalonate pathway. This pathway leads to formation of cholesterol, bile acids, dolichol, ubiquinone, steroid and retinoic hormones, and farnesylated proteins. Thus, farnesol stands at a critical step in regulating these biosynthetic pathways, and its potential role as a mediator of gene transcription is intriguing. To date, no target genes for the farnesol receptor have been identified, likely due to its recent discovery.

AUTHOR'S CONCLUSIONS AND RECOMMENDATIONS

The discovery of nutrients as regulators of gene expression in mammals is clearly a rapidly emerging field. Although such regulation was predicted over 20 years ago (Tomkins, 1975), the technology to explore this important role has developed only in the more recent past. Using these techniques, the principal components in the regulatory systems—the DNA regulatory sites and specific transcription factors—are beginning to be identified. Work to explore the mechanisms by which these components function to control gene expression will largely await identification of these key components. Clearly, this work is at a basic stage at present, and its applicability to more physiological questions of health and disease must await further advances in knowledge.

The impact of nutrients on gene transcription is likely to be imparted not in terms of short-term (seconds to minutes) control, but rather in longer-term (hours to days) adaptive responses. By changing the concentration of key enzymes and proteins that are involved in cellular processes such as metabolism, these effects will presumably allow the organism to operate more efficiently in the face of changing nutritional status. The impact of such changes is difficult to measure, as they occur within the context of changes occurring at many levels in the body. However, the conservation of these mechanisms across many species lines argues for a significant role. There is much to learn in this area in the future. Continued research efforts along these lines will help to address many of these unresolved questions.

REFERENCES

Bergot, M-O., M-J.M. Diaz-Guerra, N. Puzenat, M. Raymondjean, and A. Kahn
  1992 Cis-regulation of the L-type pyruvate kinase gene promoter by glucose, insulin and cyclic AMP. Nucleic Acids Res. 20:1871–1877.
Briggs, M.R., C. Yokoyama, X. Wang, M.S. Brown, and J.L. Goldstein
  1993 Nuclear protein that binds sterol regulatory element of low-density lipoprotein receptor promoter. I. Identification of the protein and delineation of its target nucleotide sequence. J. Biol. Chem. 268:14490–14496.
Choy, B., and M.R. Green
  1993 Eukaryotic activators function during multiple steps of preinitiation complex assembly. Nature 366:531–536.
Dreyer, C., G. Krey, H. Keller, F. Givel, G. Helftenbein, and W. Wahli
  1992 Control of the peroxisomal β-oxidation pathway by a novel family of nuclear hormone receptors. Cell 68:879–887.
Evans, R.M.
  1988 The steroid and thyroid hormone receptor superfamily. Science 240:889–895.
Forman, B.M., E. Goode, J. Chen, A.E. Oro, D.J. Bradley, T. Perlmann, D.J. Noonan, and L.T. Burka
  1995 Identification of a nuclear receptor that is activated by farnesol metabolites. Cell 81:687–693.
Fried, M., and D.M. Crothers
  1981 Equilibria and kinetics of lac repressor-operator interactions by polyacrylamide gel electrophoresis. Nucleic Acids Res. 9:6505–6525.
Goldstein, J.L., and M.S. Brown
  1990 Regulation of the mevalonate pathway. Nature 343:425–430.
Hillgartner, F.B., L.M. Salati, and A.G. Goodridge
  1995 Physiological and molecular mechanisms involved in nutritional regulation of fatty acid synthesis. Physiol. Rev. 75:47–76.
Hua, X., C. Yokoyama, J. Wu, M.R. Briggs, M.S. Brown, J.L. Goldstein, and X. Wang
  1993 SREBP-2, a second basic-helix-loop-helix-leucine zipper protein that stimulates transcription by binding to a sterol regulatory element. Proc. Natl. Acad. Sci. USA 90:11603–11607.
Issemann, I., and S. Green
  1990 Activation of a member of the steroid hormone receptor superfamily by peroxisome proliferators. Nature 347: 645–650.
Jacoby, D.B., N.D. Zilz, and H.C. Towle
  1989 Sequences within the 5'-flanking region of the S_{14} gene confer responsiveness to glucose in primary hepatocytes. J. Biol. Chem. 264:17623–17626.
Jump, D.B., A. Bell, and V. Santiago
  1990 Thyroid hormone and dietary carbohydrate interact to regulate rat liver S_{14} gene transcription and chromatin structure. J. Biol. Chem. 265:3474–3478.

Kadesch, T.
  1993 Consequences of heteromeric interactions among helix-loop-helix proteins. Cell Growth Differ. 4:49–55.
Kadonaga, J.T., and R. Tjian
  1986 Affinity purification of sequence-specific DNA binding proteins. Proc. Natl. Acad. Sci. U.S.A. 83:5889–5893.
Keller, H., C. Dreyer, J. Medin, A. Mahfoudi, K. Ozato, and W. Wahli
  1993 Fatty acids and retinoids control lipid metabolism through activation of peroxisome proliferator-activated receptor-retinoid X receptor heterodimers. Proc. Natl. Acad. Sci. USA 90:2160–2164.
Lefrancois-Martinez, A-M., M-J.M. Diaz-Guerra, V. Vallet, A. Kahn, and B. Antoine
  1994 Glucose-dependent regulation of the L-type kinase gene in a hepatoma cell line is independent of insulin and cyclic AMP. FASEB J. 8:89–96.
Liu, Z., K.S. Thompson, and H.C. Towle
  1993 Carbohydrate regulation of the rat L-type pyruvate kinase gene requires two nuclear factors: LF-A1 and a member of the c-myc family. J. Biol. Chem. 268:12787–12795.
Mariash, C.N., and J.H. Oppenheimer
  1983 Stimulation of malic enzyme formation in hepatocyte culture by metabolites: Evidence favoring a nonglycolytic metabolite as the proximate induction signal. Metabolism 33:545–552.
O'Malley, B.W., and O.M. Conneely
  1992 Orphan receptors: In search of a unifying hypothesis for activation. Mol. Endocrinol. 6:1359–1361.
Oppenheimer, J.H., H.L. Schwartz, C.N. Mariash, W.B. Kinlaw, N.C. Wong, and H.C. Freake
  1987 Advances in our understanding of thyroid hormone action at the cellular level. Endocr. Rev. 8:288–308.
Osborne, T.F.
  1991 Single nucleotide resolution of sterol regulatory region in promoter for 3-hydroxy-3-methylglutaryl Coenzyme A reductase. J. Biol. Chem. 266:13947–13951.
Sato, R., J. Yang, X. Wang, M.J. Evans, Y.K. Ho, J.L. Goldstein, and M.S. Brown
  1994 Assignment of the membrane attachment, DNA binding, and transcriptional activation domains of sterol regulatory element-binding protein-1 (SREBP-1). J. Biol. Chem. 269:17267–17273.
Shih, H-M., and H.C. Towle
  1992 Definition of the carbohydrate response element of the rat S_{14} gene. J. Biol. Chem. 267:13222–13228.
  1994 Definition of the carbohydrate response element of the rat S_{14} gene. J. Biol. Chem. 269(12):9380–9387.
Shih, H-M., Z. Liu, and H.C. Towle
  1995 Two CACGTG motifs with proper spacing dictate the carbohydrate regulation of hepatic gene transcription. J. Biol. Chem. 270:21991–21997.
Singh, H., J.H. LeBowitz, A.S. Baldwin, Jr., and P.A. Sharp
  1988 Molecular cloning of an enhancer binding protein: Isolation by screening of an expression library with a recognition site DNA. Cell 52:415–423.
Spear, D.H., J. Ericsson, S.M. Jackson, and P.A. Edwards
  1994 Identification of a 6-base pair element involved in the sterol-mediated transcriptional regulation of farnesyl diphosphate synthase. J. Biol. Chem. 269:25212–25218.
Thompson, K.S., and H.C. Towle
  1991 Localization of the carbohydrate response element of the rat L-type pyruvate kinase gene. J. Biol. Chem. 266:8679–8682.

Tomkins, G.M.
  1975   The metabolic code. Science 189:760–763.
Tugwood, J., I. Issemann, R.G. Anderson, K.R. Bundell, W.L. McPheat, and S. Green
  1992   The mouse peroxisome proliferater activated receptor recognizes a response ele-
         ment in the 5' flanking sequence of the rat acyl CoA oxidase gene. EMBO J
         11:433–439.
Wang, X., M.R. Briggs, X. Hua, C. Yokoyama, J.L. Goldstein, and M.S. Brown
  1993   Nuclear protein that binds sterol regulatory element of low density lipoprotein
         receptor promoter. II. Purification and characterization. J. Biol. Chem. 268:14497–
         14504.
Wang, X., R. Sato, M.S. Brown, X. Hua, and J.L. Goldstein
  1994   SREBP-1, a membrane-bound transcription factor released by sterol-regulated
         proteolysis. Cell 77:53–62.
Yang, J., R. Sato, J.L. Goldstein, and M.S. Brown
  1994   Sterol-resistant transcription in CHO cells caused by gene rearrangement that trun-
         cates SREBP-2. Genes Dev. 8:1910–1919.
Zawel, L., and D. Reinberg
  1993   Initiation of transcription by RNA polymerase II: A multistep process. Prog.
         Nucleic Acids Res. Mol. Biol. 44:67–108.

DISCUSSION

GUY MILLER: When the primary cells of the liver and all the zone one [periportal] hepatocytes essentially convert to zone three [perivenous] metabolism in the face of a relatively hypoxic environment, they revert from a profoundly oxidative state to a highly glycolytic state, and they are dynamically transformed as this proceeds. Clearly, that influences carbohydrate utilization as a model for what is happening *in vivo*. Do you have any suggestions for how we would start approaching that from the gene therapy or gene manipulation side of substrate utilization?

HOWARD TOWLE: That is a tough one. You are absolutely right that what we are looking at are hepatocytes, which are fairly homogeneous in their response, and, of course, in the liver there is significant zonation in terms of function, so that perivenous hepatocytes are more active in carbohydrate metabolism and lipogenesis. I really do not know how we would handle that in terms of gene therapy.

DENNIS BIER: Is this inverse effect that you mention between the induction of lipogenic enzymes by carbohydrate and the repression of these enzymes by polyunsaturated fatty acid limited to polyunsaturated fatty acids because acetyl-CoA is an allosteric regulator of pyruvate kinase and that is what happens when you take away glucose?

HOWARD TOWLE: Yes, in fact, it is quite specific for polyunsaturated fatty acids, so that saturated or monosaturated fatty acids do not show that effect at all.

DENNIS BIER: What about acetate or acetyl-CoA?

HOWARD TOWLE: Acetate does not have an effect on the hepatocytes in terms of this response, and I presume that acetate would be converted to acetyl-CoA.

ALLISON YATES: Do you see a difference between omega-3 and omega-6 fatty acids?

HOWARD TOWLE: In terms of the repression of the lipogenic enzyme expression by fatty acids? If I remember correctly, both are capable of repressing, and I am not aware of any studies showing differential actions of one group compared to another.

ROBERT NESHEIM: Thank you very much, Howard. Very interesting techniques here and it is going to be interesting to see what happens over the years. Probably, if I am around 40 years from now, I will learn a new language.

Emerging Technologies for Nutrition Research, 1997
Pp. 389–400. Washington, D.C.
National Academy Press

18

Use of Isolated-Cell and Metabolic Techniques Applied to Vitamin Transport and Disposition

Donald B. McCormick[1]

INTRODUCTION

Performance capability centrally involves the ability to acquire and utilize nutrients at the cellular level and to make such metabolic adjustments as are needed to sustain competent functioning for a specified period of time. There are well-documented changes in needs for calories, water, and replenishable electrolytes relating to alterations in exercise and in ambient temperature. The metabolic conversion of macronutrients to supply the cell's energy needs depends upon micronutrients, which are essential in the enzymatic steps involved. Yet knowledge on shifts in micronutrient intake that may be needed to optimize cellular function with changing performance is largely missing. It is known, for example, that greater utilization of carbohydrate increases the demand for thiamin, but the span of time and level of adjustment of the latter to maximize efficiency of energy utilization from the former is not fully

[1] Donald B. McCormick, Department of Biochemistry, School of Medicine, Emory University, Atlanta, GA 30322-3050

quantitated. Even less information is available on the levels of other water-soluble vitamins that may be desirable for performance enhancement. Certainly essential roles for vitamin B_6 in protein utilization and for riboflavin in general oxidative metabolism can be appreciated on the basis of known biochemical reactions, but the amounts of these and other vitamins that optimize performance with no compromise of long-term health in humans are not certain.

The gaps in information on the impact of stress or exertion on the ultimate disposition of natural derivatives of vitamins are especially great. There are few if any data on the efficiency of digestion of coenzymes within the tissues consumed as food in the face of shifting physical demands. Nothing is known about such effects on the release and recovery of vitamins from glycosides, esters, and peptides, which could account for a significant fraction of potential vitaminic material in many foods. The relationship of performance capability to micronutrient bioavailability has yet to be adequately researched.

What is known is that the metabolic pathways utilized in the molecular dissolution of nutrient compounds by *E. coli* and the human are generally similar, and among mammals even semiquantitative comparisons are usually valid. This is fortunate since it allows one to answer some questions at the cellular level with material obtained from animals (e.g., rats) that cannot ethically be accessed from humans. Cells that are freshly isolated after appropriate collagenase perfusion *in situ* of organs such as liver or kidney maintain viability for sufficient time in modified, oxygenated buffer to permit meaningful measurements of nutrient uptake and utilization. This technique allows separation of the cellular component in the overall fate of a nutrient that must undergo systemic absorption, circulatory transport, and organ dissemination. Moreover, there is no risk of cell transformation, which often occurs with the repeated transfers necessary in cell tissue culture techniques.

Considerable information has been gained regarding the mechanisms by which liver and kidney cells import and subsequently assimilate water-soluble vitamins such as riboflavin, B_6, biotin, and C (Bowman et al., 1989; McCormick and Zhang, 1993; Rose et al., 1986). Coupled with the extensive work of this laboratory on the metabolism of these vitamins and the cofactor lipoic acid (Chastain and McCormick, 1991; McCormick, 1975, 1979, 1989; McCormick and Wright, 1970), these investigators were poised to compare the means by which cells take in and differentially utilize certain natural derivatives. To illustrate this, isolated-cell and metabolic techniques recently have been used to augment understanding of the bioavailability of the glucosides of pyridoxine (Zhang et al., 1993) and of riboflavin (Joseph and McCormick, 1995).

RESULTS WITH VITAMIN GLUCOSIDES

The occurrence of natural glucosides of both vitamins B_2 (riboflavin) and B_6 has been known for some time, but their roles were less clear. The extent to which these glucosides represent forms used for storage, transport, and release of the vitamins only now is becoming evident.

Pyridoxine-5'-β-D-Glucoside

The isolation of a "bound" form of B_6 from rice bran led to its identification as 5'-O-(β-D-glucopyranosyl)pyridoxine (Yasumoto et al., 1977). The structure of this compound is shown in Figure 18-1. Only plant foods have been found to contain this compound, which can account for up to half of the total B_6 (Leklem, 1994). It may represent a storage form for higher plants, but it clearly is a less bioavailable form of B_6 for mammals. Rats absorb but poorly metabolize and largely excrete pyridoxine β-glucoside in urine (Ink et al., 1986; Trumbo and Gregory, 1988). There is apparently an inverse correlation between the percentage of glucosylated B_6 in selected foods and the bioavailability of this vitamin in humans (Kabir et al., 1983).

Since pyridoxine β-glucoside actually retards the utilization of pyridoxine in rats (Gilbert and Gregory, 1992), the possibility that the β-glucoside could inhibit uptake of pyridoxine by freshly isolated rat hepatocytes was examined first (Zhang et al., 1993). As shown by the data in Figure 18-2, the unlabeled glucoside competitively inhibits uptake of [^{3}H]pyridoxine presented to the cells. The inhibitory constant (K_i) obtained from the plot was approximately 1.4 µM. Pyridoxine β-glucoside does not inhibit uptake of glucose, however.

The β-glucoside of pyridoxine not only competes for the same plasma membrane transporter that has been shown to be relatively specific for the B_6 moiety in both liver (Kozik and McCormick, 1984) and proximal tubular cells of the kidney (Bowman and McCormick, 1989), but can be taken up in a manner reflecting saturation kinetics, as illustrated in Figure 18-3. An apparent transport constant (K_t = 13.8 µM) and a maximal velocity V_{max} = 82 pmol/10^6 cells/min can be compared to values reported earlier for pyridoxine entry into hepatocytes, with K_t = 6.3 µM and V_{max} = 28 pmol/10^6 cells/min (Kozik and McCormick, 1984; Zhang and McCormick, 1992).

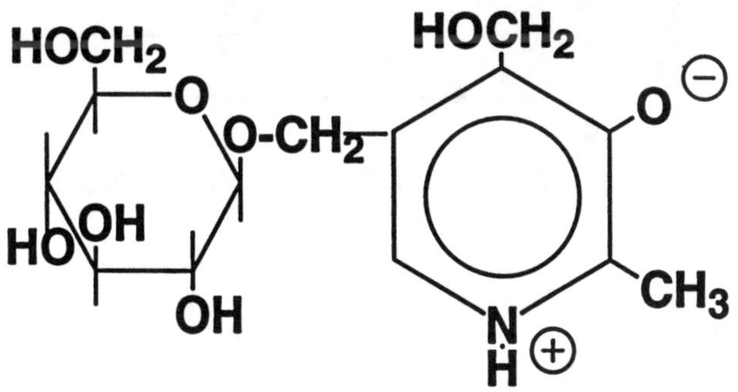

FIGURE 18-1 Structure of pyridoxine-5'-β-D-glucoside.

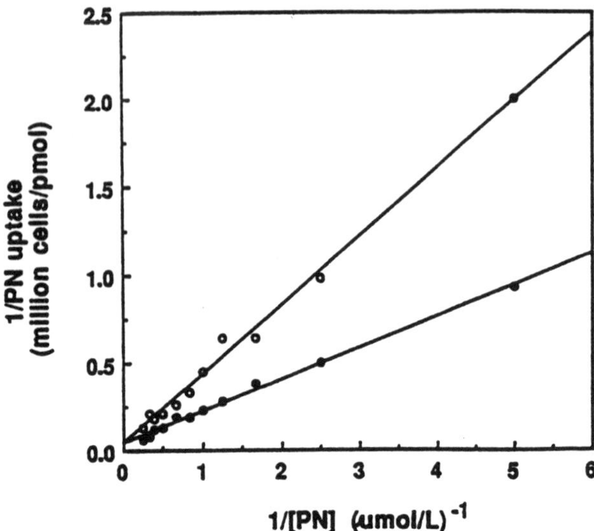

FIGURE 18-2 Double-reciprocal plots of the initial uptake rate of [³H]pyridoxine (PN) versus substrate concentration in the absence (•) and presence (o) of 2.0 μM unlabeled β-D-glucoside. SOURCE: Zhang et al. (1993) © *J. Nutr.* (123:85–89), American Society for Nutritional Sciences.

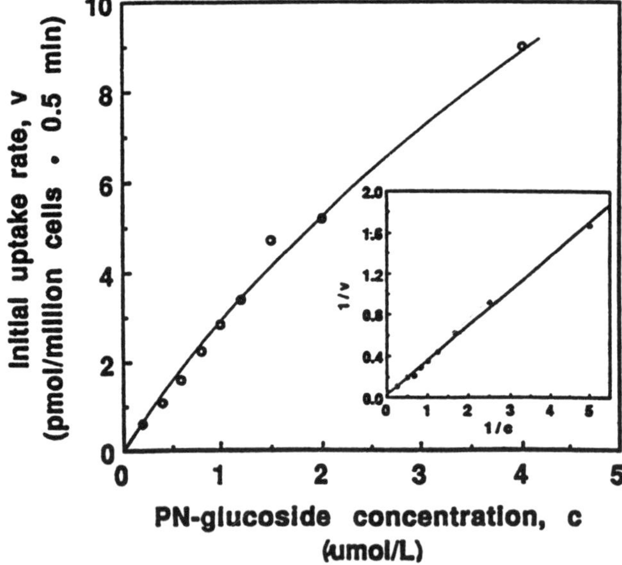

FIGURE 18-3 Dependence of initial rate of [³H]pyridoxine-5'-β-D-glucoside (PN-glucoside) uptake (0.5 minutes) on concentration. The insert presents a double-reciprocal transformation of the same curve with the straight line obtained by regression analysis. SOURCE: Zhang et al. (1993) © *J. Nutr.* (123:85–89), American Society for Nutritional Sciences..

The effect of incubation time on the transport of pyridoxine and its β-glucoside into liver cells is shown in Figure 18-4. Though the amount of transported pyridoxine increased significantly throughout the hour during which uptake was measured, the β-glucoside reached an earlier limit near 20 percent that of the free vitamin. This result is very similar to the transport of pyridoxine and its α-glucoside into rabbit erythrocytes reported by others (Kawai et al., 1972).

The intracellular distribution of transported pyridoxine β-glucoside was examined by incubating cells with the radioactive compound, then extracting and analyzing the cellular contents by chromatography. Pyridoxal 5'-phosphate (PLP) is the metabolite that has the greatest coenzyme function, ultimately arising after release of pyridoxine by a broad-specificity β-glucosidase (Trumbo et al., 1990), which must act to unfetter the 5'-hydroxymethyl group that becomes phosphorylated prior to oxidation of the 4'-hydroxymethyl function. As shown by the results in Table 18-1, the amount of PLP formed from the cellular metabolism of the β-glucoside was much less (only 0.2%) than that formed from pyridoxine. The formation of PLP also is much lower from the β-glucoside than from free vitamin in the presence of homogenate or supernatant solution enriched with the cytosolic kinase and oxidase that convert free vitamin B_6 to PLP. Hence, the rate-limiting step in metabolic utilization of pyridoxine β-glucoside is the hydrolytic release of the vitamin.

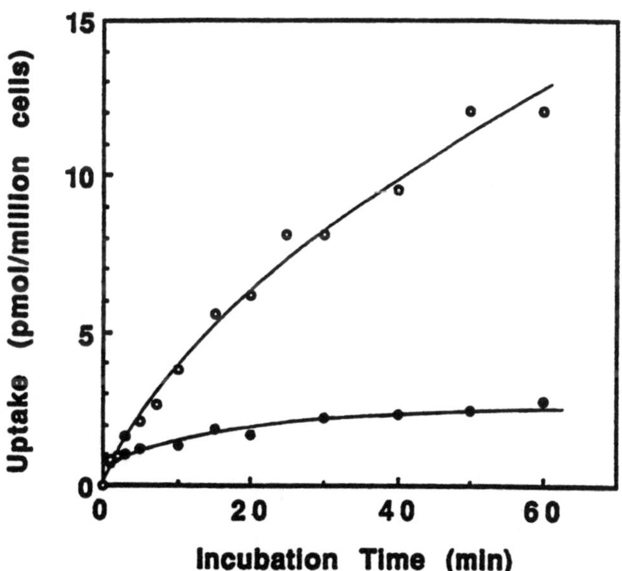

FIGURE 18-4 Effect of incubation time on the transport of pyridoxine (PN) and PN-glucoside. Isolated rat liver cells were incubated with 0.5 μM [³H]pyridoxine (o) or ³H-labeled β-D-glucoside (•). SOURCE: Zhang et al. (1993) © *J. Nutr.* (123:85–89), American Society for Nutritional Sciences.

TABLE 18-1 Results of 50-minute Uptake, Cellular Metabolism, or Enzymatic Treatments of Pyridoxine or its β-Glucoside

Compound (0.5 μM)	Uptake (pmol/10^6 cells)	Cellular Metabolism (pmol PLP/10^6 cells)	Homogenate	Supernatant
			(pmol PLP/mg protein/min)	
Pyridoxine	12	23	0.56	1.78
PN-glucoside	2.6	0.044	0.018	0.034

NOTE: PLP, pyridoxal 5'-phosphate; PN, pyridoxine.

Overall, it is clear that pyridoxine β-glucoside is less available as a source of vitamin B_6 for mammals because it enters cells less well than the free vitamin and is limited considerably in its conversion to functional coenzyme.

Riboflavin-5'-α-D-Glucoside

The formation of riboflavin-5'-α-D-glucoside was first noted to occur when riboflavin was incubated with homogenates or aqueous extracts from acetone powders of rat liver (Whitby, 1952). The structure of this α-glucoside is shown in Figure 18-5. The compound also was found in the urine of rats after oral administration of [2-^{14}C]riboflavin (Ohkawa et al., 1983). Hence, it became of interest to study disposition of the riboflavin α-glucoside with regard to its transport into and metabolic utilization by liver cells. Also since no bioavailabil-

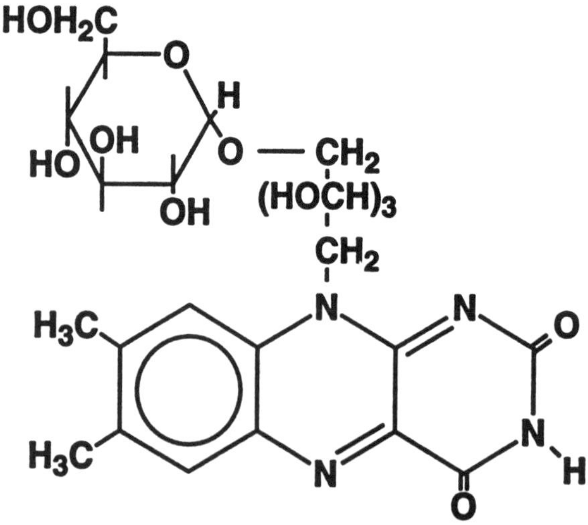

FIGURE 18-5 Structure of riboflavin-5'-α-D-glucoside.

ity studies had been done on this glucoside, its ability to replace riboflavin in the diets of young, growing rats was determined (Joseph and McCormick, 1995).

Uptake of [³H]riboflavin by freshly isolated rat hepatocytes is not affected by its unlabeled α-glucoside. This is true with comparable physiological concentrations over a period of time, as seen in Figure 18-6.

Because the solubility of riboflavin α-glucoside is much greater than that of riboflavin, it was suggested that this may be a natural derivative of importance in the transport of the relatively insoluble vitamin (Whitby, 1952). Results of a study on riboflavin α-glucoside uptake, shown in Figure 18-7, demonstrate that initial uptake of the glucoside is higher than that of riboflavin (Joseph and McCormick, 1995). However, the accumulation of α-glucoside after an hour was significantly lower.

As riboflavin α-glucoside does not inhibit uptake of riboflavin, the former probably enters the cell by an alternate route, bypassing the riboflavin transporter that has been shown to exhibit relative specificity for the flavin structure in both liver (Aw et al., 1983) and proximal tubular cells of the kidney (Bowers-Komro and McCormick, 1987). Also, the glucose transporter is not involved since uptake of riboflavin α-glucoside is not affected by glucose even when concentrations of the latter are considerably higher (Joseph and McCormick, 1995).

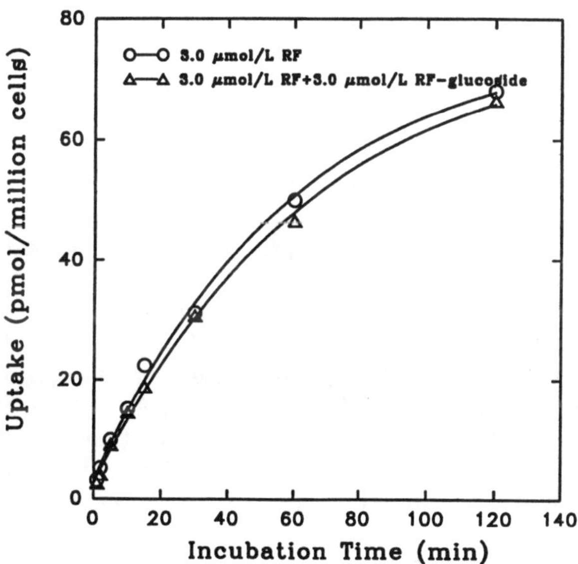

FIGURE 18-6 Time course of [³H]riboflavin (RF) uptake in the absence (o–o) and presence (Δ–Δ) of unlabeled α-D-glucoside. SOURCE: Joseph and McCormick (1995) © *J. Nutr.* (125:2194–2198), American Society for Nutritional Sciences.

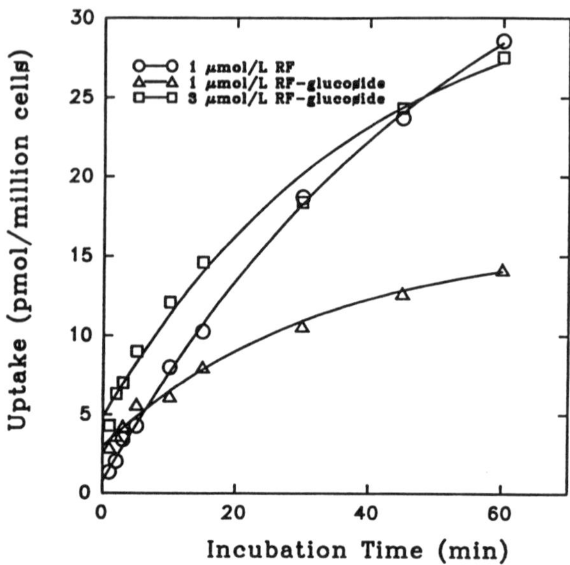

FIGURE 18-7 Effect of incubation time on the transport of [³H]riboflavin (RF) and ³H-labeled α-D-glucoside into isolated liver cells. SOURCE: Joseph and McCormick (1995) © *J. Nutr.* (125:2194–2198), American Society for Nutritional Sciences.

The effect of riboflavin α-glucoside concentration on its uptake into liver cells is shown in Figure 18-8. The process reflects saturation kinetics and exhibits an apparent K_t of 83.4 µM and a V_{max} of 207 pmol/10^6 cells/min. The uptake was significantly affected by temperature, as expected for a facilitated transport. Decreasing sodium in the incubation mixture by replacement with other cations did not affect uptake. Hence, as previously reported for riboflavin entry into liver cells (Aw et al., 1983), sodium-dependent active transport does not seem to be involved.

The metabolic conversion of riboflavin α-glucoside upon entry can be seen by representative data presented in Table 18-2. By the end of 45 minutes, approximately 45 percent of the α-glucoside had been metabolized as compared with 25 percent of riboflavin. Hydrolysis is presumably mediated by nonspecific α-glucosidases known to occur in mammalian tissues (Yamamoto et al., 1990). This is supported by the observation that rat liver α-glucosidases catalyze formation as well as hydrolysis of α-glucoside derivatives of several xenobiotics (Kamimura et al., 1992). The vitamin, whether initially free or hydrolytically released, is converted by flavokinase to flavin mononucleotide (FMN) and by FAD synthetase to flavin adenine dinucleotide (FAD). These flavocoenzymes account for most of the difference (between the initial and final concentrations of riboflavin), since only traces of other catabolites arise from enzymatic actions on riboflavin (Chastain and McCormick, 1991).

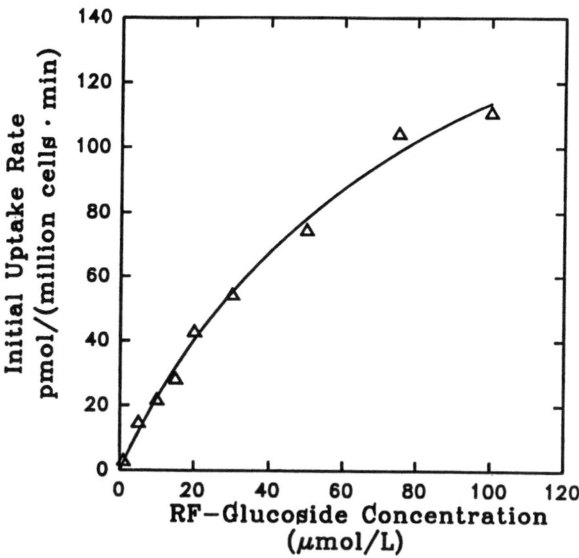

FIGURE 18-8 Dependence of initial rate of [³H]riboflavin 5'-α-D-glucoside uptake (1 minute) on its concentration. SOURCE: Joseph and McCormick (1995) © *J. Nutr.* (125:2194–2198), American Society for Nutritional Sciences.

When the effect of replacing riboflavin with its α-glucoside in the diet of weanling rats was examined (Joseph and McCormick, 1995), it was clear that the α-glucoside is at least as effective as riboflavin on an equivalent basis. Near-maximal growth rate was achieved with either 43 μg of riboflavin α-glucoside per 15 g of diet or 30 μg of the vitamin per 15 g of diet. It is probable that most of the ingested α-glucoside is hydrolyzed even before it reaches the liver since intestines are a rich source of α-glucosidases (Yamamoto et al., 1990).

Overall, it is clear that riboflavin α-glucoside is a very water-soluble form of the vitamin, which releases the vitamin after facile transport that does not involve the riboflavin transporter in the plasma membrane of cells. In fact this

TABLE 18-2 Flavins Present within Cells after a 45-minute Incubation with [³H]Riboflavin or its [³H]α-Glucoside

Initial Compound (1 μM)	Riboflavin (% initial compound)	α-Glucoside	FMN	FAD
Riboflavin	75	—	16	4
Riboflavin α-glucoside	32	55	9	2

NOTE: FMN, flavin mononucleotide; FAD, flavin adenine dinucleotide.

compound would provide an alternate way of delivering the vitamin, should there be a fault in the conventional transport system.

AUTHOR'S CONCLUSIONS AND RECOMMENDATIONS

The requirements for micronutrients as related to performance capability are arguably less well understood than requirements for calorie-yielding macronutrients. In particular, the changes in requirements that probably attend stressful conditions have not been assessed adequately for most of the water-soluble vitamins. Yet the means to acquire such information is at hand. Diverse techniques can be applied, but one that extends to animal models with the inherent potential for greater ranges of testing than ethically allowed with humans, is the isolated-cell technique. It is quite easy to project the type of experimentation outlined above with the disposition of natural glucosides of two vitamins in rat liver cells, to the more complete range of vitamins and derivatives that occurs within foods, using liver and other tissues from rats and other animals subjected to varying degrees of exertion or other stress. For example, exercising rats under controlled conditions followed by removal of cells for testing would allow information to be obtained on whether or not the increased physical demands affected uptake or metabolism of a vitamin or other essential nutrient. At present it is not clear, *a priori*, what could even be expected for some cases. Indications for work at the cellular level could then help focus what experiments might be appropriate using techniques that are often expensive, but aimed at the whole organism and, when possible, humans.

REFERENCES

Aw, T.Y., D.P. Jones, and D.B. McCormick
  1983   Uptake of riboflavin by isolated rat liver cells. J. Nutr. 113:1249–1254
Bowers-Komro, D.M., and D.B. McCormick
  1987   Riboflavin uptake by isolated rat kidney cells. Pp. 449–453 in Flavins and
          Flavoproteins, D.E. Edmondson and D.B. McCormick, eds. New York: Walter de
          Gruyter.
Bowman, B.B., and D.B. McCormick
  1989   Pyridoxine uptake by rat renal proximal tubular cells. J. Nutr. 119:745–749.
Bowman, B.B., D.B. McCormick, and I.H. Rosenberg
  1989   Epithelial transport of water-soluble vitamins. Annu. Rev. Nutr. 9:187–199.
Chastain, J.L., and D.B. McCormick
  1991   Flavin metabolites. Pp. 195–200 in Chemistry and Biochemistry of Flavoenzymes,
          vol. 1, F. Müller, ed. Boca Raton, Fla.: CRC Press.
Gilbert, J.A., and J.F. Gregory, III
  1992   Pyridoxine-5'-β-D-glucoside affects the metabolic utilization of pyridoxine in rats.
          J. Nutr. 122:1029–1035.
Ink, S.L., J.F. Gregory, and D.B. Sartain
  1986   Determination of pyridoxine β-glucoside bioavailability using intrinsic and
          extrinsic labeling in the rat. J. Agric. Food Chem. 34:857–862.

Joseph, T., and D.B. McCormick
1995   Uptake and metabolism of riboflavin-5'-α-D-glucoside by rat and isolated liver cells. J. Nutr. 125:2194–2198.

Kabir, H., J.E. Leklem, and L.T. Miller
1983   Relationship of the glycosylated vitamin B_6 content of foods to the vitamin B_6 bioavailability in humans. Nutr. Rep. Int. 28:709–715.

Kamimura, H., H. Ogata, and H. Takahara
1992   α-Glucoside formation of xenobiotics by rat liver α-glucosidases. Drug Metab. Disp. 20:309–315.

Kawai, T., H. Yamada, and K. Ogata
1972   Studies on transglucosidation to vitamin B_6 by microorganisms. VII. Transport of pyridoxine glucoside into rabbit erythrocytes. J. Vitaminol. 18:183–188.

Kozik, A., and D.B. McCormick
1984   Mechanism of pyridoxine uptake by isolated rat liver cells. Arch. Biochem. Biophys. 229:187–193.

Leklem, J.E.
1994   Vitamin B_6. Pp. 383–394 in Modern Nutrition in Health and Disease, 8th ed., vol. 1, M.A. Shils, J.A. Olson, and M. Shike, eds. Philadelphia: Lea and Febiger.

McCormick, D.B.
1975   Metabolism of riboflavin. Pp. 153–198 in Riboflavin, R.R. Rivlin, ed. New York: Plenum Press.
1979   Some aspects of the metabolism of sulfur-containing heterocyclic cofactors: Lipoic acid, biotin, and 8α-(S-L-cysteinyl)-riboflavin. Pp. 423–434 in Natural Sulfur Compounds, D. Cavallini, G.E. Gaull, and V. Zappia, eds. New York: Plenum Press.
1989   Two interconnected B vitamins: Riboflavin and pyridoxine. Physiol. Rev. 69:1170–1197.

McCormick, D.B., and L.D. Wright
1970   The metabolism of biotin and its analogues. Pp. 81–110 in Comprehensive Biochemistry, vol. 21, Metabolism of Vitamins and Trace Elements, M. Florkin and E.H. Stortz, eds. Amsterdam: Elsevier.

McCormick, D.B., and Z. Zhang
1993   Cellular assimilation of water-soluble vitamins in the mammal: Riboflavin, B_6, biotin, and C. Proc. Soc. Exp. Biol. Med. 203:265–270.

Ohkawa, H., N. Ohishi, and K. Yagi
1983   Occurrence of riboflavinyl glucoside in rat urine. J. Nutr. Sci. Vitaminol. 29:515–522.

Rose, R.C., D.B. McCormick, T-K. Li, L. Lumeng, J.G. Haddad, Jr., and R. Spector
1986   Transport and metabolism of vitamins. Fed. Proc. 45:30–39.

Trumbo, P.R., and J.F. Gregory, III
1988   Metabolic utilization of pyridoxine-β-glucoside in rats: Influence of vitamin B-6 status and route of administration. J. Nutr. 118:1336–1342.

Trumbo, P.R., M.A. Banks, and J.F. Gregory, III
1990   Hydrolysis of pyridoxine-5'-β-D-glucoside by a broad-specificity β-glucosidease from mammalian tissues. Proc. Soc. Exp. Biol. Med. 195:240–246.

Whitby, L.G.
1952   Riboflavinyl glucoside: A new derivative of riboflavin. Biochem. J. 50:433–438.

Yamamoto, I., N. Muto, E. Nagato, T. Nakamura, and Y. Suzuki
1990   Formation of a stable L-ascorbic acid α-glucoside by mammalian α-glucosidase-catalyzed transglucosylation. Biochem. Biophys. Acta 1035:44–50.

Yasumoto, K., H. Tsuji, and H. Mitsuda
  1977   Isolation from rice bran of a bound form of vitamin B_6 and its identification as 5'-O-(β-D-glucopyranosyl)-pyridoxine. Agric. Biol. Chem. 41:1061–1067.
Zhang, Z., and D.B. McCormick
  1992   Uptake and metabolism of N-(4'-pyridoxal)amines by isolated rat liver cells. Arch. Biochem. Biophys. 294:394–397.
Zhang, Z., J.F. Gregory III, and D.B. McCormick
  1993   Pyridoxine-5'-β-D-glucoside competitively inhibits uptake of vitamin B6 into isolated rat liver cells. J. Nutr. 123:85–89.

DISCUSSION

JOHN VANDERVEEN: Do you know if the traditional procedures for measuring nutrients in foods measure the glycosides as well? They are microbiological, I think, in both cases.

DONALD McCORMICK: Right. The answer to your question is "not uniformly." The results vary because the ability to measure glycosides depends on the nonspecific glucosidases that may or may not release it, and their presence varies from one microorganism to another. Some assays specifically do not do well; for instance, the streptococcal assays for B_6 apparently do not have glucosidases that can release the B_6. So no, it is no good for assessing that.

It varies, so what you are dealing with, with any biological assay, including microbiological assays, are variations on competence for releasing bound forms, meaning that there is an error in that technique, too.

Emerging Technologies for Nutrition Research, 1997
Pp. 401–414. Washington, D.C.
National Academy Press

19

Assessment of Cellular Dysfunction During Physiologic Stress

Guy Miller[1]

THE TRANSITION FROM PHYSIOLOGIC TO CELLULAR ASSESSMENT

Organ Physiology Is Derived from Cell Biochemistry

The appropriate alimentation of an individual subjected to exogenous or endogenous stress ultimately calls for the conversion of basic food elements to cellular energy. The myriad of events that combine to regulate this process effectively is controlled at many levels of the organism. Various schemes have been employed to characterize such control mechanisms (Hochachka et al., 1992, 217–348). During homeostasis, anabolism and catabolism are coupled tightly throughout the various organ systems, and hence, an almost seamless cascade of events occurs—digestion, absorption, transport, cell uptake, and utilization—directed at supplying cells with vital macro- and micronutrients to

---

[1] Guy Miller, Stanford University and Galileo Laboratories, Inc., Sunnyvale, CA 94086. gmiller@galileolabs.com

maintain and promote cell function. How this complex balance behaves when subjected to stress is a matter of great importance.

Physiologic Reserve Is a Measure of Total Cell Mass Function

The concept of physiologic reserve often is used to connote the limits of function of a particular physiologic system when a stress is brought to bear upon that system. In such a manner, a tolerance to external stressors that are, in effect, compensated for by the physiologic reserve of the system, is observed. When a stress exceeds the capability of a particular organ system to compensate adequately, physiologic dysfunction ensues. Several factors influence the magnitude of the observed physiological derangement and include: the type of stress, the prior state of the system, and the duration of the stress interval.

Physiologic Reserve often Deteriorates Unnoticed

Alterations in physiologic function are oftentimes not apparent until a critical level of function is compromised. The generalized, nonlinear deterioration of physiologic performance as related to cell function results in a disparity between the (physiologic) output signal and the (cellular) signal generator (Figure 19-1). Hence, strategies to measure physiologic function (reserve) during stress should be directed at assessing both global organ function and cellular reserve. By this means, information is obtained on the current status of the system and expectations concerning performance potential.

Measure Cell Function to Treat Cell Dysfunction

With the ultimate goal of optimization of performance during acute stress, it would be preferable to monitor cellular parameters that were causally, not associatively, related to physiologic outcome. Two advantages are derived from monitoring underlying cell function. As detailed above, early indicators of total cell function will yield information concerning organ function and will serve as an early warning system for impending failure. Additionally, the monitoring of various parameters associated with cell function affords the opportunity to design and test nutritional strategies to treat selective aspects of cell function to optimize performance.

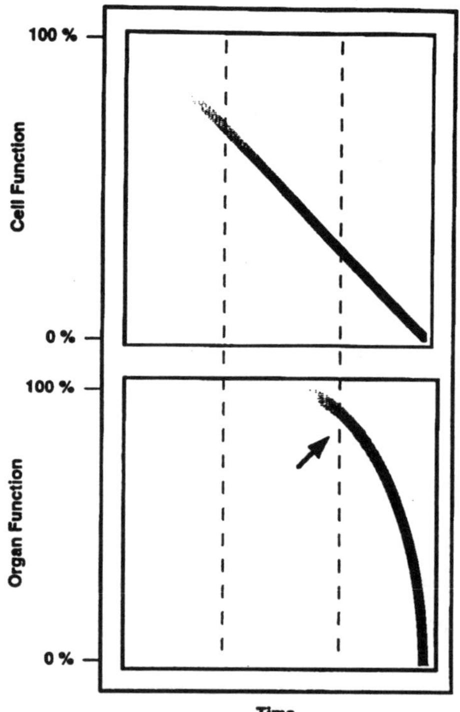

FIGURE 19-1 Organ physiology as a function of cell biochemistry. An idealized model of organ and cell function is expressed in which injury increases over a period of time. Various states are proposed that broadly reflect the severity of underlying physiologic performance as a function of progressive cellular dysfunction. Cell function can decrease by approximately one-third, with minimal decline in organ function (physiologic reserve). Further decreases in cell function are tolerated. It is often not until approximately two-thirds of total cell function are compromised that a change in traditional physiologic variables is appreciated (arrow). When a critical point is approached, attempts to improve outcome by optimizing physiologic function often fail.

CELLULAR PARAMETERS IN ACUTE CELL DYSFUNCTION

Cells Possess Multiple Responses to Stress

The cellular response to acute stress is dependent upon the cell type, the nature of the stress, and the environment of the cell. For example, intestinal epithelial cells respond differently to the effects of circulating epinephrine in comparison with myocardial myocytes. Additionally, the myocyte response depends upon the duration of epinephrine exposure (receptor downregulation). Lastly, the response of the enterocyte is dependent upon local autocrine mechanisms and is influenced by neighboring endothelial, leukocyte, and neuronal action(s). These examples illustrate not only the range of responses to be understood, but the overall complexity of the system.

Hypoxia Is a Stress that Disrupts Cell Energy Metabolism and Affects Dysfunction

Hypoxia, a disruption in normal oxygen delivery to vital tissues, occupies a central role in causing organ dysfunction and death. Tissue hypoxia involving the splanchnic viscera is of particular interest to the nutritionist concerned with performance during stress in the presence or absence of extreme environmental conditions. Hypoxia-mediated splanchnic dysfunction can lead to nutrient malabsorption, gut dysfunction, bacterial translocation, and heat stroke. For a concise review of this topic, the reader is referred to a previous text issued by the Committee on Military Nutrition Research, *Nutritional Needs in Hot Environments* (IOM, 1993). To monitor and treat hypoxia-mediated gastrointestinal dysfunction most effectively, methodologies are being fashioned that address the underlying basis of the injury: disruptions in cell energy metabolism.

Measuring Cell Energy Metabolism

Cell function is dependent upon the delicate balance between anabolism and catabolism. This process is highly regulated at the cellular level. For many cell types, the bulk of energy is derived from processes involving oxygen. Hence, in the absence of oxygen, cell function is impaired. The time course for these events is dependent upon the particular cell type. For example, highly oxidative cells such as those comprising the brain, heart, and liver have a relatively poor tolerance to hypoxia, surviving on the order of minutes. In contrast, the nonoxidative red blood cells are relatively unaffected by extended periods without oxygen and can survive stored for months.

There are various ways to measure the function of the cellular components that comprise the energetic apparatus of the cell. The challenge is in integrating the events controlling substrate utilization, cell and tissue function, and whole animal function during both normal and pathological states. Because hypoxia has a rapid and profound effect on cell energy metabolism, measurements involving cell energetic function are useful tools with which to understand and monitor the effects of hypoxia. It should be kept in mind that a single or simple measurement of energy metabolism does not exist that yields exclusive and complete information as to the health or integrity of the system. With these limitations, what information can be obtained by direct or indirect measurements involving cell energy metabolism?

PRACTICAL ISSUES IN ASSESSING CELL FUNCTION

Studies on cell energy metabolism can be performed with *in vivo* or *ex vivo* preparations. There is a general trade-off between the ability to acquire mechanistic data and the complexity of the model system. While simplified cell-model systems often allow investigators to obtain more data, the extrapolation of these results to intact organ and animal systems is fraught with many limitations. Conversely, the limited data set derived from intact organ systems oftentimes does not allow investigators to obtain certain relevant mechanistic data. The following two sections detail the advantages and limitations associated with investigating hypoxic tissue dysfunction in *ex vivo* model systems. The data and interpretation are intended both to be informative for investigators with specific interests in the field of alimentation during hypoxic cell stress, as well as to discuss the general advantages and disadvantages of transitioning from organ-based to cell-based investigations.

Identification of the Correct Cell and Model

With the goal of extrapolating events from the cell to the whole organ level and the animal level, a careful choice of cell type and model is required. In general, investigators concerned with whole organ-animal function often employ cell culture techniques to achieve one of two end points: (1) the study of a distinct process or cellular component, or (2) the study of the cell as a miniaturized model of the often complex *in vivo* counterpart. It is towards the latter that this discussion is directed.

Cell Models of Tissue Hypoxia

Using a cell system to study the more complex *in vivo* system has many advantages; however, it comes with many potential pitfalls. All too often cellular mechanisms have been elucidated that bear little resemblance to the *in vivo* context. To avoid these problems, a thorough understanding of the tissue under examination and the choice of a cellular model system is needed.

Beyond the general problems associated with cellular model systems of complex diseases, the study of hypoxia imposes its own set of limitations on the choice of cell type. The cellular response(s) to hypoxia can be divided into fast and slow responses. Included in fast responses are rapid changes in metabolic flux that occur on the order of seconds to minutes. Slow responses, more prevalent in adaptation to chronic hypoxia, appear on the order of hours and would include, for example, the synthesis of inducible nonconstituent proteins such as heat shock protein 70 (De Maio, 1995).

Because hypoxia affects the method and amount of energy a cell produces, hypoxic conditions possess the ability to alter all energy-dependent functions. In choosing a cell model to examine the fast responses associated with hypoxia, two general requirements exist: (1) the cell should derive its energy in a manner similar to the tissue of interest, and (2) the particular energy-dependent cell function of interest should possess a time-dependent decrement in function that closely parallels the modeled tissue. The following example illustrates these two points.

The Caco-2 cell is a human colonic tumor derived cell line frequently employed to study various aspects of enterocyte function. Caco-2 cells derive the bulk of their adenosine 5'-triphosphate (ATP) requirements from glycolysis, that is, substrate level phosphorylation. In contrast, intestinal function is highly dependent upon ATP-derived from oxidative phosphorylation. While removal of oxygen results in substantial intestinal (tissue) death on the order of hours, the time response for the Caco-2 cells is on the order of days (Personal communication, M. Fink, Harvard Beth Israel Hospital, Boston, Mass., 1995). The poor energy dependency and time response makes the Caco-2 cells a suboptimal model in which to study the rapid response to hypoxia.

Measurements of the Cellular Response to Hypoxia

Investigators concerned with bioenergetics have developed many techniques with which to assess cellular energy metabolism. A partial list includes the assessment of cellular energy charge by nuclear magnetic resonance spectroscopy, high-pressure liquid chromatography, or enzymatic techniques; the measurement of substrate flux; the assessment of mitochondrial function by measurement of ATP synthesis, membrane gradients, or potentials; and the examination of specific cell functions closely linked to energy supply, such as second messenger-mediated events. The choice of a particular technique is guided in part by the process under study. To examine the effects of hypoxia on splanchnic function, it was of interest to derive a measurement that was convenient and yielded generalized data on global cell energy function.

Proton Flux to Measure Rapid Responses to Change in
Cell Energy Metabolism

Cell proton production and excretion are linked closely to energy metabolism. As a first approximation, protons are derived from two metabolic pathways: glycolysis and the tricarboxylic acid (TCA) cycle. Protons produced in glycolysis are derived from the oxidation of glyceraldehyde 3-phosphate to 3-phosphoglycerate. These protons often are associated with the acid proton component of lactic acid. Additional protons are produced by the oxidation of substrates to produce carbon dioxide within the TCA cycle ($CO_2 + H_2O \rightarrow H_2CO_3 \rightarrow HCO_3^- + H^+$). These protons leave the cell by one of several mechanisms (Figure 19-2).

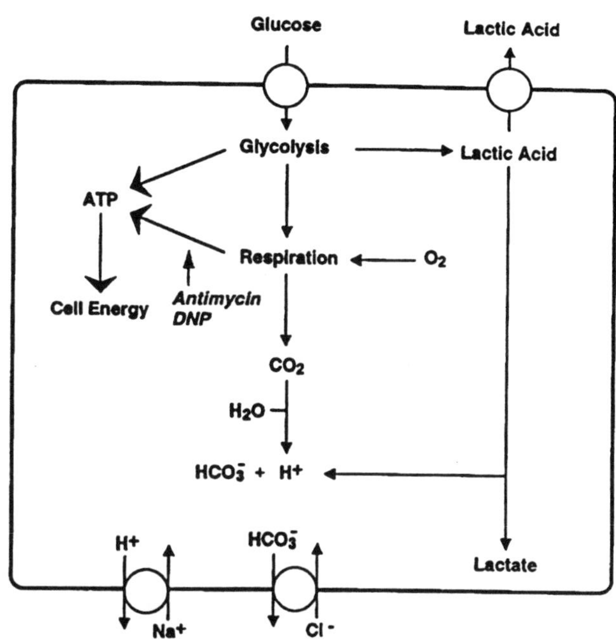

FIGURE 19-2 Cellular proton production. Protons are generated through various metabolic pathways. In this simplified scheme, protons that arise from glycolysis and respiration are shown. Protons exit the cell by one of several mechanisms, including the sodium-proton antiporter, monocarboxylate transporter, diffusion of a neutral weak acid, and diffusion of carbon dioxide-carbonic acid. Adenosine 5'-triphosphate (ATP) generated by substrate level phosphorylation and oxidative phosphorylation provides the chemical energy to power the cell. Antimycin and 2,4-dinitrophenol (DNP) inhibit the respiratory component of ATP synthesis.

Measurements of extracellular acidification can be employed to assess substrate flux through the TCA cycle or the glycolytic pathway indirectly (McConnell et al., 1992). In effect, the extracellular acidification rate can be thought of as a reflection of cellular metabolic rate expressed as proton production per minute. Changes in metabolic rate thus serve as a convenient proxy for assessing cellular energy metabolism on a more global scale.

APPLICATION: UNDERSTANDING SPLANCHNIC DYSFUNCTION DURING ISCHEMIC-HYPOXIC STRESS

Stress states arising from various conditions can lead to a reduction in blood flow to the splanchnic viscera (Gutierrez and Brown, 1996). When blood flow is reduced for critical periods of time, tissue injury can ensue, leading to cell death and/or dysfunction. With reference to the intestinal barrier function, such a sequence of events has been implicated in setting off a cascade of events associated with various systemic inflammatory responses and/or sepsis (Brinkmann et al., 1996).

Healthy and infirm individuals can be at risk for hypoperfusion of the gut. (For a detailed discussion of gut dysfunction in the critically ill, the reader is referred to the attached reference list.) Within the population of healthy individuals, splanchnic hypoperfusion has been implicated in heat stroke and bowel dysfunction secondary to dehydration and extreme stress conditions (IOM, 1993). In instances where blood flow is not promptly restored, splanchnic hypoperfusion can result in signs and symptoms ranging from generalized cramping and diarrhea to epithelial sloughing, intestinal hemorrhage, bowel perforation, and death.

To understand and design cell-based nutritional strategies to ameliorate the effects of splanchnic hypoperfusion, it is of interest to study this process with a cell-based model.

Variations in Cell Culture Lines

All enteric cells are not alike. Similarly, cells derived from the same organ and even the same (sub)population can display marked dissimilarities within cell culture conditions. For example, the susceptibility of two liver parenchymal cell types to the effects of hypoxia can differ markedly. WIF-B cells, a hepatoma-derived hybrid line, suffer near complete injury as evidenced by extensive membrane leakage of intracellular lactate dehydrogenase (LDH) after 3- to 4-h exposure to conditions modeling the effect(s) of hypoxia (Shanks et al., 1994) (Table 19-1). Hep-G2 cells, also a liver cell line obtained from a human hepatocellular carcinoma, exhibited a different pattern of injury. LDH leakage was less

TABLE 19-1 Antimycin-Mediated Cell Death

| | Percent Lactate Dehydrogenase Release | | | | | | |
| | Time (hr) | | | | | | |
Cell Type	0	1	1.5	2	3	4	5
Hep-G2	5.9	6.5	–	20.2	33.7	42.7	38.1
WIF-B	0.0	–	1.4	8.7	77.6	100.0	100.0

NOTE: WIF-B or Hep-G2 cells were grown under standard cell culture conditions and exposed to 100 nM antimycin. Aliquots of the extracellular media were removed at the indicated time points and assayed for release of cytosolic lactate dehydrogenase (LDH) into the extracellular media. Data are expressed as amount of LDH released as a percentage of total cellular LDH content.

extensive in the Hep-G2 cell line, suggesting either 100 percent injury for approximately 50 percent of one or more subpopulations, or a sublethal, approximately 50 percent injury dispersed over the entire cell population(s). In contrast, the intestinal derived Caco-2 cell line exhibits minimal enzyme leakage under similar conditions (Personal communication, M. Fink, Harvard Beth Israel Hospital, Boston, Mass., 1995).

Irrespective of the mechanism of differential cell death, the data demonstrate one limitation associated with cellular model systems: variability. The properties exhibited by the WIF-B cell line closely approximate *in vivo* events (Unpublished data, C. Kasserra, Galileo Laboratories, Inc., Sunnyvale, Calif., 1997). The Hep-G2 cells display moderate susceptibility to the effects of hypoxia, while the Caco-2 cells are almost completely resistant to hypoxic conditions. This variation in response severely affects outcome measurements. For this reason, careful consideration must be given to choosing a cell system in which to investigate the effects of hypoxia. The following general statement can be made: To maximize the utility of a given cell model, the cell type should display a pattern of and susceptibility to injury similar to that observed in the organ or tissue of interest.

Metabolic Rate Changes during Hypoxia

The dependency of the choice of cell line on variations in hypoxia-mediated LDH leakage was described in the previous section. Measurements such as enzyme (LDH) leakage assays yield information that is mostly associative, not causally related, to cell injury or death. To derive a more detailed understanding of the causal events associated with hypoxia-mediated cell injury, it was of interest to examine the effects of hypoxia on cellular energy metabolism. The specific aims included: (1) the feasibility of using proton excretion measurements to study cell-based model systems of hypoxia and (2) the use of such model systems to gain an understanding of cell function during hypoxia.

Glycolytic Cells May Upregulate Glycolysis during Hypoxia

Caco-2 cells derive the bulk of their energy supply from glycolysis and thus are relatively insensitive to the effects of agents such as dinitrophenol or antimycin that disrupt (mitochondrial) oxidative phosphorylation (Personal communication, M. Fink, Harvard Beth Israel Hospital, Boston, Mass., 1995) (see Figure 19-2). To understand the effects of hypoxic conditions more thoroughly, corresponding changes in proton flux were recorded for Caco-2 cells incubated in the presence of dinitrophenol (DNP) (Figure 19-3). Proton excretion rate increased on exposure to DNP. Removal of DNP resulted in reequilibration of the metabolic rate to baseline values, demonstrating that this process was reversible.

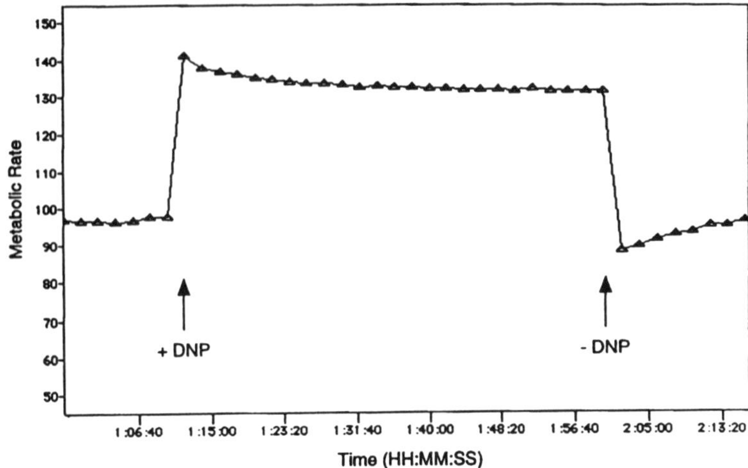

FIGURE 19-3 Effects of dinitrophenol (DNP) on metabolic rate of Caco-2 cells. Studies employing standard cell culture techniques were performed on Caco-2 cells. Cells were grown in Dulbecco's modified Eagle's medium (DMEM) plus 10 percent fetal bovine serum medium on microporous polycarbonate transwells and studied 24 hours post-seeding. Glycolytic and tricarboxylic acid (TCA) flux were assessed by quantifying proton production using a pH-sensitive silicon sensor interfaced to a 3-μL flow chamber (Owicki and Parce, 1992). Cell perfusate contained balanced salt solution, 10 mM glucose, and 100 μM DNP where indicated. Metabolic rate ($-\mu volt \times sec^{-1}$) is expressed as a percentage of basal activity obtained in balanced salt solution plus 10 mM glucose (100%).

Caco-2 cells synthesize ATP by both oxidative phosphorylation and substrate level phosphorylation. One possible explanation for the increased proton flux during DNP treatment is an increase in glycolytic flux to compensate for a decrement in ATP derived from oxidative phosphorylation. Indirect evidence for such a mechanism is derived from the known effects of variations in cellular energy charge $(EC = ATP + 0.5\ ADP/ATP + ADP + AMP)^2$ on allosteric regulation of glycolytic enzymes, for example, phosphofructokinase-1 (Atkinson, 1977, 85–107).

Oxidative Cells Decrease Metabolic Rate during Hypoxia

In contrast to Caco-2 cells, proton flux studies performed on primary rat liver hepatocytes treated with DNP had a different outcome (cf., Figures 19-3 and 19-4). The initial response recorded for hepatocytes paralleled that observed for the Caco-2 cells, namely an increase in metabolic rate. The increase in proton flux was transient and declined over the next several minutes, equal to an

---

[2] ADP, adenosine 5'-diphosphate; AMP, adenosine 5'-monophosphate.

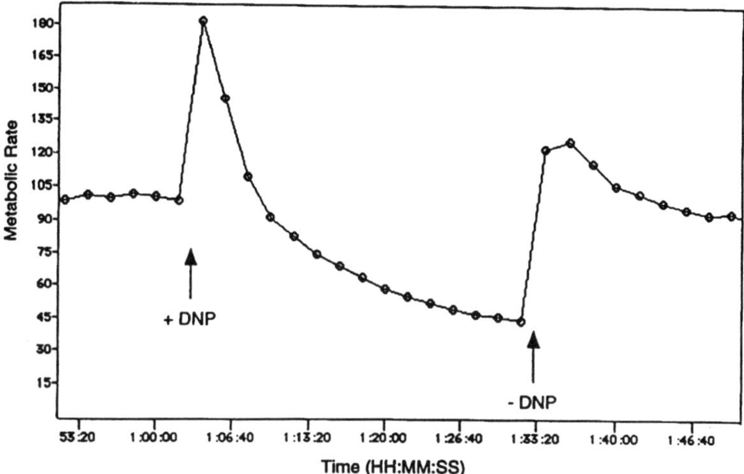

FIGURE 19-4 Effects of dinitrophenol (DNP) on metabolic rate of primary rat liver hepatocyte cells. Assessment of metabolic rate on hepatocyte cells was performed as described in the legend to Figure 19-3.

approximately 45 percent reduction in metabolic rate. Removal of DNP from the cell perfusate resulted in an approximately 20 percent overshoot of the baseline metabolic rate, followed by a trend towards reequilibration to baseline value after approximately 10 minutes.

Highly oxidative cells such as hepatocytes derive a significant portion of ATP from oxidative phosphorylation. While the effects of hypoxia-mediated ATP depletion have been studied extensively in numerous cell and organ models, an adequate explanation linking ATP depletion to a causal sequence of events leading to cell death has yet to be advanced. Proton flux data obtained from isolated hepatocytes suggest that dinitrophenol-mediated uncoupling of the mitochondrial proton gradient from ATP synthesis results in a marked reduction in net proton flux. Whether this is brought about by substrate (ATP) limitation or as a result of the triggering of a sequence of events to modulate energy consumption, is unknown. Further studies are underway to define how metabolic rate varies as a function of a graded depletion of ATP.

APPLICATIONS: FUTURE QUESTIONS TO BE ADDRESSED

The cell-based experiments described above only barely begin to address many pertinent questions of interest to nutritionists examining function during stress. The following section contains a partial list of questions whose solution(s) may be facilitated by methodologies employing cell-based assessment of cellular energy metabolism.

Substrate Flux during Hypoxic Stress

Is there a preferential use of substrates during hypoxic stress? If certain substrates are used to the exclusion of others, a nutritional formulation could be developed to potentiate beneficial metabolic pathways.

Cell Hibernation

How does the cell acutely adapt to hypoxic conditions, that is, conditions in which energy demand exceeds supply? Preliminary data suggest that the cell responds with an initial increase in metabolic rate followed by a decrease. What are the events that mediate these processes?

Metabolic Cofactors

What are the effects of metabolic cofactors such as vitamin E, glutathione, and trace minerals on conferring resistance to hypoxic stress? The antioxidants as a group have been examined extensively for nutritional efficacy during various stress circumstances. While their general role continues to be somewhat controversial, less is known about antioxidants as nutritional adjuncts during acute hypoxic stress.

Enteric Function

Will performance and outcome be improved by strategies that maintain splanchnic function during acute stress? Maintaining gut and hepatic function is critical to maintaining systemic homeostasis. The deterioration of either of these organ systems has been implicated as the causal mechanism of heat stroke and other conditions. Will strategies that are designed to use cell-based systems extrapolate to intact organ systems, and if not, how can investigators improve such model systems?

REFERENCES

Atkinson, D.
  1977   Cellular Energy Metabolism and Its Regulation. New York: Academic Press.
Brinkmann, A., C.F. Wolf, D. Berger, E. Kneitinger, B. Neumeister, M. Büchler, P. Radermacher, W. Seeling, and M. Georgieff
  1996   Perioperative endotoxemia and bacterial translocation during major abdominal surgery: Evidence for the protective effect of endogenous prostacyclin. Crit. Care Med. 24:1293–1301.
De Maio, A.
  1995   The heat shock response. New Horizons 3:198–207.

Gutierrez, G., and S. Brown
  1996   Gastrointestinal tonometry: A monitor of regional dysoxia. New Horizons 4:413–419.
Hochachka, P.W., P.L. Lutz, T. Sick, M. Rosenthal, and G. van den Thillart, eds.
  1992   Surviving Hypoxia: Mechanisms of Control and Adaptation. Tokyo: CRC Press.
IOM (Institute of Medicine)
  1993   Nutritional Needs in Hot Environments, Applications for Military Personnel in Field Operations, B.M. Marriott, ed. A report of the Committee on Military Nutrition Research, Food and Nutrition Board. Washington, D.C.: National Academy Press.
McConnell, H.M., J.C. Owicki, J.W. Parce, D.L. Miller, G.T. Baxter, H.G. Wade, and S. Pitchford
  1992   The cytosensor microphysiometer: Biological applications of silicon technology. Science 257:1906–1912.
Owicki, J.C., and J.W. Parce
  1992   Biosensors based on the energy metabolism of living cells: The physical chemistry and cell biology of extracellular acidification. Biosens. Bioelectron. 7:255–272.
Shanks, M.R., D. Cassio, O. Lecoq, and A.L. Hubbard
  1994   An improved polarized rat hepatoma hybrid cell line. J. Cell. Science 107:813–825.

DISCUSSION

DONALD McCORMICK: Fascinating. Can you use similar electrodes at the organelle level?

GUY MILLER: Yes. We have reconfigured the microphysiometer to assess cellular redox state. Specifically, we incubate cells in the presence of a redox active compound such as menadione. Menadione is taken up by the cell and couples into electron transport and undergoes a reduction reaction. Reduced menadione diffuses out of the cell and reduces an extracellular $Fe(III) \rightarrow Fe(II)$ redox couple that in turn donates an electron to the sensor producing a current.

There are several limitations to this approach that include redox and chemical perturbations affected by menadione. While I believe this to be a useful technology, improvements will have to be made to allow less cellular alterations during measurement intervals, as well as improvements in the time response of the system.

ARTHUR ANDERSON: Are the liver cells that you are growing in this system grown on a biomatrix? Or are they by themselves because liver cells will differentiate on a biomatrix, but they will not differentiate as single-cell isolates on a flat surface?

GUY MILLER: The WIF-B cells grow directly on standard 24- or 96-well cell culture plates. Your question infers the difficulty of working with primary-derived hepatocytes with specific requirements for a collagen matrix or other suitable support. One of several unique properties of the WIF-B cells is ease of propagation and convenience relative to primary cell harvesting. For your reference, these cells form a pseudo-organized liver architecture containing bile canaliculi.

DENNIS BIER: I found this very intriguing because I think it is a new, expanded way to look at sodium metabolism. I am not sure you can do some of these things in other ways. For example, people have used specifically tritiated labeled glucose molecules for years to look at the appearance rate of tritiated water to measure various steps in glycolysis outside the cell.

One can look at the TCA [tricarboxylic acid] cycle activity by looking at the rearrangement of carbons and oxaloacetate, either radio- or isotopically labeled, and that can be done outside the cell as well.

Now, people have not looked at 10-s intervals because they have not felt that that was particularly important. Maybe it is, but there are other ways to approach this. I am not sure that it should not be combined in some way with what you are doing.

GUY MILLER: I think that the idea of combining several metabolic assessment modalities to simultaneously assess both cellular and tissue metabolic variables is a good one. As I understand from Harris Lieberman, one issue to be addressed by the CMNR during this session is to examine undertaking such activities. It would be my opinion that a concerted multidisciplinary effort needs to be undertaken in the area of acute metabolic derangements during circumstances of oxygen limitation, i.e., extreme exertion or illness. While we understand a great deal about particular metabolic transformations employing single enzyme experiments, we have just begun to decipher the processes governing the dynamics of metabolic control. New technologies and approaches will also be required that take advantage of our growing understanding of functional genomics. How these methodologies are fashioned together to enhance our understanding of relevant nutritional issues will be a challenging and vital task in forging the next set of advances.

VII

Assessment of Immune Function

THE ROLE OF NUTRITION IN IMMUNE function is of considerable interest to the military. Of particular interest are the optimization and assessment of immune function in the field as well as the development of improved methods of immunization, including oral vaccines. Chapters 20 and 21 review techniques for the assessment of abnormal immune function, while Chapter 22 focuses on the development of vaccines targeted toward mucosal immunity.

In Chapter 20, the use of plasma and urinary cytokine measurements to document the presence of inflammatory stress is assessed, focusing on tumor necrosis factor-α (TNF-α), interleukin-1 (IL-1), and IL-6 because they are overlapping and distinct mediators that affect nearly every organ system in the host. The author concludes that plasma TNF-α and IL-1 are not reliable indicators of inflammation, but plasma IL-6 levels often seem to be elevated in inflammatory processes, correlating with physiologic parameters. While urinary TNF-α and IL-1 levels often are not detected in the circulation or in the urine of most surgical patients, they are increased after "eccentric" exercise. Under the same conditions, urinary IL-6 is increased. The plasma and urinary measurements of IL-6 in particular can be used for detecting metabolic stress.

Chapter 21 focuses on defining measurable, functional parameters for studying abnormalities of the immune system related to malnutrition, stress, and aging. Although the multiple components involved in immune response make this difficult, longitudinal studies incorporating measurement of serum immunoglobulin concentrations and humoral responses to vaccines and boosters, and determination of serum and urinary levels of select cytokines involved in inflammatory processes and immunoregulatory processes have shown promise. Functional assays of immune function, such as delayed hypersensitivity skin tests or natural killer cell function tests, are ideal but not always practical.

Because the effects of exposure to infectious agents and toxins can significantly impair military performance, safe and effective immunization is a priority, as the discussion of mucosal immunity in Chapter 22 indicates. The gastrointestinal and respiratory tracts are the route of entry into the body for many pathogens that may alter nutritional status, and the mucosal immune system is the point of defense against these pathogens. A better understanding of mucosal immunology, coupled with progress in biotechnology and molecular genetics, may lead to the optimization of oral vaccine administration using antibodies and antigens.

Emerging Technologies for Nutrition Research, 1997
Pp. 417–430. Washington, D.C.
National Academy Press

20

The Validity of Blood and Urinary Cytokine Measurements for Detecting the Presence of Inflammation

Lyle L. Moldawer[1]

INTRODUCTION

The purpose of this review is to assess the utility of urinary and blood cytokine measurements to document the presence of inflammatory stress, particularly as it relates to field studies and to military performance. This is a daunting challenge for two reasons. First, at least 15 different interleukins have been described, and according to Carl Nathan, there are a considerable number of additional humoral and growth factors (Nathan and Sporn, 1991). However, the focus of this discussion will be directed to the detection of three pluripotent cytokines, specifically tumor necrosis factor-α (TNF-α), interleukin-1 (IL-1), and IL-6.

The reasons to restrict this discussion to these three inflammatory mediators are severalfold. Not only have these three cytokines been implicated as the most

[1] Lyle L. Moldawer, Department of Surgery, University of Florida College of Medicine, Gainesville, FL 32610

proximal mediators in the proinflammatory cascade, but they also induce secondary inflammatory mediators such as IL-8, some of the macrophage inflammatory proteins, and the neutrophil adherence proteins (Fong et al., 1990a). Another reason to focus on TNF-α, IL-1, and IL-6 is that the actions of these three proinflammatory cytokines are both overlapping and distinct. These three cytokines affect nearly every organ system in the host. In fact, the original description of TNF-α, IL-1, and IL-6 function was due in large part to military research conducted in the 1970s by the research group at Fort Detrick, led by William R. Beisel and contributed to by Robert Wannemacher, Jr., and Michael Powanda (reviewed in Beisel, 1975, 1977, 1980). These investigators described and examined the functional group of proteins, designated leukocyte endogenous mediator (LEM), in the plasma of animals and patients after inflammatory challenges (Powanda and Beisel, 1982; Wannemacher et al., 1972).

It is now known that those mediators, originally described as LEM or as other functional monikers, including leukocytic pyrogen or endogenous pyrogen, are for the most part one or more of these three proinflammatory cytokines, TNF-α, IL-1, and IL-6. One could argue whether LEM, as originally described by Beisel's group, is IL-1 or whether it is IL-6 or TNF-α, but suffice it to say that these three cytokines are the primary mediators responsible for the induction of the proinflammatory responses to infection and inflammation. It is now recognized that the majority of innate responses to bacterial and viral pathogens, including fever, anorexia, weight loss, trace mineral redistribution, neutrophilia, and hepatic acute-phase protein synthesis among others are mediated by the release of these three proinflammatory cytokines (Beisel, 1980; Dinarello, 1994).

The second problem with discussing proinflammatory cytokines and the utility of their measurements in regard to inflammation or military performance is the dual nature of these cytokines. As several groups showed in the 1970s, the effects of these cytokines are primarily beneficial to the infected host (Kampschmidt and Pulliam, 1975; Kluger et al., 1975), including the stimulation of fever and nonspecific host immunity, the activation of macrophages, the redistribution of trace minerals, the induction of a hepatic acute-phase response, and their role as comitogens or adjuvants for cell-mediated immunity or immunoglobulin production (Beisel, 1975; Kampschmidt, 1983). Although these cytokines are inherently beneficial, they can and do often have adverse effects primarily associated with either their exaggerated production or their continued production. The former occurs in gram-negative septic shock and the disseminated intravascular coagulopathy that accompanies it (Beutler and Cerami, 1986; Dinarello and Wolff, 1993). The latter is associated with some chronic inflammatory syndromes such as AIDS or some neoplasms, or their inappropriate compartmentalized production as occurs in rheumatoid arthritis, and often can lead to devastating pathological consequences.

The challenge, therefore, is how to meaningfully interpret urinary or blood measurements of these cytokines in order to identify the presence and magnitude of an inflammatory response when it is unknown or unclear whether cytokines are mediating a beneficial or an adverse effect. The question at hand is whether blood or urinary cytokine measurements can be used to make decisions regarding therapy or performance in a field setting.

INFLAMMATION, SEPSIS, AND PLASMA CYTOKINES

Following purification and cloning of IL-1, TNF-α, and IL-6 in the early to mid-1980s, immunoassays were developed that readily could detect the presence of these proteins in the blood and tissue fluids of humans. At that time, there was a great deal of enthusiasm for the documentation of TNF-α and IL-1 in the plasma of patients with a variety of inflammatory processes. It initially was believed that these cytokines acted as endocrine factors and that they would be routinely measurable in the circulation of patients with infections or inflammation. However, these conclusions were drawn initially from studies based on patients, rodents, and primates who were administered live bacteria or endotoxin (Fong et al., 1990b; Hesse et al., 1988; Michie et al., 1988). When healthy volunteers or primates were given endotoxin or live *E. coli* bacteria, respectively, a monophasic rise in plasma TNF-α concentrations was seen, followed in some cases by a monophasic rise in IL-1 and then a later rise in plasma levels of interferon, IL-6, and other cytokines (Fong et al., 1990b; Hesse et al., 1988). The intensity of the cytokine appearance often correlated with the magnitude of the physiologic responses. These data, from patients who received small amounts of endotoxin, were first published by Douglas W. Wilmore's group in the *New England Journal of Medicine* (Michie et al., 1988). The generalized assumption, thereafter, was that these cytokines circulate frequently in the plasma in an endocrine fashion.

At the same time that these data were being presented, Anders Waage from Norway and other groups were reporting plasma cytokine measurements from septic patients and patients with other inflammatory processes (Waage et al., 1986, 1987, 1989). These investigators for the most part were only able to document an occasional appearance of TNF-α and IL-1 in the circulation of patients with acute inflammation. Unlike the observation that TNF and IL-1 are detected uniformly in animals or patients administered endotoxin or *E. coli,* these and other authors were able to detect TNF-α and IL-1β in fewer than 40 percent of patients with sepsis syndromes. This is a very important observation since it suggests that the detection of plasma TNF-α and IL-1 appearance is not essential to the manifestation of an inflammatory response. Previous studies at Cornell University by Michael Marano and Stephen Lowry examined plasma cytokine concentrations in burn patients who sustained greater than 35 percent total-body surface area thermal injury (Marano et al., 1990). Blood was collected every 4 hours from the time of admission for as long as the patients were critically ill, at times extending to periods of up to 60 or 70 days. Retrospective analyses were then performed, examining which patients became septic, which did not become septic, which survived, and which died, and these were compared with the frequency of being able to detect TNF-α in the circulation.

Statistically, there was a greater frequency of detecting TNF-α in the serum of septic patients compared with nonseptic patients. Patients who eventually died (primarily from overwhelming gram-negative sepsis) had an even higher frequency of detecting TNF-α, but a large number of patients who died from sepsis had no detectable TNF-α. In fact, in only about 40 percent of septic patients was TNF-α detected. IL-1 was detected even less frequently. Only in about 4 to 5 percent of these patients was IL-1β measurable in the circulation, despite the fact that these patients were critically ill and, in many cases, floridly septic. So, contrary to what the experimental model suggested, it was not a common finding to detect TNF-α or IL-1 in the circulation of critically ill patients, in whom increased production would be expected.

The plasma response of IL-6 to inflammatory stimuli is entirely different, however. In contrast to TNF-α or IL-1, IL-6 levels are frequently elevated in patients with inflammation, and the magnitude of the IL-6 response is often of some prognostic value. The University of Pennsylvania group (Moscovitz et al., 1994) evaluated 100 patients who were presented to the emergency room with the clinical criteria of systemic inflammatory response syndrome (SIRS) and screened them for plasma levels of TNF-α, IL-1, and IL-6. What they found was similar to what this laboratory found in burn patients, in that the frequency of detecting TNF-α and IL-1 in the circulation of patients with SIRS was very low and nonpredictive. However, all these patients had elevated plasma levels of IL-6. In fact, there was a trend toward higher concentrations of IL-6 in patients who eventually died. A retrospective analysis comparing IL-6 concentrations with the probability of the patients being septic showed that if a patient initially presented a plasma IL-6 level of greater than about 1 ng/ml, he or she had a greater than 50 percent probability of becoming septic, or in this case, bacteremic. With an IL-6 level of greater than 10 ng/ml, the likelihood increased to 90 percent. Such findings are consistent with a large body of data by several authors showing that the magnitude of the IL-6 response is often associated with the severity of the physiologic response (Calandra et al., 1991; Damas et al., 1992; Frieling et al., 1995; Rintala et al., 1995; Steinmetz et al., 1995).

The findings to date suggest that, for hospitalized patients with systemic inflammatory response syndromes, plasma TNF-α and IL-1 are not likely to be detected with any regular frequency; therefore, the utility of these plasma measurements is likely to be small. In contrast, the data suggest that IL-6 may be a reliable indicator for the presence of infection or inflammation, and levels may correlate with the severity of injury or outcome.

FACTORS INFLUENCING THE MEASUREMENT
OF PLASMA CYTOKINES

A question that arises is why plasma measurements of TNF-α and IL-1 are poor indicators of their production. It must be emphasized that the question is not really whether TNF-α and IL-1 are being produced during sepsis and systemic inflammatory response syndromes. In multiple animal models of infection or inflammation, examining organs or tissues of the reticuloendothelial system reveals evidence of up-regulation of TNF-α and IL-1 gene transcription despite an inability to detect the proteins in the circulation.

The reasons for the failure to detect TNF-α or IL-1 in the circulation are multiple and represent the inherent biology of the proteins. Foremost, the production of TNF-α and IL-1 is episodic. Macrophages exposed to continuous levels of endotoxin, for example, release TNF-α and IL-1 in a single burst over several hours and then become tolerant to repeated or continued exposure (Beutler et al., 1986). This development of tachyphylaxis (the rapid appearance of a progressive decrease in response following repetitive administration of a physiologically active substance) remains a hallmark cytokine response to exposure to bacterial cell products.

Another possible reason for failing to detect TNF-α and IL-1β is that the plasma half-lives of TNF-α and IL-1β are generally less than 60 minutes, and random sampling techniques are probably too imprecise to pick up these episodic productions. More importantly, there are inhibitors and antagonists in the blood of septic patients, which often interfere with the immunoassays or bioassays used to quantitate TNF-α and IL-1 (Engelberts et al., 1991). This becomes extremely important because the presence of these inhibitors or antagonists in the plasma may be used to document the presence of these proinflammatory cytokines indirectly (Moldawer, 1994).

Finally, the production of TNF-α and IL-1 is primarily paracrine in nature, so the appearance in the systemic circulation probably reflects those conditions when either the cytokine is being produced directly in the plasma compartment by blood monocytes and neutrophils or is being produced in large quantities in tissue compartments and is only spilling into the blood as an overflow type of phenomenon from the tissues.

The results of a study by Jean Michel Dayer's group in Geneva is extremely illustrative in this regard (Suter et al., 1992). The investigators examined TNF-α appearance in the plasma and bronchoalveolar lavage fluid (BAL) of patients with adult respiratory distress syndrome (ARDS). They evaluated three groups of patients: patients without ARDS, those with early ARDS, and those with late ARDS (24 hours later). While statistically significant plasma concentrations of TNF-α were about 100 pg/ml, BAL levels were significantly higher, on the order of 100-fold higher in early ARDS, providing evidence of compartmentalization of TNF-α in this patient population.

Unpublished data from studies that this laboratory has done with Greg Schultz's group at the University of Florida, looking at the levels of TNF-α in nonhealing wounds (decubitus ulcers or diabetic foot ulcers), are similar (Unpublished data, L. L. Moldawer, University of Florida, Gainesville, Fla., 1996). Very high levels of TNF-α were found compartmentalized in these non-healing wounds, on the order of 5 ng/ml. At the same time in the peripheral circulation of these patients, there was no detectable TNF-α (< 50 pg/ml). IL-1β levels also have been examined in these same tissues. A similar phenomenon occurred with no detectable IL-1β in the circulation of patients with nonhealing wounds, but very high levels of IL-1β in the wounds themselves.

The second reason identified above for not being able to detect TNF-α or IL-1 in the circulation is the presence of inhibitors that not only bind and inactivate the cytokines but also interfere with their detection. The most common inhibitors of TNF-α are its shed receptors, the p55 receptor and the p75 receptor. During inflammation, these receptors are shed after a protease cleaves their extracellular portions at the level of the cell membrane (Van Zee et al., 1992). The shed receptors retain the ability to bind ligand and therefore compete with remaining cellular TNF receptors for the binding of circulating TNF-α, thus making them natural inhibitors.

Studies performed in this laboratory that were published in 1992 showed that human volunteers given very small amounts of endotoxin, sufficient to produce chills and a mild tachycardia, resulted in a systemic TNF-α response (Van Zee et al., 1992). Also seen subsequent to the appearance of TNF-α (after 2 hours) was an increase in the plasma concentrations of the shed p55 and p75 receptors. Ninety minutes after the administration of endotoxin, TNF-α bioactivity and immunoactivity peaked in the plasma. Thereafter, however, plasma from such patients had net inhibitory activity for TNF-α. If recombinant TNF-α was added to the plasma, it would be bound and inactivated, due in part to the excess quantities of these shed receptors.

Where do these shed TNF receptors come from? The results of a flow cytometry study on monocytes from patients administered endotoxin, performed by Steve Calvano at Cornell University, are illustrative (van der Poll et al., 1995). After endotoxin is administered to healthy volunteers, the number of TNF binding sites on the monocytes (presumably receptors) declines. Accompanying this decline is a corresponding increase in the appearance of soluble p55 and p75 in the circulation.

Following acute inflammation secondary to endotoxin administration, there is a release of shed TNF receptors, which can bind TNF-α and act as antagonists. The same phenomenon occurs for IL-1. One of the IL-1 receptors, p68, is shed and binds to IL-1, thus inactivating it (Colotta et al., 1993). This receptor also is shed during sepsis and in major surgical procedures (Giri et al., 1994; Pruitt et al., 1995). However, the IL-1 system has another inhibitory molecule, IL-1 receptor antagonist (IL-1ra), which is a competitive antagonist for the functional type I IL-1 receptor and also is released after acute inflammation (Hannum et al., 1990).

In summary, the appearance of the TNF-α inhibitors p55 and p75 can be used as an indirect estimate of the presence and degree of inflammation. The same phenomenon holds true for the IL-1 inhibitors. It has been argued that the plasma concentration of these shed receptors or concentrations of IL-1ra can be used as an indirect estimate of the degree of inflammation present and, probably, of the induction of these cytokines at the paracrine level. Concentrations of p55 and p75 in critically ill patients are routinely elevated (Fischer et al., 1992; Rogy et al., 1994). Concentrations seen in normal volunteers are generally at the lower levels of sensitivity of this assay, while 95 percent of the patients who are critically ill, meeting the criteria for SIRS or sepsis syndrome, have elevated p55 and p75 levels (Rogy et al., 1994).

FIELD MEASUREMENT OF URINARY CYTOKINES

The problem with cytokine measurements in the field setting is that it is often difficult to obtain blood samples. The question of whether cytokine levels in the plasma or in tissue compartments can be documented through noninvasive sampling is important. At least with regard to urine measurements for cytokines, there is now good evidence to suggest that several cytokines that appear in the plasma in the high pg/ml or ng/ml range are excreted immunologically intact in the urine. Importantly, the first descriptions of many of these cytokines, and of most of the cytokine inhibitors, were based on inhibitory activity that was identified in the urine of patients with a variety of inflammatory conditions. For example, p55, p75, and IL-1ra were first purified to homogeneity and sequenced from urine samples of patients with either neoplasms, sepsis, pregnancy, or fevers (Prieur et al. 1987; Seckinger et al. 1987a, b, 1988). So it is known, at least historically, that these cytokine inhibitors can appear in the urine. What is not known is whether proinflammatory cytokines themselves are excreted in the urine and whether their detection can be used to document the presence and degree of inflammation.

Some studies done by Sprenger and colleagues in Germany, in which they looked at blood and urinary cytokine production in conditioned athletes before and after a 20-km run, have a great deal of relevance for the military (Sprenger et al., 1992). The run took about 100 minutes, so the 2-h samples actually reflect blood and urine measurements 20 minutes after the run was completed. IL-6 levels increased in the plasma, consistent with a nonspecific inflammatory response, but significant increases in urinary IL-6 also were documented. In fact, levels peaked very quickly, 2 to 3 hours after the start of the run, and then rapidly returned toward prestress values. Urinary levels were markedly higher than plasma levels, reflecting to some extent the very rapid half-life of the molecule. While conditioned athletes had measurable IL-6 in the urine, normal volunteers and unconditioned athletes did not.

The authors report a similar pattern with TNF-α (Sprenger et al., 1992). This is, in fact, one of the few published studies able to document routinely the presence of TNF-α in the urine. But the same sort of phenomenon is seen as above. TNF-α was detected in the urine of these conditioned athletes before the 20-km run, levels peaked very quickly after this, and then returned to normal. These levels of TNF-α and IL-6 in the urine are well within the range of commercial enzyme-linked immunoabsorption assays (ELISAs), so it is relatively easy to purchase an ELISA kit and measure levels in unconcentrated urine samples.

Another study of military relevance is one by Peter Stein and colleagues at the University of Medicine and Dentistry of New Jersey. These authors looked at why astronauts lose weight during spaceflight and whether it is a manifestation of a nonspecific inflammatory response. Some of these data have been published (Stein and Schluter, 1994), while the remainder are currently in preparation. To determine if urinary cytokine measurements in a setting like this would be helpful to explain some of the weight loss and immunological changes that occur during spaceflight, 24-h urine collections were obtained for 7 days preflight, during the spaceflight, and for 7 days postflight to ascertain whether differences in the urinary excretion of cytokines occurred during spaceflight and whether they would provide some insight into the metabolic changes that were occurring. During spaceflight, there was an acute phase response, indicated by increased fibrinogen synthesis. In addition, there was a remanifestation of this acute-phase response on the first recovery day after return to Earth.

Stein and Schluter (1994) showed that IL-6 excretion increased on the first flight day, and elevations in IL-6 levels corresponded very well to increases in fibrinogen synthesis during that period. This is not unexpected considering that IL-6 is thought to be a primary inducer of fibrinogen synthesis. Thereafter, levels returned to baseline (preflight) values. However, a very interesting phenomenon was seen next. As the astronauts recovered from their spaceflight and the effect of microgravity after reentry and readjusted to normal gravitational loads, there was a progressive increase in the urinary excretion of IL-6. During this recovery period, after days of microgravity (in space), the astronauts often complained of leg pain and weakness in all load-bearing muscles. This secondary increase in cytokine appearance may be due to some direct muscle injury associated with reconditioning to full gravity.

Urinary excretion of IL-1ra, p55, and p75 showed a similar pattern, with the overall profile being similar to that of IL-6. Urinary levels are again elevated on the first flight day and during the postflight recovery period.

Further evidence that urinary cytokine measurements may be used to grade the severity of the inflammatory response can be found in the results of a study that was performed by the author in collaboration with Shogo Yoshido at Kurume University (Unpublished manuscript, Department of Surgery, Kurume, Japan, 1996). Postoperative urinary cytokine levels were measured in patients undergoing either esophagectomy, which is a relatively severe inflammatory stimulus, or partial gastrectomy, which is a less severe, although still considerable, inflammatory insult. Urinary IL-6, p75, and IL-1ra excretion were significantly higher in patients undergoing esophagectomy, corresponding to the magnitude of surgical injury. The response to gastrectomy was more modest.

AUTHOR'S CONCLUSIONS

In conclusion, plasma TNF-α and IL-1 are not reliable indicators of inflammation. Elevated levels of these cytokines in septic patients, beyond a certain threshold value (about 500 pg/ml), generally are associated with adverse septic events (Waage et al., 1989). However, increased plasma concentrations of the shed TNF receptors, shed IL-1 receptor, or IL-1 receptor antagonist generally are more indicative of a local inflammatory response and can be used, with some reliability, as markers of local TNF-α and IL-1 production.

Plasma IL-6 levels, in contrast, appear to be elevated in a large number of inflammatory processes, and they seem to correlate with physiologic parameters. Urinary TNF-α and IL-1 levels are increased after eccentric exercise but cannot be detected regularly in the circulation or in the urine of a large number of patients. Conversely, urinary IL-6, IL-1ra, p55, and p75 are increased reproducibly under the same conditions.

Finally, plasma and urinary measures of IL-6, IL-1ra, and the shed TNF receptors can be used to detect the presence of metabolic stress. The urine measurements are extremely helpful in avoiding an invasive procedure and can, to some extent, be normalized for random spot collections. For example, a urinary creatinine level may be measured at the same time to achieve some level of normalization for total daily output. In contrast, plasma and urinary measures of TNF-α and IL-1 are less likely to provide meaningful information.

REFERENCES

Beisel, W.R.
    1975   Metabolic response to infection. Annu. Rev. Med. 26:9–20.
    1977   Magnitude of the host nutritional responses to infection. Am. J. Clin. Nutr. 30:1236–1247.
    1980   Endogenous pyrogen physiology. Physiologist 23:38–42.
Beutler, B., and A. Cerami
    1986   Cachectin and tumour necrosis factor as two sides of the same biological coin. Nature 320:584–588.
Beutler, B., N. Krochin, I.W. Milsark, C. Luedke, and A. Cerami
    1986   Control of cachectin (tumor necrosis factor) synthesis: Mechanisms of endotoxin resistance. Science 232:977–980.
Calandra, T., J. Gerain, D. Heumann, J.D. Baumgartner, and M.P. Glauser
    1991   High circulating levels of interleukin-6 in patients with septic shock: Evolution during sepsis, prognostic value, and interplay with other cytokines. The Swiss-Dutch J5 Immunoglobulin Study Group. Am. J. Med. 91:23–29.

Colotta, F., F. Re, M. Muzio, R. Bertini, N. Polentarutti, M. Sironi, J.G. Giri, S.K. Dower, J.E. Sims, and A. Mantovani
  1993   Interleukin-1 type II receptor: A decoy target for IL-1 that is regulated by IL-4. Science 261:472–475.
Damas, P., D. Ledoux, M. Nys, Y. Vrindts, D. De Groote, P. Franchimont, and M. Lamy
  1992   Cytokine serum level during severe sepsis in human IL-6 as a marker of severity. Ann. Surg. 215:356–362.
Dinarello, C.A.
  1994   The biological properties of interleukin-1. Eur. Cytokine Netw. 5:517–531.
Dinarello, C.A., and S.M. Wolff
  1993   The role of interleukin-1 in disease. N. Engl. J. Med. 326:106–113.
Engelberts, I., S. Stephens, G.J. Francot, C.J. van der Linden, and W.A. Buurman
  1991   Evidence for different effects of soluble TNF-receptors on various TNF measurements in human biological fluids [letter; comment]. Lancet 338:515–516.
Fischer, E., K.J. Van Zee, M.A. Marano, C.S. Rock, J.S. Kenney, D.D. Poutsiaka, C.A. Dinarello, S.F. Lowry, and L.L. Moldawer
  1992   Interleukin-1 receptor antagonist circulates in experimental inflammation and in human disease. Blood 79:2196–2200.
Fong, Y., L.L. Moldawer, G.T. Shires, and S.F. Lowry
  1990a   The biologic characteristics of cytokines and their implication in surgical injury. Surg. Gynecol. Obstet. 170:363–378.
Fong, Y.M., M.A. Marano, L.L. Moldawer, H. Wei, S.E. Calvano, J.S. Kenney, A.C. Allison, A. Cerami, G.T. Shires, and S.F. Lowry
  1990b   The acute splanchnic and peripheral tissue metabolic response to endotoxin in humans. J. Clin. Invest. 85:1896–1904.
Frieling, J.T.M., M. Van Deuren, J. Wijdenes, J.W.M. Van der Meer, C. Clement, C.J. van der Linden, and R.W. Sauerwein
  1995   Circulating interleukin-6 receptor in patients with sepsis syndrome. J. Infect. Dis. 171:469–472.
Giri, J.G., J. Wells, S.K. Dower, C.E. McCall, R.N. Guzman, J. Slack, T.A. Bird, K. Shanebeck, K. Grabstein, J.E. Sims, and M.R. Alderson
  1994   Elevated levels of shed type II IL-1 receptor in sepsis. Potential role for type II receptor regulation of IL-1 responses. J. Immunol. 153:5802–5809.
Hannum, C.H., C.J. Wilcox, W.P. Arend, F.G. Joslin, D.J. Dripps, P.L. Heimdal, L.G. Armes, A. Sommer, S.P. Eisenberg, and R.C. Thompson
  1990   Interleukin-1 receptor antagonist activity of a human interleukin-1 inhibitor. Nature 343:336–340.
Hesse, D.G., K.J. Tracey, Y. Fong, K.R. Manogue, M.A. Palladino, Jr., A. Cerami, G.T. Shires, and S.F. Lowry
  1988   Cytokine appearance in human endotoxemia and primate bacteremia. Surg. Gynecol. Obstet. 166:147–153.
Kampschmidt, R.F.
  1983   Infection, inflammation, and interleukin-1 (IL-1). Lymphokine Res. 2:97–102.
Kampschmidt, R.F., and L.A. Pulliam
  1975   Stimulation of antimicrobial activity in the rat with leukocytic endogenous mediator. J. Reticuloendothel. Soc. 17:162–169.
Kluger, M.J., D.H. Ringler, and M.R. Anver
  1975   Fever and survival. Science 188:166–168.
LeMay, L.G., A.J. Vander, and M.J. Kluger
  1990   The effects of psychological stress on plasma interleukin-6 activity in rats. Physiol. Behav. 47:957–961.

Marano, M.A., Y. Fong, L.L. Moldawer, H. Wei, S.E. Calvano, K.J. Tracey, P.S. Barie, K. Manogue, A. Cerami, G.T. Shires et al.
  1990   Serum cachectin/tumor necrosis factor in critically ill patients with burns correlates with infection and mortality. Surg. Gynecol. Obstet. 170:32–38.
Michie, H.R., K.R. Manogue, D.R. Spriggs, A. Revhaug, S. O'Dwyer, C.A. Dinarello, A. Cerami, S.M. Wolff, and D.W. Wilmore
  1988   Detection of circulating tumor necrosis factor after endotoxin administration. N. Engl. J. Med. 318:1481–1486.
Moldawer, L.L.
  1994   Biology of proinflammatory cytokines and their antagonists. Crit. Care Med. 22:S3–S7.
Moscovitz, H., F. Shofer, H. Mignott, A. Behrman, and L. Kilpatrick
  1994   Plasma cytokine determinations in emergency department patients as a predictor of bacteremia and infectious disease severity. Crit. Care Med. 22:1102–1107.
Nathan, C., and M. Sporn
  1991   Cytokines in context. J. Cell Biol. 113:981–986.
Powanda, M.C., and W.R. Beisel
  1982   Hypothesis: Leukocyte endogenous mediator/endogenous pyrogen/lymphocyte-activating factor modulates the development of nonspecific and specific immunity and affects nutritional status. Am. J. Clin. Nutr. 35:762–768.
Prieur, A.M., M.T. Kaufmann, C. Griscelli, and J.M. Dayer
  1987   Specific interleukin-1 inhibitor in serum and urine of children with systemic juvenile chronic arthritis. Lancet 2(8570):1240–1242.
Pruitt, J.H., E.M. Copeland, and L.L. Moldawer
  1995   Interleukin-1, interleukin-1 receptor antagonist and interleukin-1 receptors in sepsis, shock and the systemic inflammatory response syndrome. Shock 3:235–251.
Rintala, E., K. Pulkki, J. Mertsola, T. Nevalainen, and J. Nikoskelainen
  1995   Endotoxin, interleukin-6 and phospholipase-A2 as markers of sepsis in patients with hematological malignancies. Scand. J. Infect. Dis. 27:39–43.
Rogy, M.A., S.M. Coyle, H.S. Oldenburg, C.S. Rock, P.S. Barie, K.J. Van Zee, C.G. Smith, L.L. Moldawer, and S.F. Lowry
  1994   Persistently elevated soluble tumor necrosis factor receptor and interleukin-1 receptor antagonist levels in critically ill patients. J. Am. Coll. Surg. 178:132–138.
Seckinger, P., J.W. Lowenthal, K. Williamson, J.M. Dayer, and H.R. MacDonald
  1987a   A urine inhibitor of interleukin-1 activity that blocks ligand binding. J. Immunol. 139:1546–1549.
Seckinger, P., K. Williamson, J.F. Balavoine, B. Mach, G. Mazzei, A. Shaw, and J.M. Dayer
  1987b   A urine inhibitor of interleukin-1 activity affects both interleukin-1 alpha and -1 beta but not tumor necrosis factor alpha. J. Immunol. 139:1541–1545.
Seckinger, P., S. Isaaz, and J.M. Dayer
  1988   A human inhibitor of tumor necrosis factor alpha. J. Exp. Med. 167:1511–1516.
Sprenger, H., C. Jacobs, M. Nain, A.M. Gressner, H. Prinz, W. Wesemann, and D. Gemsa
  1992   Enhanced release of cytokines, interleukin-2 receptors, and neopterin after long-distance running. Clin. Immunol. Immunopathol. 63:188–195.
Stein, T.P., and M.D. Schluter
  1994   Excretion of IL-6 by astronauts during spaceflight. Am. J. Physiol. 266:E448–E452.
Steinmetz, H.T., A. Herbertz, M. Bertram, and V. Diehl
  1995   Increase in interleukin-6 serum level preceding fever in granulocytopenia and correlation with death from sepsis. J. Infect. Dis. 171:225–228.

Suter, P.M., S. Suter, E. Girardin, P. Roux Lombard, G.E. Grau, and J.M. Dayer
 1992 High bronchoalveolar levels of tumor necrosis factor and its inhibitors, interleukin-1, interferon, and elastase, in patients with adult respiratory distress syndrome after trauma, shock, or sepsis. Am. Rev. Respir. Dis. 145:1016–1022.
van der Poll, T., S.E. Calvano, A. Kumar, C.C. Braxton, S.M. Coyle, K. Barbosa, L.L. Moldawer, and S.F. Lowry
 1995 Endotoxin induces downregulation of tumor necrosis factor receptors on circulating monocytes and granulocytes in humans. Blood 86:2754–2759.
Van Zee, K.J., T. Kohno, E. Fischer, C.S. Rock, L.L. Moldawer, and S.F. Lowry
 1992 Tumor necrosis factor soluble receptors circulate during experimental and clinical inflammation and can protect against excessive tumor necrosis factor alpha *in vitro* and *in vivo*. Proc. Natl. Acad. Sci. USA 89:4845–4849.
Waage, A., T. Espevik, and J. Lamvik
 1986 Detection of tumour necrosis factor-like cytotoxicity in serum from patients with septicaemia but not from untreated cancer patients. Scand. J. Immunol. 24:739–743.
Waage, A., A. Halstensen, and T. Espevik
 1987 Association between tumour necrosis factor in serum and fatal outcome in patients with meningococcal disease. Lancet 1(8529):355–357.
Waage, A., P. Brandtzaeg, A. Halstensen, P. Kierulf, and T. Espevik
 1989 The complex pattern of cytokines in serum from patients with meningococcal septic shock. Association between interleukin-6, interleukin-1, and fatal outcome. J. Exp. Med. 169:333–338.
Wannemacher, R.W., Jr., H.L. DuPont, R.S. Pekarek, M.C. Powanda, A. Schwartz, R.B. Hornick, and W.R. Beisel
 1972 An endogenous mediator of depression of amino acids and trace metals in serum during typhoid fever. J. Infect. Dis. 126:77–86.

DISCUSSION

DOUGLAS WILMORE: That was a super review. I have a couple of practical questions that relate to application. You alluded to the ability to collect urine, and the issue is raised, in the military context, of people losing sweat and water by other routes, having diarrhea, or maybe not drinking as much water. I was looking at your y axes, body weight, osmolality in urine, and things like that.

Are you sure some of these measurements are not the result of urinary concentration or are not amplified because of urinary concentration? And what are some of the practical guidelines that you can give to people?

LYLE MOLDAWER: You have hit all the technical requisites for the utility of this measurement. I can tell you that the astronauts have been very well described, in that renal function is within 85 percent of normal limits during spaceflight, but that cannot explain the changes that are seen. You are correct in stating that major perturbations in renal function will affect these measurements.

We know, for example, that p55, p75, and IL-1ra are cleared predominantly by the kidney, so if there is significant renal dysfunction it will throw the validity of these measurements into question. Now, as for hydration, per se, in the

Sprenger article (Sprenger et al., 1992), they normalized for changes in the osmolality of the urine. If you look at the caveat that they discuss in the article, it really does not change the direction or the magnitude of the response.

I think if you recognize the fact that these urinary measurements are susceptible to those errors and you can incorporate that into those estimates of renal function and hydration, then they can be of value. Of course, the presence of any renal or bladder infection will invalidate the use of urine measurements for systemic production.

Sweat and saliva are other issues. Unfortunately, my feeling or bias is, and I may be corrected by people in the audience, that these secretions are from individual body compartments and are less likely to represent well-mixed whole-body pools. I think what you find is that, in burn blister fluid, cytokines are produced by keratinocytes in that local microenvironment. Whereas the stable isotope people can use saliva or sweat, you probably cannot use those compartments for cytokine measurement, because they are going to represent the cell population that produces those mediators.

DOUGLAS WILMORE: To continue this discussion, one of the things that might be very helpful, particularly in the field, if we could extrapolate it to the field, would be to measure military personnel and determine whether, in fact, they had some inflammatory component or whether it was sleep deprivation and underfeeding or something like that. Would a urinary analysis allow a sort of off-on determination, a yes-no determination, not necessarily quantitative but just "it is there or it is not there"?

LYLE MOLDAWER: I think you probably are close. There are two amazing points. One is that you do not need an infection or a tissue injury to induce these cytokines. What the Sprenger article shows and what the NASA data show—and Matt Kluger has shown this before (LeMay et al., 1990)—is that psychological stress will induce some manifestation of a proinflammatory cytokine response.

So yes, and if you read the Sprenger article, what was shown was that if you are a conditioned athlete, urinary cytokines can be measured. Unless we have an infection of some sort or some psychological stress (which is common in our field since much of our time is spent writing grant proposals), you and I do not normally exhibit the presence of urinary cytokines, although we do excrete basal quantities of cytokine inhibitors, such as IL-1ra, p55, and p75.

When I got the letter from Dr. [Bernadette] Marriott, I thought, gee, why are cytokines involved in military performance? Then I started reading these articles, and now I think it is an untouched area. The potential is there, whether the data go with the hypothesis and the theory.

DOUGLAS WILMORE: A final question. C-reactive protein[2] pretty much mirrors IL-6 and may be a much easier assay. Does it show up in the urine?

LYLE MOLDAWER: That I do not know, but you have hit on a key issue, which is that these are nonspecific indicators of inflammation. Erythrocyte sedimentation rate may be adequate. Nobody has done the sensitivity-specificity assays that are required to determine the validity of these techniques.

ROBERT NESHEIM: I think what I would like to do is move on because we do have time for discussion after the other two presentations here. It may be that all of this will come together a little bit better, so if we could do that, I would appreciate it.

LYLE MOLDAWER: Just a quick take-home message, which is that urinary cytokine measurements really are an untapped resource. We have focused predominantly on blood and tissue measurements.

---

[2] A nonspecific antibody to the C-protein of pneumococcus that is present in the serum of some individuals with inflammatory autoimmune or neoplastic disease.

Emerging Technologies for Nutrition Research, 1997
Pp. 431–450. Washington, D.C.
National Academy Press

21

New Approaches to the Study of Abnormal Immune Function

Gabriel Virella,[1] Candace Enockson, and Mariano La Via

INTRODUCTION

While the definition and diagnosis of congenital and acquired immunodeficiencies have been relatively well established for over a decade, the study of more subtle functional alterations of the immune system, which are believed (with more-or-less supporting evidence) to be associated with malnutrition or deficient nutrition, psychological stress, and aging has been slowed down by the lack of well-defined end points (Virella, 1993a). Parameters that are measurable in samples that are easy to obtain, store, and transport and that can be assayed using automated methodologies, providing highly reproducible measurements at low cost, would be ideally suited for the purpose. Unfortunately, few functional parameters related to the immune system fulfill these conditions.

[1] Gabriel Virella, Department of Microbiology and Immunology and Department of Pathology and Laboratory Medicine, Medical University of South Carolina, Charleston, SC 29407

One of the major factors complicating the selection of immune function parameters is the complexity of the immune system and the existence of regulatory networks, which tend to involve most defined cell populations and effector molecules in a complex set of interactions (Figure 21-1) and are difficult to dissect into separate measurable units with well-defined rationales. For example, classically, the effector mechanisms of the immune system are subdivided into two arms, antibody mediated and cell mediated. Antibody synthesis is a property of plasma cells that emerges after the antigenic stimulation of B-lymphocytes. The protective role of antibodies relates to (1) promoting phagocytosis or complement-mediated lysis or microorganisms and (2) blocking the interaction of microorganisms or their toxic products with their respective receptors, thus avoiding infection or the pathogenic consequences of toxin re-

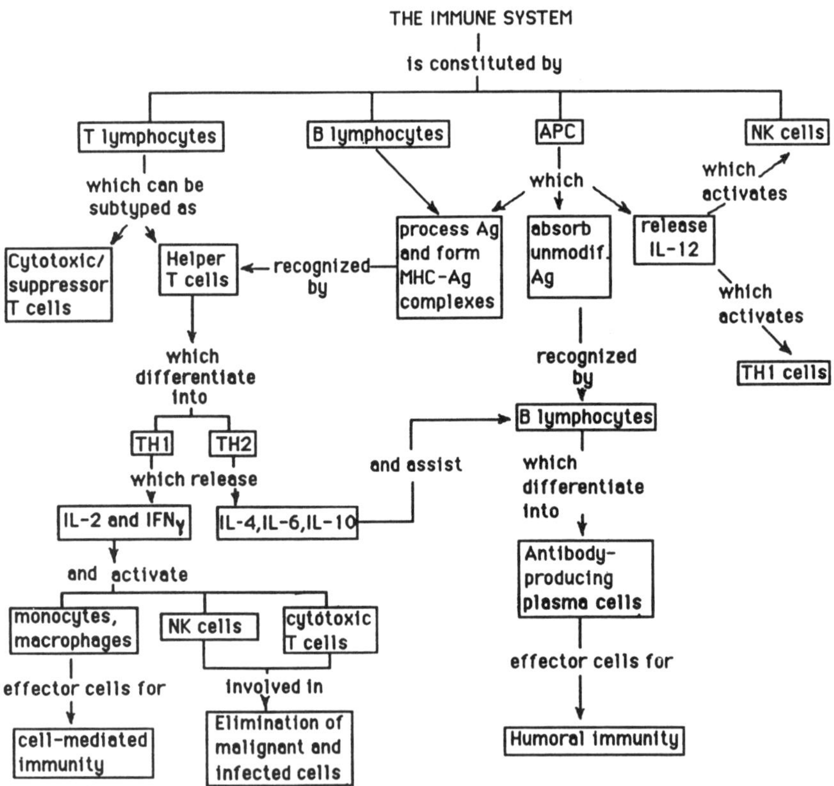

FIGURE 21-1 A simplified diagram of the main components and interactions of the human immune system. Ag, antigen; APC, antigen-presenting cell; IFNγ, interferon gamma; IL, interleukin; MHC, major histocompatability; NK, natural killer; TH1, T-helper 1 cell. SOURCE: Adapted from Virella (in press).

lease. Cell-mediated immunity is most important for the elimination of intracellular microorganisms. This can be achieved by (1) activating the intrinsic antimicrobial mechanisms of the infected cells and (2) causing the death of the infected cells (cytotoxicity, mediated primarily by CD8+ lymphocytes and natural killer [NK] cells) (Virella, 1993b). However, the direct protective effects of antibodies are limited to blocking the absorption or penetration of infective agents or of their exotoxins to the respective receptors and targets (Virella, 1993c). Other anti-infectious mechanisms primarily dependent on the synthesis of antibodies require the cooperation of other humoral systems—such as the complement system (a complex of 11 plasma proteins that interact to mediate several functions of the inflammatory response)—or of cells able to recognize target-bound antibodies through membrane Fc receptors (cell membrane receptors that interact with the terminal domains of the heavy-chain constant regions of immunoglobulin molecules), and promote the destruction of those targets (Virella, 1993c). The humoral response itself cannot be triggered without the assistance of helper T-cells and antigen-presenting cells, such as macrophages (Virella, 1993d). To add to all these problems is the fact that a great deal of uncertainty remains regarding to what extent measurements made with circulating lymphocytes or assays of circulating cytokines reflect the true physiological conditions that exist at the level of a lymphoid organ engaged in the initial stages of an active immune response.

These questions may remain unanswered for some time, but this should not stand in the way of continuing efforts to apply basic knowledge to the definition of end points that may help define subtle abnormalities of the immune system. These abnormalities are not expected to be of the magnitude associated with full-fledged immune deficiencies and may not appear to be significant by themselves. However, even relatively minor functional abnormalities are likely to play an important role as cofactors determining poor resistance to infections and malignancies.

EVALUATION OF HUMORAL IMMUNE RESPONSES

Measurement of Serum Immunoglobulin Concentrations and Antibody Levels

Humoral immune responses are the easiest and cheapest to assess, particularly when serum or secretory immunoglobulins are the parameters being measured. Serum is easy to obtain, store, and ship, and immunoglobulin levels can be measured with great accuracy using automated techniques. Thus, an immunoglobulin assay would fulfill all criteria for an ideal parameter, adequate even for field studies.

On the negative side is the exhaustive documentation of patients with normal immunoglobulin levels who fail to mount specific responses against infectious agents and are therefore classified as functionally immunocompromised

(Virella, 1993a, e; Virella and Hyman, 1991). It was a considerable surprise to researchers, in a study that was conducted on the effects of dietary fish oil supplementation in a group of healthy normal individuals, when they found that changes in serum immunoglobulin levels were the most reproducible parameter in the assessment of humoral immunity (Virella et al., 1991; Unpublished data, G. Virella, Medical University of South Carolina, Charleston, S.C., 1994). As shown in Figures 21-2 to 21-4, there was a significant reduction in the serum levels of the three major immunoglobulin classes at the end of 6 weeks of fish oil supplementation (10 g/d), which was not seen in controls who received an identical dose of olive oil. All levels measured in the participating volunteers were within the normal ranges for the respective immunoglobulin levels at all time points, and the differences between the baseline levels of volunteers receiving fish oil and those receiving olive oil also were nonsignificant due to the large individual variations in serum immunoglobulin levels. However, there was considerably less variability in any given subject when followed longitudinally. The techniques for immunoglobulin quantitation are highly reproducible, and the variations related to the technique virtually can be eliminated if all samples can be assayed on the same run. Under these circumstances, relatively small differences associated with fish oil ingestion reached statistical significance when paired analysis was performed.

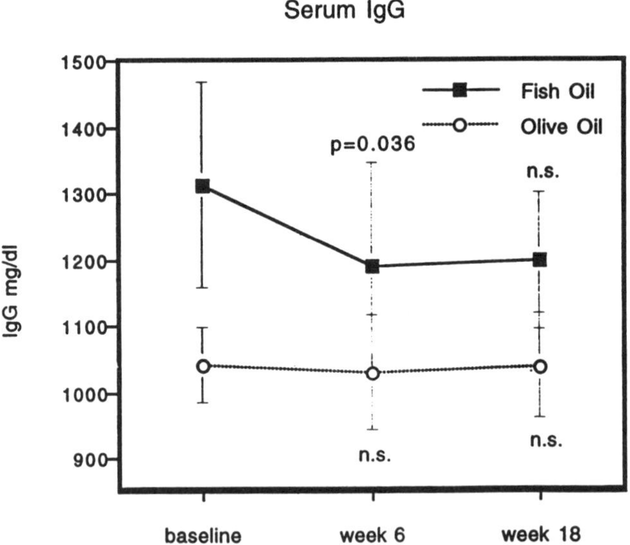

FIGURE 21-2 Longitudinal evolution of serum IgG levels in two groups of human volunteers, one whose diet was supplemented with fish oil ($n = 7$) and the other whose diet was supplemented with olive oil ($n = 6$). Statistical analysis was performed by the paired t-test, comparing week 6 and week 18 with baseline values.

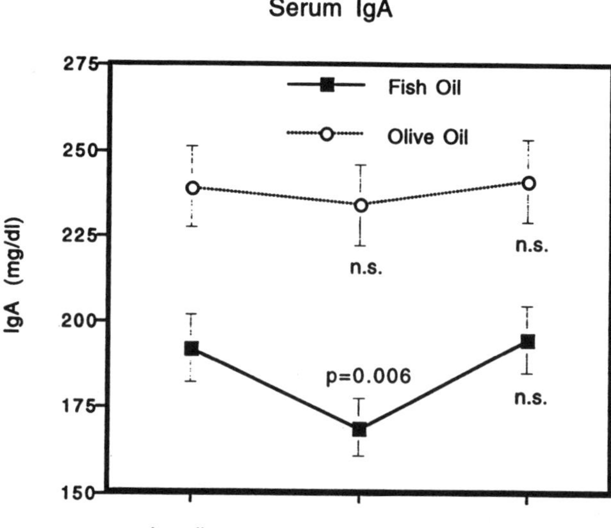

FIGURE 21-3 Longitudinal evolution of serum IgA levels in two groups of human volunteers, one whose diet was supplemented with fish oil ($n = 7$) and the other whose diet was supplemented with olive oil ($n = 6$). Statistical analysis was performed by the paired t-test, comparing week 6 and week 18 with baseline values.

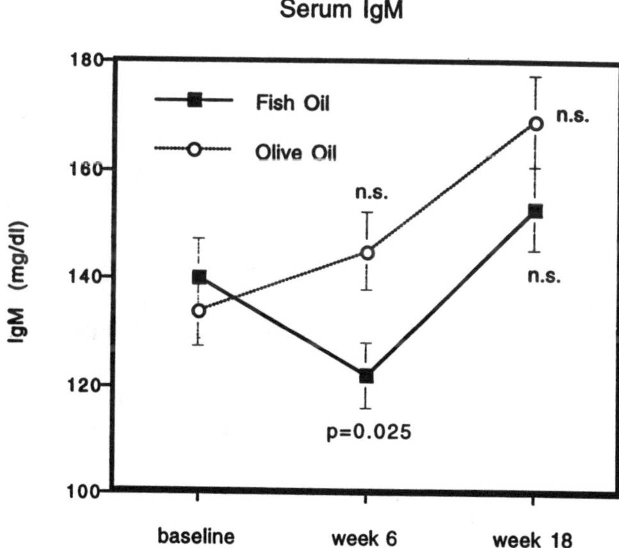

FIGURE 21-4 Longitudinal evolution of serum IgM levels in two groups of human volunteers, one whose diet was supplemented with fish oil ($n = 7$) and the other whose diet was supplemented with olive oil ($n = 6$). Statistical analysis was performed by the paired t-test, comparing week 6 and week 18 with baseline values.

When the ability to mount an immune response is evaluated, two approaches are possible. One is to study the response to an antigen that is unlikely to have been encountered previously by the subject (primary response). The other is to study the recall response to an antigen that has been experienced previously by the subject (secondary, recall, or anamnestic response). Studies in leukemia patients following bone marrow transplant have demonstrated that patients with normal immunoglobulin levels may not be able to mount either primary or secondary immune responses (Virella, 1993e; Virella and Hyman, 1991). Thus, it appears that the measurement of a specific antibody immune response should be a more sensitive end point for the assessment of functional impairment of the immune system. However, this approach also has some drawbacks. To test for a primary immune response, it is necessary to choose an antigen that is not likely to have been encountered previously by the individual, and this trivial aspect can become extremely frustrating because of previous immunizations, inapparent infections, and cross-reactions (particularly significant when polysaccharide antigens are considered as candidates for this type of study). To this day, the best candidate antigen to study the primary immune response is a phage (øX174), which has been used successfully in studies of both primary and secondary immunodeficiencies (Ochs et al., 1993; Virella, 1993e). The disadvantages of bacteriophage immunization are at least two-fold: the antigen is not easily accessible in a form approved for human use, and the assay of antibodies relies on a neutralization technique that is performed only in a few select laboratories.

Secondary immune responses to antigens, such as tetanus toxoid, are easy to assay with reproducible techniques, although these are not fully automated. The assays are carried out in serum samples collected before and after immunization. These assays are easy to apply to field studies. One aspect that needs to be considered is that, by its own dynamic nature, the response to immunization is not a parameter that can be repeatedly measured. Thus, any attempt to use an active immune response as an end point requires a proper cross-sectional design in which the response will be compared in two groups, one in which the variable with possible influence on the immune response will be applied and a control group. The timing of the immunization also needs to be considered very carefully to maximize the probabilities of observing an effect that is of sufficient magnitude so as not to be obliterated by individual variations. In addition, there are excellent data collected during the National Health and Nutrition Examination Survey III concerning the distribution of antibody titers in the general population (Gergen et al., 1995); these could allow a comparison of levels of preformed antibody or a comparison of the magnitude of response to a toxoid booster in individuals exposed to a stressor, relative to an age- and gender-matched cohort of control individuals. Of course, these participants would need to be matched for the time period elapsed since their last tetanus toxoid booster.

On the minus side, the high degree of individual variability observed in the response of humans to any kind of immunization is a significant obstacle to the use of active immune responses as parameters in studies concerned with abnormalities in immunoregulation. In the groups of healthy volunteers in which the response to immunization with tetanus toxoid has been studied, there always have been subjects who fail to respond (Virella et al., 1978, 1991), and the frequency of nonresponders seems to be relatively high, estimated between 1 and 5 percent. Also, when the studied individuals have preimmunization antibody levels in excess of 1.5 U/mL (10-fold over the lower limit of protection), there is a good chance that immunization may trigger suppressor circuits, and a reduction in the concentration of serum antitetanus antibodies may be observed after a booster (Virella and Hyman, 1991; Virella et al., 1978). There is no indication that this negative response represents a risk for those who exhibit it, but it is certainly a significant confounding factor. Probably as a consequence of all these variables, the measurement of the response to a tetanus toxoid booster in volunteers receiving fish oil or olive oil dietary supplementation failed to reveal any significant difference (Figure 21-5), while the same group had revealed a significant decline in immunoglobulin levels in association with fish oil supplementation.

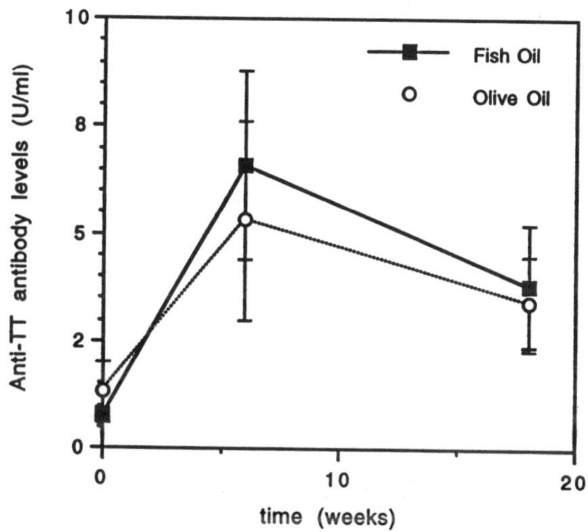

FIGURE 21-5 Longitudinal evolution of serum antitetanus toxoid antibody levels in two groups of human volunteers, one whose diet was supplemented with fish oil and the other whose diet was supplemented with olive oil. The increase in antibody concentration from baseline to week 6 was significant by the Mann-Whitney test for both groups of volunteers ($p < 0.05$), but there was no statistically significant difference between the levels of antibody reached at weeks 6 and 18 between the two groups.

Study of Humoral Immune Responses Elicited *In Vitro*

In clinical studies of patients with an unexpectedly high frequency of infectious episodes, it has been observed that a lack of *in vitro* immunoglobulin synthesis stimulation may be the only abnormality detected. However, in studies of the effects of dietary supplementation with fish oil, consistent differences could not be detected using *in vitro* immunoglobulin or antibody synthesis as end points (Virella et al., 1991). Thus, this approach may not be sensitive enough to detect low-level abnormalities in a heterogeneous population with a high degree of variability in the magnitude of their immune responses. Two additional problems with this approach are, first, the need for viable cells, which complicates sample collection, storage, and transport, and second, the nature of the assays, which are entirely manual and require specialized and experienced personnel. These factors result in higher cost and suboptimal reproducibility.

Attempts to simplify the protocols for study of mitogenic responses by using whole blood instead of mononuclear cells have the drawback of adding an additional variable—the red cells. Studies have demonstrated that adding autologous red cells to purified mononuclear cells enhances B-cell responses (Rugeles et al., 1987), probably through the delivery of costimulating signals to T-cells through cell-cell interactions that are mediated by a variety of complementary membrane molecules, including the CD2 molecule expressed by T-lymphocytes and CD58 (leukocyte function antigen-3 [LFA-3]) expressed by most nucleated cells as well as by human erythrocytes (Virella et al., 1988). The lymphocyte-erythrocyte ratio is critically important for the elicitation of this effect, and this ratio cannot be maintained absolutely constant if unfractionated blood is used in mitogenic stimulation studies. An additional problem with whole blood is that it contains plasma inhibitory compounds that interfere with cytokine activity, and these compounds are likely to vary from individual to individual.

EVALUATION OF CELL-MEDIATED IMMUNE FUNCTION

Lymphocyte Populations and Subpopulations

The parallel development of the monoclonal antibody and flow cytometry techniques has resulted in the definition of a large number of lymphocyte membrane antigens, allowing for the easy enumeration of lymphocyte subpopulations in the peripheral blood. The sample requirements are easy to fulfill—a few milliliters of unclotted blood are usually sufficient—and the techniques are semiautomated and relatively easy to perform, although both reagents and equipment are expensive and specialized personnel are essential. In spite of these limitations, the enumeration of lymphocyte subpopulations is very amenable to studies in the field.

However, the enumeration of lymphocyte subpopulations has not fulfilled the overoptimistic expectations that were raised by the studies reporting the identification of membrane markers and the definition of functional subsets based on membrane marker phenotypes. Part of the problem results from the less-than-perfect correlation between membrane markers and function. To illustrate the point, CD4+ T-cells, defined as "helper" by their phenotype, actually can have cytotoxic functions (Rahelu et al., 1993; Smyth and Ortaldo, 1993). "Help" can be mediated by CD4− cells (Locksley et al., 1993), and the clinical significance of CD4-mediated "help" has been put to test by the finding by several groups of a less-than-perfect correlation between CD4 cell counts and clinical evolution of HIV-infected patients (Dormont, 1994; Keet et al., 1994; MAPW, 1994). The extensive data concerning CD4 counts in HIV-AIDS also have illustrated a second problem with the enumeration of T-lymphocyte subpopulations, which is the variability of these subpopulations (Hughes et al., 1994). Single, isolated enumerations of CD4+ lymphocytes may have very little meaning.

Recently, the reports of the predominant role played by T-helper 1 (Th1) cells in the activation of cell-mediated immune processes, including macrophage activation (Romagnani, 1991), and the possible significance of imbalances in the activity of helper T-lymphocytes with Th1 or Th2 cytokine release patterns in the progression of HIV-infected individuals toward full-blown AIDS (Clerici and Shearer, 1993) have raised considerable interest in their assessment. Most investigators rely on the characterization of the interleukin-release pattern of T-cell clones differentiated from patients' peripheral blood lymphocytes (Romagnani, 1991; van der Pouw-Kraan et al., 1993), as well as on the assay of interleukins released by peripheral blood lymphocytes *in vitro*, spontaneously and after mitogenic stimulation (Clerici et al., 1993; van der Pouw-Kraan et al., 1993). Some reports of attempts to define membrane markers for Th1 and Th2 cells have been published recently. CD4+ and CD56+ appear to define the Th1 subpopulation (Barnaba et al., 1994) while CD4+, CD27−, and CD30+ define the Th2 subpopulation (Del Prete et al., 1995; Elson et al., 1994). Whether these preliminary reports will hold and whether the enumeration of cells with these phenotypes will be informative about the state of immune responsiveness of a given individual remain to be seen. It must be emphasized that no one can be sure about the meaning of changes in the distribution of T-lymphocyte subpopulations in the peripheral blood. It is likely that the most significant changes in lymphocyte subpopulations occur in lymphoid tissues, and sampling peripheral blood may be irrelevant.

In studies conducted in this laboratory on the effects of fish-oil dietary supplementation on lymphocyte distribution, consistent changes in lymphocyte subpopulations could not be identified, even when two-color analysis was performed to define activated subpopulations through the coexpression of CD25 (IL-2 receptor) and other markers. Others have reported changes of the NK subpopulation in association with stress and with malnutrition in cancer patients

(Schedlowski et al., 1992; Sieber et al., 1992; Villa et al., 1991). The significance of these findings is diminished by the fact that the biological significance of the NK subpopulation has been established on the basis of data obtained *in vitro*, which have yet to be corroborated by clinical data, such as the description of patients with immunodeficiency clearly related to a lack of NK cells.

Assay of Circulating Cytokines and Soluble Receptors

At the time of writing this review, a total of 15 interleukins, a large number of growth factors and cytokines, and three types of interferons have been characterized. All of them seem to play some role in the activation and/or differentiation of different types of immune cells. However, some of these soluble molecules appear to have more important roles than others: IL-1β, IL-8, and TNF-α predominantly are involved in inflammatory reactions, particularly in septic shock (Goust and Bierer, 1993). IL-12 plays a significant role in the initial activation of NK cells and helper T-cells and in the differentiation of the Th1 subpopulation, which produces large amounts of IL-2 and interferon-γ (Manetti, 1993). IL-2 plays a significant role in the expansion of the Th1 subpopulation through autocrine and paracrine circuits and, together with IL-12 and interferon-γ, activates NK cells (Goust and Bierer, 1993). Interferon-γ, in turn, activates macrophages (Virella, 1993c). Th2 cells, which mainly are involved in assisting the activation of B-lymphocytes, secrete, among others, IL-4, which activates B-cells, particularly those producing IgE (Gascan et al., 1991; Goust and Bierer, 1993) and IL-10, which downregulates Th1 cells (Fiorentino et al., 1991). One additional interleukin with major biological significance is IL-8, which is a chemotactic factor for neutrophils and lymphocytes (Ribeiro, 1994). It also has been demonstrated that upon activation, several membrane molecules are shed by lymphocytes, including IL-2 receptors (Bock et al., 1994; Campen et al., 1988) and the CD4 and CD8 molecules (Kurane et al., 1991). Some of those cytokines and receptors have been found in relatively large concentrations in the urine (Bock et al., 1994, Newstead et al., 1993).

All the above-mentioned cytokines and shed molecules can be assayed by enzyme-linked immunoabsorption (ELISA), and providing that samples are properly collected, stored, and shipped, field studies have become relatively simple. One significant problem is the cost of the assays, usually ranging from $5 to $10 per sample per cytokine or soluble molecule for reagents, plus the costs of personnel. Also, assays performed in serum tend to be less reproducible than those performed in cell culture supernatants, perhaps because of the presence of soluble molecules in circulation, which may interfere with the assays. Such interfering molecules are apparently less of a problem in urine. Assays of urinary cytokines have dual advantages: ease of sample collection and accuracy of determination. The counterpoint is the variation that may be associated with diuresis, for which reason it is necessary either to collect 24-h urine or to correct the data by expressing them as a function of urine osmolarity or some other parameter that may reflect variations in urinary volume.

Information is still somewhat limited concerning the possibility of finding significant correlations between the levels of circulating cytokines or soluble membrane receptors-markers and the status of the immune system. It also can be argued that the circulating cytokines are, in general, meaningless by-products, only a very pale reflection of the most significant lymphokine traffic that happens in lymphoid tissues. Direct interleukin traffic between cooperating cells probably involves intimate contact and even membrane fusion (Goust and Bierer, 1993). In spite of these questions, and until experimental data prove otherwise, the assay of circulating or urinary levels of selected lymphokines and lymphokine receptors, with their relatively well-established physiological roles, appears as one of the most promising avenues for functional studies of the immune system.

In Vitro Assays of Lymphocyte Function

The *in vitro* assays of lymphocyte function can be based on the incorporation of DNA precursors, expression of antigenic or mitogenic activation markers, release of lymphokines, suppression of B- or T-cell activation, and cytotoxicity (Virella et al., 1993). All the corresponding assays have the same basic problem, which is the requirement for freshly isolated cells, as discussed earlier in the chapter in the section on *in vitro* tests for B-cell function.

Mitogenic Assays

The response to mitogenic stimulation is the classic test used to evaluate lymphocyte responsiveness. In the most widely used format, the tests require incubation of mononuclear cells in the presence of mitogens for 3 days, at which time tritiated thymidine is added to the culture, and its incorporation into nascent DNA is determined 6 to 8 hours later. Other techniques have been developed that avoid the use of radioisotopes but require equally expensive technologies, such as sensitive colorimeters or flow cytometers (Huong et al., 1991; Kuhn et al., 1995). So in the end, there are few technological solutions that would allow simplification of these assays to the point of making them easy to perform in the field. Other problems faced when performing these assays are difficulties in reproducibility (changes in medium composition, source or batch of animal serum or serum replacements; incubation conditions; isolation methodology; anticoagulants; and culture vessels) and relative insensitivity.

In recent years, there has been a trend to replace DNA synthesis by what appear to be more physiological end points—such as IL-2 release or expression of IL-2 receptors—in mitogenic response assays (Virella et al., 1993). The release of IL-2 can be easily and reproducibly measured after 24 hours of incubation with pokeweed mitogen or phytohemagglutinin using standard ELISA methodology. In the authors' experience, it is not unusual to find individuals with normal or even elevated mitogenic indices when release of IL-2 is below normal (Table 21-1), suggesting that the release of IL-2 is a sensitive index of regulatory abnormalities affecting the initial stages of Th1 proliferation and differentiation.

The expression of IL-2 receptors (CD25) also has been found to be a good end point in studies evaluating the effects of stress and psychological depression on the immune system (La Via et al., 1996). As illustrated in Figure 21-6, the expression of CD25 after mitogenic stimulation was depressed significantly in a group of students tested immediately after taking their medical board examinations (Unpublished manuscript, M. F. La Via, Medical University of South Carolina, Charleston, S.C., 1994). These students also had a considerably higher

TABLE 21-1 Comparative Results of Mitogenic Responses and IL-2 Assay in Supernatants of Mitogen-Stimulated Mononuclear Cells[*]

		Mitogenic Response[†]		IL-2 Release	
Subject	Diagnosis	PHA[‡]	PWM[§]	PHA[‖]	PWM[§]
	Normal controls	33–160[*]	13–40[*]	8–60[*#]	9–39[*]
A	Immunodeficiency	**619**	**108**	7	*5*
B	BM transplant	**367**	**104**	19	*< 3*
C	BM transplant	88	**58**	*< 3*	*< 3*
D	BM transplant	138	16	7	*< 3*
E	BM transplant	121	18	*3*	*3*
F	BM transplant	151	34	10	*6*
G	Unknown	*31*	25	*< 3*	not done
H	Healthy volunteer	151	37	16	*6*

NOTE: PHA, phytohemagglutinin; PWM, pokeweed mitogen; BM, bone marrow.

[*] Values above the upper limit of normality are shown in bold; values below the lower limit of normality are shown in italics.

[†] Stimulation index [(cpm stimulated/cpm baseline) × 100].

[‡] 10 µg/ml.

[§] 1:200 dilution.

[‖] 2 µg/ml.

[#] Values expressed in U/ml.

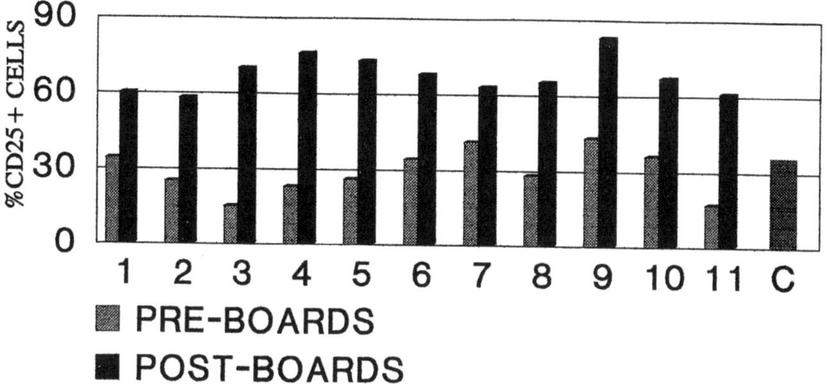

FIGURE 21-6 Comparison of the percentage of lymphocytes from 11 medical students and 10 control subjects expressing the CD25+ after 72 hours of culture in the presence of anti-CD3. The students were studied during the week before medical board examinations (cross-hatched bars) and 6 weeks after boards (black bars).The bar labeled "C" represents the average value for the 10 controls.

stress index than the respective controls. A similar depression in the percentage of cells expressing CD25 after stimulation with anti-CD3 was observed in patients with generalized anxiety disorder (La Via et al., 1996) and in another group of patients with panic disorder (PD). As shown in Table 21-2, PD patients also had a significantly higher stress intrusion score and a higher frequency of upper respiratory infections (URI) (Personal communication, G. Virella, Medical University of South Carolina, Charleston, 1997). Interestingly, a significant inverse correlation existed between the frequency of URI and CD25 expression. However, this type of study may be difficult to perform because it requires access to a sufficient number of flow cytometers to handle a large volume of samples in a short window of time, so as not to introduce significant errors due to time variations between adding the mitogen and testing for CD25 expression.

Functional Assays

In vitro mitogenic responses to antigenic stimulation using soluble proteins as antigens can be tested using thymidine incorporation as an end point. However, the results are highly variable, depending on the preceding history of exposure to the antigen in question. This variability, combined with the low magnitude of the expected responses makes this approach impractical for cross-sectional studies. A different approach that could yield interesting data would be to compare *in vitro* responses shortly after immunization in two groups of individuals, one exposed to conditions that could interfere with immunity and a

TABLE 21-2 CD25 Expression, Stress Intrusion Score, and Frequency of Upper Respiratory Infections in 19 Panic Disorder Patients and 18 Normal Controls

Variable	Control Group Mean (SD)	PD Group Mean (SD)	*p* Value[*]
% change in CD25+[†]	44.6 (24.4)	12.2 (12.2)	< 0.0005
SIS[‡]	3.7 (2.8)	9.1 (5.0)	0.0010
URI[§]	1.0 (0.6)	1.8 (1.5)	0.040

NOTE: SD, standard deviation; PD, panic disorder; SIS, stress intrusion score; URI, upper respiratory infection.

[*] Calculated by the nonpaired student's t-test.

[†] Percentage change is the difference between the percent of CD25+ cells at day 0 and day 3 after stimulation with anti-CD3 monoclonal antibody.

[‡] Stress intrusion score (La Via et al., 1996; Zilberg et al., 1982).

[§] Number of upper respiratory infections over a 6-mo period.

well-matched control group. Such studies, however, are likely to be affected by individual variations in the immune response (high responders vs. low responders) and may not have a significant advantage over the assay of serum antibodies elicited under similar circumstances, which is considerably simpler to perform.

Functional assays for helper or suppressor activity and cytotoxicity assays, although informative, are rather complex and difficult to standardize. The assay of helper/suppressor activity requires isolation of mononuclear cells and separation of T-cell- and B-cell-enriched populations and cocultures and determination of adequate end points, such as cytokine release or immunoglobulin synthesis. Cytotoxicity assays also involve isolation of lymphocytes or mononuclear cells and preparation of adequate targets. The simplest approach to studying T-cell cytotoxicity involves preparing mixed lymphocyte cultures and adding ^{51}Cr-labeled target cells to the mixed culture after 4 to 5 days of incubation (Virella et al., 1993). This becomes impractical for studies of large groups of individuals. NK-cell activity can be easily measured by exposing adequate targets (such as the K562 cell line) to NK-enriched lymphocyte preparations. A major problem with this assay is the uncertainty that surrounds the physiological role of NK cells, which has been alluded to earlier.

PHAGOCYTIC CELL ASSAYS

Most phagocytic cell function assays are carried out with polymorphonuclear (PMN) leukocytes because of their abundance in the peripheral blood and the relative ease of their isolation. As a rule, peripheral-blood PMN leukocyte preparations are constituted largely by neutrophils, and any functional tests carried out with these preparations are essentially neutrophil function tests. Acquired neutrophil abnormalities are most frequently a consequence of the depletion of this important cell population (acquired agranulocytosis). Rarely, neutrophils may be normal in number, but their function may be impaired. Neutrophil functional abnormalities have been reported in patients with severe trauma (particularly burns) and severe malnutrition (Virella, 1993a) but appear to be rather infrequent in patients with less dramatic insults to the integrity of their defenses. One of the most significant parameters of neutrophil function is the generation of superoxide and other oxygen active radicals (respiratory burst) as a consequence of the ingestion of antibody and/or complement-coated microbes or inert particles. Quantitative methodologies to measure the respiratory burst have been developed by the authors (Virella et al., 1990) and others (Metcalf, 1986, 96–114). Usually they require sophisticated equipment and trained personnel, but more importantly, they require freshly isolated cells and are not easy to adapt to the study of large numbers of individuals. Given the lack of data suggesting that the superoxide burst may be affected by physical or psychological stress, the investment in resources does not appear justified by such unlikely returns.

AUTHORS' CONCLUSIONS AND RECOMMENDATIONS

In spite of the progress that has been made in the basic knowledge of the immune system, there is a considerable gap separating that knowledge from the current methodologic approaches used to test immune abnormalities in human subjects. The choice of adequate end points for prospective studies, aimed at determining the influence of factors such as physical or psychological stress on the immune response, is particularly difficult because of the multiple components involved in a normal immune response. Pragmatic choices have to be based on the availability and reproducibility of techniques and on a good rationale supporting the decision to measure any given parameter. Longitudinal studies of serum immunoglobulin concentrations, measurement of humoral responses to vaccines and boosters, and determination of serum and urinary levels of select cytokines involved in inflammatory processes and immunoregulatory processes (particularly those cytokines that define Th1 vs. Th2 activity) are relatively easy-to-obtain parameters whose measurement can be supported by currently available basic and clinical research data. *In vitro* function assays, such as immunoglobulin synthesis, release of IL-2, or expression of CD25 in response to mitogenic stimulation, also appear to have the potential of revealing abnormalities in immunoregulation when other parameters, such as immunoglobulin levels and distribution of lymphocyte subpopulations in the peripheral blood, are within normal limits. Functional assays are more sophisticated and difficult to scale up for large population studies, but the potential rewards suggested by the authors' small-scale studies suggest that they should not be ruled out unless it is absolutely impossible to devise a protocol in which they could be incorporated.

In conclusion, many variables need to be considered when choosing the parameters to measure immune function in relation to variables such as nutritional factors. In principle, functional assays would be ideal, but practical considerations may preclude their consideration. In that case, the choice of tests should be based on their physiological relevance (e.g., expression of lymphocyte activation markers) or measurements that have been shown to be affected by dietary interventions (e.g., serum immunoglobulin levels).

REFERENCES

Barnaba, V., A. Franco, M. Paroli, R. Benvenuto, G. De Petrillo, V.L. Burgio, I. Santilio, C. Balsano, M.S. Bonavita, and G. Cappelli
   1994   Selective expansion of cytotoxic T lymphocytes with a CD4+CD56+ surface phenotype and a T helper 1 profile of cytokine secretion in the liver of patients clinically infected with hepatitis B virus. J. Immunol. 152:3074–3087.
Bock, G.H., L. Neu, C. Long, L.T. Patterson, S. Korb, J. Gelpi, and D.L. Nelson
   1994   An assessment of serum and urine soluble interleukin-2 receptor concentrations during renal transplant rejection. Am. J. Kidney Dis. 23:421–426.
Campen, D.H., D.A. Horwitz, F.P Quismorio, Jr., G.R. Ehresmann, and W.J. Martin
   1988   Serum levels of interleukin-2 receptor and activity of rheumatic diseases characterized by immune cell activation. Arthritis Rheum. 31:1358–1364.
Clerici, M., and G.M. Shearer
   1993   A Th1-Th2 switch is a critical step in the etiology of HIV infection. Immunol. Today 14:107–111.
Clerici M., F.T. Haki, D.J. Venzon, S. Blatt, C.W. Hendrix, T.A. Wynn, and G.M. Shearer
   1993   Changes in interleukin-2 and interleukin-4 production in asymptomatic, human immunodeficiency virus-seropositive individuals. J. Clin. Invest. 91:759–765.
Del Prete, G., M. De Carli, F. Almerigogna, C.K. Daniel, M.M. D'Elios, G. Zancuoghi, F. Vinante, G. Pizzolo, and S. Romagnani
   1995   Preferential expression of CD30 by human CD4+ T cells producing Th2-type cytokines. FASEB J. 9:81–86.
Dormont, J.
   1994   Future treatment strategies in HIV infection. AIDS 8 (suppl. 3):S31–S33.
Elson, L.H., S. Shaw, R.A. Van Liwer, and T.B. Nutman
   1994   T cell subpopulation phenotypes in filarial infections: CD27 negativity defines a population greatly enriched for Th2 cells. Int. Immunol. 6:1003–1009.
Fiorentino, D.F., A. Zlotnik, P. Vieira, T.R. Mosmann, M. Howard, K.W. Moore, and A. O'Garra
   1991   IL-10 acts on the antigen-presenting cell to inhibit cytokine production by Th1 cells. J. Immunol. 146:3444–3451.
Gascan, H., J.F. Gauchat, M.G. Roncarolo, H. Yssel, H. Spits, and J.E. deVries
   1991   Human B cell clones can be induced to proliferate and to switch to IgE and IgG4 synthesis by interleukin 4 and a signal provided by activated CD4+ T cell clones. J. Exp. Med. 173:747–750.

Gergen, P.J., G.M. McQuillan, M. Kiely, T.M. Ezzati-Rice, R.W. Sutter, and G. Virella
  1995   A population-based serologic survey of immunity to tetanus in the United States. N. Engl. J. Med. 332:761–766.
Goust, J.M., and B. Bierer
  1993   Cell-mediated immunity. Pp. 187–208 in Introduction to Medical Immunology, 3d ed., G. Virella, ed. New York: Marcel Dekker.
Hughes, M.D., D.S. Stein, H.M. Gundacker, F.T. Valentine, J.P. Phair, and P.A. Volberding
  1994   Within-subject variation in CD4 lymphocyte count in asymptomatic human immunodeficiency virus infection: Implications for patient monitoring. J. Infect. Dis. 169:28–36.
Huong, P.L., A.H. Kolk, T.A. Eggelte, C.P. Verstijnen, N. Gilis, and J.T. Hendriks
  1991   Measurement of antigen-specific lymphocyte proliferation using 5-bromo-deoxyuridine incorporation. An easy and low cost alternative to radioactive thymidine incorporation. J. Immunol. Meth. 140:243–248.
Keet, I.P., A. Krol, M. Koot, M.T. Roos, F. de Wolf, F. Miedema, and R.A. Coutinho
  1994   Predictors of disease progression in HIV-infected homosexual men with CD4+ cells 200×10^6/L but free of AIDS-defining clinical disease. AIDS 8:1577–1583.
Kuhn, U., U. Lempertz, J. Knop, and D. Becker
  1995   A new method for phenotyping proliferating cell nuclear antigen positive cells using flow cytometry: Implications for analysis of the immune response *in vivo*. J. Immunol. Methods 179:215–222.
Kurane, I., B.L. Innis, S. Nimmannitya, A. Nisalak, A. Meager, J. Janus, and F.A. Ennis
  1991   Activation of T lymphocytes in dengue virus infections. High levels of soluble interleukin 2 receptor, soluble CD4, soluble CD8, interleukin 2, and interferon-gamma in sera of children with dengue. J. Clin. Invest. 88:1473–1480.
La Via, M.F., J. Munno, R.B. Lydiard, E.A. Workman, J.R. Hubbard, Y. Michel, and E. Pauling
  1996   The influence of stress intrusion on immunodepression in generalized anxiety disorder patients and controls. Psychosom. Med. 58:138–142.
Locksley, R.M., S.L. Reiner, F. Hatam, D.R. Litman, and N. Killeen
  1993   Helper T-cells without CD4: Control of leishmaniasis in CD4-deficient mice. Science 261:1448–1451.
Manetti, R.
  1993   Natural killer cell stimulatory factor (interleukin 12 [IL-12]) induces T helper type 1 (Th1)-specific immune responses and inhibits the development of IL-4-producing Th cells. J. Exp. Med. 177:1199–1204.
MAPW (Multicohort Analysis Project Workshop—Part I)
  1994   Immunologic markers of AIDS progression: Consistency across five HIV-infected cohorts. AIDS 8:911–921.
Metcalf, J.A.
  1986   Laboratory Manual of Neutrophil Function. New York: Raven Press.
Newstead, C.G., W.R. Lamb, P.E. Brenchley, and C.D. Short
  1993   Serum and urine IL-6 and TNF-alpha in renal transplant recipients with graft dysfunction. Transplantation 56:831–835.
Ochs, H.D., S. Nonoyama, Q. Zhu, M. Farrington, and R.J. Wedgwood
  1993   Regulation of antibody responses: The role of complement and adhesion molecules. Clin. Immunol. Immunopathol. 67(suppl. 2):S33–S40.
Rahelu, M., G.T. Williams, D.S. Kumararatne, G.S. Eaton, and J.S. Gaston
  1993   Human CD4+ cytolitic T cells kill antigen-pulsed target T cells by induction of apoptosis. J. Immunol. 150:4856–4866.

Ribeiro, R.A.
  1994 IL-8 causes *in vivo* neutrophil migration by a cell-dependent mechanism. Immunology 73:472–477.
Romagnani, S.
  1991 Type 1 T-helper and Type 2 T-helper cells: Functions, regulation and role in protection and disease. Int. J. Clin. Lab. Res. 21:152–158.
Rugeles, M.T., M. LaVia, J-M. Goust, J.M. Kilpatrick, B. Hyman, and G. Virella
  1987 Autologous RBC potentiate antibody synthesis by unfractionated human mononuclear cell cultures. Scand. J. Immunol. 26:119–127.
Schedlowski, M., R. Jacobs, G. Stratman, S. Richter, A. Hadicke, U. Tewes, T.D. Wagner, and R.E. Schmidt
  1992 Changes in natural killer cells during acute psychological stress. J. Clin. Immunol. 13:119–126.
Sieber, B.J., J. Rodin, L. Larson, S. Ortega, N. Cummings, S. Levy, T. Whiteside, and R. Herberman
  1992 Modulation of human natural killer cell activity by exposure to uncontrollable stress. Brain Behav. Immunol. 6:141–156.
Smyth, M.J., and J.R. Ortaldo
  1993 Mechanisms of cytotoxicty used by human peripheral blood CD4+ and CD8+ T-cell subsets. The role of granule exocytosis. J. Immunol. 151:40–47.
van der Pouw-Kraan, T., R. deJong, and L. Aarden
  1993 Development of human Th1 and Th2 cytokine responses: The cytokine production profile of T cells is dictated by the primary *in vitro* stimulus. Eur. J. Immunol. 23:1–5.
Villa, M.L., E. Ferrario, F. Bergamasco, F. Bozzetti, L. Cozzaglio, and E. Clerici
  1991 Reduced natural killer cell activity and IL-2 production in malnourished cancer patients. Br. J. Cancer 63:1010–1014.
Virella, G., ed.
  1993a Immunodeficiency diseases. Pp. 543–573 in Introduction to Medical Immunology, 3d ed. New York: Marcel Dekker.
  1993b Introduction. Pp. 1–8 in Introduction to Medical Immunology, 3d ed. New York: Marcel Dekker.
  1993c Infections and immunity. Pp. 233–246 in Introduction to Medical Immunology, 3d ed. New York: Marcel Dekker.
  1993d Antigenicity and immune recognition. Pp. 49–70 in Introduction to Medical Immunology, 3d ed. New York: Marcel Dekker.
  1993e Diagnostic evaluation of humoral immunity. Pp. 275–285 in Introduction to Medical Immunology, 3d ed. New York: Marcel Dekker.
Virella, G.
  In Press Introduction to Medical Immunology, 4th ed. New York: Marcel Dekker.
Virella, G., and B. Hyman
  1991 Quantitation of anti-tetanus and anti-diphtheria antibodies by enzymoimmunoassay: Methodology and applications. J. Clin. Lab. Anal. 5:43–48.
Virella, G., H.H. Fudenberg, K.U. Kyong, J.P. Pandey, and R.M. Galbraith
  1978 A practical method for quantitation of antibody responses to tetanus and diphtheria toxoids in normal young children. Zeitschrift fur Immunitatsforschung 155:80–86.
Virella, G., M.T. Rugeles, B. Hyman, M. La Via, J.M. Goust, M. Frankis, and B.E. Bierer
  1988 The interaction of CD2 with its LFA-3 ligand expressed by autologous erythrocytes results in enhancement of B cell responses. Cell. Immunol. 116:308–319.

Virella, G., T. Thompson, and R. Haskill-Stroud
  1990   A new quantitative Nitroblue Tetrazolium Reduction Assay based on kinetic col-
         orimetry. J. Clin. Lab. Anal. 4:86–89.
Virella, G., K. Fourspring, B. Hyman, R. Haskill-Stroud, L. Long, I. Virella, M. LaVia, A.J.
         Gross, and M. Lopes-Virella
  1991   Immunosuppressive effects of fish oil in normal human volunteers: Correlation
         with the *in vitro* effects of eicosapentanoic acid on human lymphocytes. Clin.
         Immunol. Immunopathol. 61:161–176.
Virella, G., C. Patrick, and J.M. Goust
  1993   Diagnostic evaluation of lymphocyte functions and cell-mediated immunity. Pp.
         291–306 in Introduction to Medical Immunology, 3d ed., G. Virella, ed. New
         York: Marcel Dekker.
Zilberg, N.J., D.S. Weiss, and M.J. Horowitz
  1982   Impact of events scale: A cross-validation study and some empirical evidence
         supporting a conceptual model of stress response syndromes. J. Consult. Clin.
         Psychol. 50:407–414.

DISCUSSION

TIM KRAMER: I would like to direct a comment toward your last statement about using whole blood. I am the one who is responsible for those data. I think when we used the whole blood, we set it up for several reasons. One is that we wanted a physiologic response in its natural milieu.

Now, I agree with you, the red blood cell has an interaction with the T lymphocyte in its responsiveness, and that is the way it is *in vivo*.

GABRIEL VIRELLA: Well, except that *in vivo* you do not have responses in the peripheral blood. You have responses in the lymph nodes, where the number of red cells is very small.

TIM KRAMER: That is true, and I agree with you that if you take the red blood cells and if you do add them to separated mononuclear cells, you will cause the lymphocyte responses to go up.

GABRIEL VIRELLA: Not only that, but you cause an increased B-cell response that is IL-2 independent, which may reflect a predominant stimulation of Th2-type T-cells.

TIM KRAMER: This is directed to that and to your comment about recommending looking at IL-2 as being possibly better than looking at mitogenic response. I have probably run close to 7,000 to 8,000 whole-blood samples, both in the field and in the laboratory, with studies ranging from nutrition studies that are conducted in house within the U.S. Department of Agriculture, to field studies with the Army or in China, and what we have come to find out now is that if we optimize our sensitivity in a mitogen-induced whole-blood system, the CV [coefficient of variation] values are down at 17 or 20 percent in comparison to the cytokines produced from whole blood in the cultures, which are up in the 50 to 60 percent range.

Actually, we find that IL-2 gives us the poorest data in comparison with interferon gamma and IL-10. So I think when you start looking at the whole area of immunology, if you try to look at the whole big picture it becomes too complex. That is why we try to use the lymphocyte as a sort of cell from the immune system in order to look at its response *in vitro*. We have found that we get less variation when we take a CBC [complete blood count]; thus, we can calculate the data per volume of blood and also per lymphocyte. Our data actually come out tighter that way than with standard.

GABRIEL VIRELLA: It would be tighter just because you have been standardizing your technique through the years, and obviously that happens. The more we run a technique, the better trained and the more experienced our technicians are, the tighter the coefficient of variation becomes. That is fine.

But I have a problem with this being physiological. I do not think testing whole blood is a physiological way to test immune response. I mean, it does not happen in whole blood. It does not happen that way.

TIM KRAMER: That is right, but if you look at it the other way, I have a question about the physiology when you take lymphocytes and standardize them to a constant number *in vitro*. You are looking at the activity of the cells on a per cell basis, but then the differences between individuals are hard to interpret because their white blood cell counts are different. So I think you have big flaws [with both methods].

GABRIEL VIRELLA: But in the IL-2 assay, I have tighter results than you do, so each one of us has tighter results in what we like to run, you know.

(Laughter)

Emerging Technologies for Nutrition Research, 1997
Pp. 451–500. Washington, D.C.
National Academy Press

22

New Technologies for Producing Systemic and Mucosal Immunity by Oral Immunization: Immunoprophylaxis in Meals, Ready-to-Eat

Arthur O. Anderson[1]

INTRODUCTION

Immunity, inflammation, and nutrition form an interactive system that impacts on the performance of soldiers in stressful or hazardous environments. A deficiency in any component of this system diminishes the effectiveness of the others (Beisel, 1994). Decrements in performance during the first few weeks of deployment frequently are associated with illness caused by endemic infectious disease agents. This risk is enhanced by the threat of possible biological weapon attacks (Mobley, 1995). To minimize infection-induced performance decrements, troops should be immunized against recognized endemic disease and biological warfare threat agents months prior to deployment, preferably during basic training.

---

[1] Arthur O. Anderson, Department of Clinical Pathology, Diagnostics Systems Division (*formerly of* Department of Mucosal Immunology), U.S. Army Medical Research Institute of Infectious Diseases, Fort Detrick, MD 21701-5333

Promising new technologies from recombinant DNA and biodegradable polymer research will change the way vaccines are produced and will simplify how immunity is induced and maintained (Michalek et al., 1995; Walker, 1994). Two recent papers demonstrate the feasibility of large-scale agricultural production of recombinant vaccine antigens (Ma et al., 1995) and functional recombinant human antibodies (Haq et al., 1995) in quantities that would satisfy virtually any contingency requirement. Engineered human secretory antibodies could be enterically coated and incorporated into foods for passive protection of soldiers from common diarrheal diseases and enterotoxin reactions that affect nutrition and performance (Hyams et al., 1991, 1993; Sarraf et al., 1997).

The advantages of passive and active immunization[2] via the oral route are multiple. Recombinant vaccines may be encapsulated in biodegradable polymers to prolong shelf life and provide controlled-release, targeted delivery or protection from denaturation by stomach acid and intestinal enzymes until the product is absorbed in the gastrointestinal tract (Michalek et al., 1994; Morris et al., 1994). Combining encapsulated vaccines or antibodies with nutritious foods makes them more convenient and acceptable to use and removes the logistical and anxiety factors associated with the need for periodic inoculations. In addition to enhancing soldier performance and autonomy, systems for oral immunization will save time and money. It will no longer be necessary for soldiers to delay deployment so that they may assemble for vaccination. Because the new vaccines can be self-administered, they can be taken without need of medically trained personnel. Oral vaccination also eliminates dangerous medical waste and the risk of contamination, which are concerns when needles are used. Taken together, it is now feasible to provide complete passive and active protective immunity along with good nutrition in Meals, Ready-to-Eat (MREs). These new technologies should become an exciting and active area of applied research with

---

[2] Passive immunity is an unsustainable state of immunity produced by transfer of antibodies from an immunized donor (after convalescence or complete immunization regimen) to a nonimmune recipient. Protection may be sustained only if regular treatments of antibody are given. In other words, antibody from an immune donor is put into a nonimmune recipient, thus conferring a state of immunity. In this review, passive immunity is used to indicate the prevention or reduction of "traveler's diarrhea" or infections that affect soldiers within the first few days of deployment.

Active immunity is a sustainable state of immunity that results from vaccinations or recovery from an infectious illness. This kind of immunity is antigen specific and can result in logarithmically increasing amounts of antibody and other forms of immunity upon re-exposure to antigen. The most important aspect of active immunity is that immunological memory is induced. Immunological memory results from clonal expansion of lymphocytes specific for the antigen during the primary response. These lymphocytes reside in lymphatic tissues and circulate in the blood. After immunization, there may be many thousands of antigen-specific lymphocytes circulating or residing in tissues. Upon re-exposure to antigen, the rate and magnitude of the specific secondary immune response is orders of magnitude greater than the primary response. Immunological memory resulting from active immunization is more valuable for protecting soldiers than is passive immunity.

numerous opportunities for interdisciplinary collaboration and leveraging of the tasks.

CURRENT CONCEPTS AND ISSUES IN IMMUNITY

It may be useful to digress from the primary objective (i.e., that of describing the exciting new technologies) in order to explain relevant concepts and critical issues in immunology. This explanation will help establish the importance of certain new approaches to immunization and reveal how these approaches could benefit soldiers of the twenty-first century.

Concept of Compartmentalization of Immune Responses

Immune responses to vaccines are influenced by the route of immunization (injection or oral), the form of the antigen (live, killed, soluble, peptide subunit, or particulate), and the presence in the vaccine of biologically active elements, such as proteins that mediate specific tissue tropisms (components of the pathogen that enable it to attach to and replicate in specific host cells) or materials included as adjuvants (substances added to enhance antigenicity), vectors, or vehicles (Walker, 1994). For example, differences in immune responses to live versus inactivated viral vaccines may be a function of compartmentalization of immune responses, activities requiring vaccine viability like tropism, or molecular strategies for cell entry and replication (Rubin et al., 1986; Spriggs, 1996). In this review to avoid confusion, general comments about effects of route of administration or vehicles on immune responses will be restricted to responses initiated by simple, unmodified, nonreplicating protein antigens.

There is now substantial evidence supporting the existence of at least two immune systems, a "peripheral" immune system (involving the spleen, lymph nodes, and other nonepithelial tissues) and a "mucosal" immune system (involving the epithelial tissue lining the respiratory and gastrointestinal tracts) (Ogra et al., 1994). These systems operate separately and simultaneously in most species, including humans.

Protective immunity acquired during convalescence usually is referred to as "systemic immunity," but this term is imprecise. Systemic immunity might be a combination of mucosal and peripheral immunity, or it might be dominated by an incomplete form of immunity dictated by a specific pathogen (Mosmann and Sad, 1996; Salgame et al., 1991). For example, if a pathogen stimulates a cytokine cascade that favors antibody production (at the expense of endocytosis and intralysosomal killing), it would continue to prosper within a compartment in which antibodies are ineffective (Finkelman, 1995; Yamamura et al., 1991). Unless a vaccine stimulates the appropriate system or a combination of systems, protective immunity might not be complete.

The concept of anatomic compartmentalization of immunity is supported by observations from several disciplines (Kroemer et al., 1993). The anatomy of antigen uptake and the physiology and biochemistry of lymphocyte recirculation within unique tissue microenvironments may influence significantly the quality of humoral and cellular immune responses.

The way antigens are acquired by individual lymphatic tissues affects the outcome of an immune response. For example, the same antigen may produce qualitatively different immune responses in lymph nodes, spleen, or Peyer's patches (lymphoid tissue aggregates under intestinal mucosa) (Anderson, 1990). Antigens in lymph are filtered, trapped, processed, and presented at the site where lymph passes over fixed antigen-presenting cells in lymph nodes. Such antigen handling by lymph nodes most often results in peripheral immunity, characterized by the appearance of specific immunoglobulin (Ig)G in the blood. Antigens in blood are filtered, trapped, processed, and presented in strategic blood-tissue interfaces in the spleen, which also result in peripheral immunity. However, the spleen microenvironment is somewhat more complicated because it also accommodates circulating antigen-presenting cells and immunoreactive T- and B-cells from other tissues committed to either peripheral or mucosal immunity. In contrast, antigens in the lumens of enteric organs (i.e., the respiratory and gastrointestinal tracts) are nondestructively endocytosed by specialized epithelial cells called M (membraneous)-cells and transported across the cytoplasm in vacuoles onto lymphoid cells in Peyer's patches, where response to antigen presentation triggers commitment to "mucosal immunity," characterized by release of specific IgA into the secretions[3] (McGhee et al., 1992).

Lymphocyte traffic patterns, which are regulated by selective expression of adhesion proteins in peripheral or mucosal lymphatic tissues, maintain anatomic segregation of immunologic memory (that enables the immune system to mount a more vigorous and effective response whenever it is restimulated by a specific foreign antigen) by causing antigen-primed cells to return to specific anatomic destinations, where they will encounter conditions that further facilitate expression of peripheral or mucosal immunity (Butcher and Picker, 1996; Ebnet et al., 1996) (Figure 22-1). The multitude of potential conditions includes the prevalence of specific cytokines, adhesion to and costimulation by specific stromal cells, and still, unknown microenvironmental factors intrinsic to those lymphoid compartments that favor commitment of B-cells to specific immunoglobulin isotypes or T-cells to peripheral or mucosal immunity (Anderson, 1990; Rott et al., 1996).

Humoral immunity is mediated by euglobulins called antibodies that are produced locally but act at great distances from where they are made and secreted. Cellular immunity is like hand-to-hand combat. T-cells, natural killer (NK) cells, and "armed" macrophages enter into physical combat with the

---

[3] IgG binds and enables the pathogen to be ingested and destroyed by a phagocytic host cell. IgA binds the pathogen and prevents it from binding to host cells so that the luminal fluid or mucous stream will carry it away.

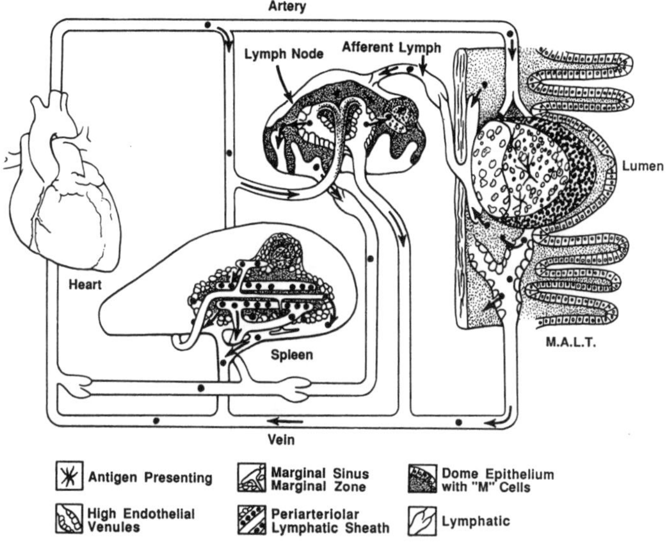

FIGURE 22-1 A simplified drawing of the structures and connections of secondary lymphatic tissues where antigen may most efficiently direct immune responses. Multiple known and unknown factors intrinsic to the microenvironments of lymph node, spleen, and mucosa-associated lymphatic tissue (here, M.A.L.T is represented by Peyer's patch) influence whether a peripheral or mucosal type of response occurs. The drawing also indicates that these tissues are integrated with each other and the rest of the individual through vascular and lymphatic connections and a system of lymphocyte recirculation. Microenvironmental structures in the drawing are identified by the symbols below the drawing.

pathogen and kill it by punching holes into its membranes or exposing it to enzymes. Cellular immunity also is associated with secretion of hormone-like molecules called cytokines and chemokines. These enable the effector cells to perform their duties actively. Many of the same cytokines also have effects on the humoral immune response by affecting B-cell division, differentiation, and maturation. The distinction between systems that regulate humoral immunity and those that regulate cellular immunity should not be confused with anatomic compartmentalization or with commitment to peripheral or mucosal immunity. There is a division of labor between cellular and humoral immunity that is parallel in both the peripheral and mucosal systems. Some of the same cell interactions and cytokines involved in cellular or humoral immunity are also involved in favoring peripheral over mucosal immunity, and vice versa (Abbas et al., 1996; Mosmann and Sad, 1996; Rocken and Shevach, 1996), as will be discussed later.

Compartmentalized Humoral Immunity

All immunoglobulins, whether peripheral or mucosal, function by binding antigen in a pocket formed by the complementarity-determining regions (CDRs) encoded by the immunoglobulin heavy (VH)- and light (VL)-chain variable region genes (Carayannopoulos and Capra, 1993). The pocket formed by the VH-VL CDRs spatially conforms to the surface shape of the antigen that binds to the antibody (Figure 22-2). The method by which the genes for antigen-specific CDRs may be obtained quickly so that recombinant protective antibodies may be produced will be discussed later in this review.

The antibody class conferred by the heavy-chain constant (C) region genes determines how the antibody will function and where it will act. Antibody C-region genes are expressed after rearrangement of the selected heavy-chain gene and attachment to the already rearranged variable, diversity, and joining region genes.[4] Thus IgM, IgD, IgG3, IgG1, IgG2a, IgG2b, IgE, and IgA each have heavy chains that control how they participate in immunity, especially with regard to third-party molecular interactions such as Fc receptor binding,[5] activation of the complement system, and endosomal transport across mucosal epithelial cells.

Peripheral Immunity and IgG

Antibodies of peripheral immunity protect the parenchymal organs and peripheral anatomic sites that are bathed in tissue fluid and supplied by the

---

[4] Immunoglobulin diversity is a function of different choices in heavy and light chain genes that may be combined to make an immunoglobulin, choices of specific variable region genes for light and heavy chains, and somatic mutations incorporated in these variable regions during B-cell development. The diversity produced by the approximately 30 human D-genes involved in V-D-J recombination during early B-cell development produces a minimal effect on overall antibody diversity. The effect of this would be realized as a change in flexibility of the antigen-combining site, which may permit binding of antigens that deviate slightly from that required for ideal fit. The approximately five J-region genes (associated V-D-J genes produced on one chromosome) are located where the recombined V-D-J may join the heavy chain genes (from another chromosome). These joining regions are not the same thing as J-chain, which is an entirely different protein that associates posttranslationally with multimers of IgM or IgA and participates in transepithelial secretion by associating the polymeric immunoglobulin with poly-Ig receptor (secretory component) expressed on epithelial cell.

[5] Immunoglobulins usually link the pathogen to a host cell or product. For example, the antigen-combining site binds to an antigen (the first party), the Fc portion (which is at the opposite end of the antibody) binds to a host cell or a product such as mucus (the second party). Other molecules, such as complement or J-chain bind to antibody near the middle of the molecule (the third party) and participate in functions that are related indirectly to that antigen-antibody interaction. Third party interactions are important modifiers of the function of antibodies and enable the antibody to perform more effectively the organ-specific function that they were designed to do.

Panel A

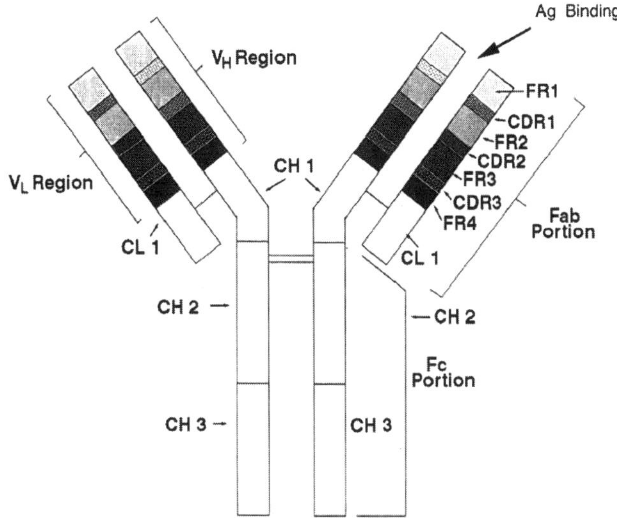

Panel B

Classic Ag Binding Pocket

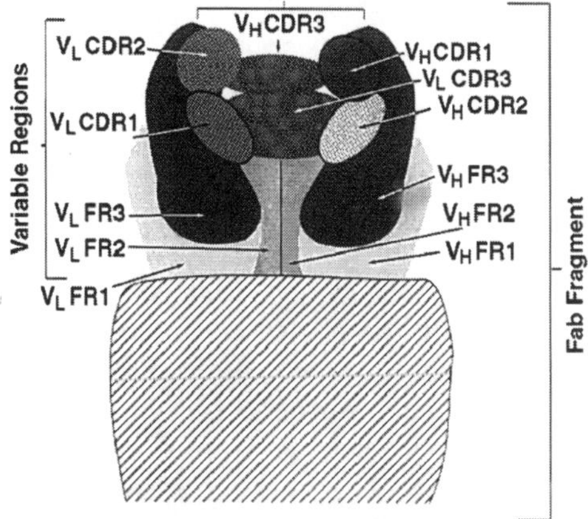

FIGURE 22-2 Diagram of an immunoglobulin molecule. The heavy and light chains of an immunoglobulin molecule are displayed linearly in Panel A, and the antigen-combining site is displayed in native configuration in Panel B. In Panel A, disulfide bonds link the light to the heavy chains, and the heavy chains to each other, to form a dimer. The light-chain constant region 1 is labeled CL 1, and the three heavy-chain constant regions are labeled CH 1–3. Although CH 2 and 3 together form the Fc portion, only the CH 3 domain binds to Fc receptors and controls (defines) the anatomic specialization of the immunoglobulin. The CH 3 region is most important in functions of specific immunoglobulin isotypes. The light- and heavy-chain variable regions are labeled VL and VH, respectively. This linear diagram helps to show the sequential location of the complementarity-determining regions (CDR 1–3) and the framework regions (FR 1–4). Framework regions are relatively conserved portions of the variable region that serve as spacers to position the antigen-binding sites properly when the variable region is folded. Panel B shows how an antigen-binding pocket forms when the VL-VH CDRs are folded into native configuration.

blood microvasculature. These antibodies maximize cellular uptake and internalization of antigens. After pathogens have breached the barriers of the skin and/or mucous membranes, antibodies of the IgM and IgG subclasses work in conjunction with the complement system. This collaboration serves to neutralize, injure, aggregate, and opsonize (to coat the pathogen with antigen-specific antibody and complement so that it can be ingested easily and destroyed by a phagocyte that is bearing receptors for Fc and complement) the pathogens so that they may be engulfed and destroyed by phagocytes.

Except in rare instances where pentameric IgM (complexed with joiner [J] chain) may be secreted across epithelium, most circulating antibodies of the IgM and IgG subclasses work in blood, lymph, and tissue fluids. They do not normally appear in mucosal secretions (Underdown and Mestecky, 1994).

Mucosal Immunity and Secretory IgA

Antibodies of mucosal immunity function outside the body at luminal surfaces of the moist epithelium lining conjunctiva; nasopharynx; oropharynx; gastrointestinal, respiratory, and urogenital tracts; and in the ducts or acini of exocrine glands. The principal antibody involved in mucosal immunity is secretory IgA (Underdown and Mestecky, 1994). This class of antibody requires the cooperation of two cell types for optimal activity *in vivo*. One cell type, the plasma cell, makes the IgA, while an epithelial cell transports it to the gut lumen where it works (Figure 22-3, Panel A). The plasma cell posttranslationally dimerizes the IgA by joining two molecules with another polypeptide, the J-chain. In addition to holding the two IgA molecules together, the J-chain facilitates binding to a poly-Ig receptor synthesized by and displayed on the abluminal side of epithelial cells. The complex is transported in endosomes to the luminal side of the epithelial cell and secreted. The portion of the poly-Ig receptor retained with secreted IgA is called the secretory component.

Pathogens adapted to infect mucosa express virulence factors that allow them to adhere, colonize, or invade epithelium. Secretory IgA prevents absorption of these viruses, bacteria, and toxins by blocking their adhesion while they are still on the external side of an epithelial barrier. This activity is opposite to that of antibodies associated with peripheral immunity, which aid the host cells to bind pathogens. By preventing cellular attachment of the antigen, IgA enables it to be flushed away in the stream of secreted fluids and mucous washing over the epithelial membranes.

IgA also may facilitate transport of pathogens and toxins out of the body by causing them to be conveyed into bile and other exocrine secretions (Mazanec et al., 1993). At sites where nondegradative endosomal transport delivers a pathogen into the host, such as across M-cells in the dome epithelium of the Peyer's patch (the region of a Peyer's patch where antigen from the gut lumen is transported into the lymphatic tissue) (Neutra and Kraehenbuhl, 1994; Owen

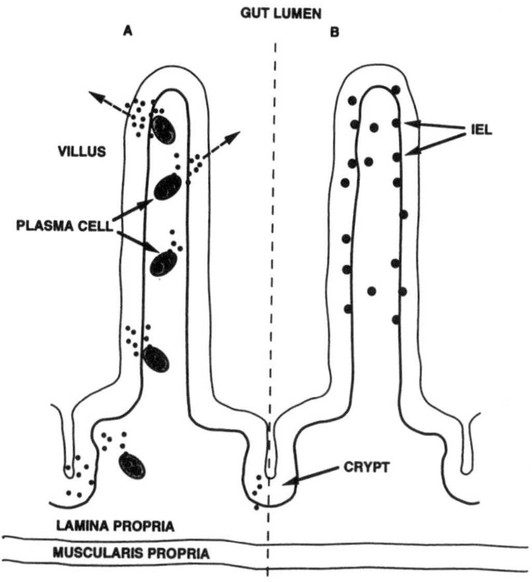

FIGURE 22-3 Diagram of small intestinal mucosa. Panel A shows the synthesis of secretory IgA by plasma cells and transport to the intestinal lumen by epithelial cells (dots and interrupted arrows). Panel B shows an intestinal villus. Large black dots represent sites where intraepithelial lymphocytes (IEL) involved in cellular prophylaxis, thymic independent T-cell maturation, or tolerance induction usually are found.

and Jones, 1974), antigen-specific IgA recently has been shown to neutralize viral pathogens while they are in the endosome (Mazanec et al., 1992).

IgA is the predominant antibody manufactured by the body. This escaped appreciation for many years because blood contains a relatively low concentration of IgA compared with other immunoglobulins. However, 75 percent of the antibody-producing cells in the body are making IgA, and most of this IgA is released on a continuous basis into gastrointestinal fluid, saliva, tears, urine, and other secretions. In humans, up to 40 mg/kg body weight of IgA is manufactured and secreted daily, which is many orders of magnitude greater than that of all other immunoglobulin isotypes (Brandtzaeg, 1994).

Compartmentalized Cell-Mediated Immunity

T-lymphocytes involved in peripheral and mucosal cell-mediated immunity compromise numerous functional subclasses of increasing diversity (Punt and Singer, 1996). Both T-helper cells (CD4) and cytotoxic T-suppressor cells (CD8) may assume immunoregulatory roles during immune responses, or they may differentiate into effector cells that exhibit segregated traffic patterns and functions (Anderson and Shaw, 1996; Ebnet et al., 1996; Salgame et al., 1991).

The profile of cytokines secreted by T-cells dictates immunoreactive cell commitment to either peripheral or mucosal immune functions. Gamma interferon from T-helper 1 (Th1) cells enhances peripheral immunity and suppresses mucosal immunity. IL-4 from T-helper 2 (Th2) cells enhances mucosal immunity and suppresses peripheral immunity. Other cytokines can further influence this divergence or lead to partial or complete compromises.

Peripheral T-Cells. T-cells committed to peripheral immunity circulate in the blood and help B- or T-cell precursors differentiate into antibody-secreting cells or cytotoxic effector cells respectively. These T-cells also release a number of cytokines that activate and arm mononuclear phagocytes and natural killer cells to destroy intracellular parasites.

Mucosal T-Cells. Mucosally committed T-cells enter Peyer's patches, the lamina propria (the layer of connective tissue underlying the mucosal epithelium), and the intraepithelial compartment (Figure 22-3, Panel B). There is considerable phenotypic diversity among these mucosal T-cells. The subclass of mucosa-homing T-cells known as intraepithelial lymphocytes is believed to play a role in protecting mucosal surfaces from being injured by infectious pathogens or parasites (London et al., 1987). However, some of the diverse cells that populate the intraepithelial compartment include thymic-independent T-cells, which enter the epithelium to complete maturation (Punt and Singer, 1996). Many of these cells display phenotypic markers that reflect intermediate stages of T-cell differentiation.

CD8 T-Cell Heterogeneity. Heterogeneity of T-cells of the suppressor-cytotoxic phenotype (CD8) has been described, especially for those cells located within the mucosal epithelium. The CD8 membrane marker is expressed as a heterodimeric complex consisting of an alpha and a beta chain (i.e., CD8$\alpha\beta$). Within the intraepithelial compartment, CD8+ cells[6] are commonly found expressing two alpha chains (CD8$\alpha\alpha$). T-cells bearing CD8$\alpha\beta$ and CD8$\alpha\alpha$ may exhibit separate traffic patterns, as suggested by the observation that they are found in peripheral and mucosal compartments in different ratios. They also may participate in regulating the balance between peripheral and mucosal immunity to specific antigens because of their nominal "suppressor" activity (Salgame et al., 1991). There is some indication from basic studies that these cells exhibit organ-selective commitments.

---

[6] CD8 is a phenotype. CD8+ indicates that a cell bears that phenotype. However, that phenotype is heterogeneous because the presence or absence of CD8β permits identification of two subtypes, one with both chains (CD8$\alpha\beta$) and the other with two α-chains (CD8$\alpha\alpha$). It is possible that these two phenotypes represent peripheral and mucosal CD8+ cells, respectively.

CD8 Homing and Cross-Regulation. When mice with severe combined immunodeficiency (SCID) (which lack mature T- or B-cells) are reconstituted with lymphocytes derived from CB17 mice (normal parent strain of SCID), the fate of cells derived from a particular tissue may be traced *in vivo* (Hilbert et al., 1994). If residence in that tissue imprints functional commitment or organ selectivity, then that will be reflected by the phenotype and homing characteristics of the cells after transfusion. Normal lymphoid cells derived from CB17 lymph nodes or Peyer's patches were transfused into syngeneic SCID mice. Donor CD8αβ T-cells, extracted from CB17 lymph nodes, lodged in lymph node paracortex and in the intestinal lamina propria of SCID recipients. The CD8αβ lymph node cells did not enter the intraepithelial compartment but remained near plasma cells in the lamina propria. The preponderant CD8+ phenotype in CB17 Peyer's patch and intraepithelial lymphocytes (IEL) is CD8αα. Infusion of Peyer's patch cells resulted in excellent reconstitution of SCID IEL, especially of CD8αα T-cells. Thus, the homing preference of these putative suppressor cell types is consistent with the possibility of their playing a role in antigen-specific cross-regulation of peripheral versus mucosal immunity as discussed later.

Functions of CD8+ Intraepithelial Lymphocytes. The exact functions of IEL subpopulations are not yet known, but animal experiments and *ex vivo* cellular cytotoxicity assays suggest that some IEL exhibit cellular cytotoxicity directed against viral antigens on infected mucosal epithelial cells (Cuff et al., 1993; London et al., 1987). IEL also are thought to be involved in initiating tolerance (Elson et al., 1995; Gelfanov et al., 1996; Sim, 1995), but it is not clear whether all IEL, or a unique subset of IEL, induce tolerance to food antigens. Presentation of antigen in a manner similar to that of nonclassical major histocompatibility (MHC) antigens[7] displayed on basolateral membranes of intestinal epithelial cells in the absence of costimulatory signals[8] (Robey and Allison, 1995) may be involved in triggering tolerogenic T-cells (T-cells that induce immunological tolerance; the concept of tolerance will be discussed later) (Matzinger, 1994). There are many basic questions to be answered in the rapidly enlarging field devoted to IEL function.

---

[7] MHC antigens are cell-surface proteins responsible for determination of tissue type and transplant compatibility. Found on antigen-presenting cells, they are divided into two classes: Class 1 MHC antigens form complexes with intracellular peptide fragments after proteosomal digestion; Class II MHC antigens form complexes with extracellular antigens after lysosomal digestion.

[8] Costimulatory signals are signals that must be provided simultaneously with the principal signals for an event to progress as expected. The immune system uses these like passwords. Presentation of an antigen to an activated lymphocyte in the absence of a costimulatory signal may cause the cell to die suddenly by apoptosis, instead of starting the process of dividing and differentiating into antibody-producing cells. Specific receptor-ligand interactions are involved.

Immune Assessment by T-Cell Phenotypes. Monoclonal antibodies are now available that enable phenotypic distinction of the class and potential function of T-cells, including their commitment to being peripheral or mucosal cells. The relative phenotypes displayed on a class of T-cells differ depending on whether they are immature, resting, activated, naive, or memory cells.[9] Other phenotypic markers make it possible to determine the percentages of T-cells committed to lodge in secondary lymphatic tissues, skin, inflammatory sites, parenchymal organs, mucosal lamina propria, or intraepithelial compartments of mucosa compared with the percentage of T-cells that will continue to circulate in the blood (Altman et al., 1996; Rott et al., 1996).

Compartmentalized Immunity and Lymphocyte Traffic

Immunity is dependent upon continuous movement of cells through blood, tissue and lymph (Anderson and Shaw, 1996). Lymphoid cells traffic to the secondary lymphoid organs of the spleen, lymph nodes, and Peyer's patches in order to encounter antigens acquired from the environment via blood, lymph, or across mucous membranes. Where, and by which cells, antigens are presented to the trafficking cells has a significant influence on the outcome of the immune response with respect to antibody isotype commitment and future homing preference of memory and effector lymphoid cells (Anderson and Shaw, 1996; Butcher and Picker, 1996; Husband and Gowans, 1978; Rott et al., 1996).

Random and segregated traffic patterns are essential for efficient operation of the two separate but overlapping immune systems operating in mammalian species. Without knowing about lymphocyte recirculation and homing, it is difficult to understand how peripheral and mucosal immune responses may be segregated yet interact for cross-regulation. An enormous number of lymphocytes are involved in this process (Ebnet et al., 1996).

The feat of coordinating the anatomically dispersed immune system comprised of mobile, circulating, individual, and extremely diverse cells depends upon movement and a system of membrane recognition and activation signals. A mixture of integrins, selectins,[10] and receptors for chemokines (chemotactic cytokines) expressed by lymphocytes and endothelial cells are involved in precipitating selective emigration of lymphoid subsets from the blood in tissues where specific counterreceptors (receptors that are also ligands) are displayed on

---

[9] Naive T-cells do not participate in an immune response, show no organ preference during recirculation, and display surface phenotypes that enable their enumeration. Memory T-cells (or their clonal predecessors) have participated in an immune response, show preference for migration through the kind of organ where they were exposed to antigen, and display a characteristic surface phenotype enabling their enumeration.

[10] Integrins are heterodimeric integral membrane proteins that mediate adhesion and signaling activity among cells and between cells and extracellular matrix. Selectins are cell-surface glycoproteins found on lymphocytes or endothelial cells, which regulate lymphocyte migration patterns.

luminal surfaces of endothelial cells. These recognition events may happen in skin, mucosa, or specific secondary lymphatic tissues, such as Peyer's patch or peripheral lymph node. Receptor-ligand interactions allow these cells to find their way around the body, as well as to determine where to adhere to endothelium, when to migrate, and how to find their site of action within tissue (Anderson and Shaw, 1996; Gretz et al., 1996; Rott et al., 1996).

A consensus hypothesis (Figure 22-4) has been offered to explain the overall process of emigration and to propose ways to explain organ-selective migration as a "combinatorial mechanism"[11] (Butcher, 1991). Circulating lymphocytes use adhesive selectins to roll on endothelial-cell luminal surfaces; they become loosely tethered using Selectin-glycam/CD34 interactions.[12] Upon activation either by receptors expressed on the endothelial surface or by chemokines, the binding characteristics of these receptors are changed very rapidly (within milliseconds) from low affinity to high affinity (Anderson and Shaw, 1993; Ebnet et al., 1996). Different specific receptor-counterreceptor interactions are responsible for each stage and mediate recognition, binding, and emigration of cells from the blood.

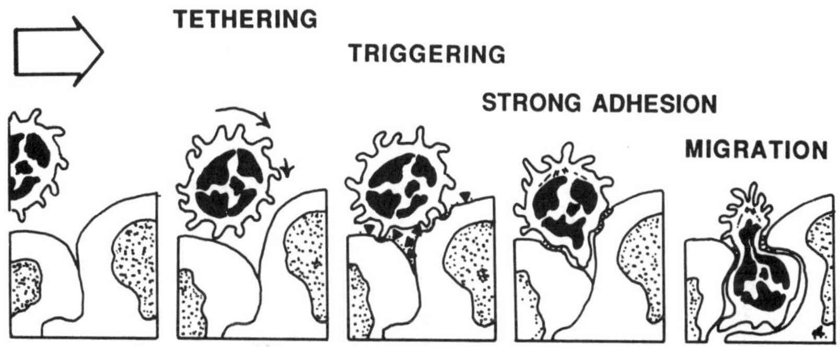

FIGURE 22-4 Diagram of the adhesion cascade. The rolling cell binds, then begins to migrate between endothelial cells and enters the tissue. SOURCE: Adapted from Anderson and Shaw (1993).

---

[11] *Combinatorial mechanism* is a term coined to explain how specificity can be created by multiple overlapping, independent, receptor-ligand interactions. The specificity is in the combination, rather than the contribution of any individual receptor-ligand pair. The previous hypothesis, that there was a specific homing receptor to explain the preference for certain cells to migrate to mucosal tissues while other cells preferred peripheral tissues, was found to be false. The phenomenon still exists, but the consensus hypothesis accepts that variable combinations of receptor-ligand pairs create this specificity.

[12] Glycam and CD34 are both mucin-like molecules expressed at endothelial cell surfaces; these molecules are highly glycosylated with sulfated proteoglycans. L-selectin molecules on lymphocyte surfaces bind to the sulfated sugars with the specificity of a C-type lectin.

Recirculation Is the Integrating Principle. Recirculation of a precursor pool of uncommitted lymphocytes, from the blood into lymph nodes or mucosal lymphatic tissues and then back to the blood again, forms the basis of immunosurveillance and integration of immune functions across the segregated systems. The magnitude of cell traffic reflected by the number of cells returned to the blood in efferent lymph is enormous. Enough lymphocytes recirculate from lymph to blood to replace the total blood lymphocyte pool from 10 to 48 times every 24 hours (Anderson and Shaw, 1996; Ebnet et al., 1996).

Compartmentalized Traffic Is Acquired. While naive lymphocytes appear to access peripheral lymphoid tissues randomly during recirculation, memory lymphocytes selectively return to the tissues where they initially were stimulated by antigen. Precursor or naive lymphocytes (those that have not seen antigen in a lymphatic tissue or participated in an immune response) enter all tissues, especially secondary lymphatic tissues, such as Peyer's patch, peripheral lymph node, or spleen, without any organ-selective bias. In the short period after activation by antigen, lymphocytes behave like inflammatory cells and avoid returning to secondary lymphoid tissues, preferring to lodge in skin, gut, or inflammatory sites as "acute memory" cells. After maturation occurs, some of these memory cells follow an organ-selective traffic route determined by the tissue in which that particular lymphocyte encountered the signals to divide, differentiate, and mature.

When activated by antigen (displayed by an antigen-presenting cell) in any secondary lymphatic tissue, lymphocytes proliferate and undergo many of the changes associated with differentiation. For a few days after their activation, they radically change their cell-surface expression of molecules involved in adhesion. When these cells emerge from lymphatic tissue as memory cells, their pattern of migration is markedly different. As new memory cells, lymphocytes preferentially home to specific nonlymphoid tissues, such as skin or gut (rather than the traffic areas of secondary lymphoid tissues). This behavior fits reasonably well with the increases seen in expression of "inflammatory" adhesion molecules, concomitant with decreases in L-selectin associated with recirculation. Memory CD4 (T-helper) cells express more VLA-4 and LFA-1 and have increased capacity to bind to their ligands VCAM-1 and ICAM-1, the expression of which is increased at sites of inflammation.

Conditions Influencing T-Cell Compartmentalization

Secondary lymphoid tissues that drain peripheral or mucosal tissues differ from each other and therefore differentially influence maturation of T-cells (Cahill et al., 1977). If lymphocytes are activated in lymph nodes that drain skin, they become specialized to migrate preferentially into skin and serve the immunologic needs of skin (Mackay, 1991; Mackay et al., 1992). Conversely, if lymphocytes are activated in lymphatic tissues sampling antigens from the gastroin-testinal (GI) tract, they become specialized to migrate preferentially into the GI tract and serve its immunologic needs (Abernethy et al., 1991; Kimpton et al., 1989).

Adhesion Molecules. Expression of specific adhesion proteins and selective secretion of cytokines in peripheral and mucosal lymphoid tissue help to create unique microenvironments (Ebnet et al., 1996). Somehow an influence of this microenvironment is imprinted on the lymphocytes differentiating therein.

Differentiation in mucosal lymph nodes results in the induction of integrins that may predispose T-cells to interact with vascular addressins[13] expressed on GI tract venular endothelium and therefore migrate into the GI tract; included are both the integrins αeβ7 for CD8+ IEL cells, which bind to E-cadherin[14] on mucosal epithelial cells (Cepek et al., 1994; Karecla et al., 1995), and α4β7 for CD4+ lymphocytes, which bind to mucosal addressin cell adhesion molecule (MADCAM)-1 on mucosal venular endothelium and splenic marginal sinus (Berlin et al., 1993; Hamann et al., 1994; Kraal et al., 1995; Lyons and Parish, 1995). Conversely, T-cells maturing in skin-draining lymph nodes preferentially retain expression of L-selectin (and the sialylated CLA [cutaneous lymphocyte-associated] antigen, recognized by HECA [human endothelial cell-associated] 452 monoclonal antibody, which binds to endothelial E-selectin). Both of these integrins appear to facilitate subsequent entry of lymphocytes into the skin or lymph node, where L-selectin binds to carbohydrates of the endothelial sia-lomucins[15] GlyCAM and CD34.

The leukocyte integrin α4 β1 (VLA-4) is activated by a signal emanating from the endothelium and mediates strong binding to VCAM-1 expressed on HEV surfaces. This is thought to facilitate leukocyte emigration between endo-thelial cells. These differences in the phenotype of emerging T-cells must reflect local differences in the microenvironment. Such differences have not been de-fined clearly; however, transforming growth factor (TGF)-β is believed to be better expressed in mucosal sites and contributes to the distinctive phenotypes of resident cells. To illustrate, TGF-β1 upregulates and maintains expression of

---

[13] Vascular addressins are molecules found on the luminal surfaces of high endothelial venules. They provide the ligand for L-selectin and α4β7 integrin expressed on lymphocytes. This molecular interaction is factored into the combinatorial system of interactions described above to confer specificity to the adhesive interaction.

[14] E (epithelial)-cadherin is an adhesion molecule requiring calcium ions that links endothelial cells to each other and to extracellular matrix, and also serves as an atypical ligand for αEβ7 integrin expressed on intraepithelial lymphocytes.

[15] Sialomucins are mucin-like molecules that are found on nonepithelial cells like lymphocytes, endothelial cells, or macrophages and are heavily sialylated, that is, the carbohydrates have a large number of sialic acid side chains. These sialomucins are strongly anionic and would be repulsive to most cells that lack lectin-like surface molecules, such as L-selectin.

αeβ7 integrin in T-cells destined to enter the intraepithelial compartment, where it anchors T-cells to E-cadherin on epithelial cells (Cepek et al., 1994).

Conditions Influencing B-Cell Compartmentalization

Primary B-cells expand rapidly in primary mucosal lymphoid follicles of very young mammals and undergo diversifying mutations in the genes encoding the antigen-binding sites during VDJ rearrangement (Weinstein et al., 1994a). They are then subject to positive selection to generate an antibody repertoire biased toward antigens prevalent in the environment; progeny that do not bind antigen in this milieu undergo apoptosis (programmed cell death). Survivors leave the follicles in efferent lymph and enter the blood where they circulate and recirculate as small precursor IgM+/IgD+ B-cells. They migrate continuously into all secondary lymphoid tissue until triggered to divide by the appropriate antigen and costimulatory signals.

The subsequent differentiation of circulating B-cells depends on whether they are first activated in peripheral lymphoid tissue (lymph nodes and spleen) or in mucosal sites (such as Peyer's patches), where they are influenced by prevalent cytokines and unique stromal and accessory cell[16] populations in the respective tissues (Weinstein and Cebra, 1991; Weinstein et al., 1991).

Some precursor B-cells will be first activated in spleen or lymph node. In that process, they are programmed toward one of the IgG isotypes (rather than IgA). Daughter cells from this clonal expansion leave the lymph node in the efferent lymph, return to the blood, and seed the spleen, bone marrow, sites of inflammation, and other lymph nodes as plasma cells and "memory" B-lymphoblasts (Cebra et al., 1977; Kantele et al., 1997; Quiding-Jarbrink et al., 1995).

Other precursor B-cells will be activated first in Peyer's patch. Those cells become committed to rearrange their immunoglobulin heavy-chain genes to express IgA (rather than IgG isotypes noted above); despite having made this commitment, the switch to IgA often is delayed for several days. These cells leave in the efferent lymph, pass through the mesenteric lymph node (where they may be subject to immunoregulation[17] by T-cells they encounter there), and return to the blood. These cells selectively migrate to the spleen, which serves as an auxiliary site for clonal expansion prior to dissemination of the daughter cells

---

[16] Stromal cells are connective tissue cells that organize the tissue and express adhesion molecules that are essential for sustaining lymphoid cells (i.e., preventing apoptosis); these cells secrete cytokines that are important in conditioning the microenvironment. Accessory cells are nonlymphoid cells like macrophages, interdigitating dendritic cells, follicular dendritic cells, and other cells that present antigens or otherwise influence immune reactions.

[17] *Immunoregulation* is a term coined to refer to the general ability of cells to increase or decrease the functions of immunoreactive cells (i.e., by enhancing, suppressing, or otherwise altering an immune response).

via the blood into mucosal lamina propria. This process takes 5 to 7 days, at least 4 trips in the blood, and 2 to 3 cell generations (Cebra et al., 1977).

Immune Assessment by B-Cell Phenotyping. Between 2 and 4 days after antigen exposure, the orderly appearance of significant quantities of recirculating (naive precursor B-cells) and nonrecirculating (memory or preplasma cells) cells in the blood varies in frequency and may provide a valid window for monitoring the status of immune responses before serum antibody can be measured (Anderson and Shaw, 1996). Analysis using a flow cytometer may be performed on cells isolated from circulating blood. Two-color FACScan (fluorescence activated cell sorter) analysis will pair red fluorochrome-labeled antigen[18] (which binds to surface immunoglobulins on specific B-cells) with green fluorochrome-labeled antibodies, which can identify whether the circulating cells are committed to peripheral or mucosal immunity or some other phenotypic marker (Quiding-Jarbrink et al., 1995).

It is relatively easy to label recombinant or highly purified antigen for use in identifying and counting antigen-specific B-cells. Numerous monoclonal antibodies are available to assist in identifying the functional commitment of cells, including whether the surface immunoglobulins include IgD (indicative of a precursor or primary B-cell), or an IgG or IgA isotype (indicative of a secondary or memory B-cell committed to peripheral or mucosal immunity, respectively). With more experience using flow cytometry, the status of an immune response will be able to be estimated as it evolves. Techniques have even been developed for detection of cytoplasmic proteins by FACScan, including cytokines secreted by T-cells that influence B-cell responses (Assenmacher et al., 1994; Openshaw et al., 1995). This is especially important for estimating the potential for mucosal IgA responses because appearance of surface IgA-positive cells in the blood precedes lodging and differentiation into antibody secretion by several days.

---

[18] In FACScan analysis, a laser beam is passed through a laminar flow fluid stream containing a dilute suspension of cells that are treated with fluorescent molecules (antibodies or antigen), which bind to certain surface phenotypic markers or membrane antibody. The laser beam excites the fluorochrome(s) to emit energy at the predetermined blue, green, yellow, or red frequency. Scatter of the light beam is used to count all cells, whether they are fluorescent or not. Light-detecting diodes exposed to light signals filtered into specific colors convert the pulses of light to electronic signals in the machine. These signals are counted and expressed as frequency distributions, signal amplitude distributions, and percentages for each group . This kind of analysis can be done with one to three different specific fluorochrome-labeled markers plus light scatter (usually one or two colors are counted). The machine can count many thousands of cells in the time it might take to count a few by eye. FACScan analysis has become a fairly routine hospital laboratory procedure.

ISSUES FOR CONVENTIONAL MODES OF VACCINATION

Complicated Diseases Require Peripheral and
Mucosal Protective Immunity

Protection from diseases that threaten military personnel requires complex forms of immunity (Mobley, 1995). The nature of the vaccine antigen and route of its administration may confer anatomic compartmentalization to the immune response, restricting it to peripheral or mucosal immunity. Some infectious disease organisms spread parenterally to involve parenchymal organs but do not infect the epithelial cells lining respiratory, gastrointestinal, or urogenital tracts. Protection against these pathogens depends on circulating IgM and IgG antibodies[19] and/or peripheral cell-mediated immunity for resolution. Other disease agents principally infect mucosal epithelium, causing serious nutritional and physiologic alterations, but in these diseases, circulating antibodies of the IgG class are not protective. Instead, secretory IgA and/or intraepithelial cytotoxic lymphocytes are needed for protection (Ogra et al., 1994).

In most biological warfare scenarios, every mucosal surface of the body could be a portal of entry for aerosol-disseminated or ingested biological agents. Once an agent enters the body through the mucosa of the eyes, nose, throat, lungs, and gastrointestinal tract, it is able to disseminate and initiate systemic parenchymal, as well as mucosal pathology. Parenteral immunization, the most common route of vaccination, usually elicits a peripheral immune response, with protective IgM-IgG antibodies and peripheral cell-mediated immunity. Parenteral immunization usually fails to stimulate mucosal lymphatic tissues to generate protective IgA antibodies or antigen-specific IEL. Many hazardous agents infect across the mucosa but spread through the systemic circulation. Protection against these agents requires vaccines that induce both peripheral and mucosal immune responses.

Cross-Regulation Is an Issue with Conventional Modes of Vaccination

Early studies suggested that the route of vaccination was crucial for determining whether protective peripheral or mucosal immunity would develop. Furthermore, immunization methods and routes for inducing mucosal immunity

---

[19] IgM and IgG are the typical kinds of antibody expected to develop during a primary peripheral immune response. IgM antibodies are pentameric macroglobulins and are very effective complement-fixing antibodies. When IgM binds to a bacterium and fixes complement, the cascade of enzymatic reactions that occur causes the complement components to punch holes in the bacterial membrane. IgM also contributes to opsonization directly and indirectly through deposition of complement molecules on the bacterium. Complement receptors and immunoglobulin Fc receptors on phagocytes are used to capture and kill bacteria. IgG also facilitates opsonization, and this isotype has been associated with targeting the pathogen for intralysosomal enzymatic destruction.

often delayed or prevented induction of peripheral immunity and vice versa (Chase, 1946; MacDonald, 1982; Mattingly and Waksman, 1978). This phenomenon, which may be termed *cross-regulation* (Figure 22-5), was first seen by Pierce and Koster (Koster and Pierce, 1983; Pierce, 1978) and Hamilton et al. (1979) when they were testing a nontoxic cholera vaccine candidate. They found that when the initial priming occurred by vaccinating via a parenteral route and the second inoculation of antigen was given by an enteric route, the ability to elicit immunity in the mucosa was reduced. But parenteral priming followed by a second parenteral dose resulted in a strong booster response.

It is important to emphasize that the vaccine alluded to above was most likely denatured cholera toxin. In contrast, recent adjuvant studies with nondenatured cholera toxin proteins (that retain the capacity to bind GM1 ganglioside, the mechanism by which cholera toxin binds to intestinal epithelial cells) show that the proteins have great promise as vaccine vehicles (Dertzbaugh and Elson, 1993a; Dertzbaugh and Van Meter, 1996; Elson and Dertzbaugh, 1994; Elson et al., 1995; Walker, 1994). Cholera toxin and its B-subunit have the special ability to overcome cross-regulation of immunity and are components of several of the new vaccine technologies that will be discussed later in this report.

When Brown et al. (1981) empirically tested the effect of route of immunization of a formalin-inactivated Rift Valley fever virus vaccine on protection from parenteral or mucosal challenge, they found that the nonreplicating vac-

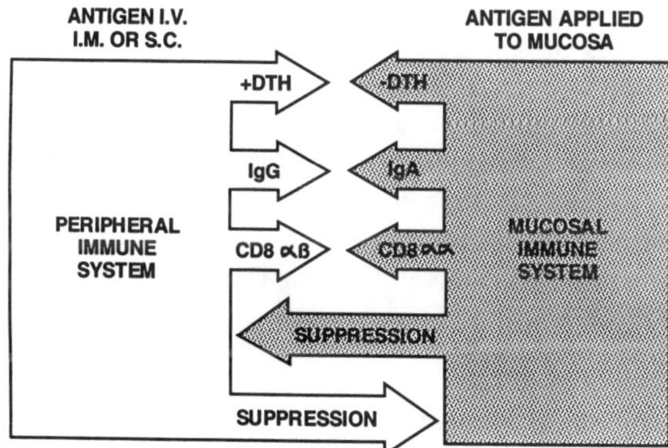

FIGURE 22-5 The dichotomy of immune systems involved in responding to vaccine antigens. Each immune system has its own stereotypical way of responding to antigen that is delivered by parenteral (left) or oral (right) routes of immunization. The predominant antibody type (IgG or IgA) and effector T-cell type (CD8αβ vs. CD8αα) are shown. Each system has the ability to suppress the other by numerous mechanisms. Delayed hypersensitivity (DTH), regulated by preponderant Th1-Th2 cytokines, is not displayed in healthy mucosal tissues.

                                          ARTHUR O. ANDERSON

cine elicited an immune response that protected mice from challenge by parenteral route but not from challenge by aerosol. This asymmetric immunity also was found for the C84 Venezuelan equine encephalitis virus vaccine (Jahrling and Stephenson, 1984). These experiments were repeated using a matrix design that tested both routes of immunization against homologous and heterologous challenge routes (Anderson et al., 1987a, b; Hart et al., 1995; Unpublished data, M. L. M. Pitt and A. O. Anderson, U.S. Army Medical Research Institute of Infectious Disease, Fort Detrick, Md., 1987). Upon heterologous challenge, viral pathogenesis (target organs affected and time course of disease evolution) was altered. Protection from encephalitis was deficient when subcutaneously immunized mice were challenged by aerosol. Moreover, when mucosally immunized mice were challenged by subcutaneous inoculation, the onset of viral infection of the liver extended over an 18-d time course, where, ordinarily, the liver is affected only during the first 3 to 6 days. The levels of specific IgA or IgG in serum and secretions corresponded to whether the challenged animals experienced protection and/or altered pathogenesis (Anderson et al., 1987b).

Oral Tolerance and Mucosal Immunity

There is no easy way to explain this phenomenon. The mucosal immune system is known to be the site of priming for two paradoxically opposite purposes, that is, tolerance (immunological nonresponsiveness or suppression to an antigen with proven immunogenicity) and mucosal immunity. The usual response of the GI tract to antigens is tolerance rather than immunity (Chen et al., 1995). The mechanisms of oral tolerance remain unclear. Tolerance could be primed in Peyer's patches or in the intraepithelial compartment, or IELs may be good candidates for communicating a toleragenic signal. Epithelial cells can present antigens, but without important costimulatory molecules, the cells that see this antigen may die or be rendered nonresponsive (Matzinger, 1994). It is thought that tolerance can occur through active suppression (cells or cytokines that induce nonresponsiveness), anergy (live nonresponsive cells), or apoptosis of antigen-reactive cells.

Tolerance Versus Cross-Regulation. The healthy GI tract is bathed in an enormously diverse collection of environmental antigens, yet only certain antigens stimulate active mucosal, peripheral, or combined mucosal and peripheral immune responses. Somehow the tissue is able to distinguish pathogens (dangerous) from normal flora (safe) and food antigens (safe) (Matzinger, 1994). Inducible chemokines may be the mucosal "danger" signal (Eckmann et al., 1993; Oppenheim et al., 1991). Pathogens that bind and/or invade mucosal epithelium cause epithelial cells to release cytokines and chemokines that attract inflammatory and/or immune cells, or cause epithelial cells to express proteins (classical and nonclassical MHC[20]) that target antigens for induction of immunity (Agace et al., 1993; Eckmann et al., 1993; McCormick et al., 1993). Mucosal antigens that lack costimulatory activity are programmed for tolerance (Bendelac, 1995; Kagnoff, 1996; Shroff et al., 1995). When tolerance results from mucosal immunization, it does not appear to diminish stimulation of B-cells committed to IgA secretion (Shroff et al., 1995); however, in contrast to cross-regulation, mucosal tolerance (Mowat, 1994) is most likely responsible for preventing systemic responses to common food antigens, but it has different conditions of triggering than that for cross-regulation.

Tolerance Versus Suppression. What some regard as mucosal or peripheral tolerance could merely represent a temporary induction of antigen-specific suppression. The suppression of systemic delayed cutaneous hypersensitivity and the reduction of IgG expression induced by mucosal priming lasts less than 3 months (Anderson et al., 1991; Koster and Pierce, 1983). In contrast, true tolerance persists until some stimulus breaks its effect. Peripheral priming with antigens in peripheral lymph nodes results in reduced mucosal immune responses comparable to that mentioned above (Anderson et al., 1987b; Anderson et al., 1991). This "yin-yang" effect on peripheral versus mucosal immunity suggests that cross-regulation might not be tolerance, but tolerance may be influenced indirectly by T-helper cells secreting cytokines that exert positive or negative feedback control (Figure 22-6). This suppression may require cell contact, or it may exert its effect through local cytokine commitment that prevents T-cell help of the required variety. For example, what is needed may be IL-4, but what is available is interferon gamma (IFNγ), and this difference is interpreted as suppression.

T-Helper Subclasses and Cross-Regulation. Because cross-regulation may influence immunity during the short period of time after oral or parenteral immunization, it is of value to discuss the possible role of T-helper cell subclasses in cross-regulation (Street and Mosmann, 1991; Swain et al., 1991; Trinchieri, 1993). T-helper cells segregate into two subsets depending on whether the cells secrete IFNγ and interleukin-2 (IL-2) (T-helper 1, Th1), or IL-4, IL-5, IL-6, and IL-10 (T-helper 2, Th2) (Mosmann and Sad, 1996). This distinction is important because the cytokines determine the kind of help provided by the respective T-helper cell types. This dualistic system, which enables the achievement of harmony between opposing cytokine influences, is illustrated graphically in Figure 22-6.

---

[20] Classical MHC antigens are encoded by the HLA gene locus in humans or the H-2 gene locus in the mouse. Nonclassical MHC antigens are a group of Fc receptors and other molecules called CD1 antigens that have been found to behave like MHC antigens, in that they can present foreign antigens as part of an immune response.

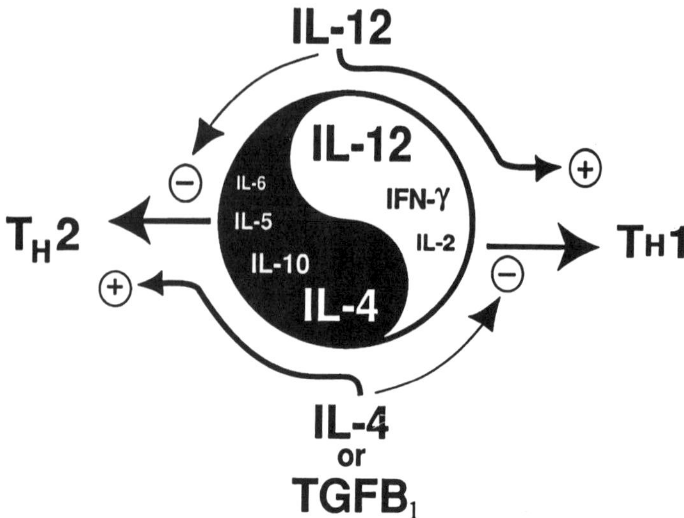

FIGURE 22-6 This diagram, resembling the oriental symbol for yin and yang, represents microenvironmental factors that stimulate T-cells to express either T-helper 1 (Th1) or T-helper 2 (Th2) cytokines, which are associated with cellular and humoral immunity, respectively. Other vectorial combinations of cytokines across this dualistic system may contribute to cross-regulation of immune responses associated with parenteral or mucosal immunization. The cytokines IL-12 and TGF-β1 are predominant influences in peripheral and mucosal lymphatic tissues. Thus, vectoral expression of these cytokines affect T- and B-cells in such a way that proliferating B-cells become committed to secrete peripheral IgG or mucosal IgA, respectively.

The central object in Figure 22-6, which resembles the symbol for yin and yang, represents the symmetric opposing effects of cytokines on lymphatic tissue microenvironments. In "peripheral" lymphoid environments, such as in lymph nodes draining the skin, IL-12 (Kang et al., 1996) secreted by Langerhans cells favors differentiation of T-cells that secrete IFNγ and IL-2. In addition to favoring cellular immunity, these Th1 cytokines favor production of IgG isotopes by B-cells. The mucosal environment in the Peyer's patch is affected by high local concentrations of TGF-β1. This cytokine favors development of T-cells that secrete IL-4 and other Th2 cytokines. IL-4 negatively affects peripheral cellular immunity at the same time that it favors development of B-cells committed to IgA secretion. Furthermore, TGF-β1 has been shown to directly affect immunoglobulin gene class switching to favor selection of α-heavy-chain genes. Thus, environmental influences, of which cytokines are a prominent few, affect the direction of the immune response toward cellular (Th1) or humoral immunity when the vector is oriented along the extreme opposites. However, intermediate vectorial orientations productive of mixed secretion of cytokines can produce mucosal or peripheral immunity when IL-4 and IFNγ moderately predominate among other microenvironmental cues. Thus, the relative concentration of T-helper types in lymph nodes or Peyer's patches influences selective expression of IgG or IgA immunoglobulin isotypes, respectively (Stavnezer, 1995). Anatomic compartmentalization of T-helper subclasses is of value in considering possible mechanisms of cross-regulation.

When Th1 responses are predominant (as they are in skin-draining lymph nodes influenced by Langerhans cells that secrete IL-12 [Kang et al., 1996]), T-helper cells secrete IL-2 and IFNγ, resulting in selective expression of IgG immunoglobulins and activation of cytotoxic T-cells and armed mononuclear phagocytes (Ariizumi et al., 1995; Kang et al., 1996; Weinstein et al., 1991). Where Th2 responses are predominant (as they are in mucosal sites), T-helper cells secrete IL-4, IL-5, IL-6, and IL-10, resulting in selective expression of different immunoglobulin isotypes, including IgA (Hiroi et al., 1995; Lebman and Coffman, 1994; Xu-Amano et al., 1993), and downregulation of peripheral cell-mediated immunity at the same time that there is increased development of cytotoxic T-cells that selectively home to mucosal intraepithelial sites (Ke and Kapp, 1996). The T-helper cell types provide positive and negative feedback control on commitment of B-cells to express specific antibody isotypes. For example, IFNγ suppresses commitment to IgA, and IL-4 suppresses commitment to IgG. Whether this is a direct effect on the B-cell or an indirect effect mediated by T-cells is a subject of great interest (Abbas et al., 1996; Finkelman, 1995; Lebman and Coffman, 1994).

Anatomic Compartmentalization of T-Helper Subclass Commitment. In mucosal sites, abundance of the cytokine TGF-β1 programs Th0 cells to develop into Th2 cells (Lebman and Coffman, 1994; Young et al., 1994). The cytokines secreted by Th2 cells contribute to expansion and differentiation of B-cells committed to IgA expression. TGF-β1 also contributes to selective expression of IgA antibodies by favoring immunoglobulin heavy-chain gene switching to IgA, and by suppressing expression of other isotypes (Lebman and Coffman, 1994; Stavnezer, 1995). TGF-β1 is not widely distributed in peripheral lymph nodes where there is selective expression of Th1 cellular responses and IgG antibodies. Recent publications suggest that Langerhans cells from the periphery may have a role in Th1 commitment by secretion of IL-12 and IL-1β-converting enzyme (Ariizumi et al., 1995; Kang et al., 1996). Other relationships of Th1-Th2 responses may be dependent upon which antigen-presenting cell type migrates into a site and conditions the microenvironment (Morikawa et al., 1995).

When this system is analyzed *in vitro* at the single-cell level, specific T-helper cell types or cytokine profiles are not sufficient to cause uncommitted IgM+, IgD+, or IgM-only B-cells to switch to IgA (Kotloff and Cebra, 1988; Schrader et al., 1990). However, when antigen-presenting cell types or stromal cells are added, switching occurs. Thus the cross-regulation is related to a sum of multiple "microenvironmental" factors unique to the tissue where the immune response is initiated (Weinstein and Cebra, 1991; Weinstein et al., 1991). Resolution of this on a molecular level awaits further research observations.

Cross-Regulation Is Incompatible with Complete Protective Immunity

Cross-regulation is not a desirable feature of conventional modes of vaccination. Effective ways to overcome the cross-regulation that prevents simultaneous induction of mucosal and peripheral immunity have been sought urgently. Not all vaccine antigens exhibit this behavior, especially those that have so-called adjuvant effects. It has been shown that modifying the vaccines with immunological adjuvants was a partial solution, but it was required that the adjuvants be used at optimal doses, which were different for each vaccine tested (Anderson, 1985; Anderson and Reynolds, 1979; Anderson and Rubin, 1985; Anderson et al., 1987b). Adjuvants were not effective with all antigens, and it was necessary to perform empirical studies to select the optimal combinations. Certain adjuvants (such as the lipoidal amine avridine) also potentiated the undesirable cross-regulation observed with native antigen (Anderson et al., 1985, 1987b). For example, if an antigen given orally elicited a good IgA response in secretions but failed to elicit or slightly depress specific IgG in serum, use of an adjuvant with the antigen would increase the IgA response and further decrease or block the IgG response in serum.

SOLUTIONS TO CROSS-REGULATION FROM
NEW TECHNOLOGIES

Although the approach of this group was to define cross-regulation, other scientists working with biodegradable microspheres and enterotoxin-derived vaccine delivery systems were finding that they could induce simultaneous peripheral and mucosal immunity. Antigens administered orally in biodegradable microspheres composed of poly(lactide/glycolide) copolymer, or antigens associated with carrier proteins derived from cholera toxin (CT) or *E. coli* heat-labile enterotoxin (LT), induced simultaneous peripheral and mucosal immunity (Eldridge et al., 1990; Elson and Ealding, 1984a, b). The same or similar antigens given without these particular vehicles yielded cross-regulation. In addition, antigens conjugated with the B-subunits of CT or LT triggered acceptable peripheral and mucosal immune responses that were unattainable when antigen was given alone (Dertzbaugh and Elson, 1991; Elson and Dertzbaugh, 1994; Holmgren et al., 1993). Taken together, this research provided evidence that cross-regulation could be overcome using nontoxic and biodegradable vaccine vehicles.

Solutions from Microencapsulation Technology

The first technology to be highlighted is microencapsulation of vaccines with biodegradable polymers for immunization of the peripheral and mucosal immune systems. There are a number of recent reviews (in new journals committed to the field) that cover all the new microencapsulation systems, polymer chemistry (Gombotz and Pettit, 1995; Langer, 1990), and biologic applications (Michalek et al., 1994; Morris et al., 1994; Walker, 1994). After reports of success in potentiating immune responses with adjuvants composed of particulate antigens, numerous particulates were tested for vaccine-enhancing activities. The chemical composition of particles that were tested included polystyrene, latex, poly(methylmethacrylate), polyacrylamide, poly(butyl-2-cyanoacrylate), alginate, ethyline-vinyl acetate copolymer, and poly(lactide glycolide) copolymer (Michalek et al., 1994). These polymers exhibited a broad range of utility, toxicity, and biodegradability. This discussion will be restricted to observations about the use of polymers comprising lactic and glycolic acids (natural products of energy metabolism) as vehicles because they have been tested for efficacy in initiating peripheral and mucosal immune responses. Poly(lactide/glycolide) copolymer originally was developed for biodegradable suture material (Morris et al., 1994). It is licensed by the U.S. Food and Drug Administration for that use and has been used with no serious adverse sequelae for many years in human subjects. During the past 10 years, there has been exponential development of microencapsulation technology for the delivery of drugs and hormones and for other uses, such as the scratch-and-sniff advertisements found in magazines.

Biodegradable Microspheres Have Adjuvant Effects

The technology was first successfully applied to parenteral and oral immunization with vaccines by John Eldridge in the early 1980s. In addition to demonstrating that encapsulation protected the antigen from deterioration or degradation in the GI tract, Eldridge revealed that microencapsulation provided an "adjuvant" effect. The same quantity of antigen in microcapsules gave more vigorous immune responses than antigen given alone (Eldridge et al., 1990; Michalek et al., 1994; Walker, 1994).

Many of Eldridge's vaccine formulations were inoculated parenterally to determine antigen-release kinetics. The rate of particle degradation (a function of molecular weight, surface area, and ratio of lactide to glycolide in polymer composition) could be utilized effectively to control the rate of antigen release. It was discovered that microcapsule formulations could be constructed that released antigens in pulses, which mimicked a multiple-inoculation schedule although the product was administered only once. This line of inquiry has prospered, and new, improved formulations have been developed that facilitate encapsulation of aqueous-phase antigens and various water-in-oil or water-in-oil-in-water emulsions (Yan et al., 1994).

Microencapsulated Vaccines Overcome Cross-Regulation

When vaccine antigen in poly(lactide/glycolide) copolymer was administered orally in various size ranges between 1 and greater than 10 μm, particles of over 10-μm diameter were not absorbed in the gut. The larger absorbable particles (diameters > 5 to < 10 μm) arrested in Peyer's patches, whereas the smaller particles (> 1 to < 5 μm) were disseminated to mesenteric lymph node and spleen (Eldridge et al., 1990). This bimodal anatomic distribution of particles was accompanied by simultaneous elicitation of IgG and IgA immune responses. Hydrophobicity, contributed by the chemical composition of the polymer, enhanced uptake of the particles in Peyer's patches, and hydrophilicity favored dissemination. Thus, the use of particles in a range of sizes appeared to be the critical determining factor that enabled simultaneous induction of peripheral and mucosal immune responses and the avoidance of cross-regulation.

Microencapsulation with biodegradable polymers is not a technology foreign to food and nutrition research (Dunne, 1994). Preparation of this manuscript brought to light that a previous meeting of the Committee on Military Nutrition Research (IOM, 1994) had included a presentation on the use of these materials for food additives. The present use of microcapsules as vaccine vehicles could fit into the area of "medical food additives." Encapsulation of antibodies for passive prophylaxis requires less technology than that for vaccines. The sole objective is to bring the antibodies past the denaturing effects of gastric acid, and for this the antibodies need only be incorporated in standard "enteric" coatings. How these recombinant human antibodies are made is another exciting technology that will be covered along with antigen-antibody expression in transgenic plants.

Solutions from Enterotoxin-Derived Vaccine Carriers

Cholera toxin (CT) has important pharmacological effects. The toxin is composed of two subunits: a toxigenic A-subunit and the B-subunit (CTB), a pentameric ring structure that mediates binding of the toxin to the surface of eukaryotic cells. This has been known since it was determined that the watery diarrhea of cholera was not caused by intestinal epithelial cell injury (Gangarosa et al., 1960). The prodigious fluid output was produced by a pharmacological effect of CT on intestinal epithelial cells. After CT binds monosialyl GM1 ganglioside on epithelial cells via the pentameric B-subunit, the toxic A-subunit enters the cell and ADP-ribosylates the adenylate cyclase regulatory protein Gs. The result is runaway adenylate cyclase activity, which causes the absorptive epithelial cells to secrete massive amounts of fluid (Holmgren, 1981; Spangler, 1992).

Adjuvant Activity of Cholera Toxin

CT is a potent immunogen regardless of route of administration (Fuhrman and Cebra, 1981; Pierce and Gowans, 1975). It is one of the few antigens that will yield a potent IgA immune response when administered orally to experimental animals. CT never induces tolerance or cross-regulation *in vivo*. Furthermore, it can prevent a tolerogenic antigen from inducing tolerance when the two are coadministered. Cholera toxin may lose its ability to increase immunogenicity of nominal antigens if its B-subunit (CTB) is denatured or blocked, adversely affecting the GM1 ganglioside-binding capacity that is essential for the adjuvant effect (Dertzbaugh and Elson, 1993a; Sun et al., 1994).

Chemical conjugation (cross-linking) of antigens to CT or CTB can cause relatively poor mucosal immunogens to stimulate peripheral and mucosal immune responses strongly (Dertzbaugh and Elson, 1991, 1993b; Elson and Dertzbaugh, 1994; Elson and Ealding, 1984 a, b; Holmgren et al., 1993). The adjuvant activity of CT can be obtained if CT is mixed with antigen (Lehner et al., 1992; Ruedl et al., 1996; Stok et al., 1994). On the other hand, nontoxic CTB must be linked to an antigen to produce an adjuvant effect. Sometimes the procedure used to link antigens to CTB chemically damages the tertiary structure of the pentameric B-subunit ring and reduces adjuvanticity. An objective of Dertzbaugh and this laboratory has been to develop a bacterial expression system that will fuse an antigenic construct genetically to CTB in such a way that it can be expressed without alteration of the native configuration of the antigen or the B-subunit. A similar approach already has been reported to have had some success (Hajishengallis et al., 1995; Wu and Russell, 1994). Dertzbaugh and this group have been focusing on the benefits of using the nontoxic B-subunit (with or without molecular spacers derived from the nontoxic A2-peptide). Using constructs that lack the A1 ADP-ribosylase will avoid the necessity of dealing with issues related to toxicity.

Immunohistochemistry (Unpublished data, A. O. Anderson and M. T. Dertzbaugh, U.S. Army Medical Research Institute of Infectious Diseases, Fort Detrick, Md., 1992) reveals that some of the increased antibody production found when CT is used as an adjuvant may result from facilitated secretion by a few plasma cells rather than an increase in the number of cells secreting antibody. It has been observed that CT induces B-cells to secrete antibody when they are still in intermediate stages of migration and differentiation. Normally, IgM- or IgG-secreting cells are seen infrequently in gut lamina propria. During the first 24 hours after oral CT treatment, IgM+, IgG+, and IgA+ cells show marked accumulation of antibodies in surrounding lamina propria, indicative of increased secretion. These effects of CT holotoxin (the complete toxin molecule, possessing all subunits) may be pharmacological rather than immunological if CT causes plasma cells to hypersecrete by a mechanism similar to that which causes diarrhea through epithelial hypersecretion.

Cholera Toxin and E. Coli *Heat-Labile Enterotoxin*

CT and heat-labile enterotoxins (LTs) of *E. coli* are very homologous in amino acid sequence (CT and LT have 80% amino acid homology [Dallas and Falkow, 1980]) and tertiary structure (Burnette, 1994; Sixma et al., 1991; Zhang et al., 1995). LT is believed to have less potent toxicity than CT, but both cause diarrhea at relatively low doses in human subjects. The LT-1 enterotoxin has been used in similar adjuvant studies and found to have effects virtually identical to those of CT (Clements et al., 1988).

One critical difference between CT and LT is that the A-subunit of CT is cleaved posttranslationally into an enzymatic A1- and a nontoxic A2-peptide, whereas the A1 and A2 of LT must be cleaved by proteases encountered in the environment for toxicity to result. A report by Lycke et al. (1992) indicated that mutations that destroy the ADP-ribosylating activities of CT or LT also destroy the adjuvanticity. However, Dickinson and Clements (1995) were able to dissociate adjuvanticity from toxicity by creating a mutant that is resistant to proteolytic activation. The R192G mutant LT has an arginine substituted for a glycine at the 192nd amino acid from the N terminus, rendering the site resistant to proteolysis. This mutant LT (mLT) retains its ability to function as an adjuvant when given orally. Furthermore, its adjuvant activity extends to the potentiation of antigen-specific IgG serum and IgA mucosal antibody responses in mice (Dickinson and Clements, 1995). It also prevented induction of tolerance (cross-regulation) to nominal antigens. This promising product is moving rapidly through preclinical and clinical safety and efficacy trials (Personal communication, CDR D. Scott, Naval Medical Research Institute, Bethesda, Md., 1996, and J. Clements, Tulane University, New Orleans, La., 1996).

Effects of CT-LT on Mucosal T-Cell Compartments

The mechanisms that enable CT or LT to overcome cross-regulation, prevent tolerance, and potentiate peripheral and mucosal immune responses are not known. *In vitro* and *in vivo* studies of the cells, cytokines, and tissues affected by CT or LT have not revealed many similarities to effects of traditional adjuvants, such as Freund's complete adjuvant[21] (Anderson, 1985; Anderson et al., 1987b; Freund, 1956). Perhaps CT and LT merely remove the effects of CD8+ cells and improve the natural immune processes described earlier in this chapter, such as antigen presentation, cytokine secretion, and lymphocyte traffic.

---

[21] A water-in-oil emulsion of antigen, to which killed mycobacteria are added to boost antigenicity.

Effect of Cholera Toxin or Cholera Toxin B-Subunit on Lymphoid Tissue Compartments

When T- and B-cell compartments in lymphatic tissues from mice that had received CT or CTB orally were examined by immunohistochemistry, there were no glaring changes in T- and B-cell populations in lymph nodes, spleen, or Peyer's patches. However, CT and CTB very quickly depleted the CD8+ cells in the intraepithelial compartment, cells that are normally very prevalent. The rapid 80 percent reduction in CD8+ IEL between 12 and 72 hours was impressive. Equally impressive was the finding that between 10 and 14 days later, the intraepithelial compartment was repopulated. Depletion of IEL primarily affected CD8+ cells, but other phenotypes also must have left the epithelium. The CD4+ cells in Peyer's patches and lamina propria stayed the same or increased in number during the drop in CD-8+ cells. The depletion of IEL was triggered by doses of CT or CTB that have been shown to be mucosal adjuvants in other studies (Elson and Ealding, 1984a, b). These anatomic findings were consistent with a hypothesis that CT-LT achieves its adjuvant effect by altering the T-cell regulatory environment in mucosal lymphoid compartments to support mucosal immunity, prevent tolerance induction, and ameliorate cross-regulation (Elson et al., 1995).

Solutions to Quantity and Cost Issues for CT-LT Vaccine Carriers

The idea of developing new vaccines that incorporate recombinant antigens and/or biologically active carriers raises a few questions. One question concerns yield. Bacteria grow rapidly, but it takes a lot of bacteria a long time to produce only a handful of product, and the cost of operating large fermenters is not trivial. Contamination of product with bacterial endotoxin also may affect the yield. The product must be purified free of endotoxin, and that could result in the loss of some of the product.

Another of the factors that might limit interest in developing recombinant vaccines and therapeutic antibodies is cost. It often has been stated that, with luck, vaccines take 10 years or more from discovery to FDA licensure. Many people start to develop vaccines, but few vaccines become licensed because anywhere along the way the product may fail. If it fails during the preclinical phase, money will be saved. Many other vaccines fail during Phase I safety trials in human volunteers, if adverse reactions are unacceptable. The worst case would be failure during field testing when a vaccine that was safe and efficacious in experimental animals failed to corroborate its efficacy in humans.

Pharmaceutical industries face these realities continually, but the public (the customers) cannot understand why every start does not necessarily translate into a new beneficial product for them. All of this costs time, personal commitment, and lots of money. This becomes an especially frustrating concept if one considers that the vaccines needed most, such as malaria vaccines, are against disease threats that are endemic in countries whose financial resources preclude any chance of buying the product.

The next section will show how both of these issues may be resolved by producing antigens or antibodies in plants.

SOLUTIONS FROM PRODUCTION IN TRANSGENIC PLANTS

Rapid progress in plant biotechnology will result in contributions to vaccine production from agriculture. Recent results suggest that genetically engineered plants may be used to produce vaccines against human diseases (Arntzen et al., 1994; Haq et al., 1995; Mason et al., 1992). A concern is that plant-produced vaccines will require purification free of alkaloids and other toxic plant materials. Two approaches may be used to resolve this. One is to use plant vectors that incorporate the protein into a tissue that lacks toxic alkyloids, for example, bananas or soybeans (Arntzen et al., 1994; McCabe et al., 1988). Another approach would be to use the same technology used to incorporate the vaccine construct into plants to remove the genes for the toxic substances genetically (Moffat, 1995; Morris et al., 1994; Personal communication, M. B. Hein, Scripps Research Institute, La Jolla, Calif., 1995).

If the potential concerns about plant alkaloids can be resolved quickly, production of vaccines in plants will be a significant improvement over current methods. Such vaccines might be cheaper than those now available because plants are easier to grow in large quantities than are cultured animal, insect, bacterial, or yeast cells now used to make most vaccines (Moffat, 1995; Morris et al., 1994).

The details of inserting antigenic constructs into plants as expression vectors have been worked out, as well as systems for the use of baculoviruses, bacteria, or yeast to produce products. The discovery that plant tumors (called galls) were produced by a bacterium called *Agrobacterium tumefasciens* is responsible for this rapid progress in developing plants as expression vectors (Horsch et al., 1988; Jefferson et al., 1987). In addition, new technologies for inserting genes into plants have been developed to overcome limited host-range specificity of *Agrobacterium* vectors (McCabe et al., 1988; Owens and Cress, 1985; Pedersen et al., 1983).

The plant biotechnology field has been working out the requirements for inserting and expressing genes in plants since the late 1970s. The recent breakthrough has been spurred by demonstration of efficient production of heterologous proteins in plants (Gasser and Fraley, 1989; Hiatt et al., 1989). This may produce a potential added benefit for worried tobacco farmers because the easiest plant vector to transform is the tobacco plant. As people progressively stop smoking, the new technology might provide important replacement crops for tobacco growers if the toxic alkaloids in tobacco leaf can be cloned out easily.

New biotechnology companies are well positioned to profit from the anticipated economic benefits because all that would be needed to scale-up production of plant-made protein to the amounts needed for a commercial vaccine is to add acreage. Cheaper vaccines that are available in large quantities make vaccination of an entire expeditionary force feasible in contingency situations. It is anticipated that use of transgenic plants as expression vectors might provide all the protein needed during one growing season, while conventional vaccine production techniques would require much more time. These vaccines potentially will be safer because production in plants virtually eliminates the problem of contamination with animal viruses.

Another line of research is the development of "edible vaccines" (Arntzen et al., 1994). These vaccines are designed with the expectation that no purification step is required, and the vaccine components are expressed in final form in the interstices of the plant. The use of a CTB or LT vaccine carrier would target the antigen construct to be taken up and processed in mucosal lymphatic tissues, where the biological effects of the carrier should program the response for peripheral and mucosal immunity.

ANTIBODY NEEDED FOR PASSIVE PROTECTION

Passive transfer of immunity by serum injection has become a routine medical practice after its original description over 100 years ago (Cohn et al., 1946; von Behring and Kitasato, 1890). Passive immunoprophylaxis by parenteral infusion (for "peripheral" protective immunity) using IgG antibodies also has become very common (Cryz, 1991). In a military scenario, the benefit of passive protection by antibodies raised by conventional means would appear to be limited by cost and availability of sufficient quantities. Except under very unusual circumstances, it would be impractical to produce industrial quantities of prophylactic antibodies in humans prospectively (DasGupta, 1993; Franz et al., 1993; Metzger and Lewis, 1979). Antibodies prepared in other species (such as horse, cow, or pig) may be given without risk for passive oral protection (Losonsky et al., 1985), but the risk of serum sickness (multiple organ damage caused by host antibodies forming complexes with the "foreign" animal proteins) (or other adverse reactions) would preclude any sequential parenteral use (Renegar and Small, 1994; Tsunemitsu et al., 1989).

Solutions for Quantities of Antibody Needed

Once again, use of transgenic plants to express recombinant human antibodies should provide a solution (Hiatt et al., 1989; Ma et al., 1995). This final section will describe how high-affinity antigen-combining sites of immunoglobulins can be obtained rapidly using recombinant DNA technology, genetically fused with human light- and heavy-chain constant regions, and expressed as functional antibodies in plants.

Preselection of "High Affinity-Ig" B-Cells for Complementarity-Determining Region Isolation and Expression in Transgenic Plants

After *in vivo* antigenic stimulation in mammals, B-cells undergo molecular and cellular changes within germinal centers of lymphoid follicles. An important change that B-cells undergo is "affinity maturation," whereby B-cells expressing specific antibodies for a given antigen undergo progressive changes that result in selection of cells capable of making antibodies with higher binding affinity (Eisen and Siskind, 1964; Gearhart, 1993).

Affinity maturation occurs through a process of somatic hypermutation, whereby single base pairs are substituted in the DNA sequence of immunoglobulin variable regions, specifically in the CDRs. The specific base substitutions occur at "hot" spots in the CDR gene sequences, which could serve as markers for immunoglobulins with increased antigen affinity (Betz et al., 1993). The DNA of such cells may be rescued selectively for development of high-affinity antibody.

After it is isolated from B-cells in tissue sections, DNA from immunoglobulin V-region genes can be cloned into filamentous phage display vectors (Winter et al., 1994). This makes it possible to study the effect of individual nucleotide changes on the affinity of antibodies from B-cells isolated at specific sites within the reactive lymphoid tissue (Bakker et al., 1995). Genomic DNA from B-cells isolated from rabbit appendix germinal centers has been cloned and sequenced, and single-point mutations in germline V-gene sequences that occurred as part of affinity maturation could be followed (Weinstein et al., 1994a, b). This procedure currently is being used to isolate antigen-specific CDRs after deliberate immunization with selected antigens including the F-1 antigen of *Yersinia pestis.*

Polymerase chain reaction (PCR) amplification and cloning of immunoglobulin VH-regions permit rapid isolation of CDRs encoding antigen-binding sites (Jacob et al., 1991, 1993; Marks et al., 1991; Weinstein et al., 1994a, b). Germinal centers are oligoclonal populations of dividing B-cells found in characteristic anatomic locations in lymphoid tissues. Sampling cells from the different regions of a germinal center (identified as specific for nominal antigen by labeled antigen-binding to surface antibody on B-cells in frozen tissue sections) will reduce the number of CDR clones that must be screened in order to select the ones encoding high-affinity antigen binding (Unpublished data, A. O. Anderson and P. D. Weinstein, U.S. Army Medical Research Institute of Infectious Diseases, Fort Detrick, Md., 1995). This is an improvement over random selection from large V-gene libraries (Marks et al., 1991). In addition, there are methods of converting low-affinity binding sites to high-affinity by directed mutagenesis (Betz et al., 1993; Griffiths et al., 1994; Wong et al., 1995).

Making Recombinant Human Antibodies in Transgenic Plants

Expression of the selected CDRs on conserved framework structures of human immunoglobulins in transgenic plants should allow production of large amounts of protective antibodies (Ma et al., 1995). The example that proved that functional antibodies could be made in plants solved many potential problems. The objective was to produce secretory IgA that was specific for a streptococcal antigen involved in dental caries.

It was a good test of feasibility because there are critical genetic and immunoglobulin structural requirements for IgA molecules to function *in vivo*. It is not sufficient to be successful in cloning a functional VH-VL CDR complex. One also must account for the fact that mammalian immunoglobulin genes are divided among different chromosomes, and the molecule is assembled posttranslationally. The assembled IgA heavy-chain structure must not interfere with dimerization because failure to dimerize interferes with secretion by epithelial cells, antibody function, or both. The dimer must link up with the J-chain so the complex can bind to the extracellular polymeric immunoglobulin receptor, which is involved in translocating the antibody across epithelium.
What Ma and his colleagues (1995) accomplished truly was amazing. They focused on conferring the ability on transgenic plants to assemble secretory IgA molecules as though they already had been secreted by the epithelial cell. They cleverly used the Mendelian genetics of their transgenic plants to divide up the task of inserting a lot of mammalian genetic material. The group made four separate transgenic plant lines, each of which received a gene for only a part of the secretory IgA. After they were certain that no genes were altered by the process, they crossed the plants the way Greggor Mendel crossed his peas. The sequence of matings is shown in Figure 22-7. Plants have a useful idiosyncrasy. The progeny efficiently produced the anticipated antibody fully assembled in functional form and in ample quantities. Where these antibodies accumulated in the transgenic plants suggested that purification of the product free of plant material should be relatively easy.

Research directed toward application of this technology will be tremendously valuable because present methods of antibody production require time-consuming immunization procedures in large animals and result in a product of limited sequential use in humans. Furthermore, the use of plants expressing a transgene that produces human antibodies would permit the quantity of antibody attainable to be limited only by the size of the crop or number of animals bred.

The sequence of development would depend upon the ease by which one rapidly could select high-affinity CDRs that bind and neutralize a pathogen, construct recombinant human antibodies of IgA or IgG isotypes using the selected CDR, and determine the affinity of the antibody constructs selected for expression in transgenic plant crops (Bakker et al., 1995; Winter et al., 1994). Depending upon the ease of isolation and purification of the product, such protective antibodies could be quickly prepared against disease threats that are en-

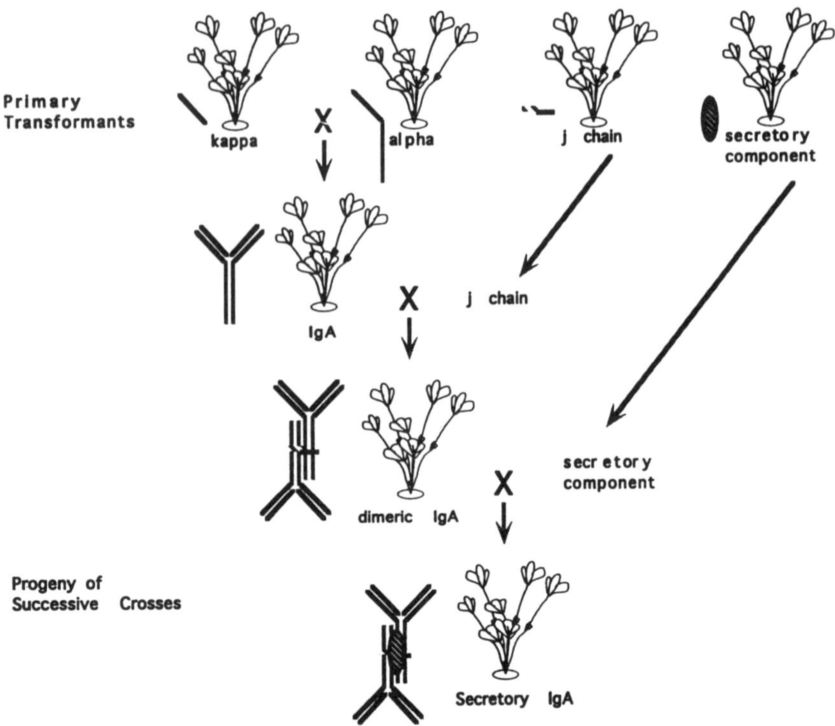

FIGURE 22-7 This schematic diagram illustrates the process for generating transgenic plants expressing assembled immunoglobulins. Individual plants were first transformed with one of four genes encoding kappa-light chain, alpha-heavy chain, J-chain, or secretory component. Plants expressing the kappa or alpha chain were first crossed to generate progeny containing assembled IgA. Successive crosses of IgA producing plants with J-chain-containing plants yielded progeny with assembled dimeric IgA. These plants were then crossed with plants expressing a truncated form of the polyimmunoglobulin receptor (secretory component) to generate progeny containing secretory IgA. SOURCE: M. Hein (Scripps Research Institute, La Jolla, Calif., 1995), used with permission.

demic worldwide. The shortened time interval and capacity for rapid scale-up should make these products inexpensive to produce in large quantities. Incorporating enterically coated recombinant antibodies in MREs could be used to bring about a significant reduction in morbidity or disease-related decrements in performance in soldiers deployed anywhere in the world.

AUTHOR'S CONCLUSIONS AND RECOMMENDATIONS

The study of mucosal immunology has contributed to the understanding of concepts and issues of host resistance that is needed for protection of the gastrointestinal tract and other mucosa that provide for optimal nutrition. An added benefit of support for this discipline has been a better understanding of how vaccines can be used more effectively.

The new technologies of vaccine microencapsulation, use of the nontoxic B-subunit of cholera or *E. coli* enterotoxin carriers for recombinant vaccine constructs, and incorporation of recombinant vaccine constructs into edible plants have become feasible, and this technology can be studied for acceptability for delivery of vaccines to military personnel.

The above technologies overcome cross-regulation and induce immune responses with circulating IgG, as well as secretory IgA. This should provide complete active prophylaxis without need for injections or time-consuming vaccine schedules.

Expression of functional recombinant human antibodies in plants has been demonstrated. This makes feasible the production of industrial quantities of protective recombinant antibody for use in passive immunoprophylaxis. Such antibody, when protected from stomach acid by enteric coatings or encapsulation, could be incorporated into meals for protection of troops from endemic causes of dysentery.

The following recommendations can be made:

• Institute a rational policy for immunizing military recruits against threat agents and selected geographic pathogens.

• Establish a Science and Technology Objective for adaptation of militarily relevant vaccines for oral administration through application of the above technology.

• To achieve this goal, encourage cooperative collaboration between the U.S. Army Research Institute of Environmental Medicine; U.S. Army Natick Research, Development and Engineering Center; and U.S. Army Medical Research Institute of Infectious Diseases.

• Increase funding support for technology development that may not be linked to specific threat agents.

REFERENCES

Abbas, A.K., K.M. Murphy, and A. Sher
  1996   Functional diversity of helper T lymphocytes. Nature 383:787–793.
Abernethy, N.J., J.B. Hay, W.G. Kimpton, E. Washington, and R.N.P. Cahill
  1991   Lymphocyte subset-specific and tissue-specific lymphocyte-endothelial cell recognition mechanisms independently direct the recirculation of lymphocytes from blood to lymph in sheep. Immunology 72:239–245.
Agace, W., S. Hedges, U. Andersson, J. Andersson, M. Ceska, and C. Svanborg
  1993   Selective cytokine production by epithelial cells following exposure to *Escherichia coli*. Infect. Immun. 61:602–609.
Altman, J.D., P.A.H. Moss, P.J.R. Goulder, D.H. Barouch, M.G. McHeyzer-Williams, J.I. Bell, A.J. McMichael, and M.M. Davis
  1996   Phenotypic analysis of antigen-specific T lymphocytes. Science 274:94–96.

Anderson, A.O.
   1985   Multiple effects of immunological adjuvants on lymphatic microenvironments. Int.
           J. Immunother. 1:185–195.
   1990   Structure and organization of the lymphatic system. Pp. 14–45 in Immunophysiol-
           ogy. The Role of Cells and Cytokines in Immunity and Inflammation, J.J.
           Oppenheim and E. Shevach, eds. New York: Oxford University Press.
Anderson, A.O., and J.A. Reynolds
   1979   Adjuvant effects of the lipid amine CP-20, 961 (on lymphoid cell traffic and anti-
           viral immunity). J. Reticuloendothel. Soc. 350:33–41.
Anderson, A.O., and D.H. Rubin
   1985   Effect of avridine on enteric antigen uptake and mucosal immunity to reovirus.
           Adv. Exp. Med. Biol. 186:579–590.
Anderson, A.O., and S. Shaw
   1993   T-cell adhesion to endothelium: The FRC conduit system and other anatomic and
           molecular features which facilitate the adhesion cascade in lymph node. Sem.
           Immunol. 5:271–282.
   1996   Lymphocyte trafficking. Pp. 39–49 in Clinical Immunology, Principles and Prac-
           tice, R.R. Rich, T.A. Fleisher, B.D. Schwartz, W.T. Shearer, and W. Strober, eds.
           St. Louis, Mo.: Mosby-Year Book, Inc.
Anderson, A.O., T.T. McDonald, and D.H. Rubin
   1985   Effect of orally administered avridine on enteric antigen uptake and mucosal im-
           munity. Int. J. Immunother. 1:107–115.
Anderson, A.O., L.F. Snyder, M.L.M. Pitt, and O.L. Wood
   1987a   Mucosal priming alters pathogenesis of Rift Valley fever. Adv. Exp. Med. Biol.
           237:727–733.
Anderson, A.O., O.L. Wood, A.D. King, and E.H. Stephenson
   1987b   Studies on anti-viral mucosal immunity using the lipoidal amine adjuvant avridine.
           Adv. Exp. Med. Biol. 216B:1781–1790.
Anderson, G.W., Jr., J.O. Lee, A.O. Anderson, N. Powell, J.A. Mangiafico, and G. Meadors
   1991   Efficacy of a Rift Valley fever virus vaccine against an aerosol infection in rats.
           Vaccine 9:710–714.
Ariizumi, K., T. Kitajima, O.R. Bergstresser, and A. Takashima
   1995   Interleukin-1β converting enzyme in murine Langerhans cells and epidermal-
           derived dendritic cell lines. Eur. J. Immunol. 25:2137–2141.
Arntzen, C.J., H.S Mason, J. Shi, T.A. Haq, M.K. Estes, and J.D. Clements
   1994   Production of candidate oral vaccines in edible tissues of transgenic plants. Pp.
           339–344 in Vaccines '94, F. Brown, R.M. Chanock, H.S. Ginsberg, and R.A.
           Lerner, eds. Cold Spring Harbor, New York: Cold Spring Harbor Laboratory.
Assenmacher, M., J. Schmitz, and A. Radbruch
   1994   Flow cytometric determination of cytokines in activated murine Th lymphocytes.
           Expression of Il-10 in IFN-gamma and in IL-4 expressing cells. Eur. J. Immunol.
           24:1097–1101.
Bakker, R., E. Lasonder, and N.A. Bos
   1995   Measurement of affinity in serum samples of antigen-free, germ-free and conven-
           tional mice after hyperimmunization with 2,4-dinitrophenyl keyhole limpet hemo-
           cyanin, using surface plasmon resonance. Eur. J. Immunol. 25:1680–1686.
Beisel, W.R.
   1994   Endocrine and immune system responses to stress. Pp. 177–207 in Food Compo-
           nents to Enhance Performance, An Evaluation of Potential Performance-Enhancing
           Food Components for Operational Rations, B.M. Marriott, ed. A report of the
           Committee on Military Nutrition Research, Food and Nutrition Board, Institute of
           Medicine. Washington, D.C.: National Academy Press.

Bendelac, A.
 1995 CD1: Presenting unusual antigens to unusual T lymphocytes. Science 269:185–192.
Berlin, C., E.L. Berg, M.J. Briskin, D.P. Andrew, P.J. Kilshaw, B. Holzmann, I.L. Weissman, A. Hamann, and E.C. Butcher
 1993 α4β7 integrin mediates lymphocyte binding to the mucosal vascular addressin MAdCAM-1. Cell 74:185–195.
Betz, A.G., M.S. Neuberger, and C. Milstein
 1993 Discriminating intrinsic and antigen-selected mutational hotspots in immunoglobulin V genes. Immunol. Today 14:405–411.
Brandtzaeg, P.
 1994 Distribution and characteristics of mucosal immunoglobulin-producing cells. Pp. 251–262 in Handbook of Mucosal Immunology, P.L. Ogra, J. Mestecky, M.E. Lamm, W. Strober, J.R. McGhee, and J. Bienenstock, eds. Boston: Academic Press, Inc.
Brown, J.L., J.W. Dominik, and R.L. Morrissey
 1981 Respiratory infectivity of a recently isolated Egyptian strain of Rift Valley fever virus. Infect. Immun. 33:848–853.
Burnette, W. Neal
 1994 AB5 ADP-ribosylating toxins: Comparative anatomy and physiology. Structure 2:151–158.
Butcher, E.C.
 1991 Leukocyte endothelial cell recognition: Three or more steps to specificity and diversity. Cell 67:1033–1036.
Butcher, E.C., and L.J. Picker
 1996 Lymphocyte homing and homeostasis. Science 272:60–66.
Cahill, R.N.P., D.C. Poskitt, H. Frost, and Z. Trnka
 1977 Two distinct pools of recirculating T lymphocytes: Migratory characteristics of nodal and intestinal T lymphocytes. J. Exp. Med. 145:420–428.
Carayannopoulos, L., and J.D. Capra
 1993 Immunoglobulins. Structure and function. Pp. 293–314 in Fundamental Immunology, 3d ed., W.E. Paul, ed. New York: Raven Press, Ltd.
Cebra, J.J., P.J. Gearhart, R. Kamat, S.M. Robertson, and J. Tseng
 1977 Origin and differentiation of lymphocytes involved in the secretory IgA responses. Cold Spring Harbor Symp. Quant. Biol. 41:201–215.
Cepek, K.L., S.K. Shaw, C.M. Parker, G.J. Russell, J.S. Morrow, D.L. Rimm, and M.B. Brenner
 1994 Adhesion between epithelial cells and T lymphocytes mediated by E-cadherin and the αEβ7 integrin. Nature 372:190–193.
Chase, M.W.
 1946 Inhibition of experimental drug allergy by prior feeding of the sensitivity agent. Proc. Soc. Exp. Biol. Med. 61:257–259.
Chen, Y., J. Inobe, R. Marks, P. Gonnella, V.K. Kuchroo, and H.L. Weiner
 1995 Peripheral deletion of antigen-reactive T-cells in oral tolerance. Nature 376:177–189.
Clements, J.D., N.M. Hartzog, and F.L. Lyon
 1988 Adjuvant activity of *Escherichia coli* heat-labile enterotoxin and effect on the induction of oral tolerance in mice to unrelated protein antigens. Vaccine 6:269–277.
Cohn, E.J., L.E. Strong, and L.W. Hughes, Jr.
 1946 Preparation and properties of serum and plasma proteins. 4. A system for the separation of fractions of proteins and lipoprotein components of biological tissues and fluids. J. Am. Chem. Soc. 8:459.

Cryz, S.J., Jr., ed.
1991 Vaccines and Immunotherapy. New York: Pergamon Press.
Cuff, C.E., C.K. Cebra, D.H. Rubin, and J.J. Cebra
1993 Developmental relationship between cytotoxic α/β T-cell receptor-positive intra-epithelial lymphocytes and Peyer's patch lymphocytes. Eur. J. Immunol. 23:1333–1339.
Dallas, W.S., and S. Falkow
1980 Amino acid sequence homology between cholera toxin and *Escherichia coli* heat-labile toxin. Nature (London) 288:499–501.
DasGupta, B.R., ed.
1993 Botulinum and Tetanus Neurotoxins, Neurotransmission and Biomedical Aspects. New York: Plenum Press.
Dertzbaugh, M.T., and C.O. Elson
1991 Cholera toxin as a mucosal adjuvant. Pp. 119–131 in Topics in Vaccine Adjuvant Research, D.R. Spriggs and W.C. Koff, eds. Boca Raton, Fla.: CRC Press.
1993a Reduction in oral immunogenicity of cholera toxin B subunit by N-terminal peptide addition. Infect. Immun. 61(2):384–390.
1993b Comparative effectiveness of the cholera toxin B subunit and alkaline phosphatase as carriers for oral vaccines. Infect. Immun. 61(1):48–55.
Dertzbaugh, M.T., and C.J. Van Meter
1996 The mucosal immunogenicity of cholera toxin B-subunit is dependent on its ability to bind to ganglioside. Unpublished manuscript. Fort Detrick, Md.: U.S. Army Medical Research Institute of Infectious Diseases.
Dickinson, B.L., and J.D. Clements
1995 Dissociation of *Escherichia coli* heat-labile enterotoxin adjuvanticity from ADP-ribosyltransferase activity. Infect. Immun. 63(5):1617–1623.
Dunne, C.P.
1994 Biochemical strategies for ration design: Concerns of bioavailability. Pp. 93–109 in Food Components to Enhance Performance, An Evaluation of Potential Performance-Enhancing Food Components for Operational Rations, B.M. Marriott, ed. A report of the Committee on Military Nutrition Research, Food and Nutrition Board, Institute of Medicine. Washington, D.C.: National Academy Press.
Ebnet, K., E.P. Kaldjian, A.O. Anderson, and S. Shaw
1996 Orchestrated information transfer underlying leukocyte endothelial interactions. Ann. Rev. Immunol. 14:155–177
Eckmann, L., M.F. Kagnoff, and J. Fierer
1993 Epithelial cells secrete the chemokine interleukin-8 in response to bacterial entry. Infect. Immun. 61:4569–4574.
Eisen, H.N., and G.W. Siskind
1964 Variations in affinities of antibodies during the immune response. Biochemistry 3:996–1008.
Eldridge, J.H., C.J. Hammond, J.A. Meulbroek, J.K. Staas, R.M. Gilley, and T.R. Tice
1990 Controlled vaccine release in the gut-associated lymphoid tissues. I. Orally administered biodegradable microspheres target the Peyer's patches. J. Controlled Release 11:205–214.
Elson, C.O., and M.T. Dertzbaugh
1994 Mucosal adjuvants. Pp. 391–401 in Handbook of Mucosal Immunology, P.L. Ogra, J. Mestecky, M.E. Lamm, W. Strober, J.R. McGhee, and J. Bienenstock, eds. Boston: Academic Press, Inc.
Elson, C.O., and W. Ealding
1984a Cholera toxin feeding did not induce oral tolerance in mice and abrogated oral tolerance to an unrelated protein antigen. J. Immunol. 133:2892–2897.

1984b Generalized systemic and mucosal immunity in mice after mucosal stimulation with cholera toxin. J. Immunol. 132:2736–2741.

Elson, C.O., S.P. Holland, M.T. Dertzbaugh, C.F. Cuff, and A.O. Anderson
1995 Morphologic and functional alterations of mucosal T-cells by cholera toxin and its B subunit. J. Immunol. 154:1032–1040.

Finkelman, F.D.
1995 Relationships among antigen presentation, cytokines, immune deviation, and autoimmune disease. J. Exp. Med. 182:279–282.

Franz, D.R., L.M. Pitt, M.A. Clayton, J.A. Hanes, and K.J. Rose
1993 Efficacy of prophylactic and therapeutic administration of antitoxin for inhalation botulism. Pp. 473–476 in Botulinum and Tetanus Neurotoxins, B.R. DasGupta, ed. New York: Plenum Press.

Freund, J.
1956 The mode of action of immunological adjuvants. Adv. Tuberc. Res. 7:130–148.

Fuhrman, J.A., and J.J. Cebra
1981 Special features of the priming process for a secretory IgA response. J. Exp. Med. 153:534–544.

Gangarosa, E.J., W.R. Beisel, C. Benyajati, H. Sprinz, and P. Piyaratn
1960 The nature of the gastrointestinal lesion in Asiatic cholera and its relation to pathogenesis: A biopsy study. Am. J. Trop. Med. Hyg. 9:125–135.

Gasser, C.S., and R.T. Fraley
1989 Genetically engineering plants for crop improvement. Science 244:1293–1299.

Gearhart, P.J.
1993 Somatic mutation and affinity maturation. Pp. 865–885 in Fundamental Immunology, 3rd ed., W.E. Paul, ed. New York: Raven Press, Ltd.

Gelfanov, V., V. Gelfanova, Y-G. Lai, and N-S. Liao
1996 Activated $\alpha\beta$-CD8+, but not $\alpha\alpha$-CD8+, TCR-$\alpha\beta$+murine intestinal intraepithelial lymphocytes can mediate perforin-based cytotoxicity, whereas both subsets are active in FAS-based cytotoxicity. J. Immunol. 156:35–41.

Gombotz, W.R., and D.K. Pettit
1995 Biodegradable polymers for protein and peptide drug delivery. Bioconjugate Chem. 6:332–351.

Gretz, J.E., E.P. Kaldjian, A.O. Anderson, and S. Shaw
1996 Sophisticated strategies for information encounter in the lymph node: The reticular network as a conduit of soluble information and a highway for cell traffic. J. Immunol. 157:495–499.

Griffiths, A.D., S.C. Williams, O. Hartley, I.M. Tomlinson, P. Waterhouse, W.L. Crosby, R.E. Kontermann, P.T. Jones, N.M. Low, T.J. Allison, T.D. Prospero, H.R. Hoogenboom, A. Nissim, J.P.L. Cox, J.L. Harrison, M. Zaccolo, E. Gherardi, and G. Winter
1994 Isolation of high affinity human antibodies directly from large synthetic repertoires. EMBO J. 13:3245–3260.

Hajishengallis, G., S.K. Hollingshead, T. Koga, and M.W. Russell
1995 Mucosal immunization with a bacterial protein antigen genetically coupled to cholera toxin A2/B subunits. J. Immunol. 154:4322–4332.

Hamann, A., D.P. Andrew, D. Jablonski-Westrich, B. Holzmann, and E.C. Butcher
1994 Role of α4-integrins in lymphocyte homing to mucosal tissues *in vivo*. J. Immunol. 152:3282–3292.

Hamilton, S.R., J.H. Yardley, and G.D. Brown
1979 Suppression of local intestinal immunoglobulin A immune response to cholera toxin by subcutaneous administration of cholera toxoids. Infect. Immun. 24:422–426.

Haq, T.A., H.S. Mason, J.D. Clements, and C.J. Arntzen
  1995   Oral immunization with a recombinant bacterial antigen produced in transgenic plants. Science 268:714–716.
Hart, M.K., W. Pratt, F. Panelo, K. Stephan, L. Aikens, R. Tammariello, and M. Dertzbaugh
  1995   Dissociation between serum neutralizing antibodies and protection from airborne VEE virus in immunized mice. Clin Immunol. Immunopathol. 76:S97
Hiatt, A., R. Cafferkey, and K. Bowdish
  1989   Production of antibodies in transgenic plants. Nature 342:76–78.
Hilbert, D.M., K.L. Holmes, A.O. Anderson, and S. Rudikoff
  1994   Long-term lymphoid reconstitution of SCID mice suggests self renewing B- and T-cell populations in peripheral and mucosal tissues. Transplantation 58:466–475.
Hiroi, T., K. Fujihashi, J.R. McGhee, and H. Kiyono
  1995   Polarized Th2 cytokine expression by both mucosal γσ and αβ T-cells. Eur. J. Immunol. 25:2743–2751.
Holmgren, J.
  1981   Actions of cholera toxin and the prevention and treatment of cholera. Nature 292:413–417.
Holmgren, J., N. Lycke, and C. Czerkinsky
  1993   Cholera toxin and cholera B subunit as oral-mucosal adjuvant and antigen vector systems. Vaccine 11(12):1179–1184.
Horsch, R.B., J. Fry, N. Hoffmann, J. Neidermeyer, S.G. Rogers, and R.T. Fraley
  1988   Leaf disc transformation. In Plant Molecular Biology Manual A5:1–9, S.B. Gelvin, R.A. Schilperoort, and D.P.S. Verma, eds. Dordrecht, Belgium: Kluwer Academic Publishers.
Husband, A.J., and J.L. Gowans
  1978   The origin and antigen-dependent distribution of IgA-containing cells in the intestine. J. Exp. Med. 148:1146–1160.
Hyams, K.C., A.L. Bourgeois, B.R. Merrell, P. Rozmajzl, J. Escamilla, S.A. Thronton, G.M. Wasserman, A. Burke, P. Echeverria, K.Y. Green, A.Z. Kapikian, and J.N. Woody
  1991   Diarrheal disease during Operation Desert Shield. N. Eng. J. Med. 325:1423–1428.
Hyams, K.C., J.D. Malone, A.Z. Kapikian, M.K. Estes, X. Jiang, A.L. Bourgeois, S. Paparello, R.E. Hawkins, and K.Y. Green
  1993   Norwalk virus infection among Desert Storm troops. J. Infect. Dis. 167:986–987.
IOM (Institute of Medicine)
  1994   Food Components to Enhance Performance, An Evaluation of Potential Performance-Enhancing Food Components for Operational Rations, B.M. Marriott, ed. A report of the Committee on Military Nutrition Research, Food and Nutrition Board. Washington, D.C.: National Academy Press.
Jacob, J., G. Kelsoe, K. Rajewsky, and U. Weiss
  1991   Intraclonal generation of antibody mutants in germinal centers. Nature 354:389–392.
Jacob, J., J. Przylepa, C. Miller, and G. Kelsoe
  1993   In situ studies of the primary immune response to (4-hydroxy-3-nitrophenyl)acetyl. III. The kinetics of V region mutation and selection in germinal center B-cells. J. Exp. Med. 178:1293–1307.
Jahrling, P.B., and E.H. Stephenson
  1984   Protective efficacies of live attenuated and formaldehyde-inactivated Venezuelan equine encephalitis virus vaccines against aerosol challenge in hamsters. J. Clin. Microbiol. 19:429–431.
Jefferson, R.A., T.A. Kavanagh, and M.W. Bevan
  1987   GUS fusions: β-glucuronidase as a sensitive and versatile gene fusion marker in higher plants. EMBO J. 6(13):3901–3907.

Kagnoff, M.F.
  1996   Mucosal immunology: New frontiers. Immunol. Today 17:57–59.
Kang, K., M. Kubin, K.D. Cooper, S.R. Lessin, G. Trinchieri, and A.H. Rook
  1996   IL-12 synthesis by human Langerhans cells. J. Immunol. 156:1402–1407.
Kantele, A., J.M. Kantele, E. Savilahti, M. Westerholm, H. Arvilommi, A. Lazarovits, E.C. Butcher, and P.H. Makela
  1997   Oral, but not parenteral, typhoid vaccination induces circulating antibody-secreting cells that all bear homing receptors directing them to the gut. J. Immunol. 158:574–579.
Karecla, P.I., S.J. Bowden, S.J. Green, and P.J. Kilshaw
  1995   Recognition of E-cadherin on epithelial cells by the mucosal T-cell integrin $\alpha_{M290}^{\beta}7$ ($\alpha E\beta7$). Eur. J. Immunol. 25:852–856.
Ke, Y., and J.A. Kapp
  1996   Oral antigen inhibits priming of CD8+ CTL, CD4+ T-cells, and antibody responses while activating CD8+ suppressor T-cells. J. Immunol. 156:916–921.
Kimpton, W.G., E.A. Washington, and R.N.P. Cahill
  1989   Recirculation of lymphocyte subsets (CD5+, CD4+, CD8+, SBU-T19+ and B-cells) through gut and peripheral lymph nodes. Immunology 66:69–75.
Koster, F.T., and N.F. Pierce
  1983   Parenteral immunization causes antigen-specific cell-mediated suppression of an intestinal IgA response. J. Immunol. 131:115–119.
Kotloff, D.B., and J.J. Cebra
  1988   Effect of TH-lines and clones on the growth and differentiation of B-cell clones in microculture. Mol. Immunol. 25:147–155.
Kraal, G., K. Schornagel, P.R. Streeter, B. Holzman, and E.C. Butcher
  1995   Expression of the mucosal vascular addressin, MAdCAM-1, on sinus-lining cells in the spleen. Am. J. Pathol. 147:763–771.
Kroemer, G., E. Cuende, and C-A. Martinez
  1993   Compartmentalization of the peripheral immune system. Adv. Immunol. 53:157–216.
Langer, R.
  1990   New methods of drug delivery. Science 249:1527–1533.
Lebman, D.A., and R.L. Coffman
  1994   Cytokines in the mucosal immune system. Pp. 243–250 in Handbook of Mucosal Immunology, P.L. Ogra, J. Mestecky, M.E. Lamm, W. Strober, J.R. McGhee, and J. Bienenstock, eds. Boston: Academic Press, Inc.
Lehner, T., L.A. Bergmeier, C. Panagiotidi, L. Tao, R. Brookes, L.S. Klavinskis, P. Walker, R.G. Ward, L. Hussain, A.J.H. Gearing, and S.E. Adams
  1992   Induction of mucosal and systemic immunity to a recombinant simian immunodeficiency viral protein. Science 258:1365–1369.
London, S.D., D.H. Rubin, and J.J. Cebra
  1987   Gut mucosal immunization with reovirus serotype 1/L stimulates virus-specific cytotoxic T-cell precursors as well as IgA memory cells in Peyer's patches. J. Exp. Med. 165:830–847.
Losonsky, G.A., J.P. Johnson, J.A. Winkelstein, and R.H. Yolken
  1985   Oral administration of human serum immunoglobulin in immunodeficient patients with viral gastroenteritis. J. Clin. Invest. 76:2362–2367.
Lycke, N., T. Tsuji, and J. Holmgren
  1992   The adjuvant effect of *Vibrio cholerae* and *Escherichia coli* heat-labile enterotoxins is linked to their ADP-ribosyltransferase activity. Eur. J. Immunol. 22:2277–2281.

Lyons, A.B., and C.R. Parish
  1995   Are murine marginal-zone macrophages the splenic white pulp analog of high endothelial venules? Eur. J. Immunol. 25:3165–3172.
Ma, J. K.-C., A. Hiatt, M. Hein, N.D. Vine, F. Wang, P. Stabila, C. van Dolleweerd, K. Mostov, and T. Lehner
  1995   Generation and assembly of secretory antibodies in plants. Science 268:716–719.
MacDonald, T.T.
  1982   Enhancement and suppression of Peyer's patch immune response by systemic priming. Clin. Exp. Immunol. 49:441–448.
Mackay, C.R.
  1991   Skin-seeking memory T-cells. Nature 349:737–738.
Mackay, C.R., W.L. Marston, L. Dudler, O. Spertini, T.F. Tedder, and W.R. Hein
  1992   Tissue-specific migration pathways by phenotypically distinct subpopulations of memory T-cells. Eur. J. Immunol. 22:887–895.
Marks, J.D., H.R. Hoogenboom, T.P. Bonnert, J. McCafferty, A.D. Griffiths, and G. Winter
  1991   By-passing immunization. Human antibodies from V-gene libraries displayed on phage. J. Mol. Biol. 222:16007–16010.
Mason, H.S., D.M. Lam, and C.J. Arntzen
  1992   Expression of hepatitis B surface antigen in transgenic plants. Proc. Natl. Acad. Sci. USA 89:11745–11749.
Mattingly, J.A., and B.H. Waksman
  1978   Immunologic suppression after oral administration of antigen. I. Specific suppressor cells formed in rat Peyer's patches after oral administration of sheep erythrocytes and their systemic migration. J. Immunol. 121:1878–1883.
Matzinger, P.
  1994   Tolerance, danger, and the extended family. Annu. Rev. Immunol. 12:991–1045.
Mazanec, M.B., C.S. Kaetzel, M.E. Lamm, D. Fletcher, and J.G. Nedrud
  1992   Intracellular neutralization of virus by immunoglobulin A antibodies. Proc. Natl. Acad. Sci. USA 89:6901–6905.
Mazanec, M.B., J.G. Nedrud, C.S. Kaetzel, and M.E. Lamm
  1993   A three-tiered view of the role of IgA in mucosal defense. Immunol. Today 14:430–435.
McCabe, D.E., W.F. Swain, B.J. Martinell, and P. Christou
  1988   Stable transformation of soybean (*Glycine max*) by particle acceleration. Bio/Tech. 6:923–926.
McCormick, B.A., S.P. Colgan, C. Delp-Archer, S.I. Miller, and J.L. Madara
  1993   *Salmonella typhimurium* attachment to human intestinal epithelial monolayers: Transcellular signaling to subepithelial neutrophils. J. Cell Biol. 123:895–907.
McGhee, J.R., J. Mestecky, M.T. Dertzbaugh, J.H. Eldridge, M. Hirasawa, and H. Kiyono
  1992   The mucosal immune system: From fundamental concepts to vaccine development. Vaccine 10:75–88.
Metzger, J.F., and G.E. Lewis, Jr.
  1979   Human-derived immune globulins for the treatment of botulism. Rev. Infect. Dis. 1:689–692.
Michalek, S.M., J.H. Eldridge, R. Curtiss III, and K.L. Rosenthal
  1994   Antigen delivery systems: New approaches to mucosal immunization. Pp. 373–380 in Handbook of Mucosal Immunology, P.L. Ogra, J. Mestecky, M.E. Lamm, W. Strober, J.R. McGhee, and J. Bienenstock, eds. Boston: Academic Press, Inc.
Michalek, S.M., N.K. Childers, and M.T. Dertzbaugh
  1995   Vaccination strategies for mucosal pathogens. Pp. 269–301 in Virulence Mechanisms of Bacterial Pathogens, 2nd ed., J.A. Roth, ed. Washington, D.C.: American Society for Microbiology.

Mobley, J.A.
1995   Biological warfare in the twentieth century: Lessons from the past, challenges for the future. Mil. Med. 160:547–553.
Moffat, A.S.
1995   Exploring transgenic plants as a new vaccine source. Science 268:658–660.
Morikawa, Y., K. Tohya, H. Ishida, N. Matsuura, and K. Kakudo
1995   Different migration patterns of antigen-presenting cells correlate with Th1/Th2-type responses in mice. Immunology 85:575–581.
Morris, W., M.C. Steinhoff, and P.K. Russell
1994   Potential of polymer microencapsulation technology for vaccine innovation. Vaccine 12:5–11.
Mosmann, T.R., and S. Sad
1996   The expanding universe of T-cell subsets: Th1, Th2 and more. Immunol. Today 17:138–146.
Mowat, A.M.
1994   Oral tolerance and regulation of immunity to dietary antigens. Pp. 185–201 in Handbook of Mucosal Immunology, P.L. Ogra, J. Mestecky, M.E. Lamm, W. Strober, J.R. McGhee, and J. Bienenstock, eds. Boston: Academic Press, Inc.
Neutra, M.R., and J-P Kraehenbuhl
1994   Cellular and molecular basis for antigen transport in the intestinal epithelium. Pp. 27–39 in Handbook of Mucosal Immunology, P.L. Ogra, J. Mestecky, M.E. Lamm, W. Strober, J.R. McGhee, and J. Bienenstock, eds. Boston: Academic Press, Inc.
Ogra, P.L., J. Mestecky, M.E. Lamm, W. Strober, J.R. McGhee, and J. Bienenstock, eds.
1994   Handbook of Mucosal Immunology. Boston: Academic Press, Inc.
Openshaw, P.J.M., E.E. Murphy, N.A. Hosken, V. Manio, K. Davis, and A. O'Garra
1995   Heterogeneity of intracellular cytokine synthesis at the single cell level in polarised T helper 1 and T helper 2 populations. J. Exp. Med. 182:1357–1367.
Oppenheim, J.J., C.O.C. Zachariae, N. Mukaida, and K. Matsushima
1991   Properties of the novel proinflammatory supergene "intercrine" cytokine family. Annu. Rev. Immunol. 9:617–648.
Owen, R.L, and A.L. Jones
1974   Epithelial cell specialization within human Peyer's patches: An ultrastructural study of intestinal lymphoid follicles. Gastroenterology 66:189–203.
Owens, L., and D.E. Cress
1985   Genotypic variability of soybean response to *Agrobacterium* strains harboring the Ti or Ri plasmids. Plant Physiol. 77:87–94.
Pedersen, H.C., J. Christiansen, and R. Wyndaele
1983   Induction and *in vitro* culture of soybean crown gall tumors. Plant Cell Rep. 2:201–204.
Pierce, N.F.
1978   The role of antigen form and function in the primary and secondary intestinal immune responses to cholera toxin and toxoid in rats. J. Exp. Med. 148:195–206.
Pierce, N.S., and J.L. Gowans
1975   Cellular kinetics of the intestinal immune response to cholera toxoid in rats. J. Exp. Med. 142:1550–1563.
Punt, J.A., and S. Singer
1996   T-cell development. Pp. 157–175 in Clinical Immunology Principles and Practice, R.R. Rich, T.A. Fleisher, B.D. Schwartz, W.T. Shearer, and W. Strober, eds. Boston: Mosby.

Quiding-Jarbrink, M., M. Lakew, I. Nordstrom, J. Bachereau, E. Butcher, J. Holmgren, and
     C. Czerkinsky
  1995 Human circulating specific antibody-forming cells after systemic and mucosal
        immunizations: Differential homing commitments and cell surface differentiation
        markers. Eur. J. Immunol. 25:322–327.
Renegar, K.B., and P.A. Small, Jr.
  1994 Passive immunization: Systemic and mucosal. Pp. 347–356 in Handbook of Mu-
        cosal Immunology, P.L. Ogra, J. Mestecky, M.E. Lamm, W. Strober, J.R.
        McGheee, and J. Bienenstock, eds. Boston: Academic Press, Inc.
Robey, E., and J.P. Allison
  1995 T-cell activation: Integration of signals from the antigen receptor and costimula-
        tory molecules. Immunol. Today 16:306–310.
Rocken, M., and E.M. Shevach
  1996 Immune deviation—The third dimension of nondeletional T-cell tolerance.
        Immunol. Rev. 149:175–194.
Rott, L.S., M.J. Briskin, D.P. Andrew, E.L. Berg, and E.C. Butcher
  1996 A fundamental subdivision of circulating lymphocytes defined by adhesion to
        mucosal addressin cell adhesion molecule-1. J. Immunol. 156:3727–3736.
Rubin, D.H., M.A. Eaton, and A.O. Anderson
  1986 Reovirus infection in adult mice: The virus hemagglutinin determines the site of
        intestinal disease. Microb. Pathog. 1:79–87.
Ruedl, C., C. Rieser, N. Kofler, G. Wick, and H. Wolf
  1996 Humoral and cellular immune responses in the murine respiratory tract following
        oral immunization with cholera toxin or *Escherichia coli* heat-labile enterotoxin.
        Vaccine 14:792–798.
Salgame, P., J.S. Abrams, C. Clayberger, H. Goldstein, J. Convit, R.L. Modlin, and B.R.
     Bloom
  1991 Differing lymphokine profiles of functional subsets of human CD4 and CD8 T cell
        clones. Science 254:279–282.
Sarraf, P., R.C. Frederich, E.M. Turner, G. Ma, N.T. Jaskowiak, D.J. Rivet III, J.S. Flier, B.B.
     Lowell, D.L. Fraker, and H.R. Alexander
  1997 Multiple cytokines and acute inflammation raise mouse leptin levels: Potential
        role in inflammatory anorexia. J. Exp. Med. 185:171–175.
Schrader, C.E., A. George, R.L. Kerlin, and J.J. Cebra
  1990 Dendritic cells support production of IgA and other non-IgM isotypes in clonal
        microculture. Int. Immunol. 2(6):563–570.
Shroff, K.E., K. Meslin, and J.J. Cebra
  1995 Commensal enteric bacteria engender a self-limiting humoral mucosal immune
        response while permanently colonizing the gut. Infect. Immun. 63:3904–3913.
Sim, G-K.
  1995 Intraepithelial lymphocytes and the immune system. Adv. Immunol. 58:297–343.
Sixma, T.K., S.E. Pronk, K.H. Kalk, E.S. Wartna, B.A.M. vanZanten, B. Witholt, and W.G.
     Hol
  1991 Crystal structure of a cholera toxin-related heat-labile enterotoxin from *E. coli*.
        Nature (London) 351:371–377.
Spangler, B.D.
  1992 Structure and function of cholera toxin and the related *Escherichia coli* heat-labile
        enterotoxin. Microbiol. Rev. 56:622–647.
Spriggs, M.K.
  1996 One step ahead of the game: Viral immunomodulatory molecules. Annu. Rev.
        Immunol. 14:101–130.

Stavnezer, J.
  1995 Regulation of antibody production and class switching by TGF-beta. J. Immunol. 155:1647–1651.
Stok, W., P.J. van der Heijden, and A.T.J. Bianchi
  1994 Conversion of orally induced suppression of the mucosal immune response to ovalbumin into stimulation by conjugating ovalbumin to cholera toxin or its B subunit. Vaccine 12:521–526.
Street, N., and T.R. Mosmann
  1991 Functional diversity of T lymphocytes due to secretion of different cytokine patterns. FASEB J. 5:171–177.
Sun, J-B., J. Holmgren, and C. Czerkinsky
  1994 Cholera toxin B subunit: An efficient transmucosal carrier-delivery system for induction of peripheral immunological tolerance. Proc. Natl. Acad. Sci. USA 91:10795–10799.
Swain, S.L., G. Huston, S. Tonkonogy, and A. Weinberg
  1991 Transforming growth factor-β and IL-4 cause helper T-cell precursors to develop into distinct effector helper cells that differ in lymphokine secretion pattern and cell surface phenotype. J. Immunol. 147:2991–3000.
Trinchieri, G.
  1993 Interleukin-12 and its role in the generation of TH1 cells. Immunol. Today 14:335–338.
Tsunemitsu, H., M. Shimizu, T. Hirai, H. Yonemichi, T. Kudo, K. Mori, and S. Onoe
  1989 Protection against bovine rotaviruses in newborn calves by continuous feeding of immune colostrum. Nippon Juigaku Zasshi 51:300–308.
Underdown, B.J., and J. Mestecky
  1994 Mucosal immunoglobulins. Pp. 79–97 in Handbook of Mucosal Immunology, P.L. Ogra, J. Mesteck, M.E. Lamm, W. Strober, J.R. McGhee, and J. Bienenstock, eds. Boston: Academic Press, Inc.
von Behring, E., and S. Kitasato
  1890 On the acquisition of immunity against diphtheria and tetanus in animals. Deutsch. Med. Wochenschr. 16:1113–1114.
Walker, R.I.
  1994 New strategies for using mucosal vaccination to achieve more effective immunization. Vaccine 12(5):387–400.
Weinstein, P.D., and J.J. Cebra
  1991 The preference for switching to IgA expression by Peyer's patch germinal center B-cells is likely due to the intrinsic influence of their microenvironment. J. Immunol. 147:4126–4135.
Weinstein, P.D., P.A. Schweitzer, J.A. Cebra-Thomas, and J.J. Cebra
  1991 Molecular genetic features reflecting the preference for isotype switching to IgA expression by Peyer's patch germinal center B-cells. Int. Immunol. 3:1253–1263.
Weinstein, P.D., A.O. Anderson, and R.G. Mage
  1994a Rabbit IgH sequences in appendix germinal centers: VH diversification by gene conversion-like and hypermutation mechanisms. Immunity 1:647–659.
Weinstein, P.D., R.G. Mage, and A.O. Anderson
  1994b The appendix functions as a mammalian bursal equivalent in the developing rabbit. Adv. Exp. Med. Biol. 355:249–254.
Winter, G., A.D. Griffiths, R.E. Hawkins, and H.R. Hoogenboom
  1994 Making antibodies by phage display technology. Annu. Rev. Immunol. 12:433–455.

Wong, Y.W., P.H. Kussie, B. Parhami-Seren, and M.N. Margolies
   1995   Modulation of antibody affinity by an engineered amino acid substitution. J. Immunol. 154:3351–3358.
Wu, H-Y., and M.W. Russell
   1994   Comparison of systemic and mucosal priming for mucosal immune responses to a bacterial protein antigen given with or coupled to cholera toxin (CT) B subunit, and effects of pre-existing anti-CT immunity. Vaccine 12(3):215–222.
Xu-Amano, J., H. Kiyono, R.J. Jackson, H.F. Staats, K. Fujihashi, P.D. Burrows, C.O. Elson, S. Pillai, and J.R. McGhee
   1993   Helper T-cell subsets for immunoglobulin A responses: Oral immunization with tetanus toxoid and cholera toxin as adjuvant selectively induces Th2 cells in mucosa-associated tissues. J. Exp. Med. 178:1309–1320.
Yamamura, M., K. Uyemura, R.J. Deans, K. Weinberg, T.H. Rea, B.R. Bloom, and R.L. Modlin
   1991   Defining protective response to pathogens: Cytokine profiles in leprosy lesions. Science 254:277–279.
Yan, C., J.H. Resau, J. Hewetson, M. West, W.L. Rill, and M. Kende
   1994   Characterization and morphological analysis of protein-loaded poly(lactide-co-glycolide) microparticles prepared by water-in-oil-in-water emulsion technique. J. Controlled Release 32:231–241.
Young, H.A., P. Ghosh, J. Ye, J. Lederer, A. Lichtman, J.R. Gerard, L. Penix, C.B. Wilson, A.J. Melvin, M.E. McGurn, D.B. Lewis, and D.D. Taub
   1994   Differentiation of the T-helper phenotypes by analysis of the methylation state of the IFN-β gene. J. Immunol. 153:3603–3610.
Zhang, R.G., M.L. Westbrook, S. Nance, B.D. Spangler, G.G. Shipley, and E.M. Westbrook
   1995   The three-dimensional crystal structure of cholera toxin. J. Mol. Biol. 251:563–573.

DISCUSSION

ROBERT NESHEIM: Are there any questions? I have a question. How stable are these antibodies in the plant materials?

ARTHUR ANDERSON: The antibodies are very stable when expressed in plant materials. The *Streptococcus* mutans-specific IgA that Ma et al. (1995) expressed in transgenic tobacco plants had been secreted into a plant compartment that made it very easy to extract. All they had to do was freeze, grind up the leaves, centrifuge at 15,000g to remove fiber and large plant molecules, and the antibodies were precipitated out of soluble proteins with 40 and 60 percent $(NH4)2SO4$.

ROBERT NESHEIM: The antibody genes can just be put into foods? What happens with heat processing?

ARTHUR ANDERSON: That could be a problem with protein antigens or antibodies expressed in plants. In the experiment of Haq et al. (1995), the mice first were given crude tobacco leaf extract. In later experiments, they ate raw potato tubers. If the tubers were cooked, as we like them, the antigen would be denatured and may not induce immunity. This is also a problem with cooking antibodies.

Everything I said about use of cholera toxin B-subunit as a carrier for oral vaccines absolutely depends on it retaining its conformational integrity. If the B-subunit pentameric ring is denatured and it cannot bind host cell membrane GM1 gangliosides, then everything I said is incorrect. However, Arntzen has been working on developing foods like transgenic bananas that could be eaten raw. Banana also could be stabilized and dried using sugars and lyophilization. This would enable it to be microencapsulated in an enteric coating to get it past the denaturing effect of stomach acid.

These are issues that people who prepare Meals, Ready-to-Eat (MREs) are most ready to test. I have not done all of the components of the vision I presented. However, the literature says that the field is ready to apply this new technology for protection of soldiers.

Obviously, I would first like to protect a soldier against the common mucosal pathogens that cause intestinal pathology. I would use recombinant antibodies from transgenic plants incorporated into every MRE to provide passive protection. At the same time, I would periodically give the soldiers "special MREs" or "vaccine candy bars" with the cholera B-subunit linked vaccines to enable development of acquired active immunity.

There is no reason to suspect that oral passive antibody would block development of immunity with encapsulated or carrier-linked antigens.

GABRIEL VIRELLA: If the ganglioside is not expressed, how does the recombinant cholera toxin B-subunit get to the right cells?

ARTHUR ANDERSON: Cholera toxin B-subunit (CTB) binds to GM1 ganglioside on all eukaryotic cells. The sialomucins on absorptive epithelial cells interfere slightly with binding, which causes the carrier to bind to M-cells over mucosal lymphatic tissues or to IEL [intraepithelial lymphocytes] cells, some of which have higher GM1 ganglioside in their membranes. The mucosal M-cells are exactly where we want the antigen to bind because this is where antigens must be taken up for a mucosal immune response to result.

The CTB binds more in the proximal small bowel than in the distal bowel because binding depletes the material before it reaches the distal bowel. However, proximal bowel binding has produced the desired results. In sheep, the distal Peyer's patches in the ileum have a different function from those in the proximal bowel. We do not know if having antigens bind to distal bowel lymphatic tissues might change the ratio of antigen priming to tolerance induction, for example.

On the other hand, there is a great deal of interest in using enterotoxin-derived carriers in stimulating immunity via intranasal route, which accesses the tonsils and adenoids as antigen-reactive mucosal lymphatic tissues.

DOUGLAS WILMORE: There is another route by which antigens can enter the gut, and that is by paracellular channels—gaps that form when the gut is underperfused and as a result of the effects of acidosis on mucosal integrity. People are now debating how the influence of endotoxin or other products affect antigens coming up those pathways. Do you see other mechanisms to protect the gut in that way?

ARTHUR ANDERSON: There has been research about particulate antigens, such as bacteria and yeast, gaining access to the blood circulation by mechanisms you referred to. Griffiss has shown that levels of IgA in the circulating blood appear to dampen the effects of bacteremia on complement activation. There is a blood threshold maintained by IgA levels, which, when exceeded, allows endotoxin to unleash its effects on cytokine cascades, complement activation, and bradykinin activation. Endotoxin and yeast and bacteria normally enter your blood during eating and eliminating and brushing one's teeth. Most people do not show any physiological reactions to this as long as their IgA levels are normal. On the other hand, IgA-deficient people are very susceptible to endotoxin-mediated shock.

Endotoxin-containing immunogens actually have been shown to down-modulate mucosal immunity. This has been confirmed by using C3H/HeN and C3H/HeJ mouse substrains. The C3H/HeJ mice lack the gene for cytokine response to endotoxin. These mice are resistant to induction of endotoxin shock. They also mount very potent IgA responses. The endotoxin-susceptible C3H/HeN mouse shows dose-related decrements in IgA production related to endotoxin added to the GI tract. There are a series of publications on this coming from Gerry McGhee's laboratory in Birmingham, Alabama.

JOHANNA DWYER: I remember that, a long time ago, one of the formula companies wanted to put antibodies in infant formulas, and I think it foundered. One of the concerns was that some infants might get leaky guts or something, which prevents complete benefit of the antibodies, and they still get sick. Does what you propose have such a danger? Can it be a two-edged sword?

ARTHUR ANDERSON: That is a good question. What I have presented about conventional modes of immunization already creates a two-edged sword. In my review, I hope I have narrowed down the alternatives to reduce this risk.

What you referred to is a phenomenon which only occurs in infants. It is called the phenomenon of gut closure. New babies do not have all the functional proteases for a while after they are born. The phenomenon relates to the fact that relatively intact proteins can be directly absorbed across the mucosa. After the mucosa matures to a point where most proteases are released, only proteins with mechanisms to resist protease degradation can get across. This, I believe, is what gut closure means. If non-IgA antibodies to pathogens are put in milk, some of those antibodies could actually enable concentration and absorption of viral pathogens in newborn babies. This would result in a paradoxical adverse effect.

Normal cow's milk already has secretory IgA against many pathogens, so adding antibodies would not really help. If the antibodies were not dimeric IgA with J-chain and secretory component, they also would not help. The added IgA was too expensive because of its method of preparation; and once you start, you have to keep giving it. I would not have done it with the technology available then, either.

I also want to comment on the double-edged sword of using enterotoxin carriers (CT/LT). Both CTB and LT/mLT have been tested in phase I trials in humans. These vaccines have been tolerated well, and dose finding studies have produced benign toxicities. I have enjoyed being a voyeur to the vaccine trials of products developed by Jan Holmgren, John Mekalanos, and John Clements and tested in the Clinical Studies unit of USAMRIID by Dave Taylor and Dan Scott, respectively. In normal unvaccinated subjects, cholera holotoxin or *Vibrio cholerae* infection is going to cause cramping and diarrhea. When CTB, with or without killed *Vibrios,* or LTB is given to unvaccinated volunteers, no signs or symptoms result. I have not referred to all the individual studies which show that oral use of CT/LT or CTB with antigen result in both IgA and IgG immune responses. I don't see a double-edged sword there, unless B-subunit loses GM1-binding activity.

DAVID SCHNAKENBERG: How often do you have to present antibodies by the oral route? You said IgA could be put in MREs. To get the effect, do you have to administer it daily?

ARTHUR ANDERSON: There is pretty wide variability in gut transit time. In the mouse, it is about 6 hours. In human beings, it can be anything from hours to days. If you use enterically coated antibodies in three meals a day, there should be sufficient antibody present all the time. IgA binds to intestinal mucin. The mucin moves more slowly than does the fecal stream, which should allow a buildup of IgA.

DAVID SCHNAKENBERG: What is the lag time from dosage to effective protection? If you are using this only to a point of deployment, is this something you start 2 weeks ahead of time?

ARTHUR ANDERSON: If you are referring to passive antibody protection, it would be adequate to give soldiers the antibodies in their meals en route. By the time they arrive, their intestines would be protected. If you are referring to active protection with vaccines, it is preferrable that the initial priming doses be given as long in advance as possible. I would say it is best to immunize troops during basic training. It is not essential that antibody levels be maintained. Desert Shield/Desert Storm taught us to trust immunological memory. There were people who got only one dose of vaccine and people who got a full series of shots before going overseas; both had sufficient antibody titers to be protective when given a booster 24 to 36 months later. Circulating memory cells will ensure that soldiers ready to deploy will have a return in protective antibody titer within 3 days of the booster. That is what I believe we need to do.

HARRIS LIEBERMAN: There is a special category of foods, I believe, of medical foods. It sounds like the kinds of things you are talking about might go into that category, a special sort of deployment ration that is essentially a medical food. I don't think you would want to put antigens in all the MREs, but you would want to have a special category.

ARTHUR ANDERSON: I agree. It is not intended that chronic enteric exposure to vaccine antigens be given. That is one of the ways tolerance to food antigens develops. However, your idea of preparing an easily identifyable MRE as a medical food, with instructions on the cover about frequency of use for optimal immunity, would be useful in assuring the proper use by deployed troops. How this would be utilized effectively is something your institute is better suited for determining.

Emerging Technologies for Nutrition Research, 1997
Pp. 501–504. Washington, D.C.
National Academy Press

VI and VII

Discussion

RONALD SHIPPEE: This has been a great session, and I think that with the focus on immunosuppression we are seeing in our Special Operations folks (and I have been talking with some people in England and with other Special Operations researchers), we need to have a workshop just on immunology. I think the climate is right.

I have two general comments; Tim Kramer has convinced me that the way for us to go is to use whole blood [to assess immune status], and I have adopted that for my lab.

But Ficoll-Hypaque, Percoll, or some of the other gradients are not without their problems, also, and I think Doug Wilmore would agree that, in the burn situation, you can get a selective collection of cells during the different degrees of burn. There are two papers on exercise in which before and after exercise, you get a selection of different cells, so you have got to be careful with that. It is not a trivial issue. Obviously, whole blood is easier for us to manipulate, too, [in addition to preventing cell selection].

I think you always have to remember, and I learned this from Dr. Good and Dr. Mason when I did 8 years in the burn unit, that when you take whole blood, you are looking at a window of the whole lymphoid system. You take 10 ccs out and that is what you are looking at right there.

With a burned rat model, if you look at a 30-percent scald burn, the peripheral blood will say the rat is immunosuppressed, based on proliferation to concanavalin A. But the draining lymph node and the spleen will say the rat is hyperresponsive.

When I look at the data from my subjects, and they increase their repertoire of immune responses, I think we always have to question whether we are trying to fix something that isn't broke here. We have to ask: are they supposed to look like this for a reason?

ARTHUR ANDERSON: You raise an important point. One of the things that happens during the induction phase of immune response is that there is a fairly large amount of apoptosis of cells that is residual from previous responses. There is a big release of thymidine and other components of cells during this digestion of apoptopic cells.

Free-thymidine could cause a cell to appear to be refractory to mitogen stimulation *in vitro* and, therefore, it would be unable to take up tritiated thymidine or other labels and would not score as an activated cell. That would not be something that would affect the CD25 assays that were discussed for interleukin-2 (IL-2) receptors.

On the other hand, immunization will cause CD25+ cells to selectively compartmentalize out of the blood, and a drop in CD25 cells in the circulation would probably be reflected by a homing of CD25+ cells to an appropriate lymphoid tissue.

GUY MILLER: I was wondering if you could comment or maybe I can take the opportunity to comment to the committee on the new class of compounds that has been rapidly identified, the meganins and defensins, and their whole role in immunological defense.

Maybe I could just give a little introduction. When folks were looking at the immunosurveillance mechanisms that amphibians use to coat all their vulnerable tissues, it turns out that if you look at a frog, every single epithelial layer, from the oral cavity and the skin down through the entire GI tract, has the potential to secrete small peptides of about 25 amino acids in length. These compounds confer significant resistance to invading microorganisms. It links to some of the thoughts that Harris Lieberman has.

These peptides are contiguous with the neuroendocrine system. They are elaborated by the neurological system and released on stimulation. In putting this little story together, you could see where the cytokines and other small peptides are also secreted in response, and one part of the response is a blood mediated one. One is a local hormonal response, and the other one, which has not yet been studied well, is the meganin-defensin system.

I think there is a significant potential to look at these very small peptides, maybe 25 [amino acids] in length, and their role in gut immunity, and whether we need to focus time and energy also on looking at that system.

ARTHUR ANDERSON: I appreciate those comments. I have seen those papers on the meganin-defensins system,[1] and they are very intriguing. I have another similar observation. It was published in *The Journal of Leukocyte Biology* in April of this year,[2] where we discovered that IL-8 is secreted in sweat collected from individuals who have run between 1 and 8 km with plastic bags taped around them.

IL-8, as a terminal cytokine in this inflammatory cytokine system, and monocyte chemotactic protein 1, which is also a terminal cytokine, represent two parts of the family of cytokines called chemokines. They are all about 8 to 10 kD in size, and they all have very similar conformation and structure. Therefore, they would be very difficult to purify unless you use special techniques.

But because they were shotgun cloned out of endotoxin-stimulated macrophages, we had libraries to work with. IL-8 is a neutrophil chemotactic factor. It is a keratinocyte chemotactic factor; it is made by keratinocytes. It has effects on fibroblastic cells and on endothelial cell angiogenesis.

At lower concentrations, it tracks lymphocytes, so when you are sweating, you are basically allowing diffusion of IL-8 into the basement membrane of your skin. So if the skin is intact, lymphocytes are already beginning to accumulate in the skin as a kind of a sentinel population. If you get a scratch, there is a higher concentration in a focal area, so neutrophils will begin to migrate out even before bacteria go across the epithelium.

This is apparently found to be true in most mucosal sites, that IL-8 is made by mucosal epithelial cells on contact between pathogenic organisms and the mucosal epithelium. It secretes in a polarized way a small puff of IL-8, which attracts neutrophils to the site before the bacterial invasion takes place.

Like the defensins that you mentioned, IL-8 is part of this first line of defense. I was happy to hear that we normally do not have IL-8 in urine. There was a study published out of Walter Reed[3]—the protocol for which I reviewed

---

[1] B.S. Schonwetter, E.D. Stolzenberg, and M.A. Zasloff. 1995. Epithelial antibiotics induced at sites of inflammation. Science 267:1645–1648.

[2] A.P. Jones, L.M.C. Webb, A.O. Anderson, E.J. Leonard, and A. Rot. 1995. Normal human sweat contains interleukin-8. J. Leukocyte Biol. 57:434–437.

P.M. Murphy. 1995. Blood, sweat, and chemotactic cytokines [commentary]. J. Leukocyte Biol. 57:438–439.

[3] K.H. Ramsey, H. Schneider, R.A. Kuschner, A.F. Trofa, A.S. Cross, and C.D. Deal. 1994. Inflammatory cytokine response to experimental human infection with *Neisseria gonorrhoeae*. Ann. N.Y. Acad. Sci. 730:322–325.

on the human use committee—where during a gonorrhea experiment, IL-8 increased tremendously in urine, showing that IL-8 in urine is probably a rational way of determining at least urinary tract infection.

LYLE MOLDAWER: We have not seen it in hospitalized patients before surgery.

C. Svanborg, W. Agace, S. Hedges, R. Lindsedt, and M.L. Svensson. 1994. Bacterial adherence and mucosal cytokine production. Ann. N.Y. Acad. Sci. 730:162–181.

VIII

Functional and Behavioral Measures of Nutritional Status

P ART VIII BEGINS WITH A DISCUSSION in Chapter 23 of the use of involuntary muscle contraction for nutritional assessment. With muscle function analysis (MFA), skeletal muscle function is measured by applying an electrical stimulus at various frequencies and then studying the resulting pattern of involuntary contractions. Studies seem to indicate that lower MFA relaxation rates indicate some nutritional abnormality, such as protein malnutrition. This method is relatively noninvasive and sensitive, but some of its disadvantages (for example, difficulty in locating the ulnar nerve) indicate that more testing is needed to establish its validity.

In Chapter 24 and 25, the focus turns to assessment of cognitive function in the military. As discussed in Chapter 24, the Army's interest in the influence of nutrition on cognitive function has focused on food deprivation in the field, underconsumption of rations, and identification of performance-optimizing ration components. There are limitations in cognitive assessment technology, and assessment has been accomplished largely through the use of observation of behavior, paper-and-pencil tests, and tests of manual dexterity or hand-eye coordination. These tests are being replaced by assessment technologies that make use of computer games or performance tracking devices.

Chapter 25 describes two electronic activity-monitoring devices for psychomotor vigilance testing: the Motionlogger Actigraph, which monitors sleeping and waking activity and collects data to calculate sleeping and waking time, and the Vigilance Monitor, which combines the aforementioned measurement capabilities with vigilance assessment and intervention capability. The Vigilance Monitor is unobtrusive, has a fairly low cost, and can be programmed to provide data on several variables concurrently while monitoring a number of subjects simultaneously.

Finally, the Iowa Driving Simulator (IDS), as described in Chapter 26, is one possible example of an interface that allows for the use of identical assessment tools in the laboratory and in the field. The IDS is a high-fidelity computational vehicle model set in a fully interactive, virtual environment. Its military applications have included the development of a virtual proving ground based on actual Army test courses, and the design and testing of new Army vehicle prototypes. The different degrees and types of fidelity required for different performance measures can be limiting, as can the extent to which subjects perceive the experience to be real.

Emerging Technologies for Nutrition Research, 1997
Pp. 507–517. Washington, D.C.
National Academy Press

23

Involuntary Muscle Contraction to Assess Nutritional Status

James S. Hayes[1]

Standard nutritional assessment techniques lack the sensitivity and specificity to identify early malnutrition and monitor short-term improvement from nutritional therapies. To improve on the available methods for nutrition assessment, Ross Products Division, Abbott Laboratories, has undertaken a research project with the goal of developing a device to study skeletal muscle function as an indication of nutritional status. The study of skeletal muscle as an indication of nutritional status was begun because of the well-known effects of malnutrition on muscle mass. Skeletal muscle function can be studied by the use of voluntary contractions (handgrip strength) or involuntary contractions (muscle contraction in response to an electrical stimulus).

Muscle function as measured by handgrip dynamometry has been shown to predict postoperative complications with a good degree of clinical accuracy (Kalfarentzos et al., 1989; Klidjian et al., 1980; Webb et al., 1989). Unfortu-

---

[1] James S. Hayes, Ross Products Division, Abbott Laboratories, Columbus, OH 43215

nately, the results of handgrip dynamometry are subject to patient effort and therefore may not be as sensitive and reliable as hoped.

The force, relaxation, and endurance characteristics of the adductor pollicis muscle in response to ulnar nerve stimulation may be a more reliable means of measuring muscle function than the measurement of voluntary muscle function. Since an electrical wave form with a standard frequency, strength, and duration is used to stimulate the ulnar nerve, the possibility that patient effort will confound the result is minimized. This technique has shown a diminution in muscle function in humans following both brief and prolonged periods of starvation (Russell et al., 1983a, b). In addition, refeeding has been shown to improve skeletal muscle function prior to appreciable changes in nitrogen status and muscle bulk (Brough et al., 1986). This improvement may occur as quickly as 4 days after the institution of nutrition support (Christie and Hill, 1990).

The basic technique that is used to study skeletal muscle function was developed in 1954 by Merton. Previous studies of ulnar nerve stimulation to assess muscle function have used strip chart recording devices to record results. The nature of this form of data collection may impair the sensitivity and possibly the specificity of the technique. This technique has been updated by the addition of a computer for collection and data analysis.

DESCRIPTION OF THE CURRENT MUSCLE FUNCTION ANALYSIS DEVICE

The current muscle function analysis (MFA) device uses a custom base plate to position the arm and force transducer, a stimulus generator with a constant current output and patient electrical isolation, and a standard IBM-compatible computer with MFA software installed. The primary factor responsible for electrical stimulation is current. However, the amount of voltage needed to produce this current is a function of the impedance presented to the source by the stimulating electrodes and the surrounding tissue. Two types of sources can be used to provide electrical stimulation, a constant voltage source or a constant current source. With a constant voltage source, the voltage waveform is sent to the electrodes, and the current waveform is dependent on the load impedance. The current value is dependent on the impedance of the tissue: the higher the impedance, the lower the current at a given voltage. A constant current source offers the advantage of being able to provide currents more independent of tissue and electrode impedance.

Figure 23-1 is a block diagram of the MFA device that illustrates the main components. The stimulus generator is a Grass Model S44 solid-state, square-wave stimulator. The stimulus pulse width, frequency, and intensity are controlled here. The isolation unit is provided to isolate the stimulus from the ground, reducing stimulus artifact, to provide a constant current for stimulation and to limit the maximum current that can be delivered to the patient to 15 mA. The patient interface consists of the base-plate assembly and force transducer.

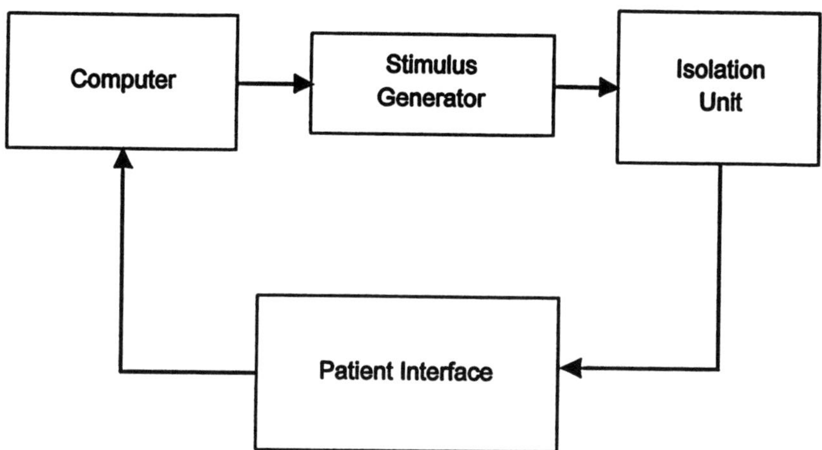

FIGURE 23-1 Block diagram of muscle function analysis device.

The force transducer provides a voltage output proportional to thumb tension. These values are sent to the computer for analysis and storage.

The base-plate assembly consists of a fiberglass-reinforced polyester plate with foam armrests and an adjustable, pivoting mount for the force transducer. There are two armrests for ambidextrous use. The armrests are designed to position the arm and hand in a palm-up position with the wrist flexed and extended. This position facilitates the search for and location of the ulnar nerve. In addition, this position aligns the thumb with the force transducer.

The force transducer is a 25-lb, tension-load cell. It is mounted on a vertical cylinder that slides over a post. The post is mounted to a slide mechanism that is controlled by a crank at the front of the base plate. The cylinder mount can swivel about the post to align itself properly in the natural plane of the force being applied. By turning the crank and moving the post and transducer assembly, the static tension applied to the load cell and thumb can be adjusted for optimal performance. When the tension is adjusted properly, the post can be locked in place by tightening the hand nut on top of the post.

The electrical signals from the force transducer are amplified and sent to the computer. The computer displays the force curve data, performs some simple computations, and displays the results with other pertinent data. The computer also controls the stimulus start and duration times by gating the stimulus generator on and off. Stimulus pulse width, frequency, and intensity are set on the stimulus generator and are not controlled by the computer at this time.

TEST PROCEDURE

With the arm of the subject placed on the base plate, the thumb loop extending from the force transducer is placed over the thumb. The hand crank is then rotated, moving the force transducer and applying a static force to the load cell. When the force is approximately 10 newtons, the post is locked into position. The electrodes from the stimulus generator are placed near the ulnar nerve, either at the wrist or elbow. A software routine that turns the stimulus on and off is initiated. This aids in locating the ulnar nerve but does not collect data. The frequency of the electrical stimulus is 1 to 5 Hz in the locate mode but can be adjusted to whatever value desired. During this location time, the electrodes are moved and gently pressed into the skin until a maximum force is elicited from the adductor pollicis muscle, as indicated on the computer screen. The computer is then switched into the data collection mode; the test sequence is started; and data is collected.

During the data collection period, contraction of the adductor pollicis muscle is caused by electrical stimulation of the ulnar nerve. The nerve is stimulated at frequencies of 10, 30, and 50 Hz at a current of up to 15 mA. The pulse duration is typically 500 μs. All of these parameters (frequency, intensity, and duration) can be varied as needed.

Contraction-relaxation curves at 10, 30, and 50 Hz are recorded by the computer. From these curves, a variety of descriptors of muscle function are obtained. These descriptors include the peak force generated at 10, 30, and 50 Hz (F_{10}, F_{30}, and F_{50}); relaxation rate at 10, 30, and 50 Hz (RR_{10}, RR_{30}, and RR_{50}), and the force frequency ratios of F_{10}/F_{50} and F_{30}/F_{50}. A typical contraction-relaxation curve is shown in Figure 23-2.

Once the stimulus is removed, the muscles will relax. The rate of relaxation has been shown to differ between adequately nourished and malnourished individuals (Lopes et al., 1982). Relaxation rate is calculated at each frequency of stimulation by:

$$RR_n = [(F_1 - F_2)/(F_p - F_B)] \cdot 100, \qquad \text{(Equation 23-1)}$$

where $F_1 - F_2$ is the 10-μs period on the relaxation portion of the curve with the greatest force difference; F_p is the peak force; and F_B is the baseline force. This calculation of relaxation rate results in a percentage of relaxation. In addition, the rate in newtons per second is calculated. The 10-μs period is based on the 100-Hz sampling rate of the analog-to-digital converter.

Force frequency ratios may be another indication of nutritional status. These are ratios of the force of contraction at a frequency not expected to produced maximal contraction (10 or 30 Hz) to the force of contraction at the frequency of maximal contraction (50 Hz). Force frequency ratios are calculated by:

$$FF_n/FF_{max} = [(F_{pn} - F_{Bn})/(F_{maxp} - F_{maxB})] \cdot 100, \qquad \text{(Equation 23-2)}$$

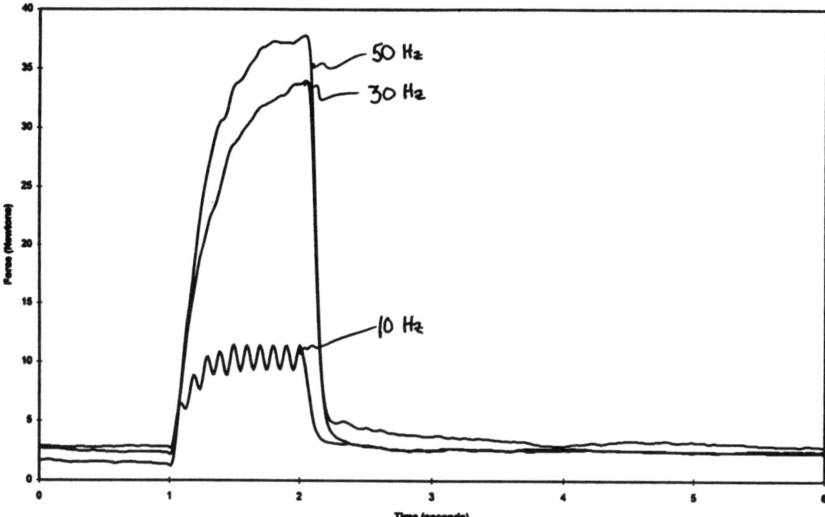

FIGURE 23-2 Typical contraction-relaxation curves at 10, 30, and 50 Hz.

where n is 10, 30, or 50 Hz; max is the maximum frequency; F_{pn} is the peak force at frequency n; F_{maxp} is the peak force at the maximum frequency; F_{Bn} is the baseline force at frequency n; and F_{maxB} is the baseline force at the maximum frequency.

In addition to these descriptors, rise time, decay time, and area under the curve are calculated.

CURRENT CLINICAL TRIALS

There are a number of papers in the literature in which muscle function has been used as an indication of nutritional status in both normal subjects and various patient populations (Berkelhammer et al., 1985; Brough et al., 1986; Christie and Hill, 1990; Lopes et al., 1982; Russell et al., 1983a, b). The MFA device used in these previous studies consisted of a stimulus generator, base plate with force transducer, and strip chart recorder to record the muscle contraction-relaxation curves. A computer was not used to calculate the muscle function descriptors. The clinical trials that are discussed in this section use the device developed by Ross Products Division, Abbott Laboratories, described earlier.

All of these studies offer proof of the concept of muscle function as an indicator of nutritional status and verify previous results of other investigators. All studies are ongoing. Populations studied include normal subjects, HIV-AIDS patients, trauma patients, renal dialysis patients, and nutritionally compromised hospitalized patients.

Normal Subjects

The purpose of this study was to establish the contractile characteristics of skeletal muscle in normal, healthy volunteers during ulnar nerve stimulation of the adductor pollicis muscle. These results potentially would pave the way for the study of muscle function in a variety of disease states.

One-hundred-four normally nourished volunteers aged 18 to 90 were recruited for this study. Subjects were distributed evenly between four age categories; 18 to 35, 36 to 55, 56 to 75, and 76 years and older. Each age group included 13 males and 13 females. A normal nutrition status was determined by a nutrition screen, which included measurements of height, weight, triceps skinfolds, midarm muscle circumference, serum albumin, and hemoglobin. Nutritional status was determined by the criteria listed in Table 23-1.

The presence of any two or more of the six factors listed in Table 23-1 was considered to place the subject in the "nutritional risk" category and therefore deemed the subject ineligible for the study. If a subject met only two criteria, these criteria had to be in two different categories for the subject to be ineligible for the study.

Each subject was tested on three separate occasions, with not more than 7 days between successive tests. Both hands were tested each time. In the 24-h period prior to each test, the subjects were asked to limit alcohol intake to the equivalent of two 12-oz beers. In addition, subjects were asked to refrain from strenuous physical exercise for 48 hours prior to each test. The effects of exercise on muscle function are not clear. However, it has been reported that moderate exercise does not alter the electrically evoked peak twitch torque (Sale et al., 1992), nor the contractile properties of muscle (Barnard et al., 1970). Disuse atrophy has been reported to result in faster relaxation (Simard et al., 1982), which is opposite of what is seen in malnutrition.

Results from this study indicate that the mean value of RR_{10} is similar to that reported in the literature. Some of the subjects in this study fell into the reported "abnormal" range. Other results included differences in:

- RR_{10} when comparing males with females older than 75 years,
- RR_{30} when comparing males with females older than 55 years,
- RR_{50} when comparing males with females 18 to 35 and older than 55 years,
- RR_{50} in males older than 75 years and males younger than 75 years, and
- RR_{30} in females older than 56 years and females younger than 56 years.

HIV-AIDS Patients

The objective of this study is to determine the ability of the MFA device to detect and monitor the effects of malnutrition and refeeding. To date, 30 patients

TABLE 23-1 Criteria for Determining Nutritional Status

Category 1: Anthropometric Criteria

  1. < 90% ideal body weight .

  2. Midarm muscle circumference < 10th percentile and/or triceps skinfold < 10th percentile.

Category 2: Nutritional Criteria

  1. Energy intake < 30–35 kcal/kg for women and 30–40 kcal/kg for men as determined from evaluation of 24-h dietary recall records.

  2. Protein intake < 0.8 g protein per kg of body weight based on ideal body weight.

Category 3: Biochemical Criteria

  1. Serum albumin < 3.5 g/dL.

  2. Hemoglobin < 14 g/dL for men and 12 g/dL for women.

---

have been studied. Nutritional assessment measurements are made at baseline and after 3 months of nutritional intervention. Results to date indicate improved nutritional status as indicated by MFA at the 3-mo visit.

Trauma Patients

The objective of this study is to determine if a peptide-based protein is better than an all amino acid-based protein in affecting the survival and nutritional status of trauma patients. Patients are studied using MFA and a variety of other techniques at baseline (admission) and at 5, 10, 15, and 21 days. Initial results indicate that the MFA relaxation rate appears to follow total body protein.

Renal Dialysis Patients

The objective of this study is to determine if long-term nutritional support can improve outcome and survival in malnourished renal dialysis patients. Patients are evaluated at baseline and at 5 and 10 months. No results have been reported as of yet.

Nutritionally Compromised Patients

The objective of this study is to determine the ability of the MFA device to detect and monitor the effects of malnutrition. In addition, the practicality of this method as a manageable, noninvasive, bedside tool is being investigated. Fifteen patients have been studied to date. Subjective global assessment is used to classify nutrition status. Patients are studied at baseline and at 10 days. Anecdotal reports indicate improved MFA parameters after feeding.

AUTHOR'S CONCLUSIONS

The potential advantages of the MFA device include:

- It may improve on currently available nutritional assessment techniques.
- It may detect early malnutrition because of its sensitivity to functional changes in feeding.
- It is noninvasive. No blood draws are required for this device.
- Results of the test are available immediately.
- It is a low-cost procedure. Neither costly equipment nor dedicated personnel are required.

The disadvantages of the current device include:

- The device is large and cumbersome.
- There is some difficulty locating the ulnar nerve.
- Once the nerve is located, there is some difficulty maintaining the location.
- There may be some voluntary component to what is supposed to be an involuntary contraction. This may be due to the subject's anticipation of or overreaction to the stimulus.
- There may be discomfort. Individual pain tolerances differ. Although the current delivered is less than 15 mA, some people find the stimulus uncomfortable.

The device is being redesigned to address the above disadvantages.

The conclusions drawn from this presentation are that prototype units are currently in use in clinical trials. The results to date are encouraging: there seems to be a correlation between muscle force descriptors and nutritional assessment parameters. The device is being redesigned to address the problems identified in the initial clinical trials.

It is hoped that this technology will offer a significant improvement over the currently available techniques because of the advantages listed above. Further clinical trials are needed to define the role of the MFA device in the assessment of nutritional status, and the trials are ongoing to validate its use in a variety of populations.

REFERENCES

Barnard, R.J., V.R. Edgerton, and J.B. Peter
  1970   Effect of exercise on skeletal muscle. II. Contractile properties. J. Appl. Physiol. 28:767–770.

Berkelhammer, C.H., L.A. Lelter, K.N. Jeejeebhoy, A.S. Detsky, D.G. Oreopoulos, P.R. Uldall, and J.P. Baker
  1985   Skeletal muscle function in chronic renal failure: An index of nutritional status. Am. J. Clin. Nutr. 42:846–864.

Brough, W., G. Horne, A. Blout, M.H. Irving, and K.N. Jeejeebhoy
  1986   Effects of nutrient intake, surgery, sepsis, and long-term administration of steroids on muscle function. Br. J. Med. 293:983–988.

Christie, P.M., and G.L. Hill
  1990   Effect of intravenous nutrition on nutrition and function in acute attacks of inflammatory bowel disease. Gastroenterology 99:730–736.

Kalfarentzos, F., J. Spiliotis, G. Velimezis, D. Dougenis, and J. Androulakis
  1989   Comparison of forearm muscle dynamometry with nutritional prognostic index as a preoperative indicator in cancer patients. J. Parenter. Enteral. Nutr. 13:34–36.

Klidjian, A.M., K.J. Foster, R.M. Kammerling, A. Cooper, and S.J. Karran
  1980   Relation of anthropometric and dynamometric variables to serious postoperative complications. Br. J. Med. 281:899–901.

Lopes, J., D.M. Russell, J. Whitwell, and K.N. Jeejeebhoy
  1982   Skeletal muscle function in malnutrition. Am. J. Clin. Nutr. 36:602–610.

Merton, P.A.
  1954   Voluntary strength and fatigue. J. Physiol. 123:553–564.

Russell, D.M., L.A. Leiter, J. Whitwell, E.B. Marliss, and K.N. Jeejeebhoy
  1983a Skeletal muscle function during hypocaloric diets and fasting: A comparison with standard nutritional assessment parameters. Am. J. Clin. Nutr. 37:133–138.

Russell, D.M, P.J. Prendergast, P.L. Darby, P.E. Garfinkel, J. Whitwell, and K.N. Jeejeebhoy
  1983b A comparison between muscle function and body composition in anorexia nervosa: The effect of refeeding. Am. J. Clin. Nutr. 38:229–237.

Sale, D.G., J.E. Martin, and D.E. Moroz
  1992   Hypertrophy without increased isometric strength after weight training. Eur. J. Appl. Physiol. 64:51–55.

Simard, C.P., S.A. Spector, and V.R. Edgerton
  1982   Contractile properties of rat hind limb muscles immobilized at different lengths. Exp. Neurology 77:467–482.

Webb, A.R., L.A. Newman, M. Taylor, and J.B. Keogh
  1989   Handgrip dynamometry as a predictor of postoperative complications: Reappraisal using age-standardized grip strengths. J. Parenter. Enteral. Nutr. 13:30–33.

DISCUSSION

JOHANNA DWYER: I have just two questions. In your first study where you were looking at the influence of sex and age, you made a comment about total body protein.

JAMES HAYES: That was in trauma [patients].

JOHANNA DWYER: How do you measure the total body protein?

JAMES HAYES: To be perfectly honest with you, I am not sure. If you want to know, I can review the protocol and let you know.

JOHANNA DWYER: You said there was no effect of age, is that right?

JAMES HAYES: As you grow older, the relaxation rates tend to decrease.

JOHANNA DWYER: Okay, they did decrease. But you were not able to associate it with the total body protein?

JAMES HAYES: No attempt was made to do that in that particular study.

GAIL BUTTERFIELD: Are you making any attempt to quantify the degree of malnutrition as evidenced by the change in . . .

JAMES HAYES: I think that one of the goals of or hopes for the device is that we will be able to quantify the degree of malnutrition rather than say that you are normally nourished or you are malnourished. That is a goal. At the current time, we are making no effort or attempt to do that. The attempt is to determine that the device works and we actually are getting results that indicate malnutrition or adequate nutrition.

ARTHUR ANDERSON: I think an important control to include in your study, especially since you made an observation that correlated muscle or body protein with delayed relaxation time, is to get thyroid function tests to correlate with that. That is a diagnostic feature of hyperthyroidism, and you would expect a low body protein or malnourished appearance in someone who is hyperthyroid.

JEFFERY ZACHWIEJA: Do you have any information on activity status and relaxation time?

JAMES HAYES: What we recommend for the studies right now is that there is no vigorous upper-body exercise for 24 hours prior to the study. I have a feeling that fatigue will affect the results, but I have not studied that. We are trying to eliminate that as a possibility. In the patient populations, they are normally not really active.

WM. CAMERON CHUMLEA: Have you thought about using some other body limb? I know the hand is easy because it is very accessible. It has been used for grip strength or for arm circumference, and those do have relationships to body composition, nutritional status, and muscle strength.

However, they do not appear to be as sensitive to the early stages and that is why a lot of the measures of those have now shifted to quadriceps strength or calf circumference because they do tend to be more sensitive to the early losses of nutrition.

JAMES HAYES: Yes, we considered any body limb to which we can attach an accelerometer or transducer that can respond to motions. One of the reasons to choose the hand is that even nonmobile patients may be using their upper bodies to transfer from bed to chair, so this muscle would be less likely to become atrophied. That is why we used that. But we could just as well use any other muscle group.

DOUGLAS WILMORE: If you think about the application of this to military personnel, you must realize that it is a functional test and that acute fluid and electrolyte changes will change muscle function, and because that is part of many states of malnutrition, this is not a malnutrition test, but it is a functional test. It may have some real advantages in that if you see muscle dysfunction, it may act as a red light as to whether you want to use personnel or not. But you do not know whether the results you see are due to electrolyte problems, you do not know whether it is salt restriction, you do not know whether it is low glucose, whether it is glycogen depletion or protein depletion.

JAMES HAYES: That is absolutely right, but one of the things, too, that we are finding is that the test is a good functional indicator of muscle function, which also may indicate nutritional status. Obviously, those things you mentioned may have an effect and we need to study those.

One of the things we wanted to do was get involved in a Ranger study so that we would able to follow those and other possible factors and have some data to support or to be more conclusive on that.

DOUGLAS WILMORE: It is just like phase angle [in bioelectrical impedance analysis], which may indicate a number of things—off or on, yes or no. This may provide another sort of measure.

Emerging Technologies for Nutrition Research, 1997
Pp. 519–532. Washington, D.C.
National Academy Press

24

Application of Cognitive Performance Assessment Technology to Military Nutrition Research

Mary Z. Mays[1]

INTRODUCTION

Military ration developers are charged with the seemingly impossible task of creating operational rations that are highly palatable, nutrient-dense, shelf-stable, lightweight, fully prepared meals. The rations must be sufficient to fuel maximum intellectual and physical performance in order to sustain combat effectiveness adequately. Thus, a substantial portion of military nutrition research literature is devoted to cognitive performance assessment.

Tests of cognitive performance attempt to quantify the measurable end points of complex intellectual behaviors. Logically, if performance were flawed on one or more of the surrogate markers, it would be an indication that more complex intellectual tasks would be done incompletely, imprecisely, or ineffectively. In a military setting, the intellectual behaviors of interest cover a

---

[1] Mary Z. Mays, Eagle Creek Research Services, San Antonio, TX 78209-5236. *Formerly of* U.S. Army Medical Research and Materiel Command, Fort Detrick, MD 21702-5012

wide spectrum, including tasks such as driving a tank, planning a covert reconnaissance operation, conducting medical triage, and handling high explosives.

The history of U.S. Army research on military nutrition can be traced easily from World War II to the present (Askew, 1994; Hirsch and Kramer, 1993; Johnson and Sauberlich, 1982; Lieberman and Shukitt-Hale, 1996; Mays, 1995; Meiselman and Kramer, 1994). Interdisciplinary teams of researchers tested rations, measuring the spectrum of biochemical, physical, psychological, and social parameters on soldiers of all ranks while they were engaged in military field operations (Crowdy et al., 1982; Hirsch et al., 1984; Johnson and Sauberlich, 1982; Shippee et al., 1994; USACDEC/USARIEM, 1986). Such settings limited the type and manner of cognitive performance assessments that were feasible. Assessments typically were made by one of three methods: observation of intact behavior, pencil and paper tests, or automated versions of pencil and paper tests. Occasionally, researchers included tests of manual dexterity and eye-hand coordination in a battery of cognitive performance tests.

In the mid-1980s, military nutrition researchers recognized the need to determine the boundary conditions within which nutritional deficits could be shown to influence cognitive performance. A report by the Committee on Military Nutrition Research (CMNR) clearly articulated the value of cognitive performance assessment in military nutrition research (NRC, 1986). It carefully reviewed methods of assessing cognitive performance by characterizing the breadth and depth of the methods available at that time for investigating the effects of nutritional deficits on memory, reasoning, decision making, and attention. The report provided a detailed discussion of specific test batteries in use in neuropsychology, neurotoxicology, psychopharmacology, and neurobiology.

The potential of the test batteries was never realized. First, the exponential growth of personal computer technology in the late 1980s rendered most of the available test batteries obsolete before they could be disseminated widely and tested for effectiveness in military nutrition research settings. New assessment technology, using computer games or performance tracking devices built into actual or simulated military vehicles and aircraft, made work on refining and tailoring batteries of cognitive performance tests seem dull and unnecessary. Second, the human and financial resources needed to lay the groundwork for a comprehensive study of the effects of nutritional deficits on cognitive performance were simply not available. Identifying those tests that were (1) psychometrically valid surrogates for cognitive components of critical military tasks, (2) appropriately reliable under adverse field conditions, and (3) extraordinarily sensitive to subtle nutritional deficiencies was well beyond the scope of the military nutrition research mission. The emphasis of the CMNR report (NRC, 1986) on the importance of using an empirically validated multivariate approach in the study of complex intellectual behavior prevented a simple choice of one method or test battery over another and left military nutrition researchers without a clearly attainable goal (Mays, 1995). Furthermore, scientific and technological breakthroughs in other disciplines were changing the focus of military nutrition research (Askew, 1994). Investigations of three different problems, food deprivation, underconsumption, and nutritional neuroscience, are typical of the role of cognitive performance assessment in military nutrition research during the decade since the CMNR report.

TYPICAL MILITARY APPLICATIONS

Behavioral scientists who collaborate with military nutrition researchers have accepted the tremendously difficult task of assessing the cognitive performance of individuals who are (1) normal, not sick; (2) highly trained and motivated, but required to perform under duress; and (3) experiencing an energy deficit, but not nutritionally deficient (Mays, 1995; Meiselman and Kramer, 1994). Under the vast majority of circumstances, the small performance decrements that can be expected to occur under such conditions would be considered inconsequential. However, combat effectiveness requires sustained vigilance, precise reasoning, and prompt decision making under stress. Subtle deficits in these intellectual behaviors can degrade military performance dramatically, resulting in significant morbidity and mortality (Belenky et al., 1994).

Food Deprivation

Several different concerns motivate military studies of food deprivation. For example, soldiers on covert missions must carry all their supplies on their backs. The operational requirement forces them to make trade-offs between ammunition, radio batteries, food, and water. Researchers must explicitly define the minimal caloric and nutrient requirements of individuals under such conditions. Similarly, the ability of survival rations to sustain intellectual and physical performance under extreme conditions must be well understood. A series of military nutrition studies in the 1960s and 1970s documented the malaise, memory lapses, and inability to concentrate that characterize semistarvation (Consolazio et al., 1967, 1968; Johnson and Sauberlich, 1982; Johnson et al., 1971). There was a renewed interest in this work in the 1990s due to concerns over the rigors of training for Special Operations soldiers (Moore et al., 1992; Shippee et al., 1994). Field research of this type requires assessment technologies that are field hardened, minimally invasive, and amenable to group administration.

Underconsumption

Military studies of underconsumption are essential to the development of improved military operational rations. Regardless of how nutritious rations may be, they will not sustain intellectual and physical performance if they are not eaten. Research has documented unequivocally the phenomenon of underconsumption of military rations (Baker-Fulco, 1995; Hirsch, 1995). Unfortunately, researchers have not tested adequately the significance of this underconsumption for cognitive performance (Mays, 1995). In this setting, cognitive performance tests must have well-established norms, very small errors in measurement, high reliability across dynamic environmental conditions, and meticulous sensitivity to nutritional manipulations in particular.

Nutritional Neuroscience

Research in the field of nutritional neuroscience over the last decade has had far-reaching implications for the engineering of military rations (Askew, 1994). It is conceivable that rations could facilitate cognitive performance by increasing or inhibiting the synthesis or destruction of neurotransmitters and receptor proteins (Wurtman, 1994). Tests of performance-enhancing ration components require yet another set of methods for assessing changes in cognitive performance. In many cases, researchers will have to test the potential of performance-enhancing ration components in controlled dose-response studies in the laboratory. They will need to borrow methods from the fields of psychopharmacology and neurotoxicology, which sample behavior over time in order to establish the time course of effects. Simulation and game technology are particularly well suited to this type of investigation.

In summary, the objective of behavioral scientists should not be to design an assessment battery that meets all the needs of military nutrition researchers. It should be to document carefully the level of sensitivity, fidelity, flexibility, field expediency, and normative data associated with the method used in a given investigation. Documenting why a method was chosen and how trade-offs among critical attributes of the method were balanced against the objectives of the investigation is an essential part of evaluating the reliability and relevance of the data. Researchers will need to judge the ability of emerging technologies to provide significant improvements in such attributes.

TWENTY-FIRST CENTURY TECHNOLOGY

The basic methods that behavioral scientists use to measure cognitive performance are not likely to change in the near future (Chouinard and Braun, 1993; Gamberale et al., 1990; Gottschalk, 1994; Iregen and Letz, 1992; Kane, 1991; Kane and Kay, 1992; Matarazzo, 1992; Reitan and Wolfson, 1994;

Retzlaff and Gibertini, 1994; Retzlaff et al., 1992; Turnage et al., 1992; White and Proctor, 1992; White et al., 1994). A thorough search of the recent civilian nutrition literature yielded some interesting data on the influence of dieting and diets on the cognitive performance of adults (Brownell and Rodin, 1994; Green et al., 1994; Heatherton et al., 1993; Riggs et al., 1996; Wing et al., 1995). Considerably more data exist on the influence of restricted diets on the cognitive performance of children and the elderly (Gold, 1995; Lopez et al., 1993; Pollitt, 1995; Rosenberg and Miller, 1992; White and Wolraich, 1995). However, none of the nutritional studies suggested that innovative cognitive performance assessment technologies might emerge in the near future. In contrast, there is little doubt that personal computer hardware and software technology will mature significantly in the early twenty-first century. Emerging technologies in automation have the potential to improve substantially the precision, timeliness, and relevance of cognitive performance assessment.

Miniaturization

One of the most productive changes in technology for behavioral scientists in military nutrition research will be the miniaturization of the personal computer's power supply and improvements in battery technology. Increases in durability, safety, and biodegradability and decreases in weight and cost are all feasible (Pen Computing, 1996a). These improvements will increase the field expediency of a number of methods and make true automation of traditional pencil and paper tests worthwhile. If the technological advances in reducing the weight, volume, and cost of power supplies were large, it would permit soldiers to carry the assessment device with them in the field. A handheld device that included a miniature cellular modem and global positioning device would allow researchers to download data from remote sites (Pen Computing, 1996a). The ability to collect data remotely would substantially reduce the invasiveness of cognitive performance assessment and improve the ability to take repeated samples of behavior over time. Having an individual soldier carry a performance assessment device with him might increase the fidelity of assessment. The assessment device could become the analog of the pilot's "black box," which records key elements of a pilot's performance in a standard format (Maitland and Mandel, 1994; Weinstein, 1995).

Interface

An area in which miniaturization will not be useful is the hardware interface between operator and computer. Anyone who has used a calculator-sized microcomputer, such as the Newton™ or the Wizard™, knows the difficulty of doing meaningful work with a tiny keyboard. However, the touch-screen and pen-based graphics interfaces of such products are quite useful (Pen Computing,

1996b). Significant increases in the speed and durability, decreases in the power and light requirements, and improvements in the resolution of the display will enable researchers to design a "natural" interface for a cognitive performance test on an appropriately sized assessment device (Sollenberger and Milgram, 1993; Trautman et al., 1995). A natural interface is one that takes advantage of the techniques humans traditionally use to interact with the world around them, such as three-dimensional imagery, spoken language, and gestures. Thus, a natural interface has two important benefits. It does not require special training, and it increases the speed of input-output processes (both for the soldier and the computer). Additionally, improvements in interfaces will permit researchers to use identical assessment techniques in the laboratory and the field, vastly increasing the relevance and usefulness of both types of investigations (Frohlich et al., 1995; Kenyon and Afenya, 1995; Massimino and Sheridan, 1994; Walker et al., 1993).

Associates

For many years, the scientists and engineers tasked with developing improved weapons platforms have been perfecting artificial intelligence software to serve as the operator's "associate" (Haas, 1995). The associate's job is to analyze information and provide it to the operator in ways that sustain optimum performance. Similarly, several personal computer software developers, including both Apple® and Microsoft®, have developed prototype operating systems that function as "intelligent agents," mimicking the attributes of "butlers" or well-trained "pets" who anticipate the needs of the user and fetch appropriate tools and information (Azar, 1995). The wide acceptance of the World Wide Web has spawned a large industry aimed at producing an "intelligent agent" to roam the Internet's Information Highway and bring back information tailored to the individual computer user's interests (Hawn, 1996; Mobilis, 1996a, b). Future associate programs based on psychological principles will be more powerful than today's clever marketing gimmicks (Doane et al., 1992; Lee and Moray, 1992; Roth et al., 1992; Stanney and Salvendy, 1995). Serious associates will permit the developers of computer-based cognitive performance tests to tailor the tasks and the manner of presentation to individual research subjects and specific research settings (Adelman et al., 1993; DeLucia and Warren, 1994; Ferri, 1995; Kirlik, 1993; Mitta and Packebush, 1995; White and Procter, 1992). Similarly, low-cost, high-speed, high-fidelity handwriting and voice recognition technologies in a handheld computer will permit behavioral science associates to conduct realistic "one-on-one interviews" with subjects in a natural language format (Gottschalk, 1994; Harrington et al., 1995; Moore, 1995; Wilpon, 1995; Wolpaw and McFarland, 1994).

TWENTY-FIRST CENTURY INCENTIVES

Military nutrition researchers are not alone in their desire to improve cognitive performance assessment technology. Vendor shows at meetings of the American Psychological Association make it clear that the development and publication of tests of cognitive performance are a highly competitive industry. Moreover, current changes in the marketplace will stimulate the growth of this industry over the next decade. One of the consequences of health care reform will be an intense interest in precisely quantifying the efficacy of treatment of neuropsychological illness and injury. A consequence of the increasing concern over occupational safety and environmental pollution will be an increased emphasis on developing and using cognitive performance tests that are extraordinarily sensitive to the neuropsychological effects of chronic sleep disturbances and the neurotoxic effects of occupational exposure to hazardous materials. A consequence of educational reform, corporate "right-sizing," and the competitive search for productive diversity in the work force will be improved methods of intelligence and achievement testing. In short, cognitive performance assessment will underlie many measurements of therapeutic efficacy and most decisions concerning job-related selection, training, promotion, and retention in the early twenty-first century.

AUTHOR'S CONCLUSIONS AND RECOMMENDATIONS

The value of cognitive performance assessment in military nutrition research has been clearly established. Military nutrition research continues to have unique needs for cost-effective, field-expedient, and automated versions of cognitive performance tests with well-established military norms and proven validity. These needs will require continued refinement of assessment devices in the twenty-first century. Predictable commercial advances in personal computer software and hardware technologies will have a significant positive impact on the devices used to conduct cognitive performance assessments. Obvious incentives exist for commercial development of emerging assessment technologies by health care corporations, occupational safety and environmental protection regulatory agencies, educational and psychological test publishers, and corporate human resource management consultants. Four conclusions can be derived from the analysis presented. First, significantly more cost-effective, practical, and relevant methods of cognitive performance assessment will be available in the next decade. Second, off-the-shelf technologies suitable for research in the field will be available for use by qualified behavioral scientists. Third, the Department of Defense can ensure that its particular needs are met in a timely fashion, if it systematically supports the development of emerging technologies by commercial firms. Finally, military nutrition researchers will continue to have unique needs for handheld assessment devices that researchers in the private sector are not likely to develop. Thus, the following recommendations seem appropriate:

- Leverage emerging technologies in the computer industry.
- Support the development of assessment technologies by commercial firms.
- Develop handheld assessment devices compatible with military field operations.

REFERENCES

Adelman, L., M.S. Cohen, T.A. Bresnick, J.O. Chinnis, and K.B. Laskey
   1993   Real-time expert systems interfaces, cognitive processes, and task performance: An empirical assessment. Hum. Factors 35(2):243–261.

Askew, E.W.
   1994   Nutritional enhancement of soldier performance at the U.S. Army Research Institute of Environmental Medicine, 1985–1992. Pp. 65–75 in Food Components to Enhance Performance, An Evaluation of Potential Performance-Enhancing Food Components for Operational Rations, B.M. Marriott, ed. A report of the Committee on Military Nutrition Research, Food and Nutrition Board, Institute of Medicine. Washington, D.C.: National Academy Press.

Azar, B.
   1995   Meet "Bob": Psychology's answer to easy computing. APA Monit. 26(4):1, 9.

Baker-Fulco, C.J.
   1995   Overview of dietary intakes during military exercises. Pp. 121–149 in Not Eating Enough, Overcoming Underconsumption of Military Operational Rations, B.M. Marriott, ed. A report of the Committee on Military Nutrition Research, Food and Nutrition Board, Institute of Medicine. Washington, D.C.: National Academy Press.

Belenky, G., D.M. Penetar, D. Thorne, K. Popp, J. Leu, M. Thomas, H. Sing, T. Balkin, N. Wesenten, and D. Redmond
   1994   The effects of sleep deprivation on performance during continuous combat operations. Pp. 127–135 in Food Components to Enhance Performance, An Evaluation of Potential Performance-Enhancing Food Components for Operational Rations, B.M. Marriott, ed. A report of the Committee on Military Nutrition Research, Food and Nutrition Board, Institute of Medicine. Washington, D.C.: National Academy Press.

Brownell, K.D., and J. Rodin
   1994   The dieting maelstrom. Is it possible and advisable to lose weight? Am. Psychol. 49(9):781–791.

Chouinard, M.J., and C.M. Braun
   1993   A meta-analysis of the relative sensitivity of neuropsychological screening tests. J. Clin. Exp. Neuropsychol. 15(4):591–607.

Consolazio, C.F., L.O. Matoush, H.L. Johnson, R.A. Nelson, and H.J. Krzywicki
   1967   Metabolic aspects of acute starvation in normal humans (10 days). Am. J. Clin. Nutr. 20:672–683.

Consolazio, C.F., L.O. Matoush, H.L. Johnson, H.J. Krzywicki, G.J. Isaac, and N.F. Witt
   1968   Metabolic aspects of calorie restriction: Hypohydration effects on body weight and blood parameters. Am. J. Clin. Nutr. 21:793–802.

Crowdy, J.P., C.F. Consolazio, A.L. Forbes, M.F. Haisman, and D.E. Worsley
  1982 The metabolic effects of a restricted food intake on men working in a tropical environment. Hum. Nutr. Appl. Nutr. 36A:325–344.

DeLucia, P.R., and R. Warren
  1994 Pictorial and motion-based depth information during active control of self-motion: Size-arrival effects on collision avoidance. J. Exp. Psychol. Hum. Percept. Perform. 20(4):783–798.

Doane, S.M., D.S. McNamara, W. Kintsch, P.G. Polson, and D.M. Clawson
  1992 Prompt comprehension in UNIX command production. Mem. Cognit. 20(4):327–343.

Ferri, F.
  1995 The medical folder as an active tool in defining the clinical decision-making process. Med. Inf. (Lond.) 20(2):97–112.

Frohlich, B., G. Grunst, W. Kruger, and G. Wesche
  1995 The responsive workbench: A virtual working environment for physicians. Comput. Biol. Med. 25(2):301–308.

Gamberale, F., A. Iregen, and A. Kjellberg
  1990 Computerized performance test in neurotoxicology. Pp. 359–395 in Behavioral Measures of Neurotoxicity, Report of a Symposium, R.W. Russell, P.E. Flattau, and A.M. Pope, eds. U.S. National Committee for the International Union of Psychological Science, Commission on Behavioral and Social Sciences and Education, National Research Council. Washington, D.C.: National Academy Press.

Gold, P.E.
  1995 Role of glucose in regulating the brain and cognition. Am. J. Clin. Nutr. 61(4 suppl.):987S–995S.

Gottschalk, L.A.
  1994 The development, validation, and applications of a computerized measurement of cognitive impairment from the content analysis of verbal behavior. J. Clin. Psychol. 50(3):349–361.

Green, M.W., P.J. Rogers, N.A. Elliman, and S.J. Gatenby
  1994 Impairment of cognitive performance associated with dieting and high levels of dietary restraint. Physiol. Behav. 55(3):447–452.

Haas, M.W.
  1995 Virtually augmented interfaces for tactical aircraft. Biol. Psychol. 40:229–238.

Harrington, M.E., R.W. Daniel, and P.J. Kyberd
  1995 A measurement system for the recognition of arm gestures using accelerometers. Eng. Med. 209(2):129–134.

Hawn, M.
  1996 Seek and ye shall find: Searching the Web. Macworld May:123–127.

Heatherton, T.F., J. Polivy, C.P. Herman, and R.F. Baumeister
  1993 Self-awareness, task failure, and disinhibition: How attentional focus affects eating. J. Pers. 61(1):49–61.

Hirsch, E.S.
  1995 Short- and long-term studies of food intake in military exercises: An overview. Pp. 151–173 in Not Eating Enough, Overcoming Underconsumption of Military Operational Rations, B.M. Marriott, ed. A report of the Committee on Military Nutrition Research, Food and Nutrition Board, Institute of Medicine. Washington, D.C.: National Academy Press.

Hirsch, E.S., and F.M. Kramer
  1993   Situational influences on food intake. Pp. 215–243 in Nutritional Needs in Hot
         Environments, Applications for Military Personnel in Field Operations, B.M.
         Marriott, ed. A report of the Committee on Military Nutrition Research, Food and
         Nutrition Board, Institute of Medicine. Washington, D.C.: National Academy
         Press.
Hirsch, E.S., H.L. Meiselman, R.D. Popper, G. Smits, B. Jezior, I. Lichton, N. Wenkham, J.
         Burt, M. Fox, S. McNutt, M.N. Thiele, and O. Dirige
  1984   The effects of prolonged feeding of Meal, Ready-to-Eat (MRE) operational rations.
         Technical report TR85/035. Natick, Mass.: U.S. Army Natick Research, Develop-
         ment and Engineering Center.
Iregen, A., and R. Letz
  1992   Computerized testing in neurobehavioral toxicology. Appl. Psychol. Int. Rev.
         41(3):247–255.
Johnson, H.L., and H.E. Sauberlich
  1982   Prolonged use of operational rations: A review of the literature. Unnumbered
         technical report. Presidio of San Francisco, Calif.: Letterman Army Institute of Re-
         search.
Johnson, H.L., C.F. Consolazio, H.J. Krzywicki, G.J. Isaac, and N.F. Witt
  1971   Metabolic aspects of calorie restriction: Nutrient balance with 500-kilocalorie
         intakes. Am. J. Clin. Nutr. 24:913–923.
Kane, R.L.
  1991   Standardized and flexible batteries in neuropsychology: An assessment update.
         Neuropsychol. Rev. 2(4):281–339.
Kane, R.L., and G.G. Kay
  1992   Computerized assessment in neuropsychology: A review of tests and test batteries.
         Neuropsychol. Rev. 3(1):1–117.
Kenyon, R.V., and M.B. Afenya
  1995   Training in virtual and real environments. Ann. Biomed. Eng. 23(4):445–455.
Kirlik, A.
  1993   Modeling strategic behavior in human-automation interaction: Why an "aid" can
         (and should) go unused. Hum. Factors 35(2):221–242.
Lee, J., and N. Moray
  1992   Trust, control strategies and allocation of function in human-machine systems.
         Ergonomics 35(10):1243–1270.
Lopez, I., I. deAndraca, C.G. Perales, E. Heresi, M. Castillo, and M. Colombo
  1993   Breakfast omission and cognitive performance of normal, wasted and stunted
         schoolchildren. Eur. J. Clin. Nutr. 47(8):533–542.
Lieberman, H.R., and B. Shukitt-Hale
  1996   Food components and other treatments that may enhance mental performance at
         high altitudes and in the cold. Pp. 453–465 in Nutritional Needs in Cold and in
         High-Altitude Environments, Applications for Military Personnel in Field Opera-
         tions, B.M. Marriott and S.J. Carlson, eds. A report of the Committee on Military
         Nutrition Research, Food and Nutrition Board, Institute of Medicine. Washington,
         D.C.: National Academy Press.
Maitland, M.E., and A.R. Mandel
  1994   A client-computer interface for questionnaire data. Arch. Phys. Med. Rehabil.
         75(6):639–642.
Massimino, M.J., and T.B. Sheridan
  1994   Teleoperator performance with varying force and visual feedback. Hum. Factors
         36(1):145–157.

Matarazzo, J.P.
1992   Psychological testing and assessment in the 21st century. Am. Psychol. 47(8):1007–1018.

Mays, M.Z.
1995   Impact of underconsumption on cognitive performance. Pp. 285–302 in Not Eating Enough, Overcoming Underconsumption of Military Operational Rations, B.M. Marriott, ed. A report of the Committee on Military Nutrition Research, Food and Nutrition Board, Institute of Medicine, Washington, D.C.: National Academy Press.

Meiselman, H.L., and F.M. Kramer
1994   The role of context in behavioral effects of foods. Pp. 137–157 in Food Components to Enhance Performance, An Evaluation of Potential Performance-Enhancing Food Components for Operational Rations, B.M. Marriott, ed. A report of the Committee on Military Nutrition Research, Food and Nutrition Board, Institute of Medicine. Washington, D.C.: National Academy Press.

Mitta, D.A., and S.J. Packebush
1995   Improving interface quality: An investigation of human-computer interaction task learning. Ergonomics 38(7):1307–1325.

Mobilis
1996a Interview with General Magic's Jim White (Part I). Mobilis 2(3) URL http://www.volksware.com /mobilis/march.96/interv1.htm.
1996b Interview with General Magic's Jim White (Part II). Mobilis 2(4) URL http://www.volksware.com/mobilis/april.96/interv1.htm.

Moore, R.C.
1995   Integration of speech with natural language understanding. Proc. Natl. Acad. Sci. USA 92(22):9983–9988.

Moore, R.J., K.E. Friedl, T.R. Kramer, L.E. Martinez-Lopez, R.W. Hoyt, R.E. Tulley, J.P. DeLany, E.W. Askew, and J.A. Vogel
1992   Changes in soldier nutritional status and immune function during the Ranger training course. Technical Report No. T13-92. Natick, Mass.: U.S. Army Research Institute of Environmental Medicine.

NRC (National Research Council)
1986   Cognitive Testing Methodology, Proceedings of a Workshop Held on June 11–12, 1984. Committee on Military Nutrition Research, Food and Nutrition Board, Commission on Life Sciences. Washington, D.C.: National Academy Press.

Pen Computing
1996a Pen computers in transportation. Pen Computing 3(10):18–33.
1996b Pen computers in healthcare. Pen Computing 3(9):18–35.

Pollitt, E.
1995   Does breakfast make a difference in school? J. Am. Diet. Assoc. 95(10):1134–1139.

Reitan, R.M., and D. Wolfson
1994   A selective and critical review of neuropsychological deficits and the frontal lobes. Neuropsychol. Rev. 4(3):161–198.

Retzlaff, P.D., and M. Gibertini
1994   Neuropsychometric issues and problems. Pp. 185–209 in Clinician's Guide to Neuropsychological Assessment, R.D. Vanderploeg, ed. Hillsdale, N.J.: Lawrence Erlbaum.

Retzlaff, P., M. Butler, and R. Vanderploeg
1992   Neuropsychological battery choice and theoretical orientation: A multivariate analysis. J. Clin. Psychol. 48(5):666–672.

Riggs, K.M., A. Spiro, K. Tucker, and D. Rush
  1996 Relationship of vitamin B_{12}, vitamin B_6, folate, and homocysteine to cognitive performance in the Normative Aging Study. Am. J. Clin. Nutr. 63(3):306–314.
Rosenberg, I.H., and J.W. Miller
  1992 Nutritional factors in physical and cognitive functions of elderly people. Am. J. Clin. Nutr. 55(6 suppl.):1237S–1243S.
Roth, E.M., D.D. Woods, and H.E. Pople
  1992 Cognitive simulation as a tool for cognitive task analysis. Ergonomics 35(10):1163–1198.
Shippee, R., K. Friedl, T. Kramer, M. Mays, K. Popp, E.W. Askew, B. Fairbrother, R. Hoyt, J. Vogel, L. Marchitelli, P. Frykman, L. Martinez-Lopez, E. Bernton, M. Kramer, R. Tulley, J. Rood, J. Delaney, D. Jezior, J. Arsenault, B. Nindl, R. Galloway, and D. Hoover
  1994 Nutritional and immunological assessment of Ranger students with increased caloric intake. Technical report T95-5. Natick, Mass: U.S. Army Research Institute of Environmental Medicine.
Sollenberger, R.L., and P. Milgram
  1993 Effects of stereoscopic and rotational displays in a three-dimensional path-tracing task. Hum. Factors 35(3):483–499.
Stanney, K.M., and G. Salvendy
  1995 Information visualization: Assisting low spatial individuals with information access tasks through the use of visual mediators. Ergonomics 38(6):1184–1198.
Trautman, E., M.A. Trautman, and P. Moskal
  1995 Preferred viewing distances for handheld and structurally fixed displays. Ergonomics 38(7):1385–1394.
Turnage, J.J., R.S. Kennedy, M.G. Smith, D.R. Baltzley, and N.E. Lane
  1992 Development of microcomputer-based mental acuity tests. Ergonomics 35(10):1271–1295.
USACDEC/USARIEM (U.S. Army Combat Developments Experimentation Center and U.S. Army Research Institute of Environmental Medicine)
  1986 Combat Field Feeding System-Force Development Test and Experimentation (CFFS-FDTE). Technical Report CDEC-TR-85-006A. Vol. 1, Basic Report; vol. 2, Appendix A; vol. 3, Appendixes B through L. Fort Ord, Calif.: U.S. Army Combat Developments Experimentation Center.
Walker, N., D.E. Meyer, and J.B. Smelcer
  1993 Spatial and temporal characteristics of rapid cursor-positioning movements with electromechanical mice in human-computer interaction. Hum. Factors 35(3):431–458.
Weinstein, C.J.
  1995 Military and government applications of human-machine communication by voice. Proc. Natl. Acad. Sci. USA 92(22):10011–10016.
White, J.W., and M. Wolraich
  1995 Effect of sugar on behavior and mental performance. Am. J. Clin. Nutr. 62(1 suppl.):242S–249S.
White, R.F., and S.P. Proctor
  1992 Research and clinical criteria for the development of neurobehavioral test batteries. J. Occup. Med. 34(2)140–148.
White, R.F., F. Gerr, R.F. Cohen, R. Green, M.D. Lezak, J. Lyberger, J. Mack, E. Silbergeld, J. Valciukas, and W. Chappell
  1994 Criteria for progressive modification of neurobehavioral batteries. Neurotoxicol. Teratol. 16(5):511–524.

Wilpon, J.G.
  1995   Voice-processing technologies—their application in telecommunications. Proc. Natl. Acad. Sci. USA 92(22):9991–9998.
Wing, R.R., J.A. Vasquez, and C.M. Ryan
  1995   Cognitive effects of ketogenic weight-reducing diets. Int. J. Obes. Relat. Metab. Disord. 19(11):811–816.
Wolpaw, J.R., and D.J. McFarland
  1994   Multichannel EEG-based brain-computer communication. Electroencephalogr. Clin. Neurophysiol. 90(6):444–449.
Wurtman, R.J.
  1994   Effects of nutrients on neurotransmitter release. Pp. 239–261 in Food Components to Enhance Performance, An Evaluation of Potential Performance-Enhancing Food Components for Operational Rations, B.M. Marriott, ed. A report of the Committee on Military Nutrition Research, Food and Nutrition Board, Institute of Medicine. Washington, D.C.: National Academy Press.

DISCUSSION

ROBERT NESHEIM: Thank you very much. I think you were concluding all the way through there, Mary.

MARY MAYS: You asked me for my opinion.

ROBERT NESHEIM: And you have never been reluctant, as I understand. Any comments or questions for Mary?

HARRIS LIEBERMAN: Thanks for that stimulating talk, as always. I have concerns about whether we are really going to be able to use commercial kinds of products most of the time for our cognitive assessment. In general, it seems to me that when we have taken things that are widely used, they get a little bit sloppy and do not exactly answer the question that we are trying to answer.

Maybe there are some large groups of people working on tests, who think about things more from the practical point of view than the theoretical, the way most performance tests and most cognitive tests have been developed up until now.

MARY MAYS: That was the interesting part of doing some homework for this presentation. I was very impressed in interviewing people—their comments were not for attribution, so I do not want to tell you the corporations—but I interviewed these people specifically about that. [I asked them] "Is there an emerging technology or is this simply an improvement on old business?"

I think that you will be really impressed, especially with this notion of managed care. There is a tremendous fight right now among psychologists who do not want to be managed by physicians [and HMOs], but who need to be a part of that HMO so that they can provide psychological services. And a part of that whole controversy and that debate is the use of diagnostic tests, but these are really performance tests.

What they are trying to diagnose is your ability to cope in the normal world, in the normal environment, and I think what we are going to see come out of this, again as a result of hardware developments, not necessarily good work by psychologists, is a field-hardened, operator-safe kind of assessment battery.

It will not be the traditional pattern, it will not be the kind of thing that the Department of Defense has always discussed. The tests will be very simple things that will be aimed at component behaviors, testing memory, testing attention, testing reasoning, testing analysis in very quick fashion. They will be, just as in a medical model they would be, surrogate markers of something else.

The point is, the commercial firms have the wherewithal and the incentive to insist that those markers are good markers. Several people at this workshop have mentioned the fact that CD4 [a cell-surface antigen on T-helper cells] is not a good marker any more, that we are starting to reject that as a marker of HIV staging and so forth. There probably will be some errors and it may be that the military researchers will discover them; for example, "This is not a very good marker of anything, I would never use this commercial test."

I do not think we should underestimate the industry's ability to put millions of dollars toward this because they expect to make billions of dollars from it.

Emerging Technologies for Nutrition Research, 1997
Pp. 533–549. Washington, D.C.
National Academy Press

25

New Techniques for Assessment of Mental Performance in the Field

Harris R. Lieberman[1] and Bryan P. Coffey

This chapter considers some of the difficulties associated with conducting behavioral research in the field, as well as more general issues regarding assessment of human performance. Although the focus is on assessing the effect of nutritional manipulations on performance in the field, the general concepts should apply to a variety of other independent variables, such as environmental factors, sleep loss, and toxic agents. After this background material has been presented, a new ambulatory monitoring technology under development at the U.S. Army Research Institute of Environmental Medicine (USARIEM) will be introduced. Finally, some recommendations regarding future research in this area will be presented.

---

[1] Harris R. Lieberman, Military Nutrition Division (*currently* Military Nutrition and Biochemical Division), U.S. Army Research Institute of Environmental Medicine, Natick, MA 01760-5007

ASSESSMENT OF HUMAN BEHAVIOR

For a number of years, many investigators have been interested in how it might be possible to measure human cognitive behavior in a more continuous and less invasive manner than is possible with conventional tests of cognitive function. Standard tests of cognitive performance usually involve filling out forms with paper and pencil, taking written tests on a computer, or using mechanical devices such as Peg-Boards or other manipulanda (items that can be manipulated). These tests measure functions like learning, memory, reaction time, vigilance, attention, manual dexterity, and sensory function. Using such tests, a very wide range of human behaviors can be assessed and, at least in theory, related to real-world performance.

Although psychologists and other scientists conducting research in this area generally are required to rely on such tests to assess performance, there are a number of problems associated with employing them, not only in the field, but also in the laboratory. One limitation is simply the difficulties associated with administering tests to people engaged in field exercises. It is generally necessary for the subject being tested to stop all ongoing activities to participate in the task. When the subjects in a research study are members of military units engaged in training exercises or other military operations, this is a particularly significant problem and often excludes behavioral assessment in field studies. Studies, nutritional or otherwise, conducted in the field generally need to be minimally intrusive with regard to use of soldiers' time. When military units agree to participate in research, they are not primarily in the field to be test subjects. Usually they are there to train. When scientists conduct research with military units, commanders generally impose significant limitations on the amount of time their soldiers will be available to the investigators. Furthermore, soldiers themselves, especially those from nonelite units, can easily become bored or frustrated with behavioral tests, and the quality of the data collected may deteriorate. Although studies cannot be conducted without prior written informed consent, soldiers often become disaffected when asked to take behavioral tests repeatedly that they regard as less than critical to their essential military duties.

Another key issue is the interpretation of data collected using formal laboratory behavioral tests. It can be difficult to relate data from performance tests to real-world performance. This is a generic problem, not just an issue of relevance to field behavioral research. There are many reasons why it is difficult to relate cognitive test performance to actual work performance. One is that a subject usually cannot engage in actual work performance and simultaneously take a behavioral test.

Another well-known problem with conducting behavioral testing is circadian variation in performance (Moore-Ede et al., 1982). Because of such variation, testing must be conducted at multiple times during the day to fully describe the daily pattern of any behavioral parameter. Alternatively, if testing is to take place once a day, each test session must be conducted at the same time. It is not appropriate to compare data collected at one time of day with data collected at another time. In field studies with military units as opposed to laboratory studies, testing at exactly the same time each day can be extremely impractical and often significantly increases the extent of disruption produced by the investigators. Furthermore, circadian variation in a specific parameter may overwhelm any differences caused by nutritional treatments or environmental conditions being evaluated. Also, individual behavioral functions appear to have different patterns of circadian rhythmicity (Moore-Ede et al., 1982).

Another critical problem is that the underlying behavioral function a performance test actually assesses is often unclear. Almost all tests, even the simplest, require the subject to use a variety of sensory systems, information processing capabilities, and motor functions. For example, visual choice reaction time requires the visual system to process sensory information, the attentional functions to focus on the critical sensory parameters, the memory functions to choose the correct stimulus, the decision-making processes to determine whether to initiate a response, and of course, the motor system to make even the simplest response. It cannot be assumed that the limiting or critical factor that any test assesses can always be defined accurately. Also, under different environmental conditions or because of the presence of some extraneous influence on performance, the critical factor in any behavioral test may change. For example, in a cold environment where substantial shivering occurs, impaired ability of the subject to make the necessary motor responses may prevent assessment of the cognitive parameter the test is actually intended to monitor.

One of the most difficult issues to address in any study of performance is determining which test or tests are optimal to answer the research question of interest. It is very difficult to determine what specific test or class of tests will be most useful to assess the effects of a particular experimental parameter. Selecting the test, particularly when only a few can be administered (as is almost always the case in field studies), presents a variety of problems to the investigator. Often, it is not known what test will be most sensitive to the effects of a nutrient, drug, or environmental condition on human performance. There is rarely agreement among scientists working in a particular area as to the best method to employ. In nutrition-behavior studies where, in most every case, the effects of nutritional manipulations are modest, this is a daunting problem. If the investigator selects the "wrong" test, it will be insensitive to the treatment being evaluated. This could then result in a Type II error—failing to detect a treatment effect that actually is present. It may not even be possible to agree on the criteria that should be used to determine the optimal test to address a specific research question. For example, for many years, there was considerable controversy about whether moderate doses of caffeine, equivalent to those found in single servings of common foods, had effects on behavior (Dews, 1984). However, when appropriate vigilance tests are employed, consistent effects of caffeine in this dose range are observed reliably (Fine et al., 1994; Lieberman, 1992).

A problem that often occurs in field studies is that subjects are inaccessible to the investigator for long periods of time. Military units frequently conduct operations in extreme and sometime dangerous environments. Often, it is not possible for investigators to accompany soldiers to administer tests. Frequently, it is these extreme environments that are of the greatest interest with regard to performance. One solution to this problem is to issue handheld computers to the soldiers participating in a study. The soldiers are then responsible for self-testing their own mental performance at designated times.

This technique, in combination with conventional tests of cognitive function, was employed in a month-long field study conducted by USARIEM and Natick Research, Development and Engineering Center (Askew et al., 1987). The study was conducted in northern Vermont in the autumn and was designed to evaluate an experimental, lightweight, 2,000 kcal/d ration (the RLW-30) in comparison with three Meals, Ready-to-Eat VI (MREs), which provide 4,000 kcal/d. Neither the conventional nor the self-administered tests of performance detected substantial changes in performance that were attributable to the RLW-30 ration, although there was some evidence of degradation of performance on some of the conventional tests among soldiers consuming the calorie-deficient ration (Askew et al., 1987; Lieberman et al., in press).

It is apparent that the problems associated with behavioral testing are substantial and magnified when testing must be conducted in the field. Several chapters in this volume provide partial solutions to some of the issues. Some require high technology and sophisticated equipment, such as simulators to collect data (see Watson and Papelis, Chapters 26 in this volume; Johnson, 1991) while others rely on simpler solutions such as paper and pencil tests (Mays, 1995; Shippee et al., 1994), or portable computers to assess performance (Banderet and Lieberman, 1989). In addition, there may be unique and innovative solutions that can be employed to provide data on soldiers in the field as they go about their daily activities without interrupting their training or other operations. Although advances in technology will provide partial solutions, no device or emerging technology will be the complete answer to these complex problems.

ACTIVITY MONITORING

One way to gather useful behavioral data in the field is by using electronic activity monitors and other passive, electronic monitoring devices such as foot strike monitors (Askew et al., 1987; Hoyt et al., 1994; Lieberman et al., 1989; Redmond and Hegge, 1985). Although such devices currently do not assess mental performance, they can be employed effectively to provide information on soldiers as they go about their typical activities in the field. Activity monitors, which were developed in part with U.S. Army sponsorship, record minute-by-minute patterns of the wearer's activity (Lieberman et al. 1989; Redmond and Hegge, 1985; Webster et al., 1982; for a comprehensive review see Tryon, 1991). The most advanced versions can record continuously for many days and are suitable for use in the field, even in extreme environmental conditions (Shippee et al., 1994). Attempts have been made to relate the levels of activity recorded on these monitors to energy expenditure. Although the relationship between activity and energy expenditure is complex, activity monitoring can improve estimates of energy expenditure provided by other methods (Hoyt et al., 1991; Patterson et al., 1993).

One sophisticated, commercially available activity monitor is manufactured by Precision Control Devices, Fort Walton Beach, Florida. The device, the Motionlogger Actigraph, model AMA-32, has been employed effectively to assess patterns of rest and activity and estimate duration and fragmentation of sleep. It has been used successfully as a supplemental measure of energy expenditure in conjunction with other techniques in military field studies (Hoyt et al., 1991). In addition, it can provide invaluable information on levels of activity and sleep patterns of volunteers. The devices are $4 \times 3.1 \times 1$ cm, weigh 57 g, and typically are worn on the wrist of the nonpreferred hand using a standard wristwatch band. Each device contains a microcomputer, 32 kilobytes of memory, an analog-to-digital converter, and a piezoelectric motion sensor and is powered by a standard wristwatch battery. Data collected by the AMA-32 can be downloaded to a laptop or other IBM-compatible computer for further analysis using a specially developed computer program (ACTION 3, Ambulatory Monitoring, Inc., Ardsley, N.Y.) or other software.

The ability of actigraphs to predict sleeping versus waking state of humans has been demonstrated by several investigators. Algorithms to classify activity patterns of individuals wearing activity monitors as representing a sleeping or waking state have been developed and validated (Cole and Kripke, 1988; Webster et al., 1982; Sadeh et al., 1989). Actigraphs are now widely employed to supplement the more accurate and detailed information provided on the extent and structure of sleep by polysomnography. Activity monitors also can be employed to assess circadian rhythms of rest and activity in normal individuals and those with disturbed rhythms because of psychiatric or other medical conditions or transmeridianal travel (Comperatore et al., 1996; Lieberman et al., 1989; Satlin et al., 1991; Teicher et al., 1986; 1988). In a study conducted at USARIEM with the Ambulatory Monitoring Inc.'s AMA-32 actigraphs, the effects on sleep quantity and quality of sleeping in a chemical protective mask were assessed. The significant degradation in sleep that the monitors documented during sleep in the mask was consistent with an observation of impaired performance the next day when soldiers were tested on computer-based performance tasks (Lieberman et al., 1994, 1996).

Figure 25-1 presents data collected with an AMA-32 activity monitor in a USARIEM nutrition field study conducted in a hot desert environment (Hotson et al., 1995). The study was designed to assess a new operational ration (the

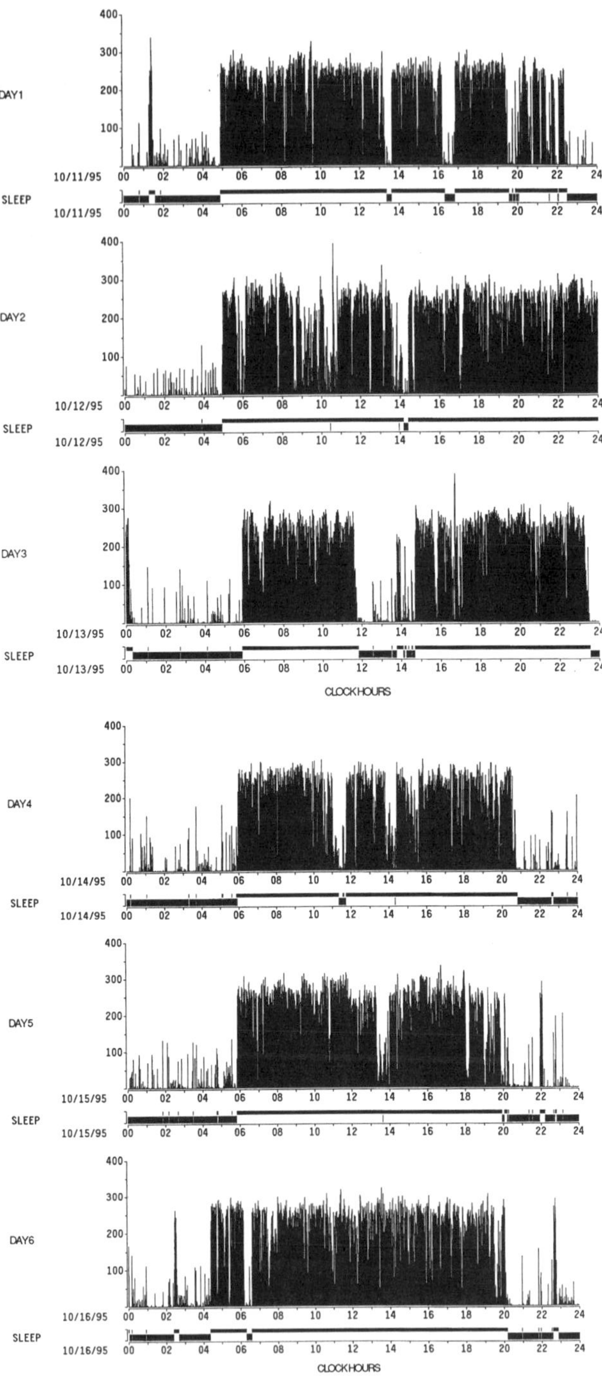

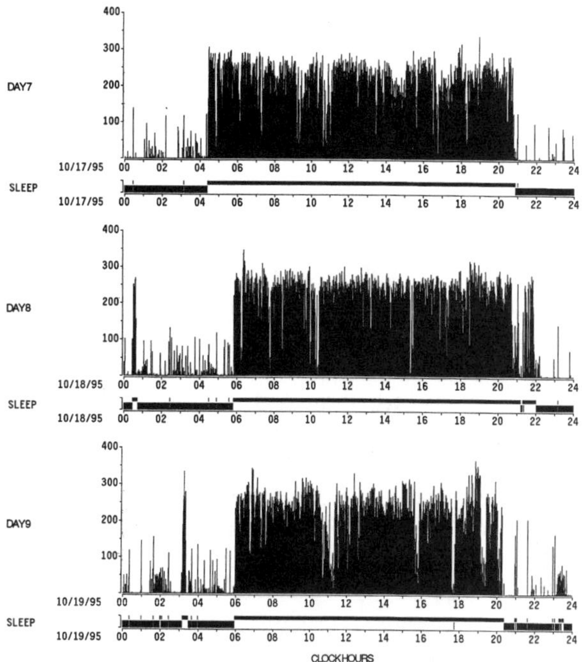

FIGURE 25-1 Daily patterns of rest and activity in a Marine volunteer wearing the AMA-32 activity monitor for 9 consecutive days. The volunteer was participating in a U.S. Army Research Institute of Environmental Medicine (USARIEM) nutrition field study in a hot desert environment. Each vertical line plotted on the x-axis represents the summed total amount of movement exhibited by the wearer in a 1-min period of time. Each individual plot represents a 24-h period starting at 0000 hours on the indicated date. Below each plot is estimated sleeping versus waking time. A thicker bar next to the x-axis indicates that the subject's activity is characteristic of sleep. SOURCE: Hotson et al. (1995).

Unified Group Ration), as well as the effects of a supplemental carbohydrate beverage on a Marine heavy artillery unit that was conducting a live-fire training exercise. As shown in Figure 25-1, which was generated by the ACTION III computer program, daily patterns of rest and activity are clearly documented over the 9 days of the study. In spite of temperatures as high as 130°F (54.5°C), subjects maintained a high level of activity on most days. Below the plots of the rest-activity pattern of each day are corresponding plots indicating the derived sleeping versus waking state of the subject at any given moment in time. The estimates of sleeping versus waking state are generated automatically by the Action III program using a validated algorithm (Figure 25-1).

One clear advantage of activity monitors over traditional cognitive tests is that they provide continuous assessment of a form of behavior, i.e., physical activity. Although activity monitors cannot assess performance *per se*, the data they collect can be related to both physical and mental state.

THE USARIEM VIGILANCE MONITOR

Based in part on the demonstrated utility of activity monitors in the laboratory, clinic, and field, USARIEM has attempted to develop new ambulatory monitoring devices that will provide additional capabilities to researchers interested in assessing behavior and performance in the field. The devices may be particularly suitable for studying soldiers as they conduct field exercises and even actual operations. The monitors combine the characteristics and capabilities of actigraphs such as the AMA-32 with the addition of performance assessment and intervention capabilities. They may be especially useful for addressing how certain nutritional and environmental variables influence mental performance and evaluating the relationship between work performance and mental state. One of the chief capabilities of these devices is the ability to assess vigilance.

Vigilance is a behavioral function that can be readily assessed and may be an important aspect of some critical areas of military performance. Obviously, there are a wide range of behavioral parameters that are critical for soldiers as they conduct their missions. Reaction time, motor skills, attention, memory, and higher-order cognitive processing are all important if soldiers are to accomplish their objectives effectively and safely. One particularly important cognitive function required for many key military duties is maintaining vigilance. It is critical that soldiers maintain vigilance under the worst circumstances, such as when they are sleep deprived; in the middle of the night or early morning when they are at the nadir of the circadian performance rhythm; and when they are physically and environmentally stressed. If a key sentry, operator of surveillance equipment like radar, truck driver, or helicopter pilot cannot maintain vigilance, the consequences can be catastrophic. Assessment of vigilance is of great practical significance since many key civilian as well as military occupations, such as operation of motor vehicles and industrial equipment, require sustained maintenance of vigilance for long periods of time (Mackie, 1987). A number of accidents, such as the Three Mile Island nuclear reactor failure and commercial aircraft crashes, have been attributed, at least in part, to the failure of human operators to detect critical stimuli (Mitler, 1988; Office of Technology Assessment, 1991). Furthermore, even at the optimal time of day, vigilance deteriorates in well-rested individuals if it must be sustained for long periods time (Koelega, 1989).

Vigilance has been reported to be a sensitive measure of the functional capability of an organism. It reflects the ability of individuals to process relevant information and respond in a timely fashion. The central mechanisms underlying vigilance performance have been investigated, and a wide variety of tasks have been used to assess the underlying process or processes (Fine et al.,

1994; Hirshkowitz et al., 1993; Koelega, 1989; Tiplady, 1992). It also has been suggested that vigilance tasks may be more relevant to the performance of everyday activities than shorter tests of cognitive performance often employed in test batteries (Koelega, 1989).

It is important to note that vigilance performance is sensitive to effects of many factors, including sleep loss, drugs, hormones, food constituents, and environmental variables (Clubley et al., 1979; Dollins et al., 1993; Koelega, 1989; Lieberman, 1992; Wilkinson, 1968). Furthermore, there is a large body of literature in this area, which makes it possible to begin to relate vigilance to real-world performance. A good example is the work on the influence of caffeine on simulated sentry duty, presented by Johnson (1991).

Given the operational importance of vigilance and its sensitivity to nutritional and other variables, a device was developed in this laboratory that is capable of continually assessing this parameter as soldiers or civilians go about their normal daily activities. The device also can measure patterns of rest and activity simultaneously and can measure several key environmental factors. As currently configured, the device contains the equivalent of a first-generation personal computer, including 128 kilobytes of memory and an 8-bit microprocessor. It also contains substantial signal processing capabilities and simple auditory and visual output capabilities. It will record continuously for more than 5 days.

The device provides a variety of information about the environment of the wearer, as well as information about the wearer's activity and performance. It can be worn on the wrist, although it is somewhat larger than state-of-the-art activity monitors, such as the AMA-32.

As discussed above, assessment of motor activity has proven to be a valuable technique for gathering information about sleep, circadian rhythms, and energy expenditure of the wearer. The vigilance monitor developed at USARIEM can simultaneously collect multiple channels of activity data. The channels can be programmed to differ in their recording characteristics. One channel might be selected to be sensitive to low-amplitude activity, while another might be sensitive to moderate- or high-amplitude accelerations. The channels also can vary with regard to their temporal characteristics so that differences in the duration of motion can be assessed.

Figure 25-2 displays data collected in the field using the USARIEM vigilance monitor (Unpublished observations, H. R. Lieberman, USARIEM, Natick, Mass., 1994). Data from three channels of activity in counts per minute are presented in the first three panels (Acc1–Acc3). Channels 1 and 2 (Acc1 and Acc2) vary with regard to amplitude of the acceleration they will sense, while Channel 3 (Acc3) has a longer time constant, so it will be more sensitive to longer-duration accelerations. It is believed that the capability to record a variety of different channels of activity simultaneously will, among other things,

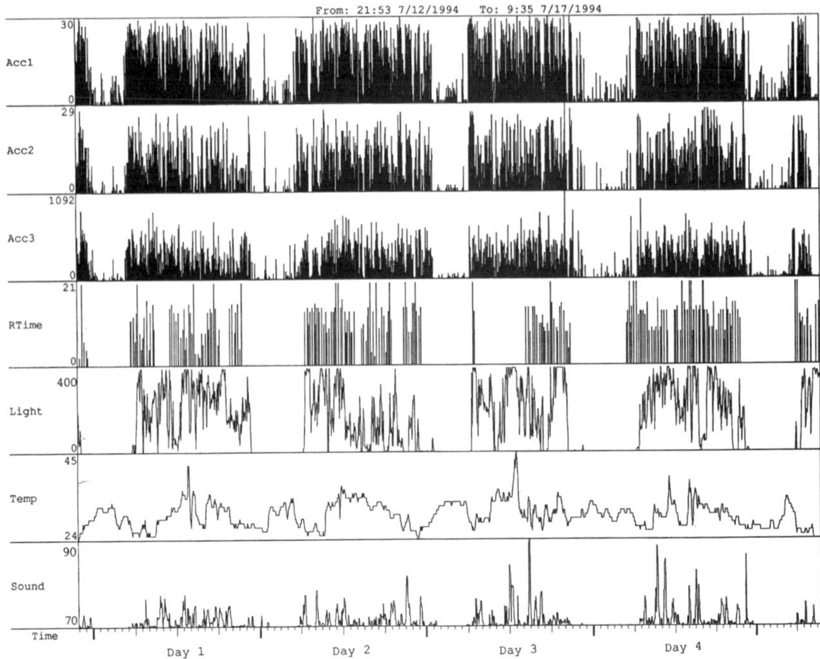

FIGURE 25-2 Four days of consecutive data collected with the vigilance monitor developed at the U.S. Army Research Institute of Environmental Medicine (USARIEM). The top three channels, Acc1 to Acc3, represent activity data collected with different sensor sensitivities. The fourth channel, labeled *Rtime*, displays the responses of the subject to the presentation of a sequence of tones at random intervals. The height of each bar represents the speed of response to the tone. The channel labeled *Light* is the illumination level recorded at the wrist of the subject. The *Temp* channel is a continuous record of ambient temperature levels, and the *Sound* channel records sound levels in decibels. SOURCE: H. R. Lieberman (Unpublished observations, USARIEM, Natick, Mass., 1994)

permit the development of improved algorithms to predict sleeping versus waking state, as well as improve the ability of monitors to predict energy expenditure.

There are, of course, a multitude of environmental factors regulating human behavior. Many cannot readily be assessed, but several can be acquired automatically with minimal difficulty because of the availability of miniature low-power sensors. Therefore, several environmental sensors have been included in the device developed at USARIEM. Specifically, the device can continuously assess and record ambient illumination, sound, and temperature levels. Although the importance of the presence or absence of light in the control of human behavior is readily apparent, it was not until a few years ago that the critical nature of bright light in the regulation of human circadian rhythms became known (Lewy et al., 1980). A light sensor has been included in the device so that information regarding the duration and amplitude of individual exposure to light can be continuously acquired (Channel 5 [Light], Figure 25-2).

Another factor influencing human rest and activity is the pattern and level of sound in the environment. Using a miniature microphone, this information also is collected continuously by the monitor (Channel 7 [Sound], Figure 25-2).

Also included is a thermistor that measures ambient temperature on the surface of the monitor (Channel 6 [Temp], Figure 25-2). The importance of ambient temperature in regulating behavior cannot be understated. When field studies are conducted, information on ambient temperature conditions to which soldiers are exposed can be difficult to collect. Furthermore, even when it is available, it does not describe the conditions an individual soldier experiences but rather the conditions at a stationary weather station (Santee and Hoyt, 1994). By individually monitoring temperature on each subject participating in a study, more accurate tracking of environmental exposure may be possible.

As configured for the study presented here (Unpublished observations, H. R. Lieberman, USARIEM, Natick, Mass., 1994), the monitor also assessed the vigilance of the wearer (Channel 4 [Rtime], Figure 25-2). On average once every 15 minutes, the monitor's speaker presented a short-duration tone. The subject was asked to respond by pushing a small switch on the monitor as soon as he or she heard the tone. If the subject did not respond to the initial tone in a few seconds, a second louder tone was presented. Finally, a third tone was presented if the subject still failed to respond. In addition to determining whether or not the subject responded to the tones, the monitor also recorded the time required for the subject to respond—his or her reaction time. Therefore, the monitor can continually assess alertness in the field as soldiers or civilians perform their daily duties. Whenever the individual wishes to turn off the behavioral task or tasks, for example to sleep, he or she can do so.

It also should be noted that because the monitor contains a user-programmable microcomputer, it can be used not only to assess vigilance but to actively intervene, if desired, to prevent degradation in performance of the wearer.

Like most other activity monitors currently available, the monitor developed at USARIEM, once programmed, will record data for many days with no investigator input. The computer program executed by the monitor is written on a standard IBM-compatible computer and is downloaded to the monitor for execution. When the experiment is complete or the memory is full, the collected data are uploaded to a standard IBM-compatible personal computer for analysis.

Some of the capabilities of the USARIEM vigilance monitor are:

• The wearer can continue with most daily activities while wearing the monitor. Of course, it will interfere somewhat with ongoing duties, but compared with stopping to take a behavioral test, responding to the monitor is a minor inconvenience.

• The monitor is suitable for field use and provides information on several environmental factors: light, sound, and ambient temperature.

• With sufficient monitors, it is possible to monitor a large number of subjects for many days in the absence of an investigator.

• The monitor is fully programmable so that it can be employed in a variety of configurations to address different experimental questions.

• The monitor may be used for the active prevention of reductions in alertness, if validated for this use.

AUTHORS' CONCLUSIONS

• There is a distinct need for innovative technologies that can be employed to assess human performance and other aspects of behavior in the field. Such technologies should assess behaviors of clear relevance to the critical duties of soldiers and other warfighters.

• Although there are currently some mature technologies, such as activity monitors, for assessment of limited aspects of behavior in the field, the development of devices with much greater functionality would significantly advance military nutrition field research.

• Personal monitoring devices are relatively inexpensive technologies to utilize in the field once the appropriate hardware and software capabilities are developed and implemented.

• There is considerable need for the development of analytic tools for processing and integrating the information collected by ambulatory monitors.

• It is recommended that laboratory or other controlled studies be conducted to relate data provided by new technologies for field assessment of performance to the information provided by standard techniques.

REFERENCES

Askew, E.W., I. Munro, M.A. Sharp, S. Siegel, R. Popper, M.S. Rose, R.W. Hoyt, K. Reynolds, H.R. Lieberman, D. Engell, and C.P. Shaw
    1987   Nutritional status and physical and mental performance of soldiers consuming the Ration, Lightweight or the Meal, Ready-to-Eat military field ration during a 30-day field training exercise (RLW-30). Technical Report T7-87. Natick, Mass.: U.S. Army Research Institute of Environmental Medicine.

Banderet L.E., and H.R. Lieberman
    1989   Treatment with tyrosine, a neurotransmitter precursor, reduces environmental stress in humans. Brain Res. Bull. 22:759–762.

Clubley, M., C.E. Bye, T.A. Henson, A.W. Peck, and C.J. Riddington
    1979   Effects of caffeine and cyclizine alone and in combination on human performance, subjective effects and EEG activity. Br. J. Clin. Pharmacol. 7:157–163.

Cole, R.J., and D.F. Kripke
 1988   Progress in automatic sleep/wake scoring by wrist actigraph. Sleep Res. 17:331.
Comperatore, C.A., H.R. Lieberman, A.W. Kirby, B. Adams, and J.S. Crowley
 1996   Melatonin efficacy in aviation missions requiring rapid deployment and night operations. Aviat. Space Environ. Med. 67(6):520–524.
Dews, P.B., ed.
 1984   Behavioral effects of caffeine. Pp. 86–100 in Caffeine. New York: Springer-Verlag.
Dollins, A.B., H.J. Lynch, M.H. Deng, K.U. Kischka, R.E. Gleason, R.J. Wurtman, and H.R. Lieberman
 1993   Effect of pharmacological daytime doses of melatonin on human mood and performance. Psychopharmacology 112:490–496.
Fine, B.J., J.L. Kobrick, H.R. Lieberman, B. Marlowe, R.H. Riley, and W.J. Tharion
 1994   Effects of caffeine or diphenhydramine on visual vigilance. Psychopharmacology 114:233–238.
Hirshkowitz, M., L. De La Cueva, and J.H. Herman
 1993   The multiple vigilance test. Behavior Research Methods, Instruments, and Computers 25(2):272–275.
Hotson, N.G., A.D. Cline, R.L. Shippee, S. McGraw, M. Kramer, W.J. Tharion, J.P. DeLany, R. Hoyt, C.J. Baker-Fulco, and H.R. Lieberman
 1995   Nutritional challenges for field feeding in a desert environment. Unpublished manuscript. Natick, Mass.: U.S. Army Research Institute of Environmental Medicine.
Hoyt, R.W., T.P. Jones, T.P. Stein, G.W. McAninch, H.R. Lieberman, E.W. Askew, and A. Cymerman
 1991   Doubly labeled water measurement of human energy expenditure during strenuous exercise. J. Appl. Physiol. 71:16–22.
Hoyt, R.W., J.J. Knapik, J.F. Lanza, B.H. Jones, and J.S. Staab
 1994   Ambulatory foot contact monitor to estimate the metabolic cost of human locomotion. J. Appl. Physiol. 76(4):1818–1822.
Johnson, R.F.
 1991   Rifle firing simulation: Effects of MOPP, heat, and medications on marksmanship. Pp. 530–535 in Proceedings of the Military Testing Association. San Antonio, Tx.: Armstrong Laboratory Resource Directorate and U.S. Air Force Occupational Measurement Squadron.
Koelega, H.S.
 1989   Benzodiazepines and vigilance performance: A review. Psychopharmacology 98:146–156.
Lewy, A.J., T.A. Wehr, F.K. Goodwin, D.A. Newsome, and S.P. Markey
 1980   Light suppresses melatonin secretion in humans. Science 210:1267–1269.
Lieberman, H.R.
 1989   Cognitive effects of various food constituents. Pp. 267–281 in Psychobiology of Human Eating and Nutritional Behavior, R. Shepard, ed. Chichester, England: Wiley.
 1992   Caffeine. Pp. 49–72 in Factors Affecting Human Performance. Volume II: The Physical Environment, D. Jones and A. Smith, eds. London: Academic Press.
Lieberman, H.R., J.J. Wurtman, and M.H. Teicher
 1989   Circadian rhythms of activity in healthy young and elderly humans. Neurobiol. Aging 10:259–265.

Lieberman H.R., M.Z. Mays, B. Shukitt-Hale, B.E. Marlowe, D.I. Welch, W.J. Tharion, P.D. Gardner, A. Pappas, and K.S.K. Chinn
   1994   Sleep in the M40 mask: Sleep quality, mask fit factor and next day performance. Technical Report T94-8. Natick, Mass.: U.S. Army Research Institute of Environmental Medicine.
Lieberman H.R., M.Z. Mays, B. Shukitt-Hale, K.S.K. Chinn, and W. J. Tharion
   1996   Effects of sleeping in a chemical protective mask on sleep quality and performance. Aviat. Space Environ. Med. 67(9):841–848.
Lieberman, H.R., E.W. Askew, and M.A. Sharp
   1997   Effects of 30 days of undernutrition on plasma neurotransmitters and other amino acids. J. Nutr. Biochem. 8(3):119–126.
Mackie, R.R.
   1987   Vigilance research—are we ready for countermeasures? Hum. Factors 29(60):707–723.
Mays, M.Z.
   1995   Impact of underconsumption on cognitive performance. Pp. 285–302 in Not Eating Enough, Overcoming Underconsumption of Military Operational Rations, B.M. Marriott, ed. A report of the Committee on Military Nutrition Research, Food and Nutrition Board, Institute of Medicine. Washington, D.C.: National Academy Press.
Mitler, M.M.
   1988   Catastrophes, sleep and public policy: Consensus report. Sleep 11(1):100–109.
Moore-Ede, M.C., F.M. Sulzman, and C.A. Fuller
   1982   The Clocks That Time Us. Physiology of the Circadian Timing System. Cambridge, Mass.: Harvard University Press.
Office of Technology Assessment, U.S. Congress
   1991   Biological rhythms: Implications for the worker. OTA-BA-463. Washington, D.C.: U.S. Government Printing Office.
Patterson, S.M., D.S. Krantz, L.C. Montgomery, P.A. Deuster, S. M. Hedges, and L.E. Nebel
   1993   Automated physical activity monitoring: Validation and comparison with physiological and self-reported measures. Psychophysiology 30(3):296–305.
Redmond, D.P., and F.W. Hegge
   1985   Observations on the design and specification of a wrist-worn human activity monitoring system. Behavior Research Methods, Instruments, and Computers 17(6):659–669.
Sadeh, A., J. Alster, D. Urbach, and P. Lavie
   1989   Actigraphically based automatic bedtime sleep-wake scoring: Validity and clinical applications. J. Ambul. Monitor 2:209–216.
Santee, W.R., and R.W. Hoyt
   1994   Recommendations for meteorological data collection during physiological field studies. Technical Report T94-9. Natick, Mass.: U.S. Army Research Institute of Environmental Medicine.
Satlin, A., M.H. Teicher, H.R. Lieberman, R.J. Baldessarini, L. Volicer, and Y. Rheaume
   1991   Circadian locomotor activity rhythms in Alzheimer's disease. Neuropsychopharmacology 5:115–126.
Shippee, R., K. Friedl, T. Kramer, M. Mays, K. Popp, E.W. Askew, B. Fairbrother, R. Hoyt, J. Vogel, L. Marchitelli, P. Frykman, L. Martinez-Lopez, E. Bernton, M. Kramer, R. Tulley, J. Rood, J. Delaney, D. Jezior, J. Arsenault, B. Nindl, R. Galloway, and D. Hoover
   1994   Nutritional and immunological assessment of Ranger students with increased caloric intake. Technical report T95-5. Natick, Mass: U.S. Army Research Institute of Environmental Medicine.

Teicher, M.H., J.M. Lawrence, N.I. Barber, S. Finkelstein, H.R. Lieberman, and R.J. Baldessarini
  1986   Altered locomotor activity in neuropsychiatric patients. Prog. Neuropsychopharmacol. Biol. Psychiatry 10:755–761.
Teicher, M.H., J.M. Lawrence, N.I. Barber, S.P. Finklestein, H.R. Lieberman, and R.J. Baldessarini
  1988   Altered circadian activity rhythms in geriatric patients with major depression. Arch. Gen. Psychiatry 45:913–917.
Tiplady, B.
  1992   Continuous attention: Rationale and discriminant variation of a test designed for use in psychopharmacology. Behavior Research Methods, Instruments, and Computers 24(1):16–21.
Tryon, W.W.
  1991   Activity Measurement in Psychology and Medicine. New York: Plenum Press.
Webster, J.B., D.F. Kripke, S. Messin, D.J. Mullaney, and G. Wyborney
  1982   An activity-based sleep monitor system for ambulatory use. Sleep 5:389–399.
Wilkinson, R.T.
  1968   Sleep deprivation: Performance tests for partial and selective sleep deprivation. Pp. 28–43 in Progress in Clinical Psychology, B.F. Reiss and L.A. Abt, eds. New York: Grune and Stratton.

DISCUSSION

JOHANNA DWYER: Knowing your wife, who is a pediatrician, I told Bill [Beisel] that you made a computerized baby that was always crying. My question is, how do you maintain the motivation to turn this thing [the vigilance monitor] off?

HARRIS LIEBERMAN: In the preliminary study that we conducted, we saw relatively stable levels of responding in the volunteers. When we test hundreds of subjects, how consistent they would be in responding to frequent stimuli is something we will just have to answer by doing the research. It is a good question.

ROBIN KANAREK: Along similar lines, it seems to me that it would depend a lot on the environment that the soldier was in at that particular time, for example if he is being shelled. Have you looked at how that would interact?

HARRIS LIEBERMAN: That is one of the nice things [about the device]. We can actually do minute-by-minute correlations, look at ambient sound levels and ambient light levels, and see if performance is affected by those particular parameters and also by some variations in temperature.

The configuration that I am showing you is fairly flexible. It would be possible to add other environmental sensors if you had a particular issue that you were concerned about, for example, exposure to a toxic gas. So you also could have that capability fairly easily, although the device would not be as field hardened with special modifications on it.

Those are experimental questions that I hope we will be able to start to address with this kind of technology. It is just the beginning.

DAVID DINGES: What you have presented is a fascinating device, and, I think a logical step to move toward, Harris. What is your best guess right now for where this will be most useful? In other words, in the back of your mind, is it that this is going to be a fall-asleep detection device? Are you going to be able to identify that the soldiers were not paying attention at the right time? What is this device going to be for?

HARRIS LIEBERMAN: In the first instance, it will be used for us to gather data for experiments in which we are testing the effects of environmental and nutritional parameters. That is really what it was built for in the first place. The capability for intervening and actually keeping people alert is a little bit far-fetched, perhaps. The only way to find out whether it is going to be useful is to get out there and try it out. I think finding the right parameters will be extremely difficult.

BERNADETTE MARRIOTT: What about another scenario where people may be concentrating on the task at hand to the point where they say, "I don't want to be bothered with this" because it is an interruption rather than a measure of lapses?

HARRIS LIEBERMAN: The device can be turned off; that is, the auditory portion of the device can simply be turned off by the subject for any length of time simply by punching it in. Yes, that is a very good question. If somebody is trying to sleep, we do not want to interrupt their sleep, and if someone is trying to do a task that requires great concentration, we do not want to be in a situation of interfering with that.

JOHN VANDERVEEN: Do you have any telemetry [monitoring] capability with this?

HARRIS LIEBERMAN: No, there is not any telemetry capability. We have sufficient memory to record all these channels of data for more than 5 days, actually. The battery, not the amount of information we can store, is the limiting factor.

For the applications that we are interested in out in the field, it is really better, I think, to collect the data this way than to do telemetry. You would have to go to a whole new device, I think, if you wanted to do telemetry with this.

PATRICK DUNNE: I was wondering if you could correlate when the subjects were eating, with the activity monitor because a real issue when you are out in the field is why the people do not take in a full caloric load if they are just not given any down time to eat it.

HARRIS LIEBERMAN: I do not think it would really tell us.

PATRICK DUNNE: There seemed to be a few low spots within a given day, and I was just wondering whether the soldiers might have gone under a shade and if that may have been when they were eating.

HARRIS LIEBERMAN: We could set up a task and simply ask them to respond by pushing a button whenever they ate. That would be one way to do it. But just looking at the data we have now, we could not tell.

Emerging Technologies for Nutrition Research, 1997
Pp. 551–567. Washington, D.C.
National Academy Press

26

The Iowa Driving Simulator: Using Simulation for Human Performance Measurement

Ginger S. Watson[1] and Yiannis E. Papelis

INTRODUCTION

This paper describes the Iowa Driving Simulator (IDS), a high-fidelity driving simulator, and relates its use to human performance measurement. This virtual reality device is currently in use for research in mechanical engineering, transportation, and medical disciplines. The IDS currently is considered one of the highest-fidelity driving simulators in the United States. Application of the device in the engineering field includes virtual prototyping, a process by which the design of new vehicles is accelerated through use of the simulator in lieu of a physical prototype. The device has been used to investigate human factors for new highway technologies, in-vehicle devices, and licensure issues, such as fitness to drive.

The paper is structured in two sections. The first section provides a technical overview of the device, along with specification for its hardware and soft-

<hr>

[1] Ginger S. Watson, Center for Computer-Aided Design, The University of Iowa, Iowa City, IA 52242

ware components. The second section discusses some of the authors' experiences with the IDS.

Driving is one of the most complex tasks with which the majority of the population is familiar. Despite its commonality, driving is a rather complex task that involves quick decision making, significant motor skills, and the ability to quickly process information from a variety of sources. To simulate this task faithfully in a simulator requires extensive realism and fidelity with respect to several factors, including the hardware providing vibration, sound, and visual stimuli involved in driving a vehicle, the performance characteristics associated with the vehicle, and the external virtual environment in which a simulation takes place. In addition to simply reproducing these cues for the driver of the simulator, several other requirements are necessary for a simulator used to conduct scientific research. These requirements include an external environment that can be customized to meet study requirements; a realistic yet repeatable set of behaviors of the surrounding area; extensive data collection and analysis capabilities; and from an engineering standpoint, strict determinism and repeatability in the execution of the overall system.

IDS TECHNICAL OVERVIEW

The IDS (Freeman et al., 1995; Kuhl et al., 1995) is a high-fidelity driving simulator located at the University of Iowa's Center for Computer-Aided Design. The IDS cueing subsystems utilize state-of-the-art technology to provide visual, motion, audio, and tactile-instrument feedback. In addition, the IDS uses a sophisticated scenario control system (Cremer et al., 1994), which includes independent simulations of multiple robot drivers that comprise the external traffic participants. The wide range of uses that has been required of IDS imposes some surprisingly challenging technical requirements. Very often, it is not only necessary to model the environment faithfully, but the environment must be modeled differently from actual life in order to test some hypotheses. For example, in order to test a new highway design, the visual database must be constructed to reflect not traditional design rules but the new rules that are under study. To test and evaluate new in-vehicle devices requires the IDS to simulate systems that are not in existence, a task perfectly fit for a simulation that is nevertheless challenging, given the lack of engineering experience in the operation of the new devices. Similarly, to research reaction to specific traffic situations, the IDS must be able to reproduce traffic scenarios faithfully that may involve multiple other robot drivers coordinated to produce interactions (such as lane incursions and sudden braking), which may or may not be able to be reproduced in real life. To achieve this level of programmability and reconfigurability, the IDS utilizes several advanced technologies associated with its cueing systems. Requirements on these systems, along with details on their design, are given below.

Visual Feedback

The IDS uses an Evans and Sutherland ESIG 2000 dedicated Image Generator (IG). The IG is capable of displaying up to 1.8 million pixels per image at rates of up to 50 images per second. The vertical field of view is 190 degrees forward, with 60 degrees in the rear view. The forward view allows the driver to observe out of both the front and side driver and passenger windows. No images are provided in the normal blind spot. The rear view is projected on a dome-shaped panel located behind the vehicle and is reflected in all three rear-view mirrors. It is possible to redesign the visual configuration of the IDS and trade the refresh rate (the rate at which the views in the rearview mirrors are changed) with resolution and/or field of view. For example, the refresh rate can be reduced in order to gain higher pixel and polygon capacity. To date, the IDS has been reconfigured with smaller field of view and higher pixel density for experiments that require higher visual fidelity. The IG supports full-color textures that can be applied to any polygon and can increase dramatically the visual detail provided to the driver. The visual system supports several sophisticated functions typical of advanced image generators, including MIP (*Multi Im Parvo*, Latin for "many things in a small place") texture (eliminates the distracting "dancing" of textures by modifying in real time the texture images based on their distance from the simulator driver), anti-aliasing (a technique that causes lines to look smoother without the jagged edges typically associated with computer-generated images), level of detail management (displaying images of varying complexity based on their distance to the eyepoint to increase the effective display capacity for complex scenes), along with a variety of special effects, such as time-of-day variation, fog, and lights. Visual databases used in the IDS are constructed with particular attention to both functional and cosmetic details associated with driving. Functional details include proper road markings, road construction consistent with highway engineering standards, proper signage, and correctly functioning traffic lights. Cosmetic issues include detailed vehicle models for the traffic participants and cultural features, such as buildings, bridges, vegetation, and a variety of structures (e.g., poles and antennas). Depending on the requirements of research studies, it is possible to construct roadways with nonstandard parameters, place features that can change adaptively based on dynamic feedback obtained during the course of a given experiment (i.e., speed limit signs that reduce or increase the speed limit based on the subject's behavior), and create numerous other special effects and customized behavior. The IDS library currently consists of numerous areas populated with rural, interstate, and town roadways with standard and nonstandard widths, markings, and signage. In addition, exact replicas of actual world locations have been constructed and used in validation studies.

Motion Feedback

Motion feedback refers to the feeling of acceleration sensed in the process of driving. The IDS uses a hexapod (six-legged) motion base with 60-in stoke hydraulic actuators that can provide a maximum of 1.1 g (unit of acceleration based on that produced by the earth's gravitational attraction) of acceleration at a frequency of about 4 Hz. A motion base such as the one used in the IDS cannot reproduce faithfully the magnitude of accelerations involved even in typical driving situations. In fact, any attempt to reproduce 100 percent of the actual acceleration involved in driving will cause the motion base to extend the hydraulic legs to their maximum followed by a sudden stop when the hard motion limits are reached. To avoid such occurrences and maximize the fidelity of the motion feedback, the IDS uses sophisticated washout algorithms that filter the input acceleration signals generated by the vehicle dynamic model and make the best use of the motion envelope available in the hexapod. The algorithms used in the IDS allow prepositioning of the motion base, a technique that maximizes the motion envelop when the behavior of the simulated vehicle can be predicted with certainty, as is often the case in prescribed scenarios. For example, if it is known that a braking maneuver always will occur at a given location, the prepositioning algorithm can shift the motion base so as to maximize actuator travel for the upcoming maneuver. The shifting of the rest point of the motion base is done at a rate that is below the human perception threshold to avoid distracting the subject. The National Advanced Driving Simulator (NADS) utilizes a more sophisticated motion base that consists of a hexapod mounted on top of an X-Y track with 20 feet of travel in each direction (Stoll and Bourne, 1996).

Audio

The audio subsystem in IDS consists of a multichannel digital sampling workstation that reproduces sounds associated with the engine, wind, and tire noise, along with sound produced by the remainder of the vehicles in the scene. The audio system will reproduce a variety of sound effects, including the Doppler shift caused by sounds generated by sources moving towards each other (as when a honking vehicle drives by another). In addition, the audio system can replay a variety of specific sounds and actually record voices under the control of the scenario system.

Tactile and Instrument Feedback

Tactile feedback is provided by a high-accuracy motor mounted on the steering wheel and a variety of additional pumps and actuators connected to the various pedals and levers. All instruments within the vehicle cab operate as in the normal car. Additional devices often are installed to provide newly designed capabilities.

Scenario Control

A virtual driving environment such as IDS requires roadway traffic simulated at the microscopic level. A microscopic level traffic simulation is one in which individual vehicles are simulated on their own and interact with each other and with the driver of the simulator (Cremer et al., 1996). In the IDS, these vehicles are aware of the rules of the road and will exhibit a rich set of behaviors similar to those in real life, including randomness and unpredictability. Whereas this behavior is attractive for casual interactions, the unpredictability contradicts the scientific requirement of repeatability necessary in controlled studies with multiple subjects. Complicating the situation even more is the fact that there are great differences among the driving habits of different subjects. Without some means to ensure that a specific interaction (such as a rear-end collision situation) occurs with the same conditions for all subjects, the results of a study may be compromised. The scenario control subsystem in the IDS utilizes an architecture in which intelligent agents within the simulator's virtual environment coordinate events and ensure that specific interactions repeat with similar conditions, despite differences because of specific drivers' habits. The scenario control system utilizes the Hierarchical Concurrent State Machine (HCSM) formalism (Cremer et al., 1995) to simulate the traffic's autonomous behavior. The HCSM formalism allows modeling of simultaneous, multiple thinking processes taking place while driving. Scenes with up to about 25 other vehicles can be simulated, and a variety of traffic situations can be forced to occur. Examples of scenarios used in IDS studies include precrash behavior, following behavior, and effectiveness of antilock brakes. An additional unique aspect of the IDS scenario system is the existence of a special database that contains all traffic participants, along with a variety of logical information about the road network, including lane positioning, signs, intersection topologies, and traffic control devices (Papelis and Bahauddin, 1995). The existence of this information is important because it allows for the collection of performance data that would otherwise be impossible to collect. For example, a simple performance measure that is often used is lane deviation. In complicated road networks (as opposed to a straight road), computing lane deviation requires some representation of the lane. The visual databases used in the IG contain textured polygonal descriptions of the virtual environment that are not useful in deriving lane information. Similarly, information on signage and road markings opens the potential for automatic evaluation tools and detailed performance analysis. In fact, the software used for scenario control in the IDS is currently in use in a simulator used for training truck drivers and utilizes the extended capabilities of the road database to provide both continuous feedback to the driver on rules-of-the-road violation, as well as other performance suggestions.

Research Issues and Limitations

While simulators of this sort provide new and interesting technologies for the measurement of human performance, they are not free of challenges and limitations for their effective use. Some of the issues include choosing and sorting through the detailed and numerous quantifiable performance measures that are possible with this technology (Bloomfield and Carroll, 1996), gathering validation evidence for those events that are safe in a simulator but not safe to test in the real world, and ensuring efficient use of the device to maximize high usage costs. While the amount of realism or fidelity required for research is assumed to be high, the degree of fidelity and associated costs necessary for sound measurement in research settings such as this are not known. Further, the amount of fidelity may vary among research study, study population, task, and experience (Alessi and Watson, 1994). Little research has been conducted to understand fidelity needs, although theoretical models do serve to guide the simulator designer and user.

Finally, simulators are known for inducing something similar to motion sickness in certain individuals. The occurrence of this phenomenon varies with simulator design (fidelity, subsystem components, and cueing congruence), individual susceptibility (gender, age, and experience), and exposure (length, time of day, and scenario interaction). Simulator designers must consider the potential for sickness and attempt to design systems that minimize its occurrence. Researchers who use these devices must understand the phenomenon and attempt to design experiments that limit the likelihood of such effects (Watson, 1995).

CONDUCTING EXPERIMENTS WITH THE IDS

The IDS is a relatively new facility that began operation in 1990. The motion-base facility was not operational until about 1993, when a new motion base was obtained. There is also a fixed-based facility in which the same computer resources are used, but a different simulation bay is set up so that there is no motion. Motion is an expensive cue to simulate, but it adds some of the additional feedback necessary to get real-world matches of driving performance between a simulated environment and that in the real world. The visual system was upgraded in 1994, which has allowed much higher visual resolution.

The IDS utilizes a six-degrees-of-freedom motion base, capable of accelerations up to 1.1 g, which is adequate for some driving maneuvers but not for all. For instance, motion cues experienced during high-speed chases and vehicle handling for a police pursuit cannot be reproduced faithfully.

Visually, the simulator utilizes a 250-degree field of view and fully textured graphics, which help images appear much more realistic and give much better sight distances. The IDS has interchangeable cabs, and vehicle modeling also can be accomplished with an engineering level of detail.

The highly reconfigurable architecture allows IDS researchers to jump between an A model car, a Ford Taurus, a HMMWV (high-mobility multipurpose wheeled vehicle), and an M1A1 tank, so different components of different vehicles can be held with that engineering level of fidelity. Researchers know that they are getting the engineering response that they should. That helps to increase the validity of measure for drivers once they are put into that environment.

There are also high-fidelity roadway models and very realistic traffic models, which help with Department of Transportation work. On-line data collection and reduction are done, and they are probably the most important elements of using simulation. The work that is done with DARPA (Defense Advanced Research Projects Agency) primarily has dealt with vehicle design and prototyping, but when a human is placed in the system, he or she must be put into a simulator. A lot of that other work can be done in a workstation on a desk without ever putting the driver in the loop. It is when the driver is put in the loop that data collection becomes important and also where high-fidelity simulation becomes important because a lower-fidelity environment cannot be immersive for certain drivers, especially experienced ones. Thus, the drivers might accept it for the first few minutes, but after those few minutes have elapsed, they no longer believe the simulation is real.

In fact, there is a lower-fidelity environment where, if the experiment goes on for very long, people start looking around at the ceiling and other things in the room. Therefore, a high-fidelity environment is necessary for data collection.

From a vehicle dynamic standpoint, the simulator utilizes multibody dynamics in real time. The power train, tires, steering, braking, and aerodynamics are simulated with multiple points so that the individual components of the vehicle, as well as the general driver performance, can be tested. All of the vehicle dynamics are at an engineering level of fidelity and take into account all the driving surface properties and elevation. For power train modeling, engine torque and speed, throttle relations, the transmission gearing, and slip are taken into account, as well as differentials and gearing. From the engineering standpoint, modeling those aspects helps with the vehicle design.

The motion system moves as the driver moves throughout the environment so that if a person makes a left-hand turn, the simulator provides the adequate cues for that situation. There are accelerometers and rate gyros hooked to the simulator. Part of the DARPA exercise for 1995 consisted of examining the responses of that motion base in particular sorts of maneuvers. In the simulator, sophisticated motion washout algorithms exist to get the motion back into a central position, so it is ready to perform the next cue.

For all visual database construction, American Association of State Highway and Transportation Officials (AASHTO) standards are utilized, which are the civil engineering standards for roadway design. Correlated terrain generation also can be done, and that is what has been done on the Churchville and Munson test courses at Aberdeen Proving Ground. Parts of these courses have been modeled with 3-in resolution. Less rough areas were modeled based on data that were gathered with profilometer.

As part of the redesign of the instrument cabs, the engine is replaced with electrical components. A Ford Taurus, a GM Saturn, and a HMMWV cab are available. A software reconfigurable cab exists for the tank simulation, which is simply a mock-up of the inside of a tank. There are several other vehicles that are not instrumented at this time, but all of the controls work, as mentioned above.

The researchers actually go out and gather audio data, which is then fed through a Musical Instrument Digital Interface (MIDI) system so that an attempt can be made to correlate it to the different engine RPMs to ensure that the audio cues are adequate. One of the things being studied right now is exaggerating the audio cues, because in the simulated environment, the sound is not 100 percent correct nor can it be. But people cannot judge their speed, and it is hoped that by exaggerating the audio cue, people might be helped to judge their speed a little bit more accurately.

The University of Iowa will host the NADS in 1999, which is sponsored by the National Highway Traffic Safety Administration. It will be much more powerful than the current IDS but will compete with the top simulator in the world, which is the Daimler-Benz driving simulator in Germany.

As of 1996, 41 studies are funded. Most funding comes from the Department of Transportation, although there is some Department of Defense (DoD) funding, and DARPA has been one of the major funding sources. Work has dealt with automated highway systems (Bloomfield et al., 1995a, b, 1996a, b) and vehicle collision warning and countermeasure devices (Hankey et al., 1996), such as "drowsy driver" countermeasures. In addition, certification of implants for intraocular lenses, examination of cognitive impairment such as Alzheimer's disease and age-related dementia (Rizzo et al., 1994a, b), and vehicle virtual prototyping (Grant and Watson, 1997) are being done.

A set of exercises was carried out last year in conjunction with the DoD project. DARPA funds two types of work at the IDS installation. One consists of pure computer-aided engineering and is performed entirely at workstations. All of the kinematically correct models are transferred to the simulation for that particular vehicle, and that is where the other part of that funding is directed.

The Aberdeen Proving Ground demonstration has been completed; the concurrent engineering is the workstation aspect of that demonstration. The Center for Computer-Aided Design is on a DIS (Distributed Interactive Simulation) network, one of the only academic nodes or sites on the network, so interactive simulation exercises can be done.

The purpose of both the 1994 and 1995 exercises is to examine vehicle virtual prototyping. The aim is to be able to establish an operator-in-the-loop design of a vehicle and redesign of the vehicle so that it is accomplished in the simulated environment prior to being mocked up. Feedback can be obtained from the driver that may be pertinent to the actual design of the vehicle to reduce the time required in the design process and to lower associated costs.

Last summer, drivers were placed on both the Munson and Churchville courses at the Aberdeen site and then brought to the simulator in Iowa City. There they drove a number of times around the simulator with a certain prescribed behavior in an effort to gather validation data from both the vehicle and the driver performance standpoint because driver performance measures were being examined extensively. An HMMWV was used to gather considerable data. It is much easier to analyze data collected in a simulated environment than those from a test course. Some of the last test course data are still being analyzed because the analysis is time-consuming due to the presence of noise in the data.

Considering the performance measures used (e.g., the velocity in miles per hour at every part of the course), it is necessary to know how challenging the course is to really understand the match of the data (how well behavior in the simulator resembles that in a real-life driving situation). The course in question has a hill with a 29 percent grade, blind turns that require the driver to "turn on a dime," and also other downhill grades; the rough part of the course has 24-in-high bumps to go over, which is difficult.

The velocity match is also very similar. People tend to overdrive a little bit in the simulator, accelerating on a few of the straight areas and maintaining high velocity in some of the areas. There is also a tendency to oversteer a bit, which could result from the lack of a motion cue; this is being examined again in the 1995 follow-up to the HMMWV study. Other parameters being measured include use of the accelerator pedal and the brake. With the accelerator pedal, there definitely is some mismatch. While a trend appears to develop in some of the areas, it is off in others. A followup study was done in October 1995 with nine HMMWV drivers.

Subjective data, workload data, and physiological data were collected from all drivers, and similar sorts of matches were obtained for all of those. A perceived realism rating also was collected in the simulator only, with a reliability of about 0.92, which is very good. Thus, an expert set of drivers, who are much harder to fool, were finding the simulator experience to be very realistic.

The IDS, as mentioned above, is DIS-compliant. This allows for the performance of interactive exercises for additional measurement sorts of settings. It allows interaction with other simulators at other installations, where synthetic battlefield exercises can be assembled or responses of the vehicles or the drivers can be examined.

The work to date has been performed primarily for realistic mobility testing and for the iterative vehicle design process[2] in which operators are included in the loop (design and testing).

---

[2] Iterative processes are those that replicate a series of operations for the purpose of successively approximating a desired result.

The IDS and the Research Community

Some of the challenges of using virtual reality for this sort of measurement include resource issues, such as billing the research community, looking at simulator effects or simulator sickness, and validation of virtual reality—in particular this driving simulator—as a measurement tool.

As part of a university, the IDS staff's first mission is to do research for the university and the Center for Computer-Aided Design at the University of Iowa. The expectation is that the IDS will be a precursor to the NADS, which is being built in Iowa City. The NADS is expected to be operational in 1999 and is funded by the National Highway Traffic Safety Administration for use by researchers throughout the nation.

With respect to educating the research community, it is not known exactly what parameters must be measured to study driving performance. Driving assessment primarily has been qualitative. It is now possible to get very precise data in the simulator; thus, attempts are being made to understand how the quantification of those data relates to the qualitative criteria that customarily are used to evaluate performance.

Also, attempts are being made to teach the research community how to use simulator technology efficiently and effectively. This technology is expensive, at least in the high-fidelity market, so not a minute is wasted on the simulator. Subjects are shuttled, and there cannot be one 30-sec down time, as a result. Experiments are run 12 hours a day. The other 12 hours of the day are used for development.

Also, attempts are being made to educate the research community on the fidelity requirements. High fidelity is not always necessary, and it is possible to use virtual reality environments that are lower in fidelity and still get very valid performance measures. However, it is necessary to understand what fidelity is required (Alessi and Watson, 1994).

Motion Sickness

The potential for motion sickness in simulator subjects is under investigation. Although it was assumed that much of the motion sickness literature from flight simulation would be applicable, that research has not been completely applicable to experiments done with driving instead of flight. The driver population is a much more generalized population than pilots, and the potential for motion sickness is therefore higher (Watson, 1995).

There is a real need for evidence regarding the validity of the simulator experience with respect to real driving, and this must be emphasized to the research community. The simulator has a very novel effect for people who have not used it before. Attempts have been made to look at experimental designs to get past that novel effect because it is necessary to know that the performance obtained is indeed real performance and that it transfers to the real world. The challenges with simulator effects are to identify those susceptible groups and the simulation in order to take care of some of those parameters. It has been possible to tune out sickness fairly well in the IDS; although there is an attrition rate of about 2 percent, up to about 8 percent of the simulator subjects report at least some symptoms.

An attempt has been made by simulator researchers to design scenes and scenarios that try to reduce the simulator effects. Sickness is always analyzed and considered as a covariant in all experiments to ensure that it is not creating performance differences.

Validation

The research community has expressed an interest in using the IDS but asks whether it is validated. Validation is an ongoing process. There is a real need to gather information for every set of tests that is run. Different validity evidence must be given to different types of tests because something that would be used for the DARPA experiments could be very different from something that might be used for the automated highways experiments. Those variables always must be examined.

Gathering on-the-road data is also a continual process, and it is time-consuming and expensive. In fact, in several studies, it has challenged the simulator rate because it is so expensive. Seven people must be out on the road in order to gather data. If it rains, the work cannot be done.

To date, a number of validation studies have been completed in addition to the DARPA study (Grant and Watson, 1997). A comparison of different age and gender groups has been done in the simulator, looking at trends from past research only (the subjects were not taken out on the road) (Romano and Watson, 1994). A recognition and detection distance of signs also has been done, taking subjects out on the road in twilight night and glare conditions and putting them in the simulator to ensure that the recognition and detection distance of signs or the supply of sign information on the simulator is a match to that in the real world.

Validation is a very important issue, and it is hoped that the appropriate validation data can be gathered with the IDS. Many other devices exist, many less expensive, and they may have real potential. However, with regard to the virtual reality environment, it is necessary to gather the validity evidence to test whether the performance measures transfer to real-world performance regardless of the simulator fidelity.

It also is necessary to test whether the perceived realism is high enough so that subjects feel they are immersed in an environment, subjects react in a similar way, and they accept that environment over a long period of time or during a number of experiments. Confounding factors such as motion sickness must be controllable, and it must be possible to take this technology to a platform[3] on which it is very cost effective, where high-fidelity simulation can be obtained for a fraction of the cost.

REFERENCES

Alessi, S.M., and G.S. Watson
  1994 Driving Simulation Research at The University of Iowa. Proceedings of the 1994 Annual Meeting of the Association for the Development of Computer-Based Instructional Systems. 16–20 February 1994, Nashville, Tenn.

Bloomfield, J.R., and S.A. Carroll
  1996 New measures of driving performance. Pp. 335–340 in Contemporary Ergonomics, S.A. Robertson, ed. London: Taylor and Francis.

Bloomfield, J.R., J.R. Buck, S.A. Carroll, M.W. Booth, R.A. Romano, D.V. McGehee, and R.A. North
  1995a Human factors aspects of the transfer of control from the automated highway system to the driver. Technical Report No. FHWA-RD-94-114. Washington, D.C.: U.S. Department of Transportation, Federal Highway Administration.

Bloomfield, J.R., J.R. Buck, J.M. Christensen, and A. Yenamandra
  1995b Human factors aspects of the transfer of control from the driver to the automated highway system. Technical Report No. FHWA-RD-94-173. Washington, D.C.: U.S. Department of Transportation, Federal Highway Administration.

Bloomfield, J.R., J.M. Christensen, S.A. Carroll, and G.S. Watson
  1996a The driver's response to decreasing vehicle separations during transitions into the automated lane. Technical Report No. FHWA-RD-95-107. Washington, D.C.: U.S. Department of Transportation, Federal Highway Administration.

Bloomfield, J.R., J.M. Christensen, A.D. Peterson, J.M. Kjaer, and A. Gault
  1996b Transferring control from the driver to the automated highway system with varying degrees of automation. Technical Report No. FHWA-RD-95-108. Washington, D.C.: U.S. Department of Transportation, Federal Highway Administration.

Cremer, J., Y.E. Papelis, J. Kearney, and R.A. Romano
  1994 The software architecture for scenario control in the Iowa Driving Simulator. Pp. 373–381 in Proceedings of the 4th Annual Computer-Generated Forces and Behavioral Representation Conference. Orlando, Fla.: Institute for Simulation and Training.

Cremer, J., J. Kearney, and Y. Papelis
  1995 HCSM: A framework for behavior and scenario control in virtual environments. ACM Trans. Modeling Comp. Simul. 5(3):242–267.

Cremer, J., J. Kearney, and Y.E. Papelis
  1996 Driving simulation: Challenges for VR technology. IEEE Comp. Graphics Appl. 16(5):16–20.

Freeman, J.S., G.S. Watson, Y.E. Papelis, A. Tayyab, R.A. Romano, and J.G. Kuhl
  1995 The Iowa Driving Simulator: An implementation and application overview. Pp. 81–90 in Proceedings of the Society for Automotive Engineers International Congress and Exposition. Detroit, Mich.: Society of Automotive Engineers.

---

[3] Platform is analogous to hardware. In the case of a device such as a simulator that is run by embedded software, the simulator is the platform.

Grant, P., and G.S. Watson
  1997   Validation of a HMMWV in the Iowa Driving Simulator. Unpublished manuscript. Iowa City: The University of Iowa.
Hankey, J.M., D.V. McGehee, T.A. Dingus, E.N. Mazzae, and W.R. Garrott
  1996   Initial driver avoidance behavior and reaction time to an unalerted intersection incursion. Pp. 896–899 in Proceedings of the 40th Annual Meeting of the Human Factors and Ergonomics Society. Santa Monica, Calif.: Human Factors and Ergonomics Society.
Kuhl, J.G., D. Evans, Y.E. Papelis, R.A. Romano, and G.S. Watson
  1995   The Iowa Driving Simulator: An immersive environment for driving-related research and development. IEEE Comput. 28(7):35–41.
Papelis, Y.E., and S. Bahauddin
  1995   Logical modeling of roadway environment to support real-time simulation of autonomous traffic. Pp. 62–71 in Proceedings of the 1st Workshop on Simulation and Interaction in Virtual Environments. Iowa City, Iowa: Department of Computer Science, University of Iowa.
Rizzo, M., G.S. Watson, D.V. McGehee, and T.A. Dingus
  1994a   Simulator driving and car crashes in aging and cognitively impaired drivers. J. Neurol. 241:526.
  1994b   Simulator driving and car crashes in Alzheimer's disease. Soc. Neurosci. Abstr. 20:439.
Romano, R.A., and G.S. Watson
  1994   Assessment of capabilities—Iowa Driving Simulator. Technical Report No. FHWA-IR-94. Washington, D.C.: U.S. Department of Transportation Federal Highway Administration.
Stoll, D., and S. Bourne
  1996   The National Advanced Driving Simulator: Potential applications to ITS and AHS research. Pp. 700–710 in Proceeding of the 6th Annual Meeting of the Intelligent Transportation Society. Washington D.C.: ITS America.
Watson, G.S.
  1995   Simulator effects in a high-fidelity driving simulator. Pp. 124–138 in Proceedings of the 1995 Driving Simulation Conference. Sophia-Antipolis, France: Neuf Associes.

DISCUSSION

JOHN VANDERVEEN: You mentioned the cost several times. What is the cost for this simulator, and what is it going to cost for the future device?

GINGER WATSON: This is part of the initial plans: It has to operate at no more than $1,000 an hour. We currently are operating loaded at the University of Iowa at $1,300, but that might drop every time computer technology gets less expensive. For instance, our previous image generator cost $1.5 million. We just bought a new one for a quarter of a million, and it has four times the capability. So every year we have to reassess those rates, and we will be doing that again in July.

BERNADETTE MARRIOTT: You mentioned physiological measures. What physiological measures do you take?

GINGER WATSON: We just took postrespiration blood pressure in that particular case. We can always correlate. We did not correlate for those experiments, and that is one of the reasons you do not see it. We did that only at the request of the PI on the project at that particular point in time. We are actually looking for some more robust measures to use and to correlate.

DAVID DINGES: That was a great presentation. I am very excited that you were candid about the validation issues and what you are doing with it. As you know probably better than anybody, this is another area where people have sold what they claim are simulators that are just utterly fraudulent. They are just nothing but a simple reaction time task.

What I wanted to ask you about was the fidelity of your crash. In NASA's aviation simulators, a crash is a serious event, and everybody works hard to avoid that. It is taken deadly seriously. What is the fidelity of the crash like in this?

GINGER WATSON: Well, we actually do not go through the full-motion simulation because we typically run people up to 85 years old. All Department of Transportation studies require that we run older populations, so we simulate only the visual aspects up to a certain point in the crash. We do not go through the full impact. But we could not do the full impact anyway with our motion base, to be very honest.

DAVID DINGES: To the extent that a crash is possible, and certain groups in the population have a tendency to drive more risky, will they take a crash event on the simulator as seriously as a real crash?

GINGER WATSON: Our sense is that they do take it very seriously in the higher-fidelity simulator, but we run a lot of studies on our lower-fidelity simulator, especially pilot work. I have to tell you, with certain populations they do not take it seriously in the less immersive environment.

Now, my question is, if you exposed somebody to the high-fidelity environment for a long period of time, would they still be as serious about it? We have actually had people cry or scream—very violent reactions.

DAVID DINGES: Finally, may I ask you statistically what is the reaction of risk-taking driving groups, such as males in their 20s. I mean, how do they behave on it?

GINGER WATSON: We have had a few that we have thrown out of studies, very few, though. We have run about 1,500 subjects now. I think we have thrown out two, and they were in the automated highways experiments.

It is a valid point because they were saying, "Oh, this is great, oh, yes." We said, "Stop; this is costing us $1,300 an hour, and you're out."

(Laughter)

PARTICIPANT: What are your instructions to the subjects?

GINGER WATSON: We tell them to drive as realistically as possible, and we try to set up a very serious situation. One of the things that we do tell them is it is very expensive to run the study. We will not pay them the full amount if we do not get the full performance from them.

Really, the only group we have ever had problems with, to tell you the truth, is young, college-age males. They are computer literate to begin with, have been in some other virtual reality environments, and do not take it quite as seriously.

DAVID DINGES: That is right; they do not take real driving seriously, either.

(Laughter)

GINGER WATSON: Yes, perhaps there is a correlation. I do not know.

PARTICIPANT: You could emphasize speed, or you could emphasize performance and you could emphasize safety, in going through the course. What is the message to the subject?

GINGER WATSON: We usually emphasize safety in subject preparation before we take them in. Then when we get them in the simulator, we always remind them what the speed limit is on a given roadway, and if it is a long drive, we will frequently remind them somewhere in the middle. We usually do not have to, though, but we do include that in the protocol quite frequently.

It has worked so far and, again, a lot of it is just anecdotal, but when we go back and review tapes, we think that people are really driving as they would. And we ask people, too—we have looked at a cross-correlation on this—what speed they normally drive on an interstate and what speed they would normally drive on a rural road. We have found some pretty decent correlations with that.

PARTICIPANT: Is your test population just from Iowa?

GINGER WATSON: No. In fact, in the DARPA experiments our test population is from Maryland. We flew those people out, but that is expensive. We are also doing a study for a company that is seeking Food and Drug Administration approval for an intraocular lens and, because of that, they have a sample population throughout the United States that will be flying in from everywhere. That is an expensive consideration. They can afford to do that; I do not know if that is cost effective for all studies.

DAVID SCHNAKENBERG: What are examples of the type of experimental variables they are trying to look at in your simulator?

GINGER WATSON: Oh, they vary. Actually, I have given a half-day presentation talking about performance variables. If it is automated highway experiments, you are looking at reaction time . . .

DAVID SCHNAKENBERG: No, what are the factors they are looking at? Is it independent variables between the driver, is it the age, is it the gender?

GINGER WATSON: That is just as complex as the dependent variables. Just to give you an idea, usually it is age; looking at different sorts of driving scenes, especially in the DARPA situation, what are the different tests that are required, and is this something that is uphill or over a rough course?

In the automated highway experiments we look at things like entry into the automated lane, is it automated, is it manual, is it partially automated (Bloomfield et al., 1996a, b)? What happens in the case of a failure, and also, we look at exit from the systems, breaking it up into those pieces, but they are looking at things like age and automation. It really varies by experiment. Every single experiment that we do has different independent and dependent variables, which really adds to our validation complexity.

JOHANNA DWYER: Have you done any experiments where you have fasted, thirsted, or sleep-deprived people or a combination thereof?

GINGER WATSON: There is a graduate student who has done a sleep-deprivation study in our low-fidelity simulator, but that is it. We have had people approach us to do that sort of work, but we have not, because, to be very honest, this is where that fidelity issue comes in for certain sorts of experiments, especially when there is a secondary task or something, you might be able to do much more cost effectively on a lower-fidelity device.

Emerging Technologies for Nutrition Research, 1997
Pp. 569–576. Washington, D.C.
National Academy Press

VIII

Discussion

DAVID DINGES: I would like to make one comment about what we have called today cognitive variables and neurobehavioral variables and alertness. From the standpoint of output, these are very far downstream. When something is wrong with them, we cannot always work backwards and figure out what caused that, which is why experiments where we use these neurobehavioral variables usually need to be structured to test a countermeasure or something. In other words, it is very hard to use these downstream variables in some logic path to figure out what part of the brain or what nutrient or what circadian phase caused the problem, and inevitably it is only correlational.

But they are, nevertheless, powerful variables from the ecological validity standpoint, and they are the functional outcomes that most people want to know about. We talked about apnea in truck drivers, and there is a huge media piece on it. I told a reporter that the public really does not care if a truck driver has hemorrhoids; they only care if hemorrhoids affect driving.

In very much the same way, in many applied scenarios, while we may care medically, what matters is that final output, that final piece, but it is hard to track back without doing assessments and careful countermeasures.

DOUGLAS WILMORE: I have sort of a broad generic question for the group of people who talked about behavioral things. It would seem to me that it would be worthwhile trying to think about how you could build a monitoring system into the actual task that the person was doing. I think Mary tipped me to this idea. If you had a computer operator, you could build the ability to shift or to spell wrong or even time variables into that particular task. And Harris, if you are looking at these guys shoving shells into that big gun that you had, it would seem to me that you could time throughout the day the speed with which they were loading the big gun or something like that.

I was wondering if that is not the evolution of all of this, that instead of asking people to stop what they are doing and do their cognitive function testing, to somehow build a monitoring system into their specific task. It may even get to the place where that foot device that looked at how many steps people take could even be programmed to do that, because you slow down and you get sore feet, and all that sort of thing.

HARRIS LIEBERMAN: Some of those things have actually been implemented, in part. Certain occupations that require the use of a computer to do a job are monitored by the supervisor or a higher level to measure individuals' efficiency on a day-to-day basis, and they are given feedback or they can even be fired if their performance does not meet the specs. What they will do is they will look at the average specs of a telephone operator because that is all automated right now, and if somebody is falling off the bottom of the distribution, that person is in significant trouble. There are some ethical questions there, certainly, but that can be done legally right now.

In terms of actually what you are asking, what is their final output, are they firing more shells? It turns out that in that particular example it is extremely difficult to get enough information to relate it back to any measure of performance, because there is so much variability in the individual unit. Some batteries are just better than other batteries, so when you try to get the individual performance data, it all gets confounded with whatever treatment you have got out there. Now, in a situation where, say, there were environmental variations over the course of a long period of time, it might be possible to relate that to some kinds of performance in a correlative kind of way and that would be valuable. That is a good idea.

MARY MAYS: Another really good example that is relatively easy to track is the motion of your eyes, where they are going and what they are looking at and so forth. We are doing some pretty nice studies of tracking the eye in doing tasks, exactly what Harris Lieberman so graphically described. Your head begins to drop, so your eyes compensate by looking up, and then the next thing you know your eyes are just rolling back in your head. One of the classic tests for drunkenness is not being able to control those saccadic movements and so forth, that are real common with sleepiness.

That is my point about behavior sampling. If we could just use our brains and we were sharp about this and smart, we ought to be able to sample the behavior that is ongoing as a part of the whole military performance. Again, sometimes that is instrumenting and eye-tracking devices, and sometimes that is just taking at face value how many shells they loaded per hour, and so forth. I think we have to move to that. We have to be ingenious about it. I also really agree with something else David Dinges said, and that is, some of the biggest charlatans are the ones who claim that they can monitor your ongoing behavior and make a sophisticated judgment about finger movements or head nods in a car and that it all means something. They can tell you exactly what it means, and they can even tell you exactly which No-Doz you need and how much you ought to take. Just based on that, we need to be very, very careful that our behavior sampling is meaningful, valid, and reliable, and that we test it out before we just take it at face value.

What I kind of disagree with is something that each of us, including me, said, that it is all that hard to determine what we should be measuring and that it is all that complex and that we really cannot do it that well. I think we are doing every bit as good a job as some of the other people are who measure interleukin (IL)-2s and IL-8s and IL-10s. I am not pointing my finger at my friends, necessarily, but we are doing as good as some other people are, but we are the first ones to always criticize ourselves. We are the first ones to point and say we do not do it well, we do not really know what it is.

JOHN VANDERVEEN: I was wondering about something. They are getting very, very light cameras now that can record for long hours. Is it possible to mount those on the individual, and see what he sees all day long and learn anything from that type of thing?

MARY MAYS: Yes and no. They can play football with cameras on their heads. The problem is, having been a graduate student in a laboratory where my major professor wanted us to do that, sitting in front of a videotape, analyzing frame by frame what went on for hours and hours and trying to reduce the data, turning them into something that you can use is tough and filled with subjectivity.

JOHN VANDERVEEN: But they are even doing computerized analysis of these types of things now.

GINGER WATSON: We actually took a year and a half to cross-validate one of our studies where we had gathered camera data out on the road. I know it was very, very time consuming, and we were always having to make qualitative judgments.

I would also like to mention that even in the case of eye-tracking, which is fairly automated, it is still not a very precise science right now. We use eye-tracking in driving to see where the person is looking, and we still are forced to go back in many, many cases to make qualitative assessments.

DAVID DINGES: We are making neurobehavioral assessments. No matter what you do, I submit that the brain is the fundamental organ of operation. Because we can technologically monitor the environment or the face of the individual or the heart rate or anything else does not mean we know what is going on.

In response to your question, we actually tried this at NASA with the pilots. We got all the pilots and all the engineers and asked whether we could find one thing that occurs in the cockpit that is an operationally relevant measure that everybody agrees on. There were zero. We tried it not one time, but three times. There is nothing that occurs in the cockpit that everybody agrees is an operationally relevant measure. So there is another way to ask the question, which is the way I ask it: Tell me the worst thing that could happen in this job. A meltdown of a reactor? Grounding a vessel on a shoal? Tell me the absolute worst thing. Now, tell me the people who would be involved in that. Now I can measure something that tells you what their capability is at any given time, and that is as close as I can come to predicting the likelihood, the probability, that they may make a fatal mistake.

JOHN VANDERVEEN: I want to ask David Dinges two questions. You said the person who could sleep anytime was in trouble, perhaps, but I want to know about the person who can sleep anywhere. I have watched crew members sleep in an airplane. When it is time for them to take their rest, they get up in the bunk and go to sleep. Is there a problem if they can just automatically go to sleep?

DAVID DINGES: No, no, I really overstated the case. Regarding that kind of prophylactic napping, we just finished a study on sleep in the cockpit bunk as opposed to the chair. Obviously, it is very adaptive. One of the nice things about having young people in the military is that they are at an age where they can turn that homeostatic drive on and allow themselves to sleep pretty quickly.

Most of us are far enough along in years that it is a lot harder to just turn that on and off; we are regulated by the clock much more. It is when you are literally falling asleep everywhere and you misattribute that to your ability that you are in trouble.

JOHANNA DWYER: I was very much taken by the self-monitoring quality that might be possible in some of these devices, both the ones we have talked about this afternoon and others, and also very much taken with the notion of prophylactic naps. In trying to put this all together into things like tanks, where there is noise and heat, people are hungry, they cannot eat, or they get six Meals, Ready-to-Eat and they are all chicken a la king for years and years, the problem is how virtual does the virtual reality of a situation like that have to be to get data that are really meaningful to the people who are supposed to be helping the enlisted people?

MARY MAYS: I am not sure I understood your question.

JOHANNA DWYER: There are multiple variables here that all have to be considered. I was taken by a comment on our last report, *Not Eating Enough*,[1] from someone who was in Vietnam for several years. He mentioned that all these things were great, but that all the factors we talked about really did not include fear and a whole bunch of other things.

MARY MAYS: At the Human Engineering Laboratory at Aberdeen Proving Ground they have a tank simulator very much like the one Ginger Watson has talked about—I think you must have worked with these people—and they do exactly that. They do not just make it move in 6 degrees of freedom, but they make it very hot, they make it very dry, they make it incredibly noisy.

I think all of us are trying to build a high-fidelity simulation. The Rangers were the perfect example. You had fear, real live fear, you had lots of performance anxiety about what was the worst thing that can happen. I can be thrown out of here, I can be humiliated, and I can die. All of those things were readily apparent every day.

Some of my data that I have not talked about very much are that their motivation levels, instead of increasing over time, went down. The more successful they were in Ranger training, the less they cared about being in Ranger training.

DAVID SCHNAKENBERG: I have sat in a lot of different meetings over the last few years where people were talking about future simulated battlefields. We are talking here about senior leaders scattered across the country doing their war games but they are doing it at a level of intensity that is very high. I've tried to talk to these folks to tell them that at some point they need to be working on a test bed to see what difference it makes if the leader is tired and sleepy versus well rested?

---

[1] Institute of Medicine. 1995. Not Eating Enough, Overcoming Underconsumption of Military Operational Rations, B.M. Marriott, ed. A report of the Committee on Military Nutrition Research, Food and Nutrition Board. Washington, D.C.: National Academy Press.

MARY MAYS: We spend a huge amount of money in the Army studying the 18 and 19 year olds. We just do not spend much time, even in our physiological studies, with our subjects (the lieutenant colonels, battalion commanders) who are 40 to 45 years of age. They are not young any more, and I do not care how good a shape they are in or what great leaders they are. They are not going to deal with all these conditions.

EDWARD HIRSCH: The Marines are much smarter.

(Laughter)

With regard to continuous operations, they have a defined policy where after X number of hours there are designated people to take over the company, to take over the command and control after X number of hours of sleep deprivation.

MARY MAYS: We had that same policy and we had lectures on it and we had signs posted on it and the first guy to violate it was the battalion commander. We had a whole daytime Tactical Operations Center (TOC) crew and a whole nighttime TOC crew. This was not an exercise. This was real live combat, and we were ready to go. But the minute that things got really exciting, the daytime TOC crew started trying to run the nighttime TOC crew because they did not trust these guys, because all during the preliminaries it was the daytime TOC crew that were the actual commanders and echelon staff.

You can have those policies, but as soon as the going gets rough, everybody wants to stay up 20 hours out of the day, and they do not go to sleep until they fall asleep.

DAVID DINGES: There was a study done at Dr. Wilmore's institution, the Brigham and Women's, that Drs. Czeisler and Richardson[2] did, where they protected the time. They had two groups of residents and they protected the time for sleep of one group but not the other. The obvious hypothesis is that the protected time guys are going to get more sleep. It was the opposite. They did not sleep when they could, because they said, "Well, I'll get my chance in protected." When they got to that point, they worked and did other things, and the net result was they actually got less sleep, which illustrates this point, the whole issue of what happens when you take a countermeasure into the field.

That is the second level of research you have got to do. You have to then check to see how people actually use it, whether it is a nutritional countermeasure or a nutritional one plus sleep. I mean, all of these energy recovery systems have got to be looked at in terms of how they were actually applied.

---

[2] Wolf, M.A., G. Richardson, and C.A. Czeisler. 1990. Improved sleep: A means of reducing the stress of internship. Trans. Am. Clin. Climatol. Assoc. 102:225–229.

GINGER WATSON: I was going to say something along that line. Virtual reality in different systems is certainly nice, but good research is good research regardless of where it is done, when you go into the lab or when you go into the virtual reality environment. You have to try to set up everything as concretely as you can to do good research, but you also have to know when to drop that sort of research and go out into the field, because it takes both.

There are people in simulation who would kill me right now, but all of the simulation and virtual reality in the world cannot replace some of that information that you gather out in the field. It has to be both.

DOUGLAS WILMORE: But you have to have buy-in, and here you have to have buy-in by commanders. You have to be court-martialed or you have to lose your pay or something like that. You have to have buy-in at an upper level if you are going to do these sorts of things.

ROBERT NESHEIM: That is the difficulty. You can have all kinds of training in that regard and all kinds of standards that are set up for it, but unless the person really buys into it and really agrees to it, and then does it when the time comes . . .

DOUGLAS WILMORE: And sets the example.

ROBERT NESHEIM: And sets the example, you do not have the control that you might like otherwise.

I think we have had a great 2 days. We have had exposure to some very interesting concepts and potential technologies, that were very thought provoking, that will generate a lot of thinking that we have to do, everybody that is here has to do, in terms of what the potential application is of these for the types of research that USARIEM and other people in the military might do and what kind of payoff we might expect from some of these and where the military should focus its effort in the near term, and maybe long term, thinking about maybe some of the things that ought to be done within the military and those things which ought to be monitored by the military but done outside by others who can bring the data better to fruition, whether it be to USARIEM or other places.

I think these are going to be some very thought-provoking times, and we as a committee have our challenge to sort through this and to come up with some way that we are going to summarize and present this in a way that will be useful to James Vogel and to the Surgeon General and to other people who will be looking at this report.

I also anticipate that the summary of all the wonderful papers that were presented here, which we are expecting all the speakers to provide in a timely manner, is going to be a report that will be in high demand, because it has brought together so many ideas, so many innovative approaches, in one place. You rarely find that much in a report like this, so I think it is going to be something that is going to be highly visible and, again, puts more of a challenge on us as a committee and staff to try to be very, very careful and innovative in how we respond to that.

The committee will be meeting tomorrow morning to start the process of figuring out how we are going to do this. I would like to thank all of the speakers and all the participants for their involvement in this. Unfortunately, a lot of our speakers have had to leave. I think this has been one of the most stimulating couple of days that I have sat through. I certainly learned a lot of vocabulary I did not know anything about 45 years ago.

Some of the concepts that are expressed here are very, very new, even in all the readings that I have been doing over recent years. So I want to thank everybody for their commitment, for their time in this.

APPENDIXES

Emerging Technologies for Nutrition Research, 1997
Pp. 579–584. Washington, D.C.
National Academy Press

A

Workshop Agenda

**EMERGING TECHNOLOGIES FOR NUTRITION RESEARCH:
POTENTIAL FOR ASSESSING MILITARY
PERFORMANCE CAPABILITY**

A Workshop Sponsored by

Committee on Military Nutrition Research

Washington, D.C

Monday, May 22, 1995

I   WELCOMES AND INTRODUCTION TO THE TOPIC

8:00 a.m.–8:15 a.m.   Welcome and Introductions
Robert O. Nesheim
Chair, Committee on Military Nutrition Research

8:15 a.m.–8:30 a.m.   Welcome on Behalf of the U.S. Army Medical
                         Research and Materiel Command
                            COL Robert Gifford
                            USAMRMC, Fort Detrick, Maryland

8:30 a.m.–8:50 a.m.   Emerging Technologies in Nutrition Research for the
                         Military: Overview of the Issues
                            James A. Vogel
                            USARIEM, Natick, Massachusetts

(There will be 5 minutes for discussion available after each presentation.)

II   BODY COMPOSITION

8:50 a.m.–9:20 a.m.   Military Application of Body Composition Assessment
                         Technologies
                            MAJ Karl E. Friedl
                            USAMRMC, Fort Detrick, Maryland

9:20 a.m.–9:50 a.m.   Imaging Techniques of Body Composition: Advantages
                         of Measurement and New Uses
                            Steven B. Heymsfield
                            St. Luke's-Roosevelt Hospital Center, New York

9:50 a.m.–10:20 a.m.   DXA: Research Issues and Equipment
                            Wendy M. Kohrt
                            Washington University School of Medicine,
                            St. Louis, Missouri

10:20 a.m.–10:35 a.m.   Coffee Break

10:35 a.m.–11:05 a.m.   Bioelectrical Impedance: A History, Research Issues,
                         and Recent Consensus
                            Wm. Cameron Chumlea
                            Wright State University School of Medicine,
                            Yellow Springs, Ohio

11:05 a.m.–11:35 a.m.   General Discussion

III ADVANCED TRACER TECHNIQUES AND METABOLISM

11:35 p.m.–12:05 p.m.	Stable Isotope Techniques: The Broad Picture, What Can and Cannot Be Done *Dennis M. Bier* Children's Nutrition Research Center, Houston, Texas
12:05 p.m.–12:35 p.m.	Energy Substrate Metabolism with Stable Isotope Tracers *Robert R. Wolfe* Shriners Burns Institute and University of Texas Medical Branch, Galveston
12:35 p.m.–1:20 p.m.	No-Host Lunch
1:20 p.m.–1:50 p.m.	Combined Stable Isotope/Positron Emission Tomography for *In Vivo* Protein Metabolism Assessment *Vernon R. Young* Massachusetts Institute of Technology, Cambridge
1:50 p.m.–2:20 p.m.	Nuclear Magnetic Resonance Studies of Carbohydrate Metabolism in Humans *Gerald I. Shulman* Yale University School of Medicine, New Haven, Connecticut
2:20 p.m.–2:50 p.m.	Doubly Labeled Water for Energy Expenditure *James P. DeLany* Pennington Biomedical Research Center, Baton Rouge, Louisiana
2:50 p.m.–3:20 p.m.	General Discussion
3:20 p.m.–3:35 p.m.	Break

IV TECHNIQUES OF ENERGY EXPENDITURE AND RESPIRATORY EXCHANGE

3:35 p.m.–4:05 p.m.	Measurement of O_2 Uptake with Portable Equipment *John F. Patton, III* USARIEM, Natick, Massachusetts

4:05 p.m.–4:35 p.m.	Advances in Ambulatory Monitoring Technologies in the Military: Electronic Sensing *Reed W. Hoyt* USARIEM, Natick, Massachusetts
4:35 p.m.–5:05 p.m.	General Discussion
5:05 p.m.–5:15 p.m.	Concluding Remarks *Robert O. Nesheim*

Tuesday, May 23, 1995

8:00 a.m.–8:15 a.m.	Opening Remarks *Robert O. Nesheim*

(There will be 5 minutes for discussion available after each presentation.)

V   MOLECULAR AND CELLULAR APPROACHES IN NUTRITION

8:15 a.m.–8:45 a.m.	Role of Metals in Gene Expression *Robert J. Cousins* Center for Nutritional Sciences University of Florida, Gainesville
8:45 a.m.–9:15 a.m.	Metabolic Regulation of Gene Expression *Howard C. Towle* University of Minnesota, Minneapolis
9:15 a.m.–9:45 a.m.	Use of Isolated Cell and Metabolic Techniques Applied to Vitamin Transport and Disposition *Donald B. McCormick* Emory University School of Medicine, Atlanta, Georgia
9:45 a.m.–10:15 a.m.	Physiologic Stress: Cellular Approaches to Nutrition *Guy M. Miller* Galileo Laboratories, Inc., Sunnyvale, California, and The Johns Hopkins University, Baltimore, Maryland
10:15 a.m.–10:30 a.m.	Break

10:30 a.m.–11:00 a.m. Urine and Blood Cytokines
                       Lyle L. Moldawer
                       University of Florida College of Medicine,
                       Gainesville

11:00 a.m.–11:30 a.m. Functional Evaluation of the Immune System in
                       Humans
                       Gabriel Virella
                       Medical University of South Carolina, Charleston

11:30 a.m.–12:00 p.m. New Advances in the Study of Immune Functions:
                       Mucosal Immunity
                       COL Arthur O. Anderson
                       USAMRIID, Fort Detrick, Maryland

12:00 p.m.–12:30 p.m. General Discussion

12:30 p.m.–1:15 p.m.   No-Host Lunch

1:15 p.m.–1:45 p.m.   Non-Invasive and Other Techniques for Assessment of
                       Plasma Metabolites
                       Donald Bodenner
                       University of Rochester, New York

VI FUNCTIONAL AND BEHAVIORAL MEASURES OF NUTRITIONAL STATUS

1:45 p.m.–2:15 p.m.   Involuntary Muscle Contraction to Assess Nutritional
                       Status
                       James S. Hayes
                       Ross Products Division, Abbott Laboratories,
                       Cleveland, Ohio

2:15 p.m.–2:45 p.m.   Application of Cognitive Performance Assessment
                       Technology to Military Nutrition Research
                       Mary Z. Mays
                       Eagle Creek Research Services, San Antonio, Texas

2:45 p.m.–3:15 p.m.   New Techniques for Laboratory Measurement of
                       Alertness in Relation to Sleep and Circadian Rhythms
                       David F. Dinges
                       University of Pennsylvania, Philadelphia

3:15 p.m.–3:45 p.m.   New Techniques for Assessment of Mental
                          Performance in the Field
                          Harris R. Lieberman
                          USARIEM, Natick, Massachusetts

3:45 p.m.–4:15 p.m.   Measurement of Soldier-Driving Performance and
                          Emerging Simulator Technologies
                          Ginger S. Watson
                          Center for Computer-Aided Design, University of
                          Iowa, Iowa City

4:15 p.m.–5:15 p.m.   Final Discussion

5:15 p.m.–5:30 p.m.   Closing Remarks
                          Robert O. Nesheim

Emerging Technologies for Nutrition Research, 1997
Pp. 585–604. Washington, D.C.
National Academy Press

B

Biographical Sketches

COMMITTEE ON MILITARY NUTRITION RESEARCH

ROBERT O. NESHEIM (*Chair*) was Vice President of Research and Development and later Science and Technology for the Quaker Oats Company. He retired in 1983 and was Vice President of Science and Technology and President of the Advanced HealthCare Division of Avadyne, Inc. before his retirement in 1992. During World War II, he served as a Captain in the U.S. Army. Dr. Nesheim has served on the Food and Nutrition Board (FNB), chairing the Committee on Food Consumption Patterns and serving as a member of several other committees. He also was active in the Biosciences Information Service (as Board Chairman), American Medical Association, American Institute of Nutrition, Institute of Food Technologists, and Food Reviews International editorial board. Dr. Nesheim's academic services included Professor and Head of the Department of Animal Science at the University of Illinois, Urbana. He is a Fellow of the American Institute of Nutrition and American Association for the Advancement of Science and a member of several

585

professional organizations. Dr. Nesheim received a B.S. in agriculture, M.S. in animal science, and Ph.D. in nutrition and animal science from the University of Illinois.

WILLIAM R. BEISEL is Adjunct Professor in the Department of Molecular Microbiology and Immunology at The Johns Hopkins University School of Hygiene and Public Health. He held several positions at the U.S. Army Medical Research Institute of Infectious Diseases at Fort Detrick, Maryland, including in turn, Chief of the Physical Sciences Division, Scientific Advisor, and Deputy for Science. He then became Special Assistant for Biotechnology to the Surgeon General. After serving in the U.S. military during the Korean War, Dr. Beisel was the Chief of Medicine at the U.S. Army Hospital in Fort Leonard Wood, Missouri, before becoming the Chief of the Department of Metabolism at the Walter Reed Army Hospital. He was awarded a Commendation Ribbon, Bronze Star for the Korean War, Hoff Gold Medal at the Walter Reed Army Institute of Research, B. L. Cohen Award of the American Society for Microbiology, the Robert Herman Award from the American Association for Clinical Nutrition, and Department of Army Decoration for Exceptional Civilian Service. He was named a Diplomate of the American Board of Internal Medicine and a Fellow of the American College of Physicians. In addition to his many professional memberships, Dr. Beisel is a *Clinical Nutrition* contributing editor and *Journal of Nutritional Immunology* associate editor. He received his A.B. from Muhlenberg College in Allentown, Pennsylvania, and M.D. from the Indiana University School of Medicine.

GAIL E. BUTTERFIELD is Director of Nutrition Research, Palo Alto Veterans Affairs Health Care System in California. Concurrently, she is Lecturer in the Department of Medicine, Stanford University Medical School; Visiting Assistant Professor in the Program of Human Biology, Stanford University; and Director of Nutrition in the Program in Sports Medicine, Stanford University Medical School. Her previous academic appointments were at the University of California, Berkeley. Dr. Butterfield belongs to the American Institute of Nutrition, American Society for Clinical Nutrition, American Dietetic Association, and American Physiological Society. As a fellow of the American College of Sports Medicine, she serves as Chair of the Pronouncements Committee and is on the Board of Trustees; she also was President and Executive Director of the Southwest Chapter of that organization. She is a member of the Respiratory and Applied Physiology Study Section of the NIH and is on the editorial boards of the following journals: *Medicine and Science in Sports and Exercise, American Journal of Clinical Nutrition, Health and Fitness Journal of ACSM, Canadian Journal of Clinical Sports Medicine,* and *International Journal of Sports Nutrition.* Dr. Butterfield received her A.B. in biological sciences, M.A. in anatomy, and M.S. and Ph.D. in nutrition from the University of California, Berkeley. Her current research interests include nutrition in exercise, effect of growth factors on protein metabolism in the elderly, and metabolic fuel use in women exposed to high altitude.

WANDA L. CHENOWETH (*from September 18, 1996*) is Professor in the Department of Food Science and Human Nutrition at Michigan State University. Previously, she held positions as Teaching Associate at the University of Iowa and University of California, Berkeley. Other work experience includes positions as Research Dietitian and Head Clinical Dietitian at University of Iowa Hospitals and as Research Dietitian at Mayo Clinic. She is a member of the American Society for Nutritional Sciences, American Dietetic Association, and Institute of Food Technology. She serves as a reviewer for several journals, including *Journal of the American Dietetic Association, American Journal of Clinical Nutrition, Journal of Nutrition*, and is a member of the associate editorial board of *Plant Foods for Human Nutrition*. She has served on a technical review committee for the Diet, Nutrition, and Cancer Program of the National Cancer Institute and as a Site Evaluator, Commission on Evaluation of Dietetic Education of the American Dietetic Association. Her research interests are in the area of mineral bioavailability and clinical nutrition. Dr. Chenoweth completed a B.S. in dietetics from the University of Iowa, dietetic internship and M.S. in nutrition at the University of Iowa, and Ph.D. in nutrition at the University of California, Berkeley.

JOHN D. FERNSTROM is Professor of Psychiatry, Pharmacology, and Behavioral Neuroscience at the University of Pittsburgh School of Medicine and Director, Basic Neuroendocrinology Program at the Western Psychiatric Institute and Clinic. He received his S.B. in biology and his Ph.D. in nutritional biochemistry from the Massachusetts Institute of Technology (M.I.T.). He was a Postdoctoral Fellow in Neuroendocrinology at the Roche Institute for Molecular Biology in Nutley, New Jersey. Before coming to the University of Pittsburgh, Dr. Fernstrom was an Assistant and then Associate Professor in the Department of Nutrition and Food Science at M.I.T. He has served on numerous governmental advisory committees. He presently is a member of the National Advisory Council of the Monell Chemical Senses Center, Chair of the Neurosciences Section of the American Society for Nutritional Sciences (ASNS), and a member of the ASNS Council. He is a member of numerous professional societies, including the American Institute of Nutrition, American Society for Clinical Nutrition, American Physiological Society, American Society for Pharmacology and Experimental Therapeutics, American Society for Neurochemistry, Society for Neuroscience, and Endocrine Society. Among other awards, Dr. Fernstrom received the Mead-Johnson Award of the American Institute of Nutrition, a Research Scientist Award from the National Institute of Mental Health, a Wellcome Visiting Professorship in the Basic Medical

Sciences, and an Alfred P. Sloan Fellowship in Neurochemistry. His current major research interest concerns the influence of the diet and drugs on the synthesis of neurotransmitters in the central and peripheral nervous systems.

G. RICHARD JANSEN is Professor Emeritus in the Department of Food Science and Human Nutrition at Colorado State University, where he was Head of the department from 1969 to 1990. He was a Research Fellow at the Merck Institute for Therapeutic Research and Senior Research Biochemist in the Electrochemical Department at E. I. DuPont de Nemours. Prior to his stint in private industry, he served in the U.S. Air Force. Dr. Jansen is a past member of the U.S. Department of Agriculture (USDA) Human Nutrition Board of Scientific Counselors and the *Journal of Nutrition*, *Nutrition Reports International*, and *Plant Foods for Human Nutrition* editorial boards. His research interests deal with protein energy relationships during lactation and new foods for LDCs based on low-cost extrusion cooking. He received the Babcock-Hart Award of the Institute of Food Technologists and a Certificate of Merit from the USDA's Office of International Cooperation and Development for his work on low-cost extrusion cooking, and he is an IFT Fellow. He is a member of the American Institute of Nutrition, Institute of Food Technologists, and American Society for Biochemistry and Molecular Biology among others. Dr. Jansen holds a B.A. in chemistry and Ph.D. in biochemistry from Cornell University in Ithaca, New York.

ROBIN B. KANAREK is Professor of Psychology and of Nutrition at Tufts University in Medford, Massachusetts, where she also is the Chair of Psychology. Her prior experience includes Research Fellow, Division of Endocrinology, UCLA School of Medicine and Research Fellow in Nutrition at Harvard University. In addition to reviewing for several journals, including *Science, Brain Research Bulletin, Journal of Nutrition, American Journal of Clinical Nutrition*, and *Annals of Internal Medicine*, she is an editorial board member of *Physiology and Behavior* and the *Tufts Diet and Nutrition Newsletter* and is a past editor-in-chief of *Nutrition and Behavior*. Dr. Kanarek has served on ad hoc review committees for the National Science Foundation, NIH, and USDA Nutrition Research, as well as the Member Program Committee of the Eastern Psychological Association. She is a Fellow of the American College of Nutrition, and her other professional memberships include the American Institute of Nutrition, New York Academy of Sciences, Society for the Study of Ingestive Behavior, and Society for Neurosciences. Dr. Kanarek received a B.A. in biology from Antioch College in Yellow Springs, Ohio and M.S. and Ph.D. in psychology from Rutgers University in New Brunswick, New Jersey.

ORVILLE A. LEVANDER is Research Leader for USDA Nutrient Requirements and Functions Laboratory in Beltsville, Maryland. He was Research Chemist at the USDA's Human Nutrition Research Center, Resident Fellow in Biochemistry at Columbia University's College of Physicians and Surgeons, and Research Associate at Harvard University's School of Public Health. Dr. Levander served on the Food and Nutrition Board's Committee on the Dietary Allowances. He also served on panels of the National Research Council's Committee on Animal Nutrition and Committee on the Biological Effects of Environmental Pollutants. He was a member of the U.S. National Committee for the International Union of Nutrition Scientists and temporary advisor to the World Health Organization's Environmental Health Criteria Document on Selenium. Dr. Levander was awarded the Osborne and Mendel Award for the American Institute of Nutrition. His society memberships include the American Institute of Nutrition, American Chemical Society, and American Society for Clinical Nutrition. Dr. Levander received his B.A. from Cornell University and his M.S. and Ph.D. in biochemistry from the University of Wisconsin-Madison.

GILBERT A. LEVEILLE (*through December 31, 1996*) recently retired as Vice President for Research and Technical Services at the Nabisco Foods Group in East Hanover, New Jersey. His other industry experience was as the Director of Nutrition and Health Science for the General Foods Corporation. He was Chair and Professor of Food Science and Human Nutrition at Michigan State University, Professor of Nutritional Biochemistry at the University of Illinois-Urbana, and a Biochemist at the U.S. Army Medical Research and Nutrition Laboratory in Colorado. Dr. Leveille was a member of the Committee on International Nutrition, a joint Food and Nutrition Board-Board on International Health project. He won a research award from the Poultry Science Association, the Mead Johnson Research Award from the American Institute of Nutrition, the Distinguished Faculty Award from Michigan State University, and the Carl R. Fellers Award from the Institute of Food Technologists. He is a member of the American Association for the Advancement of Science, American Institute of Nutrition (Past President), American Society for Clinical Nutrition, American Chemical Society, Institute of Food Technologists (Past President), and Sigma Xi. Dr. Leveille received his B.V.A. from the University of Massachusetts and M.S. and Ph.D. in nutrition and biochemistry from Rutgers University, New Jersey.

JOHN E. VANDERVEEN is the Director of the Food and Drug Administration's (FDA) Office of Plant and Dairy Foods and Beverages in Washington, D.C. His previous position at the FDA was Director of the Division of Nutrition, at the Center for Food Safety and Applied Nutrition. He also served in various capacities at the U.S. Air Force (USAF) School of Aerospace Medicine at

Brooks Air Force Base, Texas. He has received accolades for service from the FDA and the USAF. Dr. Vanderveen is a member of the American Society for Clinical Nutrition, American Institute of Nutrition, Aerospace Medical Association, American Dairy Science Association, Institute of Food Technologists, and American Chemical Society. In the past, he was the Treasurer of the American Society of Clinical Nutrition and a member of the Institute of Food Technology, National Academy of Sciences Advisory Committee. Dr. Vanderveen holds a B.S. in agriculture from Rutgers University, New Jersey and a Ph.D. in chemistry from the University of New Hampshire.

DOUGLAS W. WILMORE, the Frank Sawyer Professor of Surgery at Harvard Medical School, is a Senior Staff Scientist and Surgeon at Brigham and Women's Hospital, Boston, Massachusetts. Concurrently, he is also a consultant for the Dana-Farber Cancer Center, Children's Hospital Medical Center, the BI-Deaconess Hospital, Wrentham State School, and Youville Hospital and Rehabilitation Center. Dr. Wilmore's main interests are related to metabolic and nutritional means to support critically ill patients and enhance recovery. His basic research has been applied to patients with thermal and accidental injury, patients with infectious complications, and those with multiple organ failure. He worked with the team that developed the current method of intravenous nutrition used for patients throughout the world. This technique has been improved in Dr. Wilmore's laboratory, and new amino acid solutions have been developed utilizing the amino acid glutamine, and anabolic factors such as growth hormone have been incorporated in this new feeding program with dramatic therapeutic results. Dr. Wilmore serves on the advisory board of the Tufts Pediatric Trauma Center, international editorial committee of the *Chinese Nutritional Sciences Journal* of the Chinese Academy of Medical Sciences, and editorial boards of *Annals of Surgery* and *Journal of the American College of Surgeons*. He is senior editor of *Scientific American Surgery*, the surgical text published by the American College of Surgeons that serves as the basis for care of general surgical patients. He also has published over 300 scientific papers and 4 books. Among his professional memberships, Dr. Wilmore includes the American College of Surgeons, American Surgical Association, American Medical Association, Society of University Surgeons, and American Society for Enteral and Parenteral Nutrition. He holds a B.A. and honorary Ph.D. from Washburn University of Topeka, M.D. from the University of Kansas School of Medicine in Kansas City, and honorary M.S. from Harvard University.

JOHANNA T. DWYER (*FNB Liaison*) is the Director of the Frances Stern Nutrition Center at New England Medical Center and Professor in the Departments of Medicine and of Community Health at the Tufts Medical School and School of Nutrition Science and Policy in Boston. She is also Senior Scientist at the Jean Mayer/USDA Human Nutrition Research Center on Aging at Tufts. Dr. Dwyer is the author or coauthor of more than 100 research articles and 185 review articles published in scientific journals. Her work centers on life-cycle related concerns such as the prevention of diet-related disease in children and adolescents and maximization of quality of life and health in the elderly. She also has a longstanding interest in vegetarian and other alternative lifestyles.

Dr. Dwyer is a past President of the American Institute of Nutrition, past Secretary of the American Society for Clinical Nutrition, and past President and current Fellow of the Society for Nutrition Education. She served on the Program Development Board of the American Public Health Association from 1989 to 1992 and is a member of the Food and Nutrition Board, the Technical Advisory Committee of the Nutrition Screening Initiative, and the Board of Directors of the American Institute of Wine and Food. As a Robert Wood Johnson Health Policy Fellow (1980–1981), she served on the personal staffs of Senator Richard Lugar (R-Indiana) and Senator Barbara Mikulski (D-Maryland).

Dr. Dwyer has received numerous honors and awards for her work in the field of nutrition, including the 1996 W. O. Atwater Award of the USDA and J. Harvey Wiley Award from the Society for Nutrition Education. She gave the Lenna Frances Cooper Lecture at the annual meeting of the American Dietetic Association in 1990. Dr. Dwyer is currently on the editorial board for *Family Economics* and *Nutrition Review* and advisory board for *Clinics in Applied Nutrition*, and is a contributing editor for *Nutrition Reviews*, as well as a reviewer for the *Journal of the American Dietetic Association, American Journal of Clinical Nutrition*, and *American Journal of Public Health*. She received her D.Sc. and M.Sc. from the Harvard School of Public Health, an M.S. from the University of Wisconsin, and completed her undergraduate degree with distinction from Cornell University.

REBECCA B. COSTELLO (*FNB Staff, Project Director from July 15, 1996*) is Project Director for the Committee on Military Nutrition Research (CMNR) and Committee on Body Composition, Nutrition, and Health of Military Women (BCNH). Prior to joining the FNB staff, she served as Research Associate and Program Director for the Risk Factor Reduction Center, a referral center for the detection, modification, and prevention of cardiovascular disease through dietary and/or drug interventions at the Washington Adventist Hospital in Takoma Park, Maryland. She received her B.S. and M.S. in biology from the American University, Washington, D.C., and a Ph.D. in clinical nutrition from the University of Maryland at College Park. She has active membership in the American Institute of Nutrition, American College of Nutrition, American Dietetic Association, and American Heart Association Council on Epidemiology. Dr. Costello's areas of research interest include mineral nutrition, dietary intake methodology, and chronic disease epidemiology.

SYDNE J. CARLSON-NEWBERRY (*FNB Staff, Program Officer*) is Program Officer for the CMNR and BCNH. Prior to joining the FNB staff, she served as Project Director for the Women's Health Project and Adjunct Assistant Professor in the Department of Family Medicine, Wright State University School of Medicine; as a behavioral health educator for a hospital-based weight management program in Dayton, Ohio; and as a research associate at The Ohio State University Biotechnology Center. She received her B.A. from Brandeis University and her Ph.D. in nutritional biochemistry and metabolism from M.I.T. and completed a NIH postdoctoral fellowship in the Departments of Biochemistry and Molecular Genetics at Ohio State. Dr. Carlson-Newberry's areas of research interest include eating disorders and diabetes management.

BERNADETTE M. MARRIOTT (*FNB Staff, Project Director through November 22, 1995*) is Director of the Office of Dietary Supplements Research at NIH and was Project Director for the CMNR and Deputy Director of the FNB. She has a Ph.D. in psychology from the University of Aberdeen, Scotland, and B.Sc. in biochemistry/immunology and postdoctoral laboratory training in comparative medicine and trace mineral nutrition. She serves on the Scientific Advisory board for the Diagon Corporation and the American Health Foundation. She serves as scientific reviewer for the NIH, National Science Foundation, and National Geographic. Prior to joining the Institute of Medicine staff, she held university and medical school faculty positions at the Johns Hopkins University, University of Puerto Rico School of Medicine, and Goucher College. Her areas of research interest include bioenergetic modeling, trace mineral nutrition, and ingestive behavior in human and nonhuman primates.

AUTHORS

NATHANIEL M. ALPERT received a B.S. and Ph.D. in physics from Northeastern University. After postdoctoral training at the Massachusetts General Hospital (MGH) in the application of physics to nuclear medicine, he joined the research staff of the Department of Radiology at MGH. His research interests include tracer kinetic modeling and image processing techniques for positron emission tomography (PET). Currently, he is Director of the MGH PET Imaging Laboratory and Associate Professor of Radiology at Harvard Medical School.

ARTHUR O. ANDERSON is presently Chief, Department of Clinical Pathology, Diagnostics Systems Division at the U.S. Army Medical Research Institute of Infectious Diseases (USAMRIID), Fort Detrick, Maryland. Formerly, he was Chief, Department of Respiratory and Mucosal Immunity. His additional duties at USAMRIID include serving as the Office of Human Use and Ethics Chair of the USAMRIID IRB, referred to as the Human Use Committee.

COL Anderson earned his B.S. in biology at Wagner College, Staten Island, New York and an M.D. at the University of Maryland School of Medicine. He completed his training as a pathologist at The Johns Hopkins Hospital concomitantly with performing a postdoctoral fellowship in transplantation immunology at The Johns Hopkins University. As a Berry Plan Army reserve medical officer, COL Anderson entered active duty in 1974 at USAMRIID. It was during the period of 1974–1980 that he worked closely with committee member William R. Beisel, who was the Scientific Advisor for USAMRIID.

This 6-year period was very productive as COL Anderson studied cellular phenomena in lymphatic tissues that were responding to vaccines and adjuvants. While searching for safe and effective biological response modifiers that could be used to replace adjuvants that had unacceptable toxicity, he used lymphocyte chemotaxis and ability to affect lymphocyte recirculation rate as hypothetical indicators of adjuvant activity. This work proved insightful and revealed the complex physiology of effective immune responses.

COL Anderson was attracted away from USAMRIID in 1980 when he joined the faculty of the University of Pennsylvania in Philadelphia as an Assistant Professor of Pathology and Biology. His mentor, John J. Cebra, stimulated an interest in mucosal immunity that resulted in his searching for adjuvants that selectively stimulated development of secretory IgA. In 1982 COL Anderson presented the first study of an adjuvant that successfully enhanced secretory IgA in the intestines at the 1982 meeting of the New York Academy of Sciences meeting on the secretory immune system.

As the same time, COL Edward Stephenson at USAMRIID was discovering that parenteral immunization regimens, which completely protected mice from parenteral challenge with Venezuelan Equine Encephalitis, failed to protect similarly immunized mice from aerosol challenge. A colleague suggested that this was a problem that could be solved by a mucosal immunologist, and COL Anderson returned to set up USAMRIID's first laboratory of mucosal immunology. The review for this workshop and report represents the fruits of this department and provides insights into future adaptations of these vaccine technologies.

JOHN W. BABICH received his B.S. in pharmaceutical science from St. John's University, an M.S. in radiopharmacy from the University of Southern California, and a Ph.D. from the University of London in radiopharmaceutical chemistry. He has worked in radiopharmaceutical research at Brookhaven National Labs, the NASA-Johnson Space Center, Methodist Hospital, and Baylor College of Medicine in Houston, and in 1984 moved to England to work at the Institute of Cancer Research. In 1990 he returned to the United States to take up his current position as Principal Nuclear Pharmacist and Assistant in

Radiopharmaceutical Chemistry (Radiology) at Massachusetts General Hospital and Instructor in Radiology at Harvard Medical School. Dr. Babich has been actively involved in the clinical investigation of new radiodiagnostic agents for cancer and infection, as well as the application of positron emission tomography in drug development. His current research interests include investigations into the use of peptides and peptide mimetics for diagnosis and drug delivery.

DENNIS M. BIER is Professor of Pediatrics, Director of the USDA Children's Nutrition Research Center, and Program Director of the Pediatric Clinical Research Center at Baylor College of Medicine. He is also a Trustee of the International Pediatric Research Foundation, a Councilor of the American Pediatric Society, Associate Editor of the *Annual Review of Nutrition*, and Chair of the USDA Human Studies Review Committee. Previously, Dr. Bier was Professor of Pediatrics and Medicine at Washington University in St. Louis, where he was Director of the Mass Spectrometry Facility and Co-Director of the Pediatric Endocrinology and Metabolism Division. He has been Editor-in-Chief of *Pediatric Research*, Chair of the NIH Nutrition Study Section, Chair of the NIH General Clinical Research Centers Committee, Chair of the NIH/NICHD Expert Panel Five-Year Plan for Nutrition Research and Training, and President of the American Society for Clinical Nutrition. He also has served as a member of the various additional scientific advisory panels, including the HHS/USDA Dietary Guidelines Advisory Committee, the FNB, the FDA Food Advisory Committee, the Medical Science Advisory Board of the Juvenile Diabetes Foundation, the Steering Committee of the Pediatric Scientist Development Program, and the Advisory Board of the National Stable Isotopes Resource at Los Alamos National Laboratory.

RAYMOND K. BLANCHARD is a Postdoctoral Research Associate in Nutritional Biochemistry at the Center for Nutritional Sciences and the Food Science and Human Nutrition Department, University of Florida, where his research has focused on the regulation of genes by dietary zinc. He received his Ph.D. in biochemistry from the University of California, Riverside for research on the gene regulation of one of the components for the biosynthesis of 1,25 dihydroxyvitamin D_3. During that time, he received a Young Investigator Award from the 8th International Workshop on Vitamin D. Dr. Blanchard is also a member of Sigma Xi and an associate member of the American Society for Biochemistry and Molecular Biology.

DONALD BODENNER graduated from Harvard University. He then received his Ph.D. in chemistry, M.D., and residency training in internal medicine from the University of Minnesota. This was followed by a fellowship in endocrinology at the NIH, leading to his present position as Assistant

Professor of Medicine and Biochemistry at the University of Rochester. Dr. Bodenner currently belongs to the Endocrine Society, American Federation of Clinical Research, and American Association for the Advancement of Science.

WM. CAMERON CHUMLEA is Fels Professor of Community Health at Wright State University School of Medicine in Dayton, Ohio. His expertise is in the development of methods for nutritional assessment and measures of body composition across the age range. Dr. Chumlea is the principal investigator of numerous research projects funded by the NIH and by industry. Dr. Chumlea is the anthropometry consultant to the National Center for Health Statistics for the Health and Nutrition Examination Surveys. He also serves as a consultant for government committees and universities in the United States and Europe. Dr. Chumlea received a B.S. in pre-medicine from Washington & Lee University and an M.A. and Ph.D. in physical anthropology from the University of Texas.

BRYAN P. COFFEY is currently a member of the research staff at Riverside Research Institute, Boston Research Office, where he does research on radar systems and national defense. He has 5 years experience working on human performance and nutritional issues at the Military Performance and Neuroscience Division, U.S. Army Research Institute of Environmental Medicine (USARIEM), Natick, Massachusetts. He is a Ph.D. student in the Department of Cognitive and Neural Systems, Boston University. He received a B.E. in electrical engineering and a M.S. in computer science from Stevens Institute of Technology.

ROBERT J. COUSINS has been the Boston Family Professor of Nutrition in the Food Science and Human Nutrition Department at the University of Florida since 1982 and Director of the Center for Nutritional Sciences since 1986. From 1971 to 1982, Dr. Cousins was a Professor of Nutritional Biochemistry at Rutgers University. His research interests focus on the molecular and cell biology of zinc metabolism and function. He is the author of over 140 refereed papers in nutrition, physiology, and biochemistry journals. He has received the Mead Johnson Award (1979) and the Osborne and Mendel Award (1989) from the American Institute of Nutrition and a MERIT Award from NIH. He was Associate Editor of *The Journal of Nutrition* from 1990–1996. He was President of the Federation of American Societies for Experimental Biology, 1991–1992 and of the American Society for Nutritional Sciences (AIN), 1996–1997. He is a member of several professional organizations and honorary societies. Dr. Cousins received a B.A. in zoology/chemistry from the University of Vermont, a Ph.D. in nutritional biochemistry from the University of Connecticut, and was an NIH Postdoctoral Fellow in Biochemistry at the University of Wisconsin.

JAMES P. DeLANY is an Associate Professor at the Pennington Biomedical Research Center, Louisiana State University. He has been Director of the Stable Isotope Lab since 1989 and is involved in many studies of human metabolism, primarily in the areas of obesity and heart disease, using stable isotope tracers. He has been involved in the measurement of energy expenditure in military nutrition studies since his work as a postdoctoral fellow at the University of Chicago in 1987. Dr. DeLany received his B.S. and Ph.D. degrees in human nutrition from The Ohio State University.

CANDACE R. ENOCKSON is the Laboratory Technologist in the Clinical Laboratory of the Department of Microbiology and Immunology at the Medical University of South Carolina. Previously, she was the Chief Technologist of the Clinical Immunology Laboratory at Parkland Memorial Hospital in Dallas, Texas and has worked as a technologist in hematology and chemistry laboratories since 1972. Ms. Enockson received a B.S. in medical technology from North Dakota State University and an M.A. in religious studies from the North American Baptist Seminary and is registered by the American Society of Clinical Pathologists.

ALAN J. FISCHMAN received a B.S. in chemistry from Brooklyn College, a Ph.D. in physical biochemistry from Rockefeller University, and an M.D. from Yale University. After residency training in internal medicine at Tulane University and fellowship training in nuclear medicine at the MGH, he joined the clinical and research staff of the Department of Radiology at MGH. Currently, he is Chief of Nuclear Medicine at MGH and the Shriners Burns Institute, Director of the MGH PET Center, and Associate Professor of Radiology at Harvard Medical School. Although Dr. Fischman has maintained a broad clinical interest in general nuclear medicine, many of his clinical responsibilities have focused on infection imaging and the noninvasive evaluation of alterations in metabolism, hemodynamics, and receptor physiology in patients with neurological and cardiac disease and traumatic injuries. These clinical activities have complimented his scientific research interests, which involve the development of new radiopharmaceuticals for identifying sites of infection and inflammation, noninvasive evaluation of the pharmacokinetics and pharmacodynamics of new therapeutic agents, and the design and synthesis of new and novel probes for studying the alterations in normal physiological and biochemical function that occur in a variety of diseases.

DAVID FRAGER is currently the Deputy Director of the Department of Radiology at St. Luke's-Roosevelt Hospital Center, New York; he was formerly Section Chief of Body CT and MRI Imaging. A graduate of the University of

Pennsylvania School of Medicine, he was formerly an Associate Professor of Radiology at the Albert Einstein College of Medicine. Dr. Frager currently holds a similar appointment at the Columbia University School of Physicians and Surgeons, New York.

KARL E. FRIEDL is Deputy Director of the Army Operational Medicine Research Program at the U.S. Amy Medical Research and Materiel Command (USAMRMC), Fort Detrick, Maryland. Prior to this assignment, he was an Army Research Physiologist in the Occupational Physiology Division at USARIEM, where he specialized in physical and biochemical limits of prolonged, intensive military training. Previously, LTC Friedl worked in the Department of Clinical Investigation at Madigan Army Medical Center in Tacoma, Washington performing studies in endocrine physiology. He received his Ph.D. in physiology in 1984 from the Institute of Environmental Stress at the University of California, Santa Barbara.

SHUMEI S. GUO is Professor of Community Health at Wright State University School of Medicine in Dayton, Ohio. Her expertise is in the development of statistical models for longitudinal data related to growth, body composition, nutritional assessment, and cardiovascular disease. Dr. Guo is the principal investigator of numerous research projects funded by the NIH and by industry. She serves on the Epidemiology and Disease Control Study Section and is the statistical consultant to the National Center for Health Statistics for the Health and Nutrition Examination Surveys and other government committees and universities. Dr. Guo received a B.S. in public health from the National Taiwan University, an M.S. in applied mathematics and statistics form SUNY, Stony Brook, and a Ph.D. in biostatistics form the University of Pittsburgh.

JAMES S. HAYES is a Clinical Research Scientist at Ross Products Division, Abbott Laboratories. His research interests include methods for the determination of nutritional status, measurement of the electrical activity or the GI tract, and gastrointestinal pacing.

STEVEN B. HEYMSFIELD is Professor of Medicine at Columbia University, College of Physicians and Surgeons in New York. He also currently serves as Deputy Director of the New York Obesity Research Center and is Director of the Human Body Composition Laboratory. Dr. Heymsfield is currently President of the American Society of Parenteral and Enteral Nutrition and is an active member of the American Society of Clinical Nutrition and the North American Society for the Study of Obesity. He was recently made and honorary member of the American Dietetic Association, and he serves on the BCNH. Dr. Heymsfield received a B.S. in chemistry from Hunter College-City University of New York and an M.D. degree from Mount Sinai School of Medicine, also in New York.

REED W. HOYT is a Research Physiologist in the Altitude Physiology and Medicine Division of USARIEM. He received his Ph.D. in physiology from the University of New Mexico in 1981, and spent 5 years at the University of Pennsylvania, first as a Postdoctoral Fellow and then as a Research Assistant Professor. In 1986 he joined USARIEM. He is a member of the American Physiological Society and the American Institute of Nutrition. His research focuses on the effects of exercise and the environment on human energy, water, and fuel metabolism.

HONGBING HSU received his Ph.D. in physics from Rice University, M.A. in physics from Rice University, and a B.S. from the University of Science and Technology of China. After completing his training at Rice University, Dr. Hsu began a fellowship in medical physics at the MGH.

WENDY M. KOHRT is a Research Associate Professor in the Department of Internal Medicine, Section of Applied Physiology, Division of Geriatrics and Gerontology, at the Washington University School of Medicine in St. Louis, Missouri. She received her Ph.D. in exercise physiology from Arizona State University and completed a postdoctoral research fellowship at Washington University. Her major research efforts are directed toward identifying, characterizing, and determining, the physiological basis for adaptations to exercise that can be applied to maintenance of functional capacity and prevention of disease in middle and old age. She is currently investigating (1) the role of abdominal obesity in the glucose intolerance and insulin resistance of aging, and the extent to which exercise can restore normal glucose tolerance and insulin action, and (2) the effects of exercise and/or hormone replacement therapy on the prevention or reversal of osteoporosis.

MARIANO LA VIA is Professor Emeritus of Pathology and Laboratory Medicine at the Medical University of South Carolina, Charleston. He received an M.D. from the University of Messina in Italy, and after a pathology residency at the University of Chicago School of Medicine, was appointed an instructor at that institution. His academic career progressed with appointments as Assistant and then Associate Professor at the University of Colorado Medical Center, Professor at the Bowman Grey School of Medicine and at Emory University School of Medicine, and Professor and Director of Diagnostic Immunology at the Medical University of South Carolina. His research has dealt with cellular mechanisms of immune responses and their regulation. In the last 15 years, Dr. La Via has undertaken the investigation of the effect of stress on immunocompetence and morbidity and of its mechanism(s). He is a Fellow of the American Association for the Advancement of Science, member of several professional societies, Past President of the Clinical Cytometry Society, and Editor on Communications in *Clinical Cytometry*. He also serves on the editorial boards of several scientific journals.

HARRIS R. LIEBERMAN is currently Deputy Chief, Military Nutrition and Biochemical Division, USARIEM. He joined the civilian research staff at USARIEM in 1990. Dr. Lieberman received his Ph.D. in physiological psychology from the University of Florida. Upon completing his graduate training, he conducted postdoctoral research a the Department o Psychology and Brain Science at M.I.T. While at M.I.T., he established an interdisciplinary research program at the Department of Brain and Cognitive Science to examine the effects of various food constituents on human behavior and brain function. Key accomplishments f the laboratory included the development of appropriate methods for assessing the effects of food constituents and other subtle environmental factors on human brain function and the determination that specific foods and hormones reliably alter human behavior. He has continued this work at USARIEM, focusing on the behavioral and physiological effects of various nutritional factors on brain function and cognitive performance. He is an internationally recognized expert in the area of nutrition, neuroscience, and behavior and has published over 90 original, full-length scientific papers in scientific journals and edited books. He has been an invited lecturer at numerous national and international conferences, government research laboratories, and universities.

MARY Z. MAYS received her Ph.D. in experimental psychology with a specialization in learning and memory from the University of Oklahoma in 1977. From 1990 to 1993 she was the Director of the Military Performance and Neuroscience Division at USARIEM. Her research there focused on the impact of stress on cognitive and affective behavior. From 1993 to 1995, Dr. Mays served as the Planner for Science and Technology Programs at USAMRMC. She is currently the Director of Eagle Creek Research Services, San Antonio, Texas.

DONALD B. McCORMICK is the Fuller E. Callaway Professor of Biochemistry in the Department of Biochemistry at Emory University. He received his Ph.D. in biochemistry from Vanderbilt University and was a Postdoctoral Fellow in Biochemistry at the University of California, Berkeley.

He joined the faculty at Cornell University where he served for nearly 20 years and where he became Liberty Hyde Bailey Professor of Nutritional Biochemistry. He then went to Emory University where he has served as Chair of Biochemistry for 15 years and for part of the time as Executive Associate Dean for Science in the School of Medicine.

Dr. McCormick's research interests center around cofactors including vitamins, coenzymes, and metal ions. In particular he and his associates have isolated and characterized those enzymes that convert riboflavin and vitamin B_6 to functional coenzymes, and he has identified primary metabolites of flavins, biotin, and lipoate. Among honors and awards relating to his training and research are Bausch and Lomb and Westinghouse Science Scholarships, USPHS and Guggenheim Fellowships, Mead Johnson and the Osborne and Mendel Awards fro the American Institute of Nutrition, Wellcome Visiting Professorships, and special name lectureships at several universities.

Dr. McCormick has served on numerous committees and in functions for government and professional societies. Among these are duties as member and chair of NIH study sections and an National Cancer Institute Board of Counselors, member of the FASEB Board of Directors and Chair of the Scientific Advisory Committee for their Life Science Research Office, member and Vice Chair of the FNB, and a member of organizing committees for international conferences and symposia, especially as regards flavins and flavoproteins, vitamin B_6, and cofactors involved in carbonyl catalysis, and biofactors broadly. He is a member of several scientific societies including the American Institute of Nutrition, where he served as President; American Society of Biochemistry and Molecular Biology; American Chemical Society; and American Association for the Advancement of Science, where he is a Fellow. He has served on several editorial boards for journals in the areas of biochemical and nutritional sciences and has been an editor for "Vitamins and Coenzymes" in the *Methods of Enzymology* series, "Vitamins and Hormones," and currently the *Annual Review of Nutrition.*

GUY MILLER is founder, Chair, and Chief Executive Officer of Galileo Laboratories, Inc., Sunnyvale, California. Prior to joining Galileo, Dr. Miller was an Assistant Professor at The Johns Hopkins University School of Medicine. He obtained his Ph.D. in chemistry under the direction of Professor Sidney Hecht, John Mallet Professor of Chemistry at the University of Virginia, and his M.D. t the Medical College of Pennsylvania. After completing a surgical residency at the University of Chicago, Dr. Miller completed a residency in anesthesiology and critical care medicine at Johns Hopkins Hospital, followed by a fellowship in multidisciplinary critical care medicine. Currently, he hold an appointment as Clinical Instructor, Stanford University School of Medicine.

LYLE L. MOLDAWER is currently Professor of Surgery at the University of Florida College of Medicine. He joined the College in 1993, after serving on the faculty of Cornell University Medical College for 7 years. Dr. Moldawer currently serves on several USPHS. Scientific Advisory Committees, including Metabolic Pathology and Post-Graduate Medical Training Study Sections of the NIH and the National Institute of General Medical Sciences, respectively. He is an active member of the American Physiological Society and American Society for Leukocyte Biology. Dr. Moldawer received his Ph.D. in experimental medicine from Göteborgs Universitet in 1986.

JOHN F. PATTON is Chief of the Military Performance Division, USARIEM. He earned his Ph.D. in medical physiology from the University of Missouri, Columbia. His research interests include cold physiology, exercise physiology, physical fitness, and occupational performance. The mission of the Military Performance Division encompasses research programs in musculoskeletal injury epidemiology, occupational medicine and physiology, biomechanics, and cognitive/pschomoter performance.

ROBERT ROSS obtained a Bachelor degree in physical education form Magill University and Master's and Ph.D. in exercise physiology from the Université de Montréal. Early research interests focused on body composition methodology, in particular, the development and application of magnetic resonance imaging as a means of measuring regional adipose tissue and skeletal muscle distribution. A principal research interest is to study the separate effects of diet- and exercise-induced weight loss on adipose tissue and skeletal muscle mass, and to relate changes in these variables to concurrent changes in metabolic risk factors. Dr. Ross is currently an Assistant Professor within the School of Physical and Health Education and holds a cross-appointment in the Faculty of Medicine, Division of Endocrinology and Metabolism at Queen's University in Kingston, Ontario, Canada.

GERALD I. SHULMAN is Professor of Medicine and Cellular and Molecular Physiology at Yale University School of Medicine. He is also Associate Chief of the Endocrinology/Metabolism Section and Associate Director of the Yale Diabetes Endocrinology Research center. Dr. Shulman is a Fellow of the American College of Physicians and a member of the American Society for Clinical Investigation. He received a B.S. in biophysics form the University of Michigan and M.D.-Ph.D. (physiology) from Wayne State University. Dr. Shulman did a residency in internal medicine at Duke University Medical Center and a Fellowship in Endocrinology/Metabolism at the Massachusetts General Hospital/Harvard Medical School.

RONALD G. TOMPKINS received a B.S. in chemistry and an M.D. from Tulane University. During his surgical training at the MGH and Harvard Medical School, he received an S.M. in chemical engineering and an Sc.D. in medical and chemical engineering from the Massachusetts Institute of Technology. Following completion of his surgical training at MGH, he has been both a clinician and scientific investigator. He is the Chief of the Trauma and Burn Services at MGH, Chief of Staff at the Shriners Burns Institute in Boston, and the John Francis Burke Professor of Surgery at the Harvard Medical School. Dr. Tompkins is board-certified in surgery and in surgical critical care, and he currently serves as Director of the American Board of Surgery and the American Burn Association. Although Dr. Tompkins has maintained a broad clinical interest in surgery, many of his clinical responsibilities have focused on patients who have been injured by burns and other traumatic injuries. These clinical activities have complemented his scientific interests, which involve tissue engineering and artificial organ development, physiological transport in injury, and metabolism.

HOWARD C. TOWLE is currently Professor of Biochemistry and a member of the Institute of Human Genetics at the University of Minnesota Medical School. He received his B.A. in biological sciences and Ph.D. in biochemistry from Michigan State University. Subsequently, he did postdoctoral work in cell biology a the Baylor College of Medicine before starting his academic career at the University of Minnesota. Dr. Towle's research has focused on the influence of thyroid hormones and nutritional factors on hepatic gene expression. He has served on the NIH Study Section on Biochemistry and is a member of the editorial board for the *Journal of Biological Chemistry*. He is also a member of the Endocrine Society and American Society for Biochemistry and Molecular Biology.

GABRIEL VIRELLA received the M.D. (1967) and Ph.D. (1974) from the University of Lisbon School of Medicine in Portugal. He is Professor of Basic and Clinical Immunology and Microbiology, as well as of Pathology and Laboratory Medicine, at the Medical University of South Carolina in Charleston. he directs a special Immunology Diagnosis Laboratory in the Department of Microbiology and immunology. Previously, he was a Senior Researcher in Immunochemistry and Immunopharmacology at the Gulbenkian Institute of Science in Oeiras, Portugal, and he also held postdoctoral fellowships at the University of Birmingham Medical School and the National Institute for Medical Research, London. His research interests include immunoglobulin structure, B-lymphocyte activation, hematological malignancies, immunodeficiencies, immune complex diseases, and the role of immunological mechanisms in the pathogenesis of atherosclerosis. He has authored or coauthored 196 research articles, edited two textbooks (*Introduction* *to Clinical Immunology*, 4th ed. and *Microbiology and Infectious Diseases*, 3d ed.), is a Fellow of the American Association for the Advancement of Science and American Academy of Microbiology, a charter member of the American Board of Medical Laboratory Immunologists, and a member of the Clinical Immunology Society. Dr. Virella serves as member of the editorial board of the *Journal of Clinical Laboratory Analysis, Clinical and Diagnostic Laboratory Immunology*, and is Section Editor of *Clinical Immunology and Immunopathology*.

JAMES A. VOGEL was Director of Occupational Health and Performance at USARIEM, which encompassed research programs in occupational medicine, occupational physiology, nutrition, and behavioral performance-neuroscience. He was the principal consultant to the Department of the Army in the biomedical aspects of physical fitness and exercise physiology and chaired a NATO Research Study Group on the Biomedical Aspects of Military Physical Training. Dr. Vogel retired from federal service in September 1995. He earned a Ph.D. degree in physiology from Rutgers University, New Jersey.

ZiMIAN WANG is Senior Staff Associate, Columbia University, College of Physicians and Surgeons in New York. He formerly directed the Biochemistry Laboratory and served as Associate Research Professor at the Shanghai Research Institute of Sports Science. He is recipient of China State Sports Commission awards in 1989, 1991, and 1992. Mr. Wang is widely recognized in the body composition field for his innovative approach to multicomponent model development. He was awarded B.S. and M.S. degrees in biochemistry from Nanjing University and Shanghai Institute of Physiology, respectively. Mr. Wang is completing doctoral studies in Nutrition at Waganingen Agricultural University, The Netherlands.

PETER GREGORY WEYAND is a Postdoctoral Fellow at the Harvard University Concord Field Station in Bedford, Massachusetts. He received his B.A. in history from Bates College, Lewiston, Maine, in 1983, his M.S. in exercise physiology from Bridgewater State College, Bridgewater, Massachusetts, in 1988, and his Ph.D. in exercise physiology from the University of Georgia, Athens, Georgia, in 1992. He joined the Concord Field Station in 1992. His research interests include anaerobic energy release during exhaustive exercise, the metabolic determinants of run/walk performance in men and women, and the effects hypohydration on perceived exertion and submaximal exercise capacity.

ROBERT R. WOLFE has been Professor of Surgery and Nutritional Biochemistry at the University of Texas Medical Branch, Galveston, and Chief of Metabolism at the Shriners Burns Institute since 1983. From 1976 to 1983 he was Assistant and Associate Professor of Surgery at Harvard Medical School and the Shriners Burns Institute, Boston. Dr. Wolfe has served as associate editor of the *American Journal of Physiology, Endocrinology*, and *Metabolism* and as an editorial board member of several other journals. He has been a regular member of the Surgery, Anesthesiology, and Trauma Study Section and many other ad hoc study sections of the NIH, as well as a member of the Committee on Research Review of the American Diabetes Association. He has been an active member of the American Physiological Society and American Institute of Nutrition. Dr. Wolfe received an A.B. in biology from the University of California, Berkeley and a Ph.D. in biology from the University of California, Santa Barbara.

VERNON R. YOUNG has been at M.I.T. since 1965, where he is currently Professor of Nutritional Biochemistry. Dr. Young received a B.Sc. (agriculture) from the University of Reading, United Kingdom and a Ph.D. (nutrition) from the University of California, Davis. He later received a D.Sc. from the University of Reading for his research on various aspects of muscle and whole-body protein metabolism. He has served as President of the American Society for Nutritional Sciences (previously American Institute of Nutrition) and is currently a member of the FNB. He was elected in 1990 to the National Academy of Sciences and in 1993 to the Institute of Medicine in recognition of his research contributions, which have been focused mainly in the area of human protein and amino acid metabolism and nutritional requirements.

YONG-MING YU is an Associate Biochemist in the Department of Surgery, Trauma Service of Massachusetts General Hospital and Assistant Professor of Surgery at the Harvard Medical School. He is active in the research of metabolic response to trauma and burns using tracer methods. Dr. Yu is an active member of the American Burn Association and American Institute of Nutrition, along with other scientific societies. He received a B.S. in biology from Peking University, M.D. from Peking Union Medical College, and Ph.D. in nutritional biochemistry from M.I.T.

Emerging Technologies for Nutrition Research, 1997
Pp. 605–608. Washington, D.C.
National Academy Press

C

Abbreviations

%BF	percentage body fat
AASHATO	American Association of State Highway and Transportation Officials
Ag	antigen
APC	antigen-presenting cell
ARDS	adult respiratory distress syndrome
AT	adipose tissue
ATP	adenosine triphosphate
A-V	arteriovenous
BAL	bronchoalveolar lavage fluid
BMC	bone mineral content
BMD	bone mineral density
BMI	body mass index
BMR	basal metabolic rate
BP	base pair
BTPS	body temperature and pressure, saturated gas

CAT or CT	computed axial tomography
CDR	complementarity-determining region
CLA	cutaneous lymphocyte associated
CMNR	Committee on Military Nutrition Research
CT	cholera toxin
CTB	cholera toxin B-subunit
CV	coefficient of variation
CVD	cardiovascular disease
DARPA	Defense Advanced Research Projects Agency
DB	Douglas bag
DHHS	U.S. Department of Health and Human Services
DIS	Distributed Interactive Simulation
DLW	doubly labeled water
DPA	dual-photon absorptiometry
DTH	delayed hypersensitivity
DXA or DEXA	dual-energy x-ray absorptiometry
ECFV	extracellular fluid volume
ELISA	enzyme-linked immunoabsorption assay
EMA	effective mechanical advantage
EPI	Echo Planar Imaging
EST	expressed sequence tag
FACScan	Fluorescence Activated Cell Sorter
FCM	Foot Contact Monitor
FeO_2	fractional concentration of oxygen in expired air
$FeCO_2$	fractional concentration of carbon dioxide in expired air
F_IO_2	fractional concentration of oxygen in inspired air
FAD	flavin-adenine dinucleotide
FFA	free fatty acids
FFM	fat-free mass
FMN	flavin mononucleotide
G-6-P	glucose-6-phosphate
GC-MS	gas chromatography-mass spectrometry
HCSM	Hierarchical Concurrent State Machine
HECA	human endothelial cell associated
HMMWV	high-mobility multipurpose wheeled vehicle
HU	Hounsfield units
HW	hydrostatic weighing
I/B	intake balance
IDS	Iowa Driving Simulator
IEL	intraepithelial lymphocyte
IFNγ	interferon gamma
IG	Image Generator
IL	interleukin

IMRS	isotope ratio mass spectrometer
IOM	Institute of Medicine
J-chain	joiner-chain
kDa	kilodaltons
LDL	low-density lipoprotein
LEM	leukocyte endogenous mediator
LT	labile enterotoxin
$\dot{M}_{loco}$	metabolic cost of locomotion
MADCAM-1	mucosal addressin cell adhesion molecule-1
MFA	muscle function analysis
MHC	major histocompatibility
MIDA	mass isotopomer distribution analysis
MIDI	Musical Instrument Digital Interface
MIP	Multi Im Parvo
NIR	near-infrared
MND	Military Nutrition Division
MRE	metal response element
MREs	Meals, Ready-to-Eat
MRI	magnetic resonance imaging
MRS	magnetic resonance spectroscopy
NADS	National Advanced Driving Simulator
NHANES	National Health and Nutrition Examination Survey
NHTSA	National Highway Traffic Safety Administration
NiCd	nickel-cadmium
NIDDM	noninsulin dependent diabetes mellitus
NIH	National Institutes of Health
NK-cells	Natural Killer-cells
NMR	nuclear magnetic resonance
NRC	National Research Council
PCR	polymerase chain reaction
PCR	principal component regression
PD	Panic Disorder
PET	positron emission tomography
PHA	phytohemagglutinin
PK	pyruvate kinase
PLP	pyridoxal 5'-phosphate
PLS	partial least squares
PMN	polymorphonuclear leukocytes
PPAR	peroxisome proliferator-activated receptor
PSR	protein synthetic rate
PWM	pokeweed mitogen
FFA Ra	rate of appearance of fatty acids
RER	respiratory exchange ratio
RMR	resting metabolic rate

RF	radio-frequency
R_f	respiratory rate
RLW	Ration, Lightweight
RMSE	root mean square error
SCID	severe combined immunodeficiency
SEC	standard error of calibration
SEE	standard error of the estimate
SIRS	systemic inflammatory response syndrome
SIS	stress intrusion score
SRE	sterol response element
SREBP	SRE-binding protein
STPD	standard temperature and pressure, dry gas
TEEM 100	Total Energy Expenditure Measurement system
TBBM	total body bone mineral content
TBW	total body water
TG	triglyceride
Th1	T-helper 1 cell
TNF-α	tumor necrosis factor-alpha
URI	upper respiratory infections
USAMRMC	U.S. Army Medical Research and Materiel Command
USARIEM	U.S. Army Research Institute of Environmental Medicine
$\dot{V}CO_2$	carbon dioxide production
$\dot{V}E$	expired minute ventilation
$\dot{V}I$	inspired minute ventilation
$\dot{V}O_2max$	maximal oxygen uptake
WHO	World Health Organization
WHR	waist-to-hip circumference ratio

Emerging Technologies for Nutrition Research, 1997
Pp. 609–680. Washington, D.C.
National Academy Press

D

Emerging Technologies for Nutrition Research—A Selected Bibliography

On the following pages is a selection of references dealing with emerging technologies for nutrition research. This bibliography was compiled from the joint reference lists of the 26 chapters in this report, selected references from a limited literature search, and references recommended by the invited speakers as background reading for the workshop participants. As a result, references that are historical in nature are included in this listing with the most current studies.

Abate, N., D. Burns, R.M. Peshock, A. Garg, and S.M. Grundy
  1994 Estimation of adipose tissue mass by magnetic resonance imaging: Validation against dissection in human cadavers. J. Lipid Res. 35:1490–1496.
Abbas, A.K., K.M. Murphy, and A. Sher
  1996 Functional diversity of helper T lymphocytes. Nature 383:787–793.
Abernethy, N.J., J.B. Hay, W.G. Kimpton, E. Washington, and R.N.P. Cahill
  1991 Lymphocyte subset-specific and tissue-specific lymphocyte-endothelial cell recognition mechanisms independently direct the recirculation of lymphocytes from blood to lymph in sheep. Immunology 72:239–245.
Adelman, L., M.S. Cohen, T.A. Bresnick, J.O. Chinnis, and K.B. Laskey
  1993 Real-time expert systems interfaces, cognitive processes, and task performance: An empirical assessment. Hum. Factors 35(2):243–261.
Agace, W., S. Hedges, U. Andersson, J. Andersson, M. Ceska, and C. Svanborg
  1993 Selective cytokine production by epithelial cells following exposure to *Escherichia coli*. Infect. Immun. 61:602–609.
Akers, R., and E.R. Buskirk
  1969 An underwater weighing system utilizing "force cube" transducers. J. Appl. Physiol. 2:649–652.
Akiyama, T., and Y. Yamauchi
  1994 Use of near infrared reflectance spectroscopy in the screening for biliary atresia. J. Pediatr. Surg. 29(5):645–647.
Alessi, S.M., and G.S. Watson
  1994 Driving Simulation Research at The University of Iowa. Proceedings of the 1994 Annual Meeting of the Association for the Development of Computer-Based Instructional Systems. 16–20 February 1994, Nashville, Tenn.
Alexander, R. McN., A.S. Jayes, G.M.O. Maloiy, and E.M. Wathuta
  1981 Allometry of the leg muscles of mammals. J. Zool. (Lond.) 194:539–552.
Allen, T.H., B.E. Welch, T.T. Trujilo, and J.E. Roberts
  1959 Fat, water and tissue solids of the whole body less its bone mineral. J. Appl. Physiol. 14:1009–1012.
Altman, J.D., P.A.H. Moss, P.J.R. Goulder, D.H. Barouch, M.G. McHeyzer-Williams, J.I. Bell, A.J. McMichael, and M.M. Davis
  1996 Phenotypic analysis of antigen-specific T lymphocytes. Science 274:94–96.
Anderson, A.O.
  1985 Multiple effects of immunological adjuvants on lymphatic microenvironments. Int. J. Immunother. 1:185–195.
  1990 Structure and organization of the lymphatic system. Pp. 14–45 in Immunophysiology. The Role of Cells and Cytokines in Immunity and Inflammation, J.J. Oppenheim and E. Shevach, eds. New York: Oxford University Press.
Anderson, A.O., and J.A. Reynolds
  1979 Adjuvant effects of the lipid amine CP-20, 961 (on lymphoid cell traffic and antiviral immunity). J. Reticuloendothelial Soc. 350:33–41.
Anderson, A.O., and D.H. Rubin
  1985 Effect of avridine on enteric antigen uptake and mucosal immunity to reovirus. Adv. Exp. Med. Biol. 186:579–590.
Anderson, A.O., and S. Shaw
  1993 T-cell adhesion to endothelium: The FRC conduit system and other anatomic and molecular features which facilitate the adhesion cascade in lymph node. Sem. Immunol. 5:271–282.

1996   Lymphocyte trafficking. Pp. 39–49 in Clinical Immunology, Principles and Practice, R.R. Rich, T.A. Fleisher, B.D. Schwartz, W.T. Shearer, and W. Strober, eds. St. Louis, Mo.: Mosby-Year Book, Inc.

Anderson, A.O., A. Plotner, and D.H. Rubin
1983   Effect of enteric priming with reovirus and lipoidal amine adjuvant on mucosal lymphatic tissue and anti-viral IgA secretion. Ann. N.Y. Acad. Sci. 409:769–775.

Anderson, A.O., T.T. McDonald, and D.H. Rubin
1985   Effect of orally administered avridine on enteric antigen uptake and mucosal immunity. Int. J. Immunother. 1:107–115.

Anderson, A.O., L.F. Snyder, M.L.M. Pitt, and O.L. Wood
1987   Mucosal priming alters pathogenesis of Rift Valley fever. Adv. Exp. Med. Biol. 237:727–733.

Anderson, A.O., O.L. Wood, A.D. King, and E.H. Stephenson
1987   Studies on anti-viral mucosal immunity using the lipoidal amine adjuvant avridine. Adv. Exp. Med. Bio. 216B:1781–1790.

Anderson, G.W., Jr., J.O. Lee, A.O. Anderson, N. Powell, J.A. Mangiafico, and G. Meadors
1991   Efficacy of a Rift Valley fever virus vaccine against an aerosol infection in rats. Vaccine 9:710–714.

AR (Army Regulation) 600-9
1986   *See* U.S. Department of the Army, 1986.

Ariizumi, K., T. Kitajima, O.R. Bergstresser, and A. Takashima
1995   Interleukin-1β converting enzyme in murine Langerhans cells and epidermal-derived dendritic cell lines. Eur. J. Immunol. 25:2137–2141.

Armstrong, R.B., and M.H. Laughlin
1985   Metabolic indicators of fibre recruitment in mammalian muscles during locomotion. J. Exp. Biol. 115:201–213.

Arner, P., and J. Ostman
1974   Mono and di-acyl glycerols in human adipose tissue. Biochem. Biophys. Acta 369:209–221.

Arnold, M.A., and G.W. Small
1990   Determination of physiological levels of glucose in an aqueous matrix with digitally filtered Fourier transform near-infrared spectra. Anal. Chem. 62:1457–1464.

Arntzen, C.J., H.S Mason, J. Shi, T.A. Haq, M.K. Estes, and J.D. Clements
1994   Production of candidate oral vaccines in edible tissues of transgenic plants. Pp. 339–344 in Vaccines '94, F. Brown, R.M. Chanock, H.S. Ginsberg, and R.A. Lerner, eds. New York: Cold Spring Harbor Laboratory, Cold Spring Harbor.

Askew, E.W.
1994   Nutritional enhancement of soldier performance at the U.S. Army Research Institute of Environmental Medicine, 1985–1992. Pp. 65–75 in Food Components to Enhance Performance, An Evaluation of Potential Performance-Enhancing Food Components for Operational Rations, B.M. Marriott, ed. A report of the Committee on Military Nutrition Research, Food and Nutrition Board, Institute of Medicine. Washington, D.C.: National Academy Press.

Askew, E.W., I. Munro, M.A. Sharp, S. Siegel, R. Popper, M.S. Rose, R.W. Hoyt, J.W. Martin, K. Reynolds, H.R. Lieberman, D. Engell, and C.P. Shaw
1987   Nutritional status and physical and mental performance of Special Operations soldiers consuming the Ration, Lightweight or the Meal, Ready-to-Eat military field ration during a 30-day field training exercise (RLW-30). Technical Report T7-87. Natick, Mass.: U.S. Army Research Institute of Environmental Medicine.

Assenmacher, M., J. Schmitz, and A. Radbruch
  1994   Flow cytometric determination of cytokines in activated murine Th lymphocytes. Expression of Il-10 in IFN-gamma and in IL-4 expressing cells. Eur. J. Immunol. 24:1097–1101.
Ästrand, P.O., and K. Rodahl
  1986   Textbook of Work Physiology, Physiological Bases of Exercise, 3d ed. New York: McGraw-Hill Book Co.
Astrup, A., and N.J. Christensen
  1992   Role of the sympathetic nervous system in obese and post-obese subjects. Pp. 299–309 in Energy Metabolism: Tissue Determinants and Cellular Corollaries, J.M. Kinney and H.G. Tucker, eds. New York: Raven Press.
Atkinson, D.
  1977   Cellular Energy Metabolism and Its Regulation. New York: Academic Press.
Aw, T.Y., D.P. Jones, and D.B. McCormick
  1983   Uptake of riboflavin by isolated rat liver cells. J. Nutr. 113:1249–1254
Azar, B.
  1995   Meet "Bob": Psychology's answer to easy computing. APA Monit. 26(4):1, 9.
Azcue, M., D. Wesson, M. Neuman, and P. Pencharz
  1993   What does bioelectrical impedance spectroscopy (BIS) measure? Basic Life Sci. 60:121–123.
Baker, D., and K.H. Norris
  1985   Near-infrared reflectance measurement of total sugar content of breakfast cereals. Appl. Spec. 39(4):618–621.
Baker, L.E.
  1989   Principles of the impedance technique. IEEE Eng. Med. Biol. Mag. 3:11–15.
Baker-Fulco, C.J.
  1995   Overview of dietary intakes during military exercises. Pp. 121–149 in Not Eating Enough, Overcoming Underconsumption of Military Operational Rations, B.M. Marriott, ed. A report of the Committee on Military Nutrition Research, Food and Nutrition Board, Institute of Medicine. Washington, D.C.: National Academy Press.
Baker-Fulco, C.J., S.A. Torri, J.E. Arsenault, and J.C. Buchbinder
  1994   Impact of menu changes designed to promote a training diet [abstract]. J. Am. Diet. Assoc. 94(4 suppl.):A9.
Bakker, R., E. Lasonder, and N.A. Bos
  1995   Measurement of affinity in serum samples of antigen-free, germ-free and conventional mice after hyperimmunization with 2,4-dinitrophenyl keyhole limpet hemocyanin, using surface plasmon resonance. Eur. J. Immunol. 25:1680–1686.
Ballal, M.A., and I.A. MacDonald
  1982   An evaluation of the Oxylog as a portable device with which to measure oxygen consumption. Clin. Phys. Physiol. Meas. 3:57–65.
Ballor, D.L., and V.L. Katch
  1989   Validity of anthropometric regression equations for predicting changes in body fat of obese females. Am. J. Hum. Biol. 1:97–101.
Banderet, L.E., and H.R. Lieberman
  1989   Treatment with tyrosine, a neurotransmitter precursor, reduces environmental stress in humans. Brain Res. Bull. 22:759–762.
Barnaba, V., A. Franco, M. Paroli, R. Benvenuto, G. De Petrillo, V.L. Burgio, I. Santilio, C. Balsano, M.S. Bonavita, and G. Cappelli
  1994   Selective expansion of cytotoxic T lymphocytes with a CD4+CD56+ surface phenotype and a T helper 1 profile of cytokine secretion in the liver of patients clinically infected with hepatitis B virus. J. Immunol. 152:3074–3087.

Barnard, R.J., V.R. Edgerton, and J.B. Peter
  1970 Effect of exercise on skeletal muscle. II. Contractile properties. J. Appl. Physiol. 28:767–770.
Barnett, A.
  1937 The basic factors in proposed electrical methods for measuring thyroid function, III. The phase angle and the impedance of the skin. West. J. Surg. Obstet. Gynecol. 45:540–554.
Barnett, A., and S. Bagno
  1936 The physiological mechanisms involved in the clinical measure of phase angle. Am. J. Physiol. 114:366–382.
Barrett, E.J., J.H. Revkin, L.H. Young, B.L. Zavel, R. Jacob, and R.A. Gelfand
  1987 An isotopic method for measurement of muscle protein synthesis and degradation *in vivo*. Biochem. J. 245:223–228.
Barstow, T.J., D.M. Cooper, E.M. Sobel, E.M. Landau, and S. Epstein
  1990 Influence of increased metabolic rate on ^{13}C-bicarbonate washout kinetics. Am. J. Physiol. 259:R163–R171.
Baumgartner, R.N., W.C. Chumlea, and A.F. Roche
  1988 Bioelectric impedance phase angle and body composition. Am. J. Clin. Nutr. 48:16–23.
  1989 Estimation of body composition from bioelectric impedance of body segments. Am. J. Clin. Nutr. 50:221–226.
Baumgartner, R.N., R.L. Rhyne, C. Troup, S. Wayne, and P.J. Garry
  1992 Appendicular skeletal muscle areas assessed by magnetic resonance imaging in older persons. J. Gerontol. 47:M67–72.
Baumgartner, R.N., S.B. Heymsfield, and A.F. Roche
  1995 Human body composition and the epidemiology of chronic disease. Obes. Res. 3:73–95.
Beckett, M.B., and J.A. Hodgdon
  1987 Lifting and carrying capacities relative to physical fitness measures. Technical Report No. 87-26. San Diego, Calif.: Naval Health Research Center.
Bedell, G.N., R. Marshall, A.B. DuBois, and J.H. Harris
  1956 Measurement of the volume of gas in the gastrointestinal tract. Values in normal subjects and ambulatory patients. J. Clin. Invest. 35:336–345.
Beebe, K.R., and B.R. Kowalske
  1987 An introduction to multivariate calibration and analysis. Anal. Chem. 59:1007a–1017a.
Behnke, A.R., and J.H. Wilmore
  1974 Evaluation and Regulation of Body Build and Composition. Englewood Cliffs, N.J.: Prentice-Hall, Inc.
Behnke, A.R., Jr., F.G. Feen, and W.C. Welham
  1942 The specific gravity of healthy men: Body weight divided by volume as an index of obesity. J. Am. Med. Assoc. 118:495–498.
Beisel, W.R.
  1975 Metabolic response to infection. Annu. Rev. Med. 26:9–20.
  1977 Magnitude of the host nutritional responses to infection. Am. J. Clin. Nutr. 30:1236–1247.
  1980 Endogenous pyrogen physiology. Physiologist 23:38–42.
  1994 Endocrine and immune system responses to stress. Pp. 177–207 in Food Components to Enhance Performance, An Evaluation of Potential Performance-Enhancing Food Components for Operational Rations, B.M. Marriott, ed. A report of the Committee on Military Nutrition Research, Food and Nutrition Board, Institute of Medicine. Washington, D.C.: National Academy Press.

Belenky, G., D.M. Penetar, D. Thorne, K. Popp, J. Leu, M. Thomas, H. Sing, T. Balkin, N. Wesenten, and D. Redmond
  1994 The effects of sleep deprivation on performance during continuous combat operations. Pp. 127–135 in Food Components to Enhance Performance, An Evaluation of Potential Performance-Enhancing Food Components for Operational Rations, B.M. Marriott, ed. A report of the Committee on Military Nutrition Research, Food and Nutrition Board, Institute of Medicine. Washington, D.C.: National Academy Press.

Bendelac, A.
  1995 CD1: Presenting unusual antigens to unusual T lymphocytes. Science 269:185–192.

Bergot, M-O., M-J.M. Diaz-Guerra, N. Puzenat, M. Raymondjean, and A. Kahn
  1992 Cis-regulation of the L-type pyruvate kinase gene promoter by glucose, insulin and cyclic AMP. Nucleic Acids Res. 20:1871–1877.

Berkelhammer, C.H., L.A. Lelter, K.N. Jeejeebhoy, A.S. Detsky, D.G. Oreopoulos, P.R. Uldall, and J.P. Baker
  1985 Skeletal muscle function in chronic renal failure: An index of nutritional status. Am. J. Clin. Nutr. 42:846–864.

Berlin, C., E.L. Berg, M.J. Briskin, D.P. Andrew, P.J. Kilshaw, B. Holzmann, I.L. Weissman, A. Hamann, and E.C. Butcher
  1993 $\alpha 4\beta 7$ integrin mediates lymphocyte binding to the mucosal vascular addressin MAdCAM-1. Cell 74:185–195.

Berthold, H.K., D.L. Hachey, P.J. Reeds, O.P. Thomas, S. Hoeksema, and P.D. Klein
  1991 Uniformly ^{13}C-labeled algal protein used to determine amino acid essentiality *in vivo*. Proc. Natl. Acad. Sci. USA 88:8091–8095.

Berthold, H.K., L.J. Wykes, F. Jahoor, P.D. Klein, and P.J. Reeds
  1994 The use of uniformly labelled substrates and mass isotopomer analysis to study intermediary metabolism. Proc. Nutr. Soc. 53:345–354.

Berthold, H.K., P.F. Crain, I. Gouni, P.J. Reeds, and P.D. Klein
  1995 Evidence for incorporation of intact dietary pyrimidine (but not purine) nucleosides into hepatic RNA. Proc. Natl. Acad. Sci. USA 92(2):10123–10127.

Best, W.R., and W.J. Kuhl
  1955 Physical, roentgenologic and chemical anthropometry in basic trainees. Technical Report No. 157. Denver, Colo.: Medical Nutrition Laboratory.

Betz, A.G., M.S. Neuberger, and C. Milstein
  1993 Discriminating intrinsic and antigen-selected mutational hotspots in immunoglobulin V genes. Immunol. Today 14:405–411.

Beutler, B., and A. Cerami
  1986 Cachectin and tumour necrosis factor as two sides of the same biological coin. Nature 320:584–588.

Beutler, B., N. Krochin, I.W. Milsark, C. Luedke, and A. Cerami
  1986 Control of cachectin (tumor necrosis factor) synthesis: Mechanisms of endotoxin resistance. Science 232:977–980.

Beylot, M.
  1994 The use of stable isotopes and mass spectrometry in studying lipid metabolism. Proc. Nutr. Soc. 53:355–362.

Bier, D.M.
  1987 The use of stable isotopes in metabolic investigation. Bailliere's Clin. Endocrinol. Metab. 1(4):817–836.

Biewener, A.A.
  1989 Scaling body support in mammals: Limb posture and muscle mechanics. Science 245:45–48.

Biewener, A., R.M. Alexander, and N.C. Heglund
 1981   Elastic energy storage in the hopping of kangaroo rats (*Dipodomys spectabilis*). J.
        Zool. (Lond.) 195:369–383.
Biolo, G., D. Chinkes, X-J. Zhang, and R.R. Wolfe
 1992   A new model to determine *in vivo* the relationship between amino acid transmem-
        brane transport and protein kinetics in muscle. J. Parenter. Enteral Nutr. 16:305–
        315.
Biolo, G., A. Gastaldelli, X-J. Zhang, and R.R. Wolfe
 1994   Protein synthesis and breakdown in skin and muscle: A leg model of amino acid
        kinetics. Am. J. Physiol. 267:E467–E474.
Biolo, G., R.Y.D. Fleming, and R.R. Wolfe
 1995   Physiologic hyperinsulinemia stimulates protein synthesis and enhances transport
        of selected amino acids in human skeletal muscle. J. Clin. Invest. 95:811–819.
Björntorp, P.
 1986   Adipose tissue distribution and morbidity. Pp. 60–65 in Recent Advances in Obe-
        sity Research, V.E.M. Berry, S.H. Blundheim, H.E. Eliahou, and E. Shafrir, eds.
        London: John Libby.
 1990   Obesity and adipose tissue distribution as risk factors for the development of dis-
        ease. Infusiontherapie 17:24–27.
Blair, H.A., R.J. Dern, and P.L. Bates
 1947   The measurement of volume of gas in the digestive tract. Am. J. Physiol. 149:688–
        707.
Blair, S.N.
 1993   Evidence for success of exercise in weight loss and control. Ann. Intern. Med.
        119:702–706.
Blair, S.N., H.W. Kohl, N.F. Gordon, and R.S. Paffenbarger, Jr.
 1992   How much physical activity is good for health? Annu. Rev. Public Health 13:99–
        126.
Blake, G.M., J.C. Parker, F.M.A. Buxton, and I. Fogelman
 1993   Dual x-ray absorptiometry: A comparison between fan beam and pencil beam
        scans. Br. J. Radiol. 66:902–906.
Blanchard, R.K., and R.J. Cousins
 1996   Differential display of intestinal mRNAs regulated by dietary zinc. Proc. Natl.
        Acad. Sci. USA 93:6863–6868.
Blickhan, R.
 1989   The spring-mass model for running and hopping. J. Biomech. 22:1217–1227.
Bloch, F., W.W. Hansen, and M.E. Packard
 1946   Nuclear introduction. Phys. Rev. 70:460–474.
Bloomfield, J.R., and S.A. Carroll
 1996   New measures of driving performance. Pp. 335–340 in Contemporary Ergonomics,
        S.A. Robertson, ed. London: Taylor and Francis.
Bloomfield, J.R., J.R. Buck, S.A. Carroll, M.W. Booth, R.A. Romano, D.V. McGehee, and
        R.A. North
 1995   Human factors aspects of the transfer of control from the automated highway sys-
        tem to the driver. Technical Report No. FHWA-RD-94-114. Washington, D.C.:
        U.S. Department of Transportation, Federal Highway Administration.
Bloomfield, J.R., J.R. Buck, J.M. Christensen, and A. Yenamandra
 1995   Human factors aspects of the transfer of control from the driver to the automated
        highway system. Technical Report No. FHWA-RD-94-173. Washington, D.C.:
        U.S. Department of Transportation, Federal Highway Administration.

Bloomfield, J.R., J.M. Christensen, S.A. Carroll, and G.S. Watson
  1996   The driver's response to decreasing vehicle separations during transitions into the automated lane. Technical Report No. FHWA-RD-95-107. Washington, D.C.: U.S. Department of Transportation, Federal Highway Administration.
Bloomfield, J.R., J.M. Christensen, A.D. Peterson, J.M. Kjaer, and A. Gault
  1996   Transferring control from the driver to the automated highway system with varying degrees of automation. Technical Report No. FHWA-RD-95-108. Washington, D.C.: U.S. Department of Transportation, Federal Highway Administration.
Bock, G.H., L. Neu, C. Long, L.T. Patterson, S. Korb, J. Gelpi, and D.L. Nelson
  1994   An assessment of serum and urine soluble interleukin-2 receptor concentrations during renal transplant rejection. Am. J. Kidney Dis. 23:421–426.
Bolot, J-F., G. Fournier, A. Bertoye, J. Lenior, P. Jenin, and A. Thomasset
  1977   Determination of lean body mass by the electrical impedance measure. Presse Med. 6:2249–2251.
Borkan, G.A., S.G. Gerzof, A.H. Robbins, D.E. Hults, C.K. Silbert, and J.E. Silbert
  1982   Assessment of abdominal fat content by computerized tomography. Am. J. Clin. Nutr. 36:172–177.
Boulier, A., J. Fricker, A.L. Thomasset, and M. Apfelbaum
  1990   Fat-free mass estimation by the two electrode impedance method. Am. J. Clin. Nutr. 52:581–585.
Boutton, T.W.
  1991   Stable carbon isotope ratios of natural materials: I. Sample preparation and mass spectrometric analysis. Pp. 155–171 in Carbon Isotope Techniques, D.C. Coleman and D.M. Jones, eds. San Diego: Academic Press, Inc.
Bowers-Komro, D.M., and D.B. McCormick
  1987   Riboflavin uptake by isolated rat kidney cells. Pp. 449–453 in Flavins and Flavoproteins, D.E. Edmondson and D.B. McCormick, eds. New York: Walter de Gruyter.
Bowman, B.B., and D.B. McCormick
  1989   Pyridoxine uptake by rat renal proximal tubular cells. J. Nutr. 119:745–749.
Bowman, B.B., D.B. McCormick, and I.H. Rosenberg
  1989   Epithelial transport of water-soluble vitamins. Annu. Rev. Nutr. 9:187–199.
Brandtzaeg, P.
  1994   Distribution and characteristics of mucosal immunoglobulin-producing cells. Pp. 251–262 in Handbook of Mucosal Immunology, P.L. Ogra, J. Mestecky, M.E. Lamm, W. Strober, J.R. McGhee, and J. Bienenstock, eds. Boston: Academic Press, Inc.
Bray, G.A., F.L. Greenway, M.E. Molitch, W.T. Dahms, R.L. Atkinson, and K. Hamilton
  1978   Use of anthropometric measures to assess weight loss. Am. J. Clin. Nutr. 31:769–773.
Briggs, M.R., C. Yokoyama, X. Wang, M.S. Brown, and J.L. Goldstein
  1993   Nuclear protein that binds sterol regulatory element of low-density lipoprotein receptor promoter. I. Identification of the protein and delineation of its target nucleotide sequence. J. Biol. Chem. 268:14490–14496.
Brinkmann, A., C.F. Wolf, D. Berger, F. Kneitinger, B. Neumeister, M. Büchler, P. Radermacher, W. Seeling, and M. Georgieff
  1996   Perioperative endotoxemia and bacterial translocation during major abdominal surgery: Evidence for the protective effect of endogenous prostacyclin. Crit. Care Med. 24:1293–1301.
Brough, W., G. Horne, A. Blout, M.H. Irving, and K.N. Jeejeebhoy
  1986   Effects of nutrient intake, surgery, sepsis, and long-term administration of steroids on muscle function. Br. J. Med. 293:983–988.

Brown, J.L., J.W. Dominik, and R.L. Morrissey
  1981   Respiratory infectivity of a recently isolated Egyptian strain of Rift Valley fever virus. Infect. Immun. 33:848–853.
Brownell, K.D., and J. Rodin
  1994   The dieting maelstrom. Is it possible and advisable to lose weight? Am. Psychol. 49(9):781–791.
Brownell, K.D., A.A. Stunkard, and J.M. Albaun
  1980   Evaluation and modification of exercise patterns in the natural environment. Am. J. Psychiatry 137:1540–1545.
Brozék, J., and A. Keys
  1951   The evaluation of leanness-fatness in man: Norms and interrelationships. Br. J. Nutr. 5:194–206.
Brozék, J., F. Grande, J.T. Anderson, and A. Keys
  1963   Densitometric analysis of body composition: Revision of some quantitative assumptions. Ann. N.Y. Acad. Sci. 110:113–140.
Bruce, R.A., F. Kusumi, and D. Hosmer
  1973   Maximal oxygen intake and nomographic assessment of functional aerobic impairment in cardiovascular disease. Am. Heart J. 85:546–562.
Brugnera, E., O. Georgiev, F. Radtke, R. Heuchel, E. Baker, G.R. Sutherland, and W. Schaffner
  1994   Cloning, chromosomal mapping and characterization of the human metal-regulatory transcription factor MTF-1. Nucleic Acids Res. 22:3167–3173.
Brummer, R.J.M., L. Lonn, U.L. Grangard, B.A. Bengtsson, H. Kvist, and L. Sjöström
  1993   Adipose tissue and muscle volume determinations by computed tomography in acromegaly, before and one year after adenectomy. Eur. J. Clin. Invest. 23:199–205.
Brusilow, S.W., and A.L. Horwich
  1989   Urea cycle enzymes. Pp. 629–663 in The Metabolic Basis of Inherited Disease, C.R. Scriver, A.L. Beaudet, W.S. Sly, and D. Valle, eds. New York: McGraw-Hill Info. Services Co., Health Professions Division.
Bunt, J.C., T.G. Lohman, and R.A. Boileau
  1989   Impact of total body water fluctuations on estimation of body fat from body density. Med. Sci. Sports Exerc. 21:96–100.
Burger, G.C.E., J.C. Drummond, and H.R. Sanstead
  1948   Malnutrition and Starvation in Western Netherlands, Part I. The Hague, Netherlands: General State Printing Office.
Burnett, K.R., C.B. Taylor, and W.S. Agras
  1985   Ambulatory computer-assisted therapy for obesity: A new frontier for behavior therapy. J. Consult. Clin. Psychol. 53:698–703.
Burnette, W. Neal
  1994   AB5 ADP-ribosylating toxins: Comparative anatomy and physiology. Structure 2:151–158.
Bustany, P., M. Chatel, J.M. Derlon, P. Sgouropoulos, F. Soussaline, and A. Syrota
  1986   Brain tumor protein synthesis and histological grades; a study by positron emission tomography (PET) with C-11-L-methionine. J. Neurooncol. 3:397–404.
Butcher, E.C.
  1991   Leukocyte endothelial cell recognition: Three or more steps to specificity and diversity. Cell 67:1033–1036.
Butcher, E.C., and L.J. Picker
  1996   Lymphocyte homing and homeostasis. Science 272:60–66.

Butcher, E.C., R.C. Scollay, and I.L. Weissman
  1980   Organ specificity of lymphocyte migration: Mediation by highly selective lymphocyte interaction with organ-specific determinants on high endothelial venules. Eur. J. Immunol. 10:556—561.
Byers, T.
  1995   Body weight and mortality [editorial]. New Engl. J. Med. 333:723–724.
Cahill, R.N.P., D.C. Poskitt, H. Frost, and Z. Trnka
  1977   Two distinct pools of recirculating T lymphocytes: Migratory characteristics of nodal and intestinal T lymphocytes. J. Exp. Med. 145:420–428.
Calandra, T., J. Gerain, D. Heumann, J.D. Baumgartner, and M.P. Glauser
  1991   High circulating levels of interleukin-6 in patients with septic shock: Evolution during sepsis, prognostic value, and interplay with other cytokines. The Swiss-Dutch J5 Immunoglobulin Study Group. Am. J. Med. 91:23–29.
Calder, A.G., S.E. Anderson, I. Grant, M.A. McNurlan, and P.J. Garlick
  1992   The determination of low d_5-phenylalanine enrichment (0.001–0.09 atoms percent excess), after conversion to phenylethylamine, in relation to protein turnover studies by gas chromatography/mass spectrometry. Rapid Commun. Mass Spectrom. 6:421–424.
Campen, D.H., D.A. Horwitz, F.P Quismorio, Jr., G.R. Ehresmann, and W.J. Martin
  1988   Serum levels of interleukin-2 receptor and activity of rheumatic diseases characterized by immune cell activation. Arthritis Rheum. 31:1358–1364.
Carayannopoulos, L., and J.D. Capra
  1993   Immunoglobulins. Structure and function. Pp. 293–314 in Fundamental Immunology, 3rd ed., W.E. Paul, ed. New York: Raven Press, Ltd.
Carney, J.M., W. Landrum, L. Mayes, Y. Zou, and R.A. Lodder
  1993   Near-infrared spectrophotometric monitoring of stroke-related changes in the protein and lipid composition of whole gerbil brains. Anal. Chem. 65(10):1305–1313.
Cavagna, G.A., F.P. Sabiene, and R. Margaria
  1964   Mechanical work in running. J. Appl. Physiol. 19:249–256.
Cavanaugh, P.R., and K.R. Williams
  1982   The effect of stride length variation on oxygen uptake during distance running. Med. Sci. Sports Exerc. 14:30–35.
Cebra, J.J., P.J. Gearhart, R. Kamat, S.M. Robertson, and J. Tseng
  1977   Origin and differentiation of lymphocytes involved in the secretory IgA responses. Cold Spring Harbor Symp. Quant. Biol. 41:201–215.
Ceesay, S.M., A.M. Prentice, K.C. Day, P.R. Murgatroyd, G.R. Goldberg, and W. Scott
  1989   The use of heart rate monitoring in the estimation of energy expenditure: A validation study using indirect whole-body calorimetry. Br. J. Nutr. 61:175–186.
Cepek, K.L., S.K. Shaw, C.M. Parker, G.J. Russell, J.S. Morrow, D.L. Rimm, and M.B. Brenner
  1994   Adhesion between epithelial cells and T lymphocytes mediated by E-cadherin and the $\alpha E\beta 7$ integrin. Nature 372:190–193.
Cha, K., E.F. Brown, and D.W. Wilmore
  1994   A new bioelectrical impedance method for measurement of the erythrocyte sedimentation rate. Physiol. Meas. 15:499–508.
Cha, K., R.G. Faris, E.F. Brown, and D.W. Wilmore
  1994   An electronic method for rapid measurement of haematocrit in blood samples. Physiol. Meas. 15:129–137.
Chase, M.W.
  1946   Inhibition of experimental drug allergy by prior feeding of the sensitivity agent. Proc. Soc. Exp. Biol. Med. 61:257–259.

Chastain, J.L., and D.B. McCormick
  1991 Flavin metabolites. Pp. 195–200 in Chemistry and Biochemistry of Flavoenzymes, vol. 1, F. Müller, ed. Boca Raton, Fla.: CRC Press.
Chen, Y., J. Inobe, R. Marks, P. Gonnella, V.K. Kuchroo, and H.L. Weiner
  1995 Peripheral deletion of antigen-reactive T-cells in oral tolerance. Nature 376:177–189.
Cheng, K.N., F. Dworzak, G.C. Ford, M.J. Rennie, and D. Halliday
  1985 Direct determination of leucine and protein metabolism in humans using L-[1-^{13}C,^{15}N]-leucine and the forearm model. Eur. J. Clin. Invest. 15:349–354.
Chiplonkar, S.A., V.V. Agte, M.K. Gokhale, V.V. Kulkarni, and S.T. Mane
  1992 Energy intake and resting metabolic rate of young Indian men and women. Indian J. Med. Res. 96:250–254.
Chouinard, M.J., and C.M. Braun
  1993 A meta-analysis of the relative sensitivity of neuropsychological screening tests. J. Clin. Exp. Neuropsychol. 15(4):591–607.
Chowdhury, B., L. Sjöström, M. Alpsten, J. Kostanty, H. Kvist, and R. Löfgren
  1994 A multicompartment body composition technique based on computerized tomography. Int. J. Obes. 18:219–234.
Choy, B., and M.R. Green
  1993 Eukaryotic activators function during multiple steps of preinitiation complex assembly. Nature 366:531–536.
Christensen, C.C., H.M.M. Frey, E. Foenstelien, E. Aadland, and H.E. Refsum
  1983 A critical evaluation of energy expenditure estimates based on individual O_2 consumption/heart rate curves and average daily heart rate. Am. J. Clin. Nutr. 37:468–472.
Christian, P.E.
  1994 Physics of nuclear medicine. Pp. 35–52 in Nuclear Medicine. Technology and Techniques, 3d ed., D.R. Bernier, P.E. Christian, and J.K. Langan, eds. St. Louis, Mo.: Mosby.
Christensen, P., B. Eriksen, and S.W. Henneberg
  1993 Precision of a new bedside method for estimation of the circulating blood volume. Acta Anaesthesiol. Scand. 37(6):622–627.
Christie, P.M., and G.L. Hill
  1990 Effect of intravenous nutrition on nutrition and function in acute attacks of inflammatory bowel disease. Gastroenterology 99:730–736.
Chumlea, W.C., and R.N. Baumgartner
  1990 Bioelectrical impedance methods for the estimation of body composition. Can. J. Sport Sci. 15(3):172–179.
Chumlea, W.C., and S.S. Guo
  1994 Bioelectrical impedance and body composition: Present status and future directions. Nutr. Rev. 52(4):123–131.
Chumlea, W.C., A.F. Roche, S. Guo, and B. Woynarowska
  1987 The influence of physiologic variables and oral contraceptives on bioelectric impedance. Hum. Biol. 59:257–270.
Chumlea, W.C., S.S. Guo, D.B. Cockram, and R.M. Siervogel
  1996 Mechanical and physiologic modifiers and bioelectrical impedance spectrum determinants of body composition. Am. J. Clin. Nutr. 64(suppl.):413S–422S.
Clark, M.G., E.Q. Colquhoun, S. Rattigon, K.A. Dora, T.P.D. Eldershaw, J.L. Hall, and J. Ye
  1995 Vascular and endocrine control of muscle metabolism. Am. J. Physiol. 268:E797–E812.

Clark, R.R., J.M. Kuta, and J.C. Sullivan
  1993   Prediction of percent body fat in adult males using dual energy x-ray absorptiometry, skinfolds, and hydrostatic weighing. Med. Sci. Sports Exerc. 25:528–535.

Clausen, J.P
  1977   Effects of physical training on cardiovascular adjustments to exercise in man. Physiol. Rev. 57:779–816.

Clemens, J.D., D.A. Sack, J.R. Harris, F. Van Loon, J. Chakraborty, F. Ahmed, M.R. Rao, M.R. Kahn, M. Yunus, N. Huda et al.
  1990   Field trial of oral cholera vaccines in Bangladesh: Results from three-year follow-up. Lancet 335(8684):270–273.

Clements, J.D., N.M. Hartzog, and F.L. Lyon
  1988   Adjuvant activity of *Escherichia coli* heat-labile enterotoxin and effect on the induction of oral tolerance in mice to unrelated protein antigens. Vaccine 6:269–277.

Clerici, M., and G.M. Shearer
  1993   A TH_1-TH_2 switch is a critical step in the etiology of HIV infection. Immunol. Today 14:107–111.

Clerici M., F.T. Haki, D.J. Venzon, S. Blatt, C.W. Hendrix, T.A. Wynn, and G.M. Shearer
  1993   Changes in interleukin-2 and interleukin-4 production in asymptomatic, human immunodeficiency virus-seropositive individuals. J. Clin. Invest. 91:759–765.

Clubley, M., C.E. Bye, T.A. Henson, A.W. Peck, and C.J. Riddington
  1979   Effects of caffeine and cyclizine alone and in combination on human performance, subjective effects and EEG activity. Br. J. Clin. Pharmacol. 7:157–163.

Clure, C., P.B. Watts, P. Gallagher, R. Hill, S. Humphreys, and B. Wilkins
  1995   Accuracy of the TEEM 100 metabolic analyzer during maximum oxygen uptake testing of Nordic skiers [abstract]. Med. Sci. Sports Exerc. 27:S86.

Cobelli, C., G. Toffolo, D.M. Bier, and R. Nosadini
  1987   Models to interpret kinetic data in stable isotope tracer studies. Am. J. Physiol. 253:E551–E564.

Cobelli, C., G. Toffolo, and D.M. Foster
  1992   Tracer-to-tracee ratio for analysis of stabie isotope tracer data: Link with radioactive kinetic formalism. Am. J. Physiol. 262:E968–E975.

Cohn, E.J., L.E. Strong, and L.W. Hughes, Jr.
  1946   Preparation and properties of serum and plasma proteins. 4. A system for the separation of fractions of proteins and lipoprotein components of biological tissues and fluids. J. Am. Chem. Soc. 8:459.

Cohn, S.H., D. Vartsky, S. Yasamura, A. Sawitsky, I. Zoni, A. Vaswani, and K.J. Ellis
  1980   Compartmental body composition based on total-body nitrogen, potassium and calcium. Am. J. Physiol. 239:E524–E530.

Cole, R.J., and D.F. Kripke
  1988   Progress in automatic sleep/wake scoring by wrist actigraph. Sleep Res. 17:331.

Cole, T.J., and W.A. Coward
  1992   Precision and accuracy of doubly labeled water energy expenditure by multipoint and two-point methods. Am. J. Physiol. 263 (26):E965–E973.

Colotta, F., F. Re, M. Muzio, R. Bertini, N. Polentarutti, M. Sironi, J.G. Giri, S.K. Dower, J.E. Sims, and A. Mantovani
  1993   Interleukin-1 type II receptor: A decoy target for IL-1 that is regulated by IL-4. Science 261:472–475.

Comperatore, C.A., H.R. Lieberman, A.W. Kirby, B. Adams, and J.S. Crowley
  1996   Melatonin efficacy in aviation missions requiring rapid deployment and night operations. Aviat. Space Environ. Med. 67(6):520–524.

Consolazio, C.F.
  1971   Energy expenditure studies in military populations using Kofranyi-Michaelis respirometers. Am. J. Clin. Nutr. 24:1431–1437.
Consolazio, C.F., L.O. Matoush, H.L. Johnson, R.A. Nelson, and H.J. Krzywicki
  1967   Metabolic aspects of acute starvation in normal humans (10 days). Am. J. Clin. Nutr. 20:672–683.
Consolazio, C.F., L.O. Matoush, H.L. Johnson, H.J. Krzywicki, G.J. Isaac, and N.F. Witt
  1968   Metabolic aspects of calorie restriction: Hypohydration effects on body weight and blood parameters. Am. J. Clin. Nutr. 21:793–802.
Conway, J.M., and K.H. Norris
  1987   Non-invasive body composition in humans by near infrared interactance. Pp. 163–170 in *In Vivo* Body Composition Studies, K.J. Ellis, S. Yasumura, and W.D. Morgan, eds. London: The Institute of Physical Sciences in Medicine.
Conway, J.M., K.H. Norris, and C.E. Bodwell
  1984   A new approach for the estimation of body composition: Infrared interactance. Am. J. Clin. Nutr. 40:1123–1130.
Conway, J.M., S.Z. Yanovski, N.A. Avila, and V.S. Hubbard
  1995   Visceral adipose tissue differences in black and white women. Am. J. Clin. Nutr. 61:765–771.
Cormack, M.M.
  1980   Early two-dimensional reconstruction and recent topics stemming from it. Med. Phys. 7:277–281.
Cote, K., and W.C. Adams
  1993   Effect of bone density on body composition estimates in young adult black and white women. Med. Sci. Sports Exerc. 25:290–296.
Cousins, R.J.
  1994   Metal elements and gene expression. Annu. Rev. Nutr. 14:449–469.
  1995   Trace element micronutrients. Pp. 898–901 in Molecular Biology and Biotechnology: A Comprehensive Desk Reference, R.A. Meyers, ed. New York: VCH Publishers.
Coward, A.
  1990   The doubly labeled water method for measuring energy expenditure. Technical recommendations for use in humans. Calculation of pool sizes and flux rates. Pp. 48–68 in NAHRES-4, A Consensus Report by the IDECG Working Group, A.M. Prentice, ed. Vienna: IAEA.
Coward, W.A.
  1988   The doubly labeled water ($^2H_2^{18}O$) method: Principles and practice. Proc. Nutr. Soc. 47:209–218.
Coward, W.A., P. Ritz, and T.J. Cole
  1994   Revision of calculations in the doubly labeled water method for measurement of energy expenditure in humans. Am. J. Physiol. 267 (30):E805–E807.
Coyle, E.F.
  1991   Carbohydrate feedings: Effects on metabolism, performance and recovery. Pp. 1–14 in Advances in Nutrition and Top Sport. Basel: Karger.
Crandall, C.G., S.L. Taylor, and P.B. Raven
  1994   Evaluation of the COSMED K2 portable telemetric oxygen uptake analyzer. Med. Sci. Sports Exerc. 26:108–111.
Cremer, J., Y.E. Papelis, J. Kearney, and R.A. Romano
  1994   The software architecture for scenario control in the Iowa Driving Simulator. Pp. 373–381 in Proceedings of the 4th Annual Computer-Generated Forces and Behavioral Representation Conference. Orlando, Fla.: Institute for Simulation and Training.

Cremer, J., J. Kearney, and Y. Papelis
  1995   HCSM: A framework for behavior and scenario control in virtual environments. ACM Trans. Modeling Comp. Simul. 5(3):242–267.
Cremer, J., J. Kearney, and Y.E. Papelis
  1996   Driving simulation: Challenges for VR technology. IEEE Comp. Graphics Appl. 16(5):16–20.
Crews, H.M., V. Ducros, J. Eagles, F.A. Mellon, P. Kastenmayer, J.B. Luten, and B.A. McGaw
  1994   Mass spectrometric methods for studying nutrient mineral and trace element absorption and metabolism in humans using stable isotopes. A review. Analyst 119:2491–2514.
Crowdy, J.P., C.F. Consolazio, A.L. Forbes, M.F. Haisman, and D.E. Worsley
  1982   The metabolic effects of a restricted food intake on men working in a tropical environment. Hum. Nutr. Appl. Nutr. 36A:325–344.
Cryz, S.J., Jr., ed.
  1991   Vaccines and Immunotherapy. Pp. 1–463. New York: Pergamon Press.
Cuff, C.E., C.K. Cebra, D.H. Rubin, and J.J. Cebra
  1993   Developmental relationship between cytotoxic α/β T-cell receptor-positive intraepithelial lymphocytes and Peyer's patch lymphocytes. Eur. J. Immunol. 23:1333–1339.
Daghighian, F., R. Sumida, and M.E. Phelps
  1990   PET imaging: An overview and instrumentation. J. Nucl. Med. Technol. 18:5–15.
Dallas, W.S., and S. Falkow
  1980   Amino acid sequence homology between cholera toxin and *Escherichia coli* heat-labile toxin. Nature (London) 288:499–501.
Damadian, R.
  1971   Tumor detection by nuclear magnetic resonance. Science 171:1151–1153.
Damas, P., D. Ledoux, M. Nys, Y. Vrindts, D. De Groote, P. Franchimont, and M. Lamy
  1992   Cytokine serum level during severe sepsis in human IL-6 as a marker of severity. Ann. Surg. 215:356–362.
Dansgaard, W.
  1964   Stable isotopes in precipitation. Tellus 16:436–468.
DasGupta, B.R., ed.
  1993   Botulinum and Tetanus Neurotoxins, Neurotransmission and Biomedical Aspects. New York: Plenum Press.
da Silva, J.J.R., and R.J.P. Williams, eds.
  1991   The Biological Chemistry of the Elements: The Inorganic Chemistry of Life. Oxford: Clarendon Press.
Dausch, J.G.
  1992   The problem of obesity: Fundamental concepts of energy metabolism gone awry. Crit. Rev. Food Sci. Nutr. 31:271–298.
Dawid, I.B., R. Toyama, and M. Taira
  1995   LIM domain proteins. C. R. Acad. Sci. Paris 318:295–306.
De Blasi, R.A., M. Ferrari, A. Natali, G. Conti, A. Mega, and A. Gasparetto
  1994   Noninvasive measurement of forearm blood flow and oxygen consumption by near-infrared spectroscopy. J. Appl. Physiol. 76(3):1388–1393.
DeFronzo, R.A., R.C. Bonadonna, and E. Ferrannini
  1992   Pathogenesis of NIDDM: A precarious balance between insulin action and insulin secretion. Pp. 569–663 in International Textbook of Diabetes Mellitus, vol. 1, K.G.M.M. Alberti, R.A. DeFronzo, H. Keen, and P. Zimmet, eds. Chichester: John Wiley and Sons.

Del Prete, G., M. De Carli, F. Almerigogna, C.K. Daniel, M.M. D'Elios, G. Zancuoghi, F. Vinante, G. Pizzolo, and S. Romagnani
   1995   Preferential expression of CD30 by human CD4+ T cells producing TH2-type cytokines. FASEB J. 9:81–86.

DeLany, J.P., D.A. Schoeller, R.W. Hoyt, E.W. Askew, and M.A. Sharp
   1989   Field use of $D_2^{18}O$ to measure energy expenditure of soldiers at different energy intakes. J. Appl. Physiol. 67(5):1922–1929.

DeLany, J.P., R.J. Moore, and R.W. Hoyt
   1991   Use of doubly labeled water for measurement of energy of soldiers during training exercises in a cold environment and at high altitude [abstract]. Int. J. Obes. 15:48.

DeLucia, P.R., and R. Warren
   1994   Pictorial and motion-based depth information during active control of self-motion: Size-arrival effects on collision avoidance. J. Exp. Psychol. Hum. Percept. Perform. 20(4):783–798.

De Maio, A.
   1995   The heat shock response. New Horizons 3:198–207.

Denton, R.M., and J.M. Tavaré
   1992   Action of insulin on intracellular processes. Pp. 385–408 in International Textbook of Diabetes Mellitus, vol. 1, K.G.M.M. Alberti, R.A. DeFronzo, H. Keen, and P. Zimmet, eds. Chichester: John Wiley and Sons.

de Ridder, C.M., R.M. de Boer, J.C. Seidell, C.M. Nieuwenhoff, J.A.L. Jeneson, C.J.G. Bakker, M.L. Zonderland, and W.B.M. Erich
   1992   Body fat distribution in pubertal girls quantified by magnetic resonance imaging. Int. J. Obes. 16:443–449.

Dertzbaugh, M.T., and C.O. Elson
   1991   Cholera toxin as a mucosal adjuvant. Pp. 120–131 in Topics in Vaccine Adjuvant Research, D.R. Spriggs and W.C. Koff, eds. Boca Raton, Fla.: CRC Press, Inc.
   1993a Comparative effectiveness of the cholera toxin B subunit and alkaline phosphatase as carriers for oral vaccines. Infect. Immun. 61(1):48–55.
   1993b Reduction in oral immunogenicity of cholera toxin B subunit by N-terminal peptide addition. Infect. Immun. 61(2):384–390.

Despres, J-P., C. Bouchard, A. Tremblay, R. Savard, and M. Marcotte
   1985   Effects of aerobic training on fat distribution in male subjects. Med. Sci. Sports Med. 17:113–118.

Despres, J-P., M-C. Pouliot, S. Moorjani, A. Nadeau, A. Tremblay, P.J. Lupien, G. Theriault, and C. Bouchard
   1991   Loss of abdominal fat and metabolic response to exercise training in obese women. Am. J. Physiol. 261:E159–E167.

Despres, J-P., D. Prud'homme, M-C. Pouliot, A. Tremblay, and C. Bouchard
   1991   Estimation of deep abdominal adipose-tissue accumulation from simple anthropometric measurements in men. Am. J. Clin. Nutr. 54:471–477.

Des Rosiers, C., L. Di Donato, B. Comte, A. Laplante, C. Marcoux, F. David, C.A. Fernandez, and H. Brunengraber
   1995   Isotopomer analysis of citric acid cycle and gluconeogenesis in rat liver. Reversibility of isocitrate dehydrogenase and involvement of ATP-citrate lyase in gluconeogenesis. J. Biol. Chem. 270:10027–10036.

Deurenberg, P., and F.J.M. Schouten
   1992   Loss of total body water and extracellular water assessed by multifrequency impedance. Eur. J. Clin. Nutr. 46:247–255.

Deurenberg, P., K.V.D. Kooy, A. Paling, and P. Withagen
   1989   Assessment of body composition in 8–11 year old children by bioelectrical impedance. Eur. J. Clin. Nutri. 43:623–629.

Deurenberg, P., J.A. Weststrate, and J.G.A.J. Hautvast
  1989 Changes in fat-free mass during weight loss measured by bioelectrical impedance and by densitometry. Am. J. Clin. Nutr. 49:33–36.
Deurenberg, P., F.J.M. Schouten, A. Andreoli, and A. de Lorenzo
  1993 Assessment of changes in extracellular water and total body water using multifrequency bio-electrical impedance. Pp. 129–132 in Human Body Composition, K.J. Ellis and J.D. Eastman, eds. New York: Plenum Press.
Deurenberg, P., E. Van Malkenhorst, and T. Schoen
  1995 Distal versus proximal electrode placement in the prediction of total body water and extracellular water from multifrequency bioelectrical impedance. Am. J. Hum. Biol. 7:77–83.
Dews, P.B., ed.
  1984 Behavioral effects of caffeine. Pp. 86–100 in Caffeine. New York: Springer-Verlag.
DHHS (U.S. Department of Health and Human Services)
  1988 The Surgeon General's Report on Nutrition and Health—Summary and Recommendations. DHHS (PHS) Publ. No. 88-50211. Public Health Service, U.S. Department of Health and Human Services. Washington, D.C.: U.S. Government Printing Office.
Dickinson, B.L., and J.D. Clements
  1995 Dissociation of *Escherichia coli* heat-labile enterotoxin adjuvanticity from ADP-ribosyltranserase activity. Infect. Immun. 63(5):1617–1623.
Dinarello, C.A.
  1994 The biological properties of interleukin-1. Eur. Cytokine Netw. 5:517–531.
Dinarello, C.A., and S.M. Wolff
  1993 The role of interleukin-1 in disease. N. Engl. J. Med. 326:106–113.
Dinges, D.F.
  1992 Probing the limits of functional capability: The effects of sleep loss on short-duration tasks. Pp. 176–188 Sleep, Arousal and Performance, R.J. Broughton and R. Ogilvie, eds. Cambridge, Mass.: Birkhauser-Boston, Inc.
Dinges, D.F., and N.B. Kribbs
  1991 Performing while sleepy: Effects of experimentally induced sleepiness. Pp. 97–128 in Sleep, Sleepiness, and Performance, T.H. Monk, ed. New York: John Wiley & Sons, Ltd.
Dinges, D.F., and J.W. Powell
  1985 Microcomputer analyses of performance on a portable, simple visual RT task during sustained operations. Behav. Res. Meth. Instr. Comput. 17:652–655.
Dixon, M., and E.L. Webb
  1979 Enzymes. New York: Academic.
Doane, S.M., D.S. McNamara, W. Kintsch, P.G. Polson, and D.M. Clawson
  1992 Prompt comprehension in UNIX command production. Mem. Cognit. 20(4):327–343.
Dollins, A.B., H.J. Lynch, M.H. Deng, K.U. Kischka, R.E. Gleason, R.J. Wurtman, and H.R. Lieberman
  1993 Effect of pharmacological daytime doses of melatonin on human mood and performance. Psychopharmacology 112:490–496.
Dormont, J.
  1994 Future treatment strategies in HIV infection. AIDS 8 (suppl. 3):S31–S33.
Dreyer, C., G. Krey, H. Keller, F. Givel, G. Helftenbein, and W. Wahli
  1992 Control of the peroxisomal β-oxidation pathway by a novel family of nuclear hormone receptors. Cell 68:879–887.

Ducimetiere, P., J. Richard, and F. Cambien
  1986 The pattern of subcutaneous fat distribution in middle-aged men and the risk of coronary heart disease: The Paris Prospective Study. Int. J. Obes. 10:229–240.
Ducrot, H., A. Thomasset, R. Jolz, P. Jungers, C. Eyraud, and J. Lenior
  1970 Determination of extracellular fluid volume in man by measurement of whole body impedance. Presse Med. 51:2269–2272.
Dunne, C.P.
  1994 Biochemical strategies for ration design: Concerns of bioavailability. Pp. 93–109 in Food Components to Enhance Performance, An Evaluation of Potential Performance-Enhancing Food Components for Operational Rations, B.M. Marriott, ed. A report of the Committee on Military Nutrition Research, Food and Nutrition Board, Institute of Medicine. Washington, D.C.: National Academy Press.
Durnin, J.V.G.A., and Satwanti
  1982 Variations in the assessment of the fat content of the human body due to experimental technique in measuring body density. Ann. Hum. Biol. 9:221–225.
Durnin, J.V.G.A., and J. Womersley
  1974 Body fat assessed from total body density and its estimation from skinfold thickness: Measurements on 481 men and women aged from 16 to 72 years. Br. J. Nutr. 32:77–97.
Duyn, J.H., V.S. Mattay, R.H. Sexton,G.S. Sobering, F.A. Barrios, G. Liu, J.A. Frank, D.R. Weinberger, and C.T. Moonen
  1994 Three-dimensional functional imaging of human brain using echo-shifted FLASH MRI. Magn. Reson. Med. 32:150.
Ebnet, K., E.P. Kaldjian, A.O. Anderson, and S. Shaw
  1996 Orchestrated information transfer underlying leukocyte endothelial interactions. Ann. Rev. Immunol. 14:155–177
Eckmann, L., M.F. Kagnoff, and J. Fierer
  1993 Epithelial cells secrete the chemokine interleukin-8 in response to bacterial entry. Infect. Immun. 61:4569–4574.
Edwards, J.S.A., E.W. Askew, N. King, C.S. Fulco, R.W. Hoyt, and J.P. DeLany
  1991 An assessment of the nutritional intake and energy expenditure of unacclimatized U.S. Army soldiers living and working at high altitude. Technical Report No. T10-91. Natick, Mass.: U.S. Army Research Institute of Environmental Medicine.
Eiken, P., O. Bärenholdt, L. Bjorn Jensen, J. Gram, and S. Pors Nielsen
  1994 Switching from DXA pencil-beam to fan-beam. I: Studies *in vitro* at four centers. Bone 15:667–670.
Eiken, P., N. Kolthoff, O. Bärenholdt, F. Hermansen, and S. Pors Nielsen
  1995 Switching from DXA pencil-beam to fan-beam. II: Studies *in vivo*. Bone 15:671–676.
Eisen, H.N., and G.W. Siskind
  1964 Variations in affinities of antibodies during the immune response. Biochemistry 3:996–1008.
Eldridge, J.H., C.J. Hammond, J.A. Meulbroek, J.K. Staas, R.M. Gilley, and T.R. Tice
  1990 Controlled vaccine release in the gut-associated lymphoid tissues. I. Orally administered biodegradable microspheres target the Peyer's patches. Journal of Controlled Release 11:205–214.
Elia, M.
  1995 General integration and regulation of metabolism at the organ level. Proc. Nutr. Soc. (London) 54:213–232.

Elson, C.O., and M.T. Dertzbaugh
  1994   Mucosal adjuvants. Pp. 391–401 in Handbook of Mucosal Immunology, P.L. Orga, J. Mestecky, M.E. Lamm, W. Strober, J.R. McGhee, and J. Bienestock, eds. New York: Academic Press, Inc.
Elson, C.O., and W. Ealding
  1984a Cholera toxin feeding did not induce oral tolerance in mice and abrogated oral tolerance to an unrelated protein antigen. J. Immunol. 133:2892–2897.
  1984b Generalized systemic and mucosal immunity in mice after mucosal stimulation with cholera toxin. J. Immunol. 132:2736–2741.
Elson, C.O., S.P. Holland, M.T. Dertzbaugh, C.F. Cuff, and A.O. Anderson
  1995   Morphologic and functional alterations of mucosal T-cells by cholera toxin and its B subunit. J. Immunol. 154:1032–1040.
Elson, L.H., S. Shaw, R.A. Van Liwer, and T.B. Nutman
  1994   T cell subpopulation phenotypes in filarial infections: CD27 negativity defines a population greatly enriched for TH_2 cells. Int. Immunol. 6:1003–1009.
Engelberts, I., S. Stephens, G.J. Francot, C.J. van der Linden, and W.A. Buurman
  1991   Evidence for different effects of soluble TNF-receptors on various TNF measurements in human biological fluids [letter; comment]. Lancet 338:515–516.
Engell, D.B., D.E. Roberts, E.W. Askew, M.S. Rose, J. Buchbinder, and M.A. Sharp
  1987   Evaluation of the Ration, Cold Weather during a 10-day cold weather field training exercise. Technical Report TR87/030. Natick, Mass.: U.S. Army Natick Research, Development and Engineering Center.
Engstrom, C.M., G.E. Loeb, J.R. Reid, W.J. Forrest, and L. Avruch
  1991   Morphometry of the human thigh muscles. A comparison between anatomical sections and computer tomographic and magnetic resonance images. J. Anat. 176:139–156.
Essen, P., M.A. McNurlan, J. Wernerman, E. Vinnars, and P.J. Garlick
  1992   Uncomplicated surgery, but not general anesthesia, decreases muscle protein synthesis. Am. J. Physiol. 262:E253–E260.
Ettinger, W.H., Jr., and R.F. Afable
  1994   Physical disability from knee osteoarthritis: The role of exercise as an intervention. Med. Sci. Sports Exerc. 26:1435–1440.
Evans, D.J., R.G. Hoffmann, R.K. Kalkhoff, and A.H. Kissebah
  1983   Relationship of androgenic activity to body fat topography, fat cell morphology, and metabolic aberrations in premenopausal women. J. Clin. Endocrinol. Metab. 57:304–310.
Evans, R.M.
  1988   The steroid and thyroid hormone receptor superfamily. Science 240:889–895.
Faris, F., M. Doyle, Y. Wickramasinghe, R. Houston, P. Rolfe, and S. O'Brien
  1994   A non-invasive optical technique for intrapartum fetal monitoring: Preliminary clinical studies. Med. Eng. Phys. 16(4):287–291.
Farley, C.T., and O. Gonzalez
  1996   Leg stiffness and stride frequency in human running. J. Biomech. 29(2):181–186.
Farley, C.T., and T.A. McMahon
  1992   Energetics of walking and running: Insights from reduced gravity. J. Appl. Physiol. 73:2709–2712.
Farley, C.T., R. Blickhan, J. Saito, and C.R. Taylor
  1991   Hopping frequency in humans: A test of how springs set stride frequency in bouncing gaits. J. Appl. Physiol. 71:2127–2132.
Farley, C.T., J. Glasheen, and T.A. McMahon
  1993   Running springs: Speed and animal size. J. Exp. Biol. 185:71–87.

Faulkner, D.B., K.J. Kearfott, and R.G. Manning
  1991   Planning a clinical PET center. J. Nucl. Med. Technol. 19:5–19.
Ferri, F.
  1995   The medical folder as an active tool in defining the clinical decision-making process. Med. Inf. (Lond.) 20(2):97–112.
Fine, B.J., J.L. Kobrick, H.R. Lieberman, B. Marlowe, R.H. Riley, and W.J. Tharion
  1994   Effects of caffeine or diphenhydramine on visual vigilance. Psychopharmacology 114:233–238.
Finkelman, F.D.
  1995   Relationships among antigen presentation, cytokines, immune deviation, and autoimmune disease. J. Exp. Med. 182:279–282.
Finkelstein, J.D.
  1990   Methionine metabolism in mammals. J. Nutr. Biochem. 1:228–237.
Fiorentino, D.F., A. Zlotnik, P. Vieira, T.R. Mosmann, M. Howard, K.W. Moore, and A. O'Garra
  1991   IL-10 acts on the antigen-presenting cell to inhibit cytokine production by TH_1 cells. J. Immunol. 146:3444–3451.
Fischer, E., K.J. Van Zee, M.A. Marano, C.S. Rock, J.S. Kenney, D.D. Poutsiaka, C.A. Dinarello, S.F. Lowry, and L.L. Moldawer
  1992   Interleukin-1 receptor antagonist circulates in experimental inflammation and in human disease. Blood 79:2196–2200.
Fishman, E.K.
  1994   Spiral imaging methods assure survival of CT. Diagn. Imaging. (November): 59–67.
Fitzgerald, P.I., J.A. Vogel, W.L. Daniels, J.E. Dziados, M.A. Teves, R.P. Mello, and P.J. Reich
  1986   The Body Composition Project: A summary report and descriptive data. Technical Report T5-87. Natick, Mass.: U.S. Army Research Institute of Environmental Medicine.
Fliederbaum, J., A. Heller, K. Zweibaum, and J. Zarchi
  1979   Clinical aspects of hunger disease in adults. Pp 13–36 in Hunger Disease–Studies by the Jewish Physicians in the Warsaw Ghetto, M. Wynick, ed. New York: John Wiley and Sons.
Fong, Y.M., M.A. Marano, L.L. Moldawer, H. Wei, S.E. Calvano, J.S. Kenney, A.C. Allison, A. Cerami, G.T. Shires, and S.F. Lowry
  1990a The acute splanchnic and peripheral tissue metabolic response to endotoxin in humans. J. Clin. Invest. 85:1896–1904.
Fong, Y., L.L. Moldawer, G.T. Shires, and S.F. Lowry
  1990b The biologic characteristics of cytokines and their implication in surgical injury. Surg. Gynecol. Obstet. 170:363–378.
Forbes, G.B.
  1987   Human Body Composition. Growth, Aging, Nutrition and Activity. New York: Springer-Verlag.
Forbes, G.B., W. Simon, and J.M. Amatruda
  1992   Is bioimpedance a good predictor of body composition change? Am. J. Clin. Nutr. 56:4–6.
Forbes-Ewan, C.H., B.L.L. Morrissey, G.C. Gregg, and D.R. Waters
  1989   Use of doubly labeled water technique in soldiers training for jungle warfare. J. Appl. Physiol. 67(1):14–18.

Forman, B.M., E. Goode, J. Chen, A.E. Oro, D.J. Bradley, T. Perlmann, D.J. Noonan, and L.T. Burka
 1995   Identification of a nuclear receptor that is activated by farnesol metabolites. Cell 81:687–693.
Formica, C., M.G. Atkinson, I. Nyulasi, J. McKay, W. Heale, and E. Seeman
 1993   Body composition following hemodialysis: Studies using dual-energy x-ray absorptiometry and bioelectrical impedance analysis. Osteoporos. Int. 3:192–197.
Forsyth, R., M.J. Plyley, and R.J. Shephard
 1988   Residual volume as a tool in body fat prediction. Ann. Nutr. Metab. 32:62–67.
Foster, M.A., J.M.S. Hutchison, J.R. Mallard, and M. Fuller
 1984   Nuclear magnetic resonance pulse sequence and discrimination of high- and low-fat tissues. Mag. Reson. Imaging 2:187–192.
Fowler, J.S., and A.P. Wolf
 1986   Positron emitter-labeled compounds: Priorities and problems. Pp. 391–450 in Positron Emission Tomography and Autoradiography: Principles and Applications for the Brain, M.E. Phelps, T.C. Mazziotta, and H.R. Schelbert, eds. New York: Raven Press.
Fowler, P.A., M.F. Fuller, C.A. Glasby, M.A. Foster, G.G. Cameron, G. McNiel, and R.J. Maughan
 1991   Total and subcutaneous AT distribution in women: The measurement of distribution and accurate prediction of quantity by using magnetic resonance imaging. Am. J. Clin. Nutr. 54:18–25.
Fowler, P.A., M.F. Fuller, C.A. Glasbey, G.G. Cameron, and M.A. Foster
 1992   Validation of the *in vivo* measurement of adipose tissue by magnetic resonance imaging of lean and obese pigs. Am. J. Clin. Nutr. 56:7–13.
Franz, D.R., L.M. Pitt, M.A. Clayton, J.A. Hanes, and K.J. Rose
 1993   Efficacy of prophylactic and therapeutic administration of antitoxin for inhalation botulism. Pp. 473–476 in Botulinum and Tetanus Neurotoxins, B.R. DasGupta, ed. New York: Plenum Press.
Frayn, K.N.
 1983   Calculation of substrate oxidation rates *in vivo* from gaseous exchange. J. Appl. Physiol. 55:628–634.
Freeman, J.S., G.S. Watson, Y.E. Papelis, A. Tayyab, R.A. Romano, and J.G. Kuhl
 1995   The Iowa Driving Simulator: An implementation and application overview. Pp. 81–90 in Proceedings of the Society for Automotive Engineers International Congress and Exposition. Detroit, Mich.: Society of Automotive Engineers.
Freeman, S., J.H. Last, D.T. Petty, and I.L. Faller
 1955   Total body water in man: Adaptation of measurement of total body water to field studies. Technical Report EP-11. NTIS AD-067 598. Natick, Mass.: Quartermaster Research and Development Center.
Freund, J.
 1956   The mode of action of immunological adjuvants. Adv. Tuberc. Res. 7:130–148.
Fried, M., and D.M. Crothers
 1981   Equilibria and kinetics of lac repressor-operator interactions by polyacrylamide gel electrophoresis. Nucleic Acids Res. 9:6505–6525.
Friedl, K.E.
 1992   Body composition and military performance: Origins of the Army standards. Pp. 31–55 in Body Composition and Physical Performance, Applications for the Military Services, B.M. Marriott and J. Grumstrup-Scott, eds. A report of the Committee on Military Nutrition Research, Food and Nutrition Board, Institute of Medicine. Washington D.C.: National Academy Press.

Friedl, K.E., and S.R. Plymate
  1985   Effect of obesity on reproduction in the female. J. Obes. Weight Regul. 4(2):129–145.
Friedl, K.E., and J.A. Vogel
  1992   Looking for a few good generalized body-fat equations. Am. J. Clin. Nutr. 53:795–796.
  1997   Validity of percent body fat predicted from circumferences: Classification of men for weight control regulations. Mil. Med. 162:194–200.
Friedl, K.E., C.M. DeWinne, and R.L. Taylor
  1987   The use of the Durnin-Womersley generalized equations for body fat estimation and their impact on the Army Weight Control Program. Mil. Med. 152:150–155.
Friedl, K.E., J.A. Vogel, M.W. Bovee, and B.H. Jones
  1989   Assessment of body weight standards in male and female Army recruits. Technical Report 15-90. Natick, Mass.: U.S. Army Research Institute of Environmental Medicine.
Friedl, K.E., J.P. DeLuca, L.J. Marchitelli, and J.A. Vogel
  1992   Reliability of body-fat estimations from a four-compartment model by using density, body water, and bone mineral measurements. Am. J. Clin. Nutr. 55:764–770.
Friedl, K.E., L.J. Marchitelli, S. Carson, K.A. Westphal, and W. Berkowitz
  1993   Validity of body water estimations by dual-energy x-ray absorptiometry and by bioelectrical impedance spectroscopy before and after isotonic dehydration. Research Protocol A-5827. Natick, Mass.: U.S. Army Research Institute of Environmental Medicine.
Friedl, K.E., J.A. Vogel, L.J. Marchitelli, and S.L. Kubel
  1993   Assessment of regional body composition changes by dual-energy x-ray absorptiometry. Pp. 99–103 in Human Body Composition, K.J. Ellis and J.D. Eastman, eds. New York: Plenum Press.
Friedl, K.E., R.J. Moore, L.E. Martinez-Lopez, J.A. Vogel, E.W. Askew, L.J. Marchitelli, R.W. Hoyt, and C.C. Gordon
  1994   Lower limits of body fat in healthy active men. J. Appl. Physiol. 77:933–940.
Friedl, K.E., K.A. Westphal, L.J. Marchitelli, and J.F. Patton
  1994   Effect of fat patterning on body composition changes in young women during U.S. Army basic training [abstract]. Int. J. Obes. 18(suppl. 2):69.
Friedl, K.E., M.V. Klicka, N. King, L.J. Marchitelli, and E.W. Askew
  1995   Effects of reduced fat intake on serum lipids in healthy young men and women at the U.S. Military Academy. Mil. Med. 160:527–533.
Frieling, J.T.M., M. Van Deuren, J. Wijdenes, J.W.M. Van der Meer, C. Clement, C.J. van der Linden, and R.W. Sauerwein
  1995   Circulating interleukin-6 receptor in patients with sepsis syndrome. J. Infect. Dis. 171:469–472.
Frohlich, B., G. Grunst, W. Kruger, and G. Wesche
  1995   The responsive workbench: A virtual working environment for physicians. Comput. Biol. Med. 25(2):301–308.
Fuhrman, J.A., and J.J. Cebra
  1981   Special features of the priming process for a secretory IgA response. J. Exp. Med. 153:534–544.
Fulco, C.S., K.E. Friedl, and A. Cymerman
  1991   The use of dual-energy x-ray absorptiometry for the assessment of body composition before and after an altitude exposure. FASEB J. 5:#4386.

Fulco, C.S., R.W. Hoyt, C.J. Baker-Fulco, J. Gonzalez, and A. Cymerman
1992   Use of bioelectrical impedance to assess body composition changes at high altitude. J. Appl. Physiol. 72:2181–2187.

Fuller, N.J., and M. Elia
1989   Potential use of bioelectrical impedance of the "whole body" and of body segments for the assessment of body composition: Comparison with densitometry and anthropometry. Eur. J. Clin. Nutr. 43:779–791.

Gadian, D.G.
1982   Nuclear Magnetic Resonance and Its Application to Living Systems. New York: Oxford University Press.

Gamberale, F., A. Iregen, and A. Kjellberg
1990   Computerized performance test in neurotoxicology. Pp. 359–395 in Behavioral Measures of Neurotoxicity, Report of a Symposium, R.W. Russell, P.E. Flattau, and A.M. Pope, eds. U.S. National Committee for the International Union of Psychological Science, Commission on Behavioral and Social Sciences and Education, National Research Council. Washington, D.C.: National Academy Press.

Gangarosa, E.J., W.R. Beisel, C. Benyajati, H. Sprinz, and P. Piyaratn
1960   The nature of the gastrointestinal lesion in Asiatic cholera and its relation to pathogenesis: A biopsy study. Am. J. Trop. Med. Hyg. 9:125–135.

Garard, E.L., R.C. Snow, D.N. Kennedy, R.E. Frisch, A.R. Guimaraes, R.L. Barbieri, A.G. Sorenson, T.K. Egglin, and B.R. Rosen
1991   Overall body fat and regional fat distribution in young women: Quantification with MR imaging. Am. J. Radiol. 157:97–104.

Garg, A., J.L. Fleckenstein, R.M. Peshock, and S.M. Grundy
1992   Peculiar distribution of adipose tissue in patients with congenital generalized lipodystrophy. J. Clin. Endocrinol. Metab. 75:358–361.

Garlick, P.J., and M.A. McNurlan
1994   Isotopic methods for studying protein turnover. Pp. 29–47 in Protein Metabolism During Infancy, N.C.R. Räihä, ed. New York: Raven Press.

Garn, S.M.
1957   Roentgenogrammetric determination of body composition. Hum. Biol. 29:337.
1961   Radiographic analysis of body composition. Pp. 36–58 in Techniques for Measuring Body Composition, Proceedings of a Conference, Quartermaster Research and Engineering Center, Natick, Mass., January 22–23, 1959, J. Broézek and A. Henschel, eds. Washington, D.C.: National Academy of Sciences/National Research Council.

Gascan, H., J.F. Gauchat, M.G. Roncarolo, H. Yssel, H. Spits, and J.E. deVries
1991   Human B cell clones can be induced to proliferate and to switch to IgE and IgG4 synthesis by interleukin 4 and a signal provided by activated CD4+ T cell clones. J. Exp. Med. 173:747–750.

Gasser, C.S., and R.T. Fraley
1989   Genetically engineering plants for crop improvement. Science 244:1293–1299.

Gearhart, P.J.
1993   Somatic mutation and affinity maturation. Pp. 865–885 in Fundamental Immunology, 3rd ed., W.E. Paul, ed. New York: Raven Press, Ltd.

Gelfanov, V., V. Gelfanova, Y-G. Lai, and N-S. Liao
1996   Activated $\alpha\beta$-CD8+, but not $\alpha\alpha$-CD8+, TCR-$\alpha\beta$+murine intestinal intraepithelial lymphocytes can mediate perforin-based cytotoxicity, whereas both subsets are active in Fas-based cytotoxicity. J. Immunol. 156:35–41.

Genant, H.K., S. Grampp, C.C. Glüer, K.G. Faulkner, M. Jergas, K. Engelke, S. Hagiwara, and C. Van Kuijk
1994   Universal standardization for dual x-ray absorptiometry: Patient and phantom cross-calibration results. J. Bone Miner. Res. 9:1503–1514.
Gergen, P.J., G.M. McQuillan, M. Kiely, T.M. Ezzati-Rice, R.W. Sutter, and G. Virella
1995   A population-based serologic survey of immunity to tetanus in the United States. N. Engl. J. Med. 332:761–766.
Gilbert, J.A., and J.F. Gregory III
1992   Pyridoxine-5'-β-D-glucoside affects the metabolic utilization of pyridoxine in rats. J. Nutr. 122:1029–1035.
Giri, J.G., J. Wells, S.K. Dower, C.E. McCall, R.N. Guzman, J. Slack, T.A. Bird, K. Shanebeck, K. Grabstein, J.E. Sims, and M.R. Alderson
1994   Elevated levels of shed type II IL-1 receptor in sepsis. Potential role for type II receptor regulation of IL-1 responses. J. Immunol. 153:5802–5809.
Glickman-Weiss, E.L., F.L. Goss, R.J. Robertson, K.F. Meets, and D.A. Cassinelli
1991   Physiological and thermal responses of males with varying body compositions during immersion in moderately cold water. Aviat. Space Environ. Med. 62:1063–1067.
Going, S.B., M.P. Massett, M.C. Hall, L.A. Bare, P.A. Root, D.P. Williams, and T.G. Lohman
1993   Detection of small changes in body composition by dual-energy x-ray absorptiometry. Am. J. Clin. Nutr. 57:845–850.
Gold, P.E.
1995   Role of glucose in regulating the brain and cognition. Am. J. Clin. Nutr. 61(4 suppl.):987S–995S.
Goldberg, A.L., and A. St. John
1976   Intracellular protein degradation in mammalian and bacterial cells. Annu. Rev. Biochem. 45:747–802.
Goldman, R.F., and E.R. Buskirk
1961   Body volume measurement by underwater weighing: Description of a method. Pp. 78–89 in Techniques for Measuring Body Composition, Proceedings of a Conference, Quartermaster Research and Engineering Center, Natick, Mass., January 22–23, 1959, J. Brozék and A. Henschel, eds. Washington D.C.: National Academy of Sciences/National Research Council.
Goldstein, J.L., and M.S. Brown
1990   Regulation of the mevalonate pathway. Nature 343:425–430.
Gombotz, W.R., and D.K. Pettit
1995   Biodegradable polymers for protein and peptide drug delivery. Bioconjugate Chem. 6:332–351.
Goodman, K.J., and J.T. Brenna
1992   High sensitivity tracer detection using high-precision gas chromatography-combustion isotope ratio mass spectrometry and highly enriched [U-^{13}C]-labeled precursors. Anal. Chem. 64:1088–1095.
Goodman, M.N.
1991   Tumor necrosis factor induces skeletal muscle protein breakdown in rats. Am. J. Physiol. 260:E727–E730.
Goodsitt, M.M.
1992   Evaluation of a new set of calibration standards for the measurement of fat content via DPA and DXA. Med. Phys. 19:35–44.
Gordon, C.C., and K.E. Friedl
1994   Anthropometry in the U.S. Armed Forces. Pp. 178–210 in Anthropometry: The Individual and the Population, S.J. Ulijaszek and C.G.N. Mascie-Taylor, eds. Cambridge, U.K.: Cambridge University Press.

Gottschalk, L.A.
  1994 The development, validation, and applications of a computerized measurement of cognitive impairment from the content analysis of verbal behavior. J. Clin. Psychol. 50(3):349–361.
Gould, B.A.
  1869 Investigations in the Military and Anthropological Statistics of American Soldiers. New York: Hurd and Houghton. (Also available in reprint from Arno Press, New York, 1979).
Goust, J.M., and B. Bierer
  1993 Cell-mediated immunity. Pp. 187–208 in Introduction to Medical Immunology, 3d ed., G. Virella, ed. New York: Marcel Dekker.
Graham, T.E., J.W.E. Rush, and M.H. van Soeren
  1994 Caffeine and exercise: Metabolism and performance. Can. J. Appl. Physiol. 19:111–138.
Gray, D., K. Fujioka, P.M. Colletti, H. Kim, W. Devine, T. Cuyegkeng, and T. Pappas
  1991 Magnetic-resonance imaging used for determining fat distribution in obesity and diabetes. Am. J. Clin. Nutr. 54:623–627.
Green, M.W., P.J. Rogers, N.A. Elliman, and S.J. Gatenby
  1994 Impairment of cognitive performance associated with dieting and high levels of dietary restraint. Physiol. Behav. 55(3):447–452.
Gretz, J.E., E.P. Kaldjian, A.O. Anderson, and S. Shaw
  1996 Sophisticated strategies for information encounter in the lymph node: The reticular network as a conduit of soluble information and a highway for cell traffic. J. Immunol. 157:495–499.
Griffiths, A.D., S.C. Williams, O. Hartley, I.M. Tomlinson, P. Waterhouse, W.L. Crosby, R.E. Kontermann, P.T. Jones, N.M. Low, T.J. Allison, T.D. Prospero, H.R. Hoogenboom, A. Nissim, J.P.L. Cox, J.L. Harrison, M. Zaccolo, E. Gherardi, and G. Winter
  1994 Isolation of high affinity human antibodies directly from large synthetic repertoires. EMBO J. 13:3245–3260.
Grove, G., and A.A. Jackson
  1995 Measurement of protein turnover in normal man using the end-product method with oral [^{15}N]glycine: Comparison of single-dose and intermittent-dose regimens. Brit. J. Nutr. 74:491–507.
Gunga, H-Chr., K. Kirsch, F. Baartz, H-J. Steiner, P. Wittels, and L. Röcker
  1995 Fluid distribution and tissue thickness changes in 29 men during 1 week at moderate altitude (2,315 m). Eur. J. Appl. Physiol. 70:1–5.
Guo, S.S., and W.C. Chumlea
  1996 Statistical methods for the development and testing of predictive equations. Pp. 191–202 in Human Body Composition: Methods and Findings, A.F. Roche, S.B. Heymsfield, and T.G. Lohman, eds. Champaign, Ill.: Human Kinetics Press.
Gutierrez, G., and S. Brown
  1996 Gastrointestinal tonometry: A monitor of regional dysoxia. New Horizons 4:413–419.
Haaland, D.M.
  1990 Multivariate calibration methods applied to quantitative FT-IR analyses. Pp. 395–468 in Practical Fourier Transform Infrared Spectroscopy, J.R. Ferraro and K. Krishnan, eds. New York: Academic Press.
  1992 Multivariate calibration methods applied to the quantitative analysis of infrared spectra. Pp. 1–30 in Computer-Enhanced Analytical Spectroscopy, vol. 3, P-C. Jurs, ed. New York: Plenum Press.

Haarbo, J., A. Gotfredsen, C. Hassager, and C. Christiansen
  1991 Validation of body composition by dual energy x-ray absorptiometry (DEXA). Clin. Physiol. 11:331–341.
Haas, M.W.
  1995 Virtually augmented interfaces for tactical aircraft. Biol. Psychol. 40:229–238.
Hajishengallis, G., S.K. Hollingshead, T. Koga, and M.W. Russell
  1995 Mucosal immunization with a bacterial protein antigen genetically coupled to cholera toxin A2/B subunits. J. Immunol. 154:4322–4332.
Hakala, P.
  1994 Weight reduction programmes at a rehabilitation centre and a health centre based on group counselling and individual support: Short- and long-term follow-up study. Int. J. Obes. 18:483–489.
Hall, J.W., and A. Pollard
  1993 Near-infrared spectroscopic determination of serum total proteins, albumin, globulins, and urea. Clin. Biochem. 26(6):483–490.
Halliday, D., and M.J. Rennie
  1982 The use of stable isotopes for diagnosis and clinical research. Clin. Sci. 63:485–496.
Hamann, A., D.P. Andrew, D. Jablonski-Westrich, B. Holzmann, and E.C. Butcher
  1994 Role of α4-integrins in lymphocyte homing to mucosal tissues *in vivo*. J. Immunol. 152:3282–3292.
Hamilton, S.R., J.H. Yardley, and G.D. Brown
  1979 Suppression of local intestinal immunoglobulin A immune response to cholera toxin by subcutaneous administration of cholera toxoids. Infect. Immun. 24:422–426.
Hankey, J.M., D.V. McGehee, T.A. Dingus, E.N. Mazzae, and W.R. Garrott
  1996 Initial driver avoidance behavior and reaction time to an unalerted intersection incursion. Pp. 896–899 in Proceedings of the 40th Annual Meeting of the Human Factors and Ergonomics Society. Santa Monica, Calif.: Human Factors and Ergonomics Society.
Hannan, W.J., S.J. Cowen, K.C.H. Fearon, C.E. Plester, and J.S. Falconer
  1994 Evaluation of multi-frequency bio-impedance analysis for the assessment of extracellular and total body water in surgical patients. Clin. Sci. 86:479–485.
Hannum, C.H., C.J. Wilcox, W.P. Arend, F.G. Joslin, D.J. Dripps, P.L. Heimdal, L.G. Armes, A. Sommer, S.P. Eisenberg, and R.C. Thompson
  1990 Interleukin-1 receptor antagonist activity of a human interleukin-1 inhibitor. Nature 343:336–340.
Hansen, N.J., T.G. Lohman, S.B. Going, M.C. Hall, R.W. Pamenter, L.A. Bare, T.W. Boyden, and L.B. Houtkooper
  1993 Prediction of body composition in premenopausal females from dual-energy x-ray absorptiometry. J. Appl. Physiol. 75(4):1637–1641.
Haq, T.A., H.S. Mason, J.D. Clements, and C.J. Arntzen
  1995 Oral immunization with a recombinant bacterial antigen produced in transgenic plants. Science 268:714–716.
Harman, E.A., and P.N. Frykman
  1992 The relationship of body size and composition to the performance of physically demanding military tasks. Pp. 105–118 in Body Composition and Physical Performance, Applications for the Military Services, B.M. Marriott and J. Grumstrup-Scott, eds. A report of the Committee on Military Nutrition Research, Food and Nutrition Board, Institute of Medicine. Washington, D.C.: National Academy Press.

Harrington, M.E., R.W. Daniel, and P.J. Kyberd
  1995   A measurement system for the recognition of arm gestures using accelerometers. Eng. Med. 209(2):129–134.
Harris, J.A., and F.G. Benedict
  1919   A biometric study of basal metabolism in man. Publication no. 279. Washington, D.C.: Carnegie Institute of Washington.
Harris, R.C., K. Soderlund, and E. Hultman
  1992   Elevation of creatine in resting and exercised muscle of normal subjects by creatine supplementation. Clin. Sci. Colch. 83:367–374.
Harrison, M.H., G.A. Brown, and A.J. Belyavin
  1982   The "Oxylog": An evaluation. Ergonomics 25:809–820.
Hart, M.K., W. Pratt, F. Panelo, K. Stephan, L. Aikens, R. Tammariello, and M. Dertzbaugh
  1995   Dissociation between serum neutralizing antibodies and protection from airborne VEE virus in immunized mice. Clin Immunol. Immunopathol. 76:S97
Hartz, A.J., D.C. Rupley, and A.A. Rimm
  1984   The association of girth measurements with disease in 32,856 women. Am. J. Epidemiol. 119:71–80.
Haskell, W.L., M.C. Yee, A. Evans, and P.J. Irby
  1993   Simultaneous measurement of heart rate and body motion to quantitate physical activity. Med. Sci. Sports Exerc. 25:109–115.
Hattori, K., N. Numata, M. Ikoma, A. Matsuzaka, and R.R. Danielson
  1991   Sex differences in the distribution of subcutaneous and internal fat. Hum. Biol. 63:53–63.
Hawkins, R.A., S-C. Huang, J.R. Barrio, R.E. Keen, D. Feng, J.C. Mazziotta, and M.E. Phelps
  1989   Estimation of local cerebral protein synthesis rates with 1-[1-^{11}C]leucine and PET: Methods, model and results in animals and humans. J. Cereb. Blood Flow Metab. 9:446–460.
Hawn, M.
  1996   Seek and ye shall find: Searching the Web. Macworld May:123–127.
Hayes, P.A., P.J. Sowood, A. Belyavin, J.B. Cohen, and F.W. Smith
  1988   Subcutaneous fat thickness measured by magnetic resonance imaging, ultrasound, and calipers. Med. Sci. Sports Exerc. 20:303–309.
Heatherton, T.F., J. Polivy, C.P. Herman, and R.F. Baumeister
  1993   Self-awareness, task failure, and disinhibition: How attentional focus affects eating. J. Pers. 61(1):49–61.
Hediger, M.L., and S.H. Katz
  1986   Fat patterning, overweight, and adrenal androgen interactions in black adolescent females. Hum. Biol. 58:585–600.
Heglund, N.C., and C.R. Taylor
  1988   Speed, stride frequency, and energy cost per stride: How do they change with body size and gait? J. Exp. Biol. 108:429–439.
Heglund, N.C., M.A. Fedak, C.R. Taylor, and G.A. Cavagna
  1982   Energetics and mechanics of terrestrial locomotion. IV. Total mechanical energy changes as a function of speed and body size in birds and mammals. J. Exp. Biol. 97:57–66.
Hehir, P.
  1922   Effects of chronic starvation during the siege of Kut. Br. Med. J. 1:865–868.
Heise, H.M., R. Marbach, T. Koschinsky, and F.A. Gries
  1994   Noninvasive blood glucose sensors based on near-infrared spectroscopy. Artif. Organs 18(6):439–447.

Hellerstein, M.K., and R.A. Neese
  1992   Mass isotopomer distribution analysis: A technique for measuring biosynthesis and turnover of polymers. Am. J. Physiol. 263:E998–E1001.
Hellerstein, M.K., J-M. Schwarz, and R. Neese
  1996   Regulation of hepatic *de novo* lipogenesis in humans. Ann. Rev. Nutr. 16:523–527.
Henneman, E., G. Somjen, and D.C. Carpenter
  1965   Functional significance of cell size in spinal motoneurons. J. Neurophysiol. 28:581–598.
Hesse, D.G., K.J. Tracey, Y. Fong, K.R. Manogue, M.A. Palladino, Jr., A. Cerami, G.T. Shires, and S.F. Lowry
  1988   Cytokine appearance in human endotoxemia and primate bacteremia. Surg. Gynecol. Obstet. 166:147–153.
Heymsfield, S.B.
  1987   Human body composition: Analysis by computerized axial tomography and nuclear magnetic resonance. Pp. 92–96 in AIN Symposim Proceedings. Nutrition '87, O.A. Levander, ed. Bethesda, Md.: American Institute of Nutrition.
Heymsfield, S.B., and R. Noel
  1981   Radiographic analysis of body composition by computerized axial tomography. Nutr. Cancer 17:161–172.
Heymsfield, S.B., T. Fulenwider, B. Nordlinger, R. Balow, P. Sones, and M. Kutner
  1979   Accurate measurement of liver, kidney, and spleen volume and mass by computerized axial tomography. Ann. Intern. Med. 90:185–187.
Heymsfied, S.B., R. Noel, M. Lynn, and M. Kutner
  1979   Accuracy of soft tissue density predicted by CT. J. Comput. Assist. Tomogr. 3:859–860.
Heymsfield, S.B., R.P. Olafson, M.H. Kutner, and D.W. Nixon
  1979   A radiographic method of quantifying protein-calorie undernutrition. Am. J. Clin. Nutr. 32:693–702.
Heymsfield, S.B., J. Wang, S. Heshka, J.J. Kehayias, and R.N. Pierson, Jr.
  1989   Dual-photon absorptiometry: Comparison of bone mineral and soft tissue mass measurements *in vivo* with established methods. Am. J. Clin. Nutr. 49:1282–1289.
Heymsfield, S.B., S. Lichtman, R.N. Baumgartner, J. Wang, Y. Kamen, A. Aliprantis, R.N. Pierson, Jr.
  1990   Body composition of humans: Comparison of two improved four-compartment models that differ in expense, technical complexity, and radiation exposure. Am. J. Clin. Nutr. 52:52–58.
Heymsfield, S.B., R. Smith, M. Aulet, B. Bensen, S. Lichtman, J. Wang, and R.N. Pierson, Jr.
  1990   Appendicular skeletal muscle mass: Measurement by dual-photon absorptiometry. Am. J. Clin. Nutr. 52:214–218.
Hiatt, A., R. Cafferkey, and K. Bowdish
  1989   Production of antibodies in transgenic plants. Nature 342:76–78.
Hilbert, D.M., K.L. Holmes, A.O. Anderson, and S. Rudikoff
  1994   Long term lymphoid reconstitution of SCID mice suggests self renewing B and T-cell populations in peripheral and mucosal tissues. Transplantation 58:466–475.
Hill, A.V.
  1950   The dimensions of animals and their muscular dynamics. Sci. Prog. 38:209–230.
Hill, G.L.
  1992   Disorders in Nutrition and Metabolism in Clinical Surgery. Edinburgh: Churchill Livingstone.
Hillgartner, F.B., L.M. Salati, and A.G. Goodridge
  1995   Physiological and molecular mechanisms involved in nutritional regulation of fatty acid synthesis. Physiol. Rev. 75:47–76.

Hiroi, T., K. Fujihashi, J.R. McGhee, and H. Kiyono
  1995   Polarized Th2 cytokine expression by both mucosal $\gamma\sigma$ and $\alpha\beta$ T-cells. Eur. J. Immunol. 25:2743–2751.
Hirsch, E.S.
  1995   Short- and long-term studies of food intake in military exercises: An overview. Pp. 151–173 in Not Eating Enough, Overcoming Underconsumption of Military Operational Rations, B.M. Marriott, ed. A report of the Committee on Military Nutrition Research, Food and Nutrition Board, Institute of Medicine. Washington, D.C.: National Academy Press.
Hirsch, E.S., and F.M. Kramer
  1993   Situational influences on food intake. Pp. 215–243 in Nutritional Needs in Hot Environments, Applications for Military Personnel in Field Operations, B.M. Marriott, ed. A report of the Committee on Military Nutrition Research, Food and Nutrition Board, Institute of Medicine. Washington, D.C.: National Academy Press.
Hirsch, E.S., H.L. Meiselman, R.D. Popper, G. Smits, B. Jezior, I. Lichton, N. Wenkham, J. Burt, M. Fox, S. McNutt, M.N. Thiele, and O. Dirige
  1984   The effects of prolonged feeding of Meal, Ready-to-Eat (MRE) operational rations. Technical report TR85/035. Natick, Mass.: U.S. Army Natick Research, Development and Engineering Center.
Hirshkowitz, M., L. De La Cueva, and J.H. Herman
  1993   The multiple vigilance test. Behavior Research Methods, Instruments, and Computers 25(2):272–275.
Hochachka, P.W., P.L. Lutz, T. Sick, M. Rosenthal, and G. van den Thillart, eds.
  1992   Surviving Hypoxia: Mechanisms of Control and Adaptation. Tokyo: CRC Press.
Hodgdon, J.A.
  1992   Body composition in military services: Standards and methods. Pp. 57–70 in Body Composition and Physical Performance, Applications for the Military Services, B.M. Marriott and J. Grumstrup-Scott, eds. A report of the Committee on Military Nutrition Research, Food and Nutrition Board, Institute of Medicine. Washington D.C.: National Academy Press.
Hodgdon, J.A., and M.B. Beckett
  1984   Prediction of body fat for U.S. Navy women from body circumferences and height. Technical Report 84-29. San Diego, Calif.: Naval Health Research Center.
Hodgdon, J.A., and P.I. Fitzgerald
  1987   Validity of impedance predictions at various levels of fatness. Hum. Biol. 59:281–298.
Hodgdon, J.A., P.I. Fitzgerald, and J.A. Vogel
  1990   Relationships between body fat and appearance ratings of U.S. soldiers. Technical Report 12-90. Natick, Mass.: U.S. Army Research Institute of Environmental Medicine.
Hodgdon, J.A., K.E. Friedl, M.B. Beckett, K.A. Westphal, and R.L. Shippee
  1996   Use of bioelectrical impedance analysis measurements as predictors of physical performance. Am. J. Clin. Nutr. 64(suppl.):463S–468S.
Hoffer, E.C., C.K. Meador, and D.C. Simpson
  1969   Correlation of whole-body impedance with total body water volume. J. Appl. Physiol. 27:531–534.
Hoffman, E.J., and M.E. Phelps
  1986   Positron emission tomography: Principles and quantitation. Pp. 237–286 in Positron Emission Tomography and Autoradiography: Principles and Applications for the Brain, M.E. Phelps, J.S. Mazziotta, and H.R. Schelbert, eds. New York: Raven Press.

Holmgren, J.
 1981 Actions of cholera toxin and the prevention and treatment of cholera. Nature 292:413–417.
Holmgren, J., N. Lycke, and C. Czerkinsky
 1993 Cholera toxin and cholera B subunit as oral-mucosal adjuvant and antigen vector systems. Vaccine 11(12):1179–1184.
Honigs, D.E., J.M. Freelin, G.M. Hieftje, and T.B. Hirschfeld
 1983 Near-infrared reflectance analysis by Gauss-Jordan linear algebra. Appl. Spec. 37(6):491–497.
Horber, F.F., F. Thomi, J.P. Casez, J. Fonteille, and P. Jaeger
 1992 Impact of hydration status on body composition as measured by dual energy x-ray absorptiometry in normal volunteers and patients on haemodialysis. Br. J. Radiol. 65(778):895–900.
Hounsfield, G.N.
 1973 Computerized transverse axial scanning (tomography). Br. J. Radiol. 46:1016.
Hovell, M.F., C.R. Hofstetter, J.F. Sallis, M.J.D. Rauh, and E. Barrington
 1992 Correlates of change in walking for exercise: An exploratory analysis. Res. Q. Exerc. Sport 63:425–434.
Hoyt, R.W., and A. Honig
 1996 Environmental influences on body fluid balance during exercise: Altitude. Pp. 187–200 in Body Fluid Balance in Exercise and Sport, E.R. Buskirk and S.M. Puhl, eds. Boca Raton, Fla.: CRC Press, Inc.
Hoyt, R.W., T.E. Jones, T.P. Stein, G.W. McAninch, H.R. Lieberman, E.W. Askew, and A. Cymerman
 1991 Doubly labeled water measurement of human energy expenditure during strenuous exercise. J. Appl. Physiol. 71(1):16–22.
Hoyt, R.W., T.E. Jones, C.J. Baker-Fulco, D.A. Schoeller, R.B. Schoene, R.S. Schwartz, E.W. Askew, and A. Cymerman
 1994 Doubly labeled water measurement of human energy expenditure during exercise at high altitude. Am. J. Physiol. 266:R966–R971.
Hoyt, R.W., J.J. Knapik, J.F. Lanza, B.H. Jones, and J.S. Staab
 1994 Ambulatory foot contact monitor to estimate the metabolic cost of human locomotion. J. Appl. Physiol. 76(4):1818–1822.
Hruschka, W.R., and K.H. Norris
 1982 Least-squares curve fitting of near-infrared spectra predicts protein and moisture content of ground wheat. Appl. Spec. 36(3):261–264.
Hsu, H., Y-M. Yu, J.W. Babich, J.F. Burke, E. Livini, R.G. Tompkins, V.R. Young, N.M. Alpert, and A.J. Fischman
 1996 Measurement of muscle protein synthesis by positron emission tomography with L-[methyl^{11}C]methionine. Proc. Natl. Acad. Sci. USA 93:1841–1846.
Hua, X., C. Yokoyama, J. Wu, M.R. Briggs, M.S. Brown, J.L. Goldstein, and X. Wang
 1993 SREBP-2, a second basic-helix-loop-helix-leucine zipper protein that stimulates transcription by binding to a sterol regulatory element. Proc. Natl. Acad. Sci. USA 90:11603–11607.
Huang, S-C., and M.E. Phelps
 1986 Principles of tracer kinetic modeling in positron emission tomography and autoradiography. Pp. 287–346 in Positron Emission Tomography and Autoradiography: Principles and Applications for the Brain and Heart, M. Phelps, J. Mazziotta, and H. Schelbert, eds. New York: Raven Press.

Huang, S-C., R.E. Carson, E.J. Hoffman, J. Carson, N. MacDonald, J.R. Barrio, and M.E.
    Phelps
  1983 Quantitative measurement of local cerebral blood flow in humans by positron
        computed tomography and O-15 water. J. Cereb. Blood Flow Metab. 3:141–153.
Huang, S-C, D.G. Feng, and M.E. Phelps
  1986 Model dependency and estimation reliability in measurement of cerebral oxygen
        utilization rate with oxygen-15 and dynamic positron emission tomography. J.
        Cereb. Blood Flow Metab. 6:105–119.
Hughes, M.D., D.S. Stein, H.M. Gundacker, F.T. Valentine, J.P. Phair, and P.A. Volberding
  1994 Within-subject variation in CD4 lymphocyte count in asymptomatic human immu-
        nodeficiency virus infection: Implications for patient monitoring. J. Infect. Dis.
        169:28–36.
Humphrey, S.J.E., and H.S. Wolff
  1977 The Oxylog. J. Physiol. 267:12P.
Huong, P.L., A.H. Kolk, T.A. Eggelte, C.P. Verstijnen, N. Gilis, and J.T. Hendriks
  1991 Measurement of antigen-specific lymphocyte proliferation using 5-bromo-de-
        oxyuridine incorporation. An easy and low cost alternative to radioactive
        thymidine incorporation. J. Immunol. Methods 140:243–248.
Husband, A.J., and J.L. Gowans
  1978 The origin and antigen-dependent distribution of IgA-containing cells in the intes-
        tine. J. Exp. Med. 148:1146–1160.
Hyams, K.C., A.L. Bourgeois, B.R. Merrell, P. Rozmajzl, J. Escamilla, S.A. Thronton, G.M.
    Wasserman, A. Burke, P. Echeverria, K.Y. Green, A.Z. Kapikian, and J.N. Woody
  1991 Diarrheal disease during Operation Desert Shield. N. Eng. J. Med. 325:1423–1428.
Hyams, K.C., J.D. Malone, A.Z. Kapikian, M.K. Estes, X. Jiang, A.L. Bourgeois, S.
    Paparello, R.E. Hawkins, and K.Y. Green
  1993 Norwalk virus infection among Desert Storm troops. J. Infect. Dis. 167:986–987.
Ikegami, Y., S. Hiruta, H. Ikegami, and M. Miyamura
  1988 Development of a telemetry system for measuring oxygen uptake during sports
        activities. Eur. J. Appl. Physiol. 57:622–626.
Ink, S.L., J.F. Gregory, and D.B. Sartain
  1986 Determination of pyridoxine β-glucoside bioavailability using intrinsic and extrin-
        sic labeling in the rat. J. Agric. Food Chem. 34:857–862.
IOM (Institute of Medicine)
  1992 A Nutritional Assessment of U.S. Army Ranger Training Class 11/91. A brief re-
        port of the Committee on Military Nutrition Research, Food and Nutrition Board.
        March 23, 1992. Washington, D.C.
  1993 Nutritional Needs in Hot Environments, Applications for Military Personnel in
        Field Operations, B.M. Marriott, ed. A report of the Committee on Military Nutri-
        tion Research, Food and Nutrition Board. Washington, D.C.: National Academy
        Press.
  1993b Review of the Results of Nutritional Intervention, U.S. Army Ranger Training
        Class 11/92 (Ranger II), B.M. Marriott, ed. A report of the Committee on Military
        Nutrition Research, Food and Nutrition Board. Washington, D.C.: National Acad-
        emy Press.
  1994 Food Components to Enhance Performance, An Evaluation of Potential Perform-
        ance-Enhancing Food Components for Operational Rations, B.M. Marriott, ed. A
        report of the Committee on Military Nutrition Research, Food and Nutrition Board.
        Washington, D.C.: National Academy Press.

1996	Nutritional Needs in Cold and in High-Altitude Environments, Applications for Military Personnel in Field Operations, B.M. Marriott and S.J. Carlson, eds. A report of the Committee on Military Nutrition Research, Food and Nutrition Board. Washington, D.C.: National Academy Press.

Iregen, A., and R. Letz
1992	Computerized testing in neurobehavioral toxicology. Appl. Psychol. Int. Rev. 41(3):247–255.

Ishiwata, K., W. Vaalburg, P.H. Elsinga, A.M.J. Paana, and M.G. Waldreng
1988	Comparison of L-[1-^{11}C]methionine and L-methyl-[^{11}C]methionine for measuring *in vitro* protein synthesis rates with PET. J. Nucl. Med. 29:1419–1427.

Israel, R.G., J.A. Houmard, K.F. O'Brien, M.R. McCammon, B.S. Zamora, and A.W. Eaton
1989	Validity of a near-infrared spectrophotometry device for estimating human body composition. Res. Q. Exerc. Sport 60:379–383.

Issemann, I., and S. Green
1990	Activation of a member of the steroid hormone receptor superfamily by peroxisome proliferators. Nature 347: 645–650.

Jackson, A.S., and M.L. Pollock
1978	Generalized equations for predicting body density of men. Br. J. Nutr. 40:497–504.

Jackson, A.S., M.L. Pollock, and A. Ward
1980	Generalized equations for predicting body density in women. Med. Sci. Sports Exerc. 12:175–182.

Jacob, J., G. Kelsoe, K. Rajewsky, and U. Weiss
1991	Intraclonal generation of antibody mutants in germinal centers. Nature 354:389–392.

Jacob, J., J. Przylepa, C. Miller, and G. Kelsoe
1993	In situ studies of the primary immune response to (4-hydroxy-3-nitrophenyl)acetyl. III. The kinetics of V region mutation and selection in germinal center B cells. J. Exp. Med. 178:1293–1307.

Jacoby, D.B., N.D. Zilz, and H.C. Towle
1989	Sequences within the 5'-flanking region of the S_{14} gene confer responsiveness to glucose in primary hepatocytes. J. Biol. Chem. 264:17623–17626.

Jahrling, P.B., and E.H. Stephenson
1984	Protective efficacies of live attenuated and formaldehyde-inactivated Venezuelan equine encephalitis virus vaccines against aerosol challenge in hamsters. J. Clin. Microbiol. 19:429–431.

James, W.P.T., J.P. Haggarty, and B.A. McGaw
1988	Recent progress in studies on energy expenditure: Are the new methods providing answers to old questions? Proc. Nutr. Soc. 47:195–208.

Jardetzky, O., and G.C.K. Roberts
1981	NMR in Molecular Biology. New York: Academic Press.

Jebb, S.A., G.R. Goldberg, and E. Marinos
1993	DXA measurements of fat and bone mineral density in relation to depth and adiposity. Pp. 115–119 in Human Body Composition, K.J. Ellis and J.D. Eastman, eds. New York: Plenum Press.

Jebb, S.A., P.R. Murgatroyd, G.R. Goldberg, A.M. Prentice, and W.A. Coward
1993	*In vivo* measurement of changes in body composition: Description of methods and their validation against 12-d continuous whole-body calorimetry. Am. J. Clin. Nutr. 58:455–462.

Jefferson, R.A., T.A. Kavanagh, and M.W. Bevan
1987	GUS fusions: β-glucuronidase as a sensitive and versatile gene fusion marker in higher plants. EMBO J. 6(13):3901–3907.

Jenin, P., J. Lenoir, C. Roullet, A. Thomasset, and H. Ducrot
1975 Determination of body fluid compartments by electrical impedance measurements. Aviat. Space Environ. Med. 46:152–155.

Jensen, L.B., F. Quaade, and O.H. Sorensen
1994 Bone loss accompanying voluntary weight loss in obese humans. J. Bone Miner. Res. 9:459–463.

Jensen, M.D., J.A. Kanaley, L.R. Roust, P.C. O'Brien, J.S. Braun, W.L. Dunn, and H.W. Wahner
1993 Assessment of body composition with use of dual-energy x-ray absorptiometry: Evaluation and comparison with other methods. Mayo Clin. Proc. 68:867–873.

Jensen, M.D., J.A. Kanaley, J.E. Reed, and P.F. Sheedy
1995 Measurement of abdominal and visceral fat with computed tomography and dual-energy x-ray absorptiometry. Am. J. Clin. Nutr. 61:274–278.

Jergas, M., M. Breitenseher, C.C. Glüer, W. Yu, and H.K. Genant
1995 Estimates of volumetric bone density from projectional measurements improve the discriminatory capability of dual x-ray absorptiometry. J. Bone Miner. Res. 10:1101–1110.

Jobe, J.B., and L.E. Banderet
1986 Cognitive testing in military performance research. Pp. 181–193 in Cognitive Testing Methodology: Application to Military Nutrition Research. Proceedings of a workshop of the Committee on Military Nutrition Research, Food and Nutrition Board, Commission on Life Sciences, National Research Council. Washington, D.C.: National Academy Press.

Jobsis, F.F.
1977 Noninvasive, infrared monitoring of cerebral and myocardial oxygen sufficiency and circulatory parameters. Science 198:1264–1267.

Johansson, A.G., A. Forslund, A. Sjodin, H. Mallmin, L. Hambraeus, and S. Ljunghall
1993 Determination of body composition—a comparison of dual-energy x-ray absorptiometry and hydrodensitometry. Am. J. Clin. Nutr. 57:323–326.

Johnson, H.L., and H.E. Sauberlich
1982 Prolonged use of operational rations: A review of the literature. Unnumbered technical report. Presidio of San Francisco, Calif.: Letterman Army Institute of Research.

Johnson, H.L., C.F. Consolazio, H.J. Krzywicki, G.J. Isaac, and N.F. Witt
1971 Metabolic aspects of calorie restriction: Nutrient balance with 500-kilocalorie intakes. Am. J. Clin. Nutr. 24:913–923.

Johnson, M.J., K.E. Friedl, P.N. Frykman, and R.J. Moore
1994 Loss of muscle mass is poorly reflected in grip strength performance in healthy young men. Med. Sci. Sports Exerc. 26:235–240.

Johnson, R.F.
1991 Rifle firing simulation: Effects of MOPP, heat, and medications on markmanship. Pp. 530–535 in Proceedings of the Military Testing Association. San Antonio, Tx.: Armstrong Laboratory Resource Directorate and U.S. Air Force Occupational Measurement Squadron.

Jolesz, F.A.
1992 Fast spin-echo technique extends versatility of MR. Diagn. Imaging 14:78.

Jones, A.P., L.M.C. Webb, A.O. Anderson, E.J. Leonard, and A. Rot
1995 Normal human sweat contains interleukin-8. J. Leukocyte Biol. 57:434–437.

Jones, P.J.H., A. Winthrop, D.A. Schoeller, R.M. Filler, P.R. Swyer, J.Smith, and T. Heim
1988 Evaluation of doubly labeled water for measuring energy expenditure during changing nutrition. Am. J. Clin. Nutr. 47:799–804.

Jones, T.E., R.W. Hoyt, J.P. DeLany, R.L Hesslink, and E.W. Askew
  1993 A comparison of two methods of measuring water intake of soldiers in the field [abstract]. FASEB J. 7:A610.
Joseph, T., and D.B. McCormick
  1995 Uptake and metabolism of riboflavin-5'-α-D-glucoside by rat and isolated liver cells. J. Nutr. 125:2194–2198.
Jump, D.B., A. Bell, and V. Santiago
  1990 Thyroid hormone and dietary carbohydrate interact to regulate rat liver S_{14} gene transcription and chromatin structure. J. Biol. Chem. 265:3474–3478.
Kabir, H., J.E. Leklem, and L.T. Miller
  1983 Relationship of the glycosylated vitamin B_6 content of foods to the vitamin B_6 bioavailability in humans. Nutr. Rep. Int. 28:709–715.
Kadesch, T.
  1993 Consequences of heteromeric interactions among helix-loop-helix proteins. Cell Growth Differ. 4:49–55.
Kadonaga, J.T., and R. Tjian
  1986 Affinity purification of sequence-specific DNA binding proteins. Proc. Natl. Acad. Sci. U.S.A. 83:5889–5893.
Kagnoff, M.F.
  1996 Mucosal immunology: New frontiers. Immunol. Today 17:57–59.
Kalfarentzos, F., J. Spiliotis, G. Velimezis, D. Dougenis, and J. Androulakis
  1989 Comparison of forearm muscle dynamometry with nutritional prognostic index as a preoperative indicator in cancer patients. J. Parenter. Enteral. Nutr. 13:34–36.
Kamimura, H., H. Ogata, and H. Takahara
  1992 α-Glucoside formation of xenobiotics by rat liver α-glucosidases. Drug Metab. Disp. 20:309–315.
Kampschmidt, R.F.
  1983 Infection, inflammation, and interleukin 1 (IL-1). Lymphokine Res. 2:97–102.
Kampschmidt, R.F., and L.A. Pulliam
  1975 Stimulation of antimicrobial activity in the rat with leukocytic endogenous mediator. J. Reticuloendothel. Soc. 17:162–169.
Kanai, H., M. Haeno, and K. Sakamoto
  1987 Electrical measurement of fluid distribution in legs and arms. Med. Prog. Technol. 12:159–170.
Kane, R.L.
  1991 Standardized and flexible batteries in neuropsychology: An assessment update. Neuropsychol. Rev. 2(4):281–339.
Kane, R.L., and G.G. Kay
  1992 Computerized assessment in neuropsychology: A review of tests and test batteries. Neuropsychol. Rev. 3(1):1–117.
Kang, K., M. Kubin, K.D. Cooper, S.R. Lessin, G. Trinchieri, and A.H. Rook
  1996 IL-12 synthesis by human Langerhans cells. J. Immunol. 156:1402–1407.
Kantele, A., J.M. Kantele, E. Savilahti, M. Westerholm, H. Arvilommi, A. Lazarovits, E.C. Butcher, and P.H. Makela
  1997 Oral, but not parenteral, typhoid vaccination induces circulating antibody-secreting cells that all bear homing receptors directing them to the gut. J. Immunol. 158:574–579.
Kappagoda, C.T., R.J. Linden, and J.P. Newell
  1979 Effect of the Canadian Air Force training programme on a submaximal exercise test. Q. J. Exp. Physiol. 64:185–204.

Karecla, P.I., S.J. Bowden, S.J. Green, and P.J. Kilshaw
  1995　Recognition of E-cadherin on epithelial cells by the mucosal T-cell integrin $\alpha_{M290}\beta7$ ($\alpha E\beta7$). Eur. J. Immunol. 25:852–856.
Karpinos, B.D.
  1961　Current height and weight of youths of military age. Hum. Biol. 33:335–354.
Kashiwazaki, H., T. Inaoka, T. Suzuki, and Y. Kondo
  1986　Correlations of pedometer readings with energy expenditure in workers during free-living daily activities. Eur. J. Appl. Physiol. 54:585–590.
Katch, F., E.D. Michael, and S.M. Horvath
  1967　Estimation of body volume by underwater weighing: Description of a simple method. J. Appl. Physiol. 23:811–813.
Katch, V.L., B. Champaigne, P. Freedson, S. Sady, F.I. Katch, and A.R. Behnke
  1980　Contribution of breast volume and weight to body fat distribution in females. Am. J. Phys. Anthropol. 53:93–100.
Katz, J., and W-NP. Lee
  1991　Application of mass isotopomer analysis for determination of pathways of glycogen synthesis. Am. J. Physiol. 261:E332–E336.
Kawai, T., H. Yamada, and K. Ogata
  1972　Studies on transglucosidation to vitamin B_6 by microorganisms. VII. Transport of pyridoxine glucoside into rabbit erythrocytes. J. Vitaminol. 18:183–188.
Kawakami, Y. D. Nozake, A. Matsuo, and T. Fukunaga
  1992　Reliability of measurement of oxygen uptake by a portable telemetric system. Eur. J. Appl. Physiol. 65:409–414.
Kay C.F., P.T. Bothwell, and E.L. Foltz
  1954　Electrical resistivity of living body tissues at low frequencies. J. Physiol. 13:131–136.
Ke, Y., and J.A. Kapp
  1996　Oral antigen inhibits priming of CD8+ CTL, CD4+ T-cells, and antibody responses while activating CD8+ suppressor T-cells. J. Immunol. 156:916–921.
Keet, I.P., A. Krol, M. Koot, M.T. Roos, F. de Wolf, F. Miedema, and R.A. Coutinho
  1994　Predictors of disease progression in HIV-infected homosexual men with CD4+ cells 200×10^6/L but free of AIDS-defining clinical disease. AIDS 8:1577–1583.
Keller, H., C. Dreyer, J. Medin, A. Mahfoudi, K. Ozato, and W. Wahli
  1993　Fatty acids and retinoids control lipid metabolism through activation of peroxisome proliferator-activated receptor-retinoid X receptor heterodimers. Proc. Natl. Acad. Sci. USA 90:2160–2164.
Kendall, S.D., and M.J. Christensen
  1995　Modified differential display identifies genes in rat liver differentially regulated by selenium [abstract]. FASEB J. 9:A158.
Kenyon, R.V., and M.B. Afenya
  1995　Training in virtual and real environments. Ann. Biomed. Eng. 23(4):445–455.
Ker, R.F., M.B. Bennett, S.R. Bibby, R.C. Kester, and R.M. Alexander
  1987　The spring in the arch of the human foot. Nature 325:147–149.
Kerr, M.H., R.D. Forsyth, and M.J. Plyley
  1992　Cold water and hot iron: Trial by ordeal in England. J. Interdisciplin. History 22:573–595.
Keys, A., H.L. Taylor, O. Mickelsen and A. Henschel
  1946　Famine edema and the mechanism of its formation. Science 103:669–670.
Keys, A., J. Brozék, A. Henschel, O. Mickelsen, and H.L. Taylor
  1950　The Biology of Human Starvation, vol. 1. Minneapolis: University of Minnesota Press.

Kimpton, W.G., E.A. Washington, and R.N.P. Cahill
1989 Recirculation of lymphocyte subsets (CD5+, CD4+, CD8+, SBU-T19+ and B-cells) through gut and peripheral lymph nodes. Immunology 66:69–75.

King, A.C., S.N. Blair, D.E. Bild, R.K. Dishman, P.M. Dubbert, R.H. Marcus, N.B. Oldridge, R.S. Paffenbarger, Jr., K.E. Powell, and K.K. Yeager
1992 Determinants of physical activity and interventions in adults. Med. Sci. Sports Exerc. 24:S221–S236.

King, M.A., and F.I. Katch
1986 Changes in body density, fatfolds and girths at 2.3 kg increments of weight loss. Hum. Biol. 58:709–718.

King, N., S.H. Mutter, D.E. Roberts, E.W. Askew, A.J. Young, T.E. Jones, M.Z. Mays, M.R. Sutherland, J.P. DeLany, B.E. Cheema, and R. Tulley
1992 Nutrition and hydration status of soldiers consuming the 18-Man Arctic Tray Pack Ration Module with either the Meal, Ready-to-Eat or the Long Life Ration Packet during a cold weather field training exercise. Technical Report T4-92. Natick, Mass.: U.S. Army Research Institute of Environmental Medicine.

King, N., J.E. Arsenault, S.H. Mutter, C. Champagne, T.G. Murphy, K.A. Westphal, and E.W. Askew
1994 Nutritional intake of female soldiers during the U.S. Army basic combat training. Technical Report T17-94. Natick, Mass.: U.S. Army Research Institute of Environmental Medicine.

Kinney, J.M.
1995 Metabolic responses of the critically ill patient. Crit. Care Clin. 11:569–585.

Kinney, J.M., and D.H. Elwyn
1983 Protein metabolism and injury. Annu. Rev. Nutr. 3:433–466.

Kirlik, A.
1993 Modeling strategic behavior in human-automation interaction: Why an "aid" can (and should) go unused. Hum. Factors 35(2):221–242.

Kirschner, M.A., E. Samojlik, M. Drejka, E. Szmal, and G. Schneider
1990 Androgen and estrogen metabolism in women with upper body versus lower body obesity. J. Clin. Endocrinol. Metab. 70:473–479.

Kitai, T., A. Tanaka, A. Tokuka, K. Tanaka, Y. Yamaoka, K. Ozawa, and K. Hirao
1993 Quantitative detection of hemoglobin saturation in the liver with near-infrared spectroscopy. Hepatology 18(4):926–936.

Klicka, M.V., D.E. Sherman, N. King, K.E. Friedl, and E.W. Askew
1993 Nutritional assessment of cadets at the U.S. Military Academy: Part 2. Assessment of nutritional intake. Technical Report T1-94. Natick, Mass.: U.S. Army Research Institute of Environmental Medicine.

Klidjian, A.M., K.J. Foster, R.M. Kammerling, A. Cooper, and S.J. Karran
1980 Relation of anthropometric and dynamometric variables to serious postoperative complications. Br. J. Med. 281:899–901.

Klug, A., and J.W.R. Schwabe
1995 Zinc fingers. FASEB J. 9:597–604.

Kluger, M.J., D.H. Ringler, and M.R. Anver
1975 Fever and survival. Science 188:166–168.

Koelega, H.S.
1989 Benzodiazepines and vigilance performance: A review. Psychopharmacology 98:146–156.

Kohrt, W.M.
1995 Body composition by DXA: Tried and true? Med. Sci. Sports Exerc. 27(10):1349–1353.

Kohrt, W.M., and S.J. Birge, Jr.
1995   Differential effects of estrogen treatment on bone mineral density of the spine, hip, wrist, and total body in late postmenopausal women. Osteoporos. Int. 5(3):150–155.

Koster, F.T., and N.F. Pierce
1983   Parenteral immunization causes antigen-specific cell-mediated suppression of an intestinal IgA response. J. Immunol. 131:115–119.

Kotloff, D.B., and J.J. Cebra
1988   Effect of TH-lines and clones on the growth and differentiation of B-cell clones in microculture. Mol. Immunol. 25:147–155.

Kozik, A., and D.B. McCormick
1984   Mechanism of pyridoxine uptake by isolated rat liver cells. Arch. Biochem. Biophys. 229:187–193.

Kraal, G., K. Schornagel, P.R. Streeter, B. Holzman, and E.C. Butcher
1995   Expression of the mucosal vascular addressin, MAdCAM-1, on sinus-lining cells in the spleen. Am. J. Pathol. 147:763–771.

Kram, R., and C.R. Taylor
1990   Energetics of running: A new perspective. Nature 346(6281):265–267.

Kraning, K.K. II
1991   A computer simulation for predicting the time course of thermal and cardiovascular responses to various combinations of heat stress, clothing and exercise. Technical Report T13-91. Natick, Mass.: U.S. Army Research Institute of Environmental Medicine.

Kribbs, N.B., and D. Dinges
1994   Vigilance decrement and sleepiness. Pp. 113–125 in Sleep Onset Mechanisms, J.R. Harsh and R.D. Ogilvie, eds. Washington, D.C.: American Psychological Association.

Kroemer, G., E. Cuende, and C. Martinez-A.
1993   Compartmentalization of the peripheral immune system. Adv. Immunol. 53:157–216.

Krotkiewski, M., and P. Björntorp
1986   Muscle tissue in obesity with different distribution of adipose tissue: Effects of physical training. Int. J. Obes. 10:331–341.

Kubota, K., T. Matsuzawa, M. Ito, K. Ito, T. Fujiwara, Y. Abe, S. Toshioka, H. Fukuda, J. Hatazawa, R. Iwata, S. Watanuki, and T. Ido
1985   Lung tumor imaging by positron emission tomography using C-11-L-methionine. J. Nucl. Med. 26:37–42.

Kuhl, J.G., D. Evans, Y.E. Papelis, R.A. Romano, and G.S. Watson
1995   The Iowa Driving Simulator: An immersive environment for driving-related research and development. IEEE Comp. 28(7):35–41.

Kuhn, U., U. Lempertz, J. Knop, and D. Becker
1995   A new method for phenotyping proliferating cell nuclear antigen positive cells using flow cytometry: Implications for analysis of the immune response *in vivo*. J. Immunol. Methods 179:215–222.

Kurane, I., B.L. Innis, S. Nimmannitya, A. Nisalak, A. Meager, J. Janus, and F.A. Ennis
1991   Activation of T lymphocytes in dengue virus infections. High levels of soluble interleukin 2 receptor, soluble CD4, soluble CD8, interleukin 2, and interferon-gamma in sera of children with dengue. J. Clin. Invest. 88:1473–1480.

Kushner, R.F., and D.A. Schoeller
1986   Estimation of total body water by bioelectrical impedance analysis. Am. J. Clin. Nutr. 44:417–424.

Kushner, R.F., G. Gudivaka, and D.A. Schoeller
  1996   Clinical characteristics influencing bioelectrical impedance analysis measurements. Am. J. Clin. Nutr. 64(3S):423S–427S.
Kvist, H., L. Sjöström, and U. Tylen
  1986   Adipose tissue volume determinations in women by computed tomography: Technical considerations. Int. J. Obes. 10:53–67.
Kvist, H., B. Chowdhury, U. Grangard, U. Tyler, and L. Sjöström
  1988   Total and visceral adipose-tissue volumes derived from measurements with computed tomography in adult men and women: Predictive equations. Am. J. Clin. Nutr. 48:1351–1361.
Kvist, H., B. Chowdhury, L. Sjöström, U. Tyler, and Å. Cederblad
  1988   Adipose tissue volume determination in males by computed tomography and ^{40}K. Int. J. Obes. 12:249–266.
La Via, M.F., J. Munno, R.B. Lydiard, E.A. Workman, J.R. Hubbard, Y. Michel, and E. Pauling
  1996   The influence of stress intrusion on immunodepression in generalized anxiety disorder patients and controls. Psychosom. Med. 58:138–142.
LaFrance, N.D., L. O'Tauma, V. Villemagne, J. Williams, K. Douglas, R.F. Dannals, H. Ravert, A. Wilson, H. Drew, J. Links, D. Wong, B. Carson, H. Brem, L. Strauss, and H.N. Wagner
  1987   Quantitative imaging and follow-up experience of C-11-L-methionine accumulation in brain tumors with positron emission tomography. J. Nucl. Med. 26:37–42.
Lai, K.C., M.M. Goodsitt, R. Murano, and C.H. Chesnut III
  1992   A comparison of two dual-energy x-ray absorptiometry systems for spinal bone mineral measurement. Calcif. Tissue Int. 50:203–208.
Landau, B.R., V. Chandramouli, W.C. Schumann, K. Ekberg, K. Kumaran, S.C. Kalhan, and J. Wahren
  1995   Estimates of Krebs cycle activity and contributions of gluconeogenesis to hepatic glucose production in fasting healthy subjects and IDDM patients. Diabetologia 38:831–838.
Lands, L.C., G.J.F. Heigenhauser, C. Gordon, N.L. Jones, and C.E. Webber
  1991   Accuracy of measurements of small changes in soft tissue mass by use of dual-photon absorptiometry. J. Appl. Physiol. 71:698–702.
Langer, R.
  1990   New methods of drug delivery. Science 249:1527–1533.
LaPorte, R.E., H.J. Montoye, and C.J. Casperson
  1985   Assessment of physical activity in epidemiologic research: Problems and prospects. Public Health Rep. 100:131–146.
Larsson, B., K. Svardsudd, L. Welin, L. Wilhelmsen, P. Björntorp, and G. Tibblin
  1984   Abdominal adipose tissue distribution, obesity, and risk of cardiovascular disease and death: 13 year follow up to participants in the study of men born in 1913. Br. Med. J. 288:1401–1404.
Laskey, M.A., K.D. Lyttle, M.E. Flaxman, and R.W. Barber
  1992   The influence of tissue depth and composition on the performance of the Lunar dual-energy x-ray absorptiometer whole-body scanning mode. Eur. J. Clin. Nutr. 46:39–45.
Lauterber, P.C.
  1973   Image formation by induced local interactions: Examples employing nuclear magnetic resonance. Nature 242:190–191.

Lawes, J.B., and J.H. Gilbert
   1859   Experimental inquiry into the composition of some of the animals fed and slaughtered as human food. Philos. Trans. R. Soc. London 149:493–680.
Lebman, D.A., and R.L. Coffman
   1994   Cytokines in the mucosal immune system. Pp. 243–250 in Handbook of Mucosal Immunology, P.L. Ogra, J. Mestecky, M.E. Lamm, W. Strober, J.R. McGhee, and J. Bienenstock, eds. Boston: Academic Press, Inc.
Lee, J., and N. Moray
   1992   Trust, control strategies and allocation of function in human-machine systems. Ergonomics 35(10):1243–1270.
Leenon, R., K. van der Kooy, J.C. Seidell, and P. Durenberg
   1992   Visceral fat accumulation measured by magnetic resonance imaging in relation to serum lipids in obese men and women. Atherosclerosis 94:171–181.
Lefrancois-Martinez, A-M., M-J.M. Diaz-Guerra, V. Vallet, A. Kahn, and B. Antoine
   1994   Glucose-dependent regulation of the L-type kinase gene in a hepatoma cell line is independent of insulin and cyclic AMP. FASEB J. 8:89–96.
Lehner, T., L.A. Bergmeier, C. Panagiotidi, L. Tao, R. Brookes, L.S. Klavinskis, P. Walker, R.G. Ward, L. Hussain, A.J.H. Gearing, and S.E. Adams
   1992   Induction of mucosal and systemic immunity to a recombinant simian immunodeficiency viral protein. Science 258:1365–1369.
Leitch, C.A., and P.J.H. Jones
   1993   Measurement of human lipogenesis using deuterium incorporation. J. Lipid Res. 34:157–163.
Leklem, J.E.
   1994   Vitamin B_6. Pp. 383–394 in Modern Nutrition in Health and Disease, 8th ed., vol. 1, M.A. Shils, J.A. Olson, and M. Shike, eds. Philadelphia: Lea and Febiger.
LeMay, L.G., A.J. Vander, and M.J. Kluger
   1990   The effects of psychological stress on plasma interleukin-6 activity in rats. Physiol. Behav. 47:957–961.
Lemieux, S., D. Prud'homme, C. Bouchard, A. Tremblay, and J-P. Despres
   1993   Sex differences in the relation of visceral adipose tissue accumulation to total body fatness. Am. J. Clin. Nutr. 58:463–367.
   1996   A single threshold value of waist girth identifies normal-weight and overweight subjects with excess visceral adipose tissue. Am. J. Clin. Nutr. 64:685–693.
Lewin, B.
   1994   Genes V. Oxford: Oxford University Press.
Lewy, A.J., T.A. Wehr, F.K. Goodwin, D.A. Newsome, and S.P. Markey
   1980   Light suppresses melatonin secretion in humans. Science 210:1267–1269.
Ley, C.J., B. Lees, and J.C. Stevenson
   1992   Sex- and menopause-associated changes in body fat distribution. Am. J. Clin. Nutr. 55:950–954.
Liang, P., L. Averboukh, and A.B. Pardee
   1993   Distribution and cloning of eukaryotic mRNAs by means of differential display: Refinements and optimization. Nucl. Acids Res. 21:3269–3275.
Liao, Z., J.H. Tu, C.B. Small, S.M. Schnipper, and D.L. Rosentreich
   1993   Increased urine interleukin-1 levels in aging. Gerontology 39:19–27.
Lieberman, H.R.
   1989   Cognitive effects of various food constituents. Pp. 267–281 in Psychobiology of Human Eating and Nutritional Behavior, R. Shepard, ed. Chichester, England: Wiley.

Lieberman, H.R.
  1992   Caffeine. Pp. 49–72 in Factors Affecting Human Performance. Volume II: The
         Physical Environment, D. Jones and A. Smith, eds. London: Academic Press.
Lieberman, H.R., and B. Shukitt-Hale
  1996   Food components and other treatments that may enhance mental performance at
         high altitudes and in the cold. Pp. 453–465 in Nutritional Needs in Cold and in
         High-Altitude Environments, Applications for Military Personnel in Field Opera-
         tions, B.M. Marriott and S.J. Carlson, eds. A report of the Committee on Military
         Nutrition Research, Food and Nutrition Board, Institute of Medicine. Washington,
         D.C.: National Academy Press.
Lieberman, H.R., J.J. Wurtman, and M.H. Teicher
  1989   Circadian rhythms of activity in healthy young and elderly humans. Neurobiol.
         Aging 10:259–265.
Lieberman H.R., M.Z. Mays, B. Shukitt-Hale, B.E. Marlowe, D.I. Welch, W.J. Tharion, P.D.
         Gardner, A. Pappas, and K.S.K. Chinn
  1994   Sleep in the M40 mask: Sleep quality, mask fit factor and next day performance.
         Technical Report T94-8. Natick, Mass.: U.S. Army Research Institute of Environ-
         mental Medicine.
Lieberman H.R., M.Z. Mays, B. Shukitt-Hale, K.S.K. Chinn, and W. J. Tharion
  1996   Effects of sleeping in a chemical protective mask on sleep quality and perform-
         ance. Aviat. Space Environ. Med. 67(9):841–848.
Lifson, N., and R. McClintock
  1966   Theory of use of turnover rates of body water for measuring energy and material
         balance. J. Theor. Biol. 12:46–74.
Lifson, N., G.B. Gordon, and R. McClintock
  1955   Measurement of total carbon dioxide production by means of D_2O^{18}. J. Appl.
         Physiol. 7:705–710.
Lifson, N., W.S. Little, D.G. Levitt, and R.M. Henderson
  1975 $D_2^{18}O$ method for CO_2 output in small mammals and economic feasibility in man.
         J. Appl. Physiol. 39(4):657–664.
Lilley, J., B.G. Walters, D.A. Heath, and Z. Drolc
  1991   *In vivo* and *in vitro* precision for bone density measured by dual-energy x-ray ab-
         sorption. Osteoporos. Int. 1:141–146.
Links, J.M.
  1994   Instrumentation. Pp. 53–85 in Nuclear Medicine Technology, D.R. Bernier, P.E.
         Christian, and J.K. Langan, eds. St. Louis, Mo.: Mosby.
Liu, Z., K.S. Thompson, and H.C. Towle
  1993   Carbohydrate regulation of the rat L-type pyruvate kinase gene requires two nu-
         clear factors: LF-A1 and a member of the c-*myc* family. J. Biol. Chem.
         268(17):12787–12795.
Locksley, R.M., S.L. Reiner, F. Hatam, D.R. Litman, and N. Killeen
  1993   Helper T cells without CD4: Control of leishmaniasis in CD4-deficient mice. Sci-
         ence 261:1448–1451.
Lohman, T.G.
  1986   Applicability of body composition techniques and constants for children and
         youths. Exerc. Sports Sci. Rev. 14:325–357.
  1996   Dual energy x-ray absorptiometry. Pp. 63–78 in Human Body Composition, A.F.
         Roche, S.B. Heymsfield, and T.G. Lohman, eds. Champaign, Ill.: Human Kinetics.
London, S.D., D.H. Rubin, and J.J. Cebra
  1987   Gut mucosal immunization with reovirus serotype 1/L stimulates virus-specific
         cytotoxic T-cell precursors as well as IgA memory cells in Peyer's patches. J. Exp.
         Med. 165:830–847.

Lopes, J., D.M. Russell, J. Whitwell, and K.N. Jeejeebhoy
  1982   Skeletal muscle function in malnutrition. Am. J. Clin. Nutr. 36:602–610.
Lopez, I., I. deAndraca, C.G. Perales, E. Heresi, M. Castillo, and M. Colombo
  1993   Breakfast omission and cognitive performance of normal, wasted and stunted schoolchildren. Eur. J. Clin. Nutr. 47(8):533–542.
Losonsky, G.A., J.P. Johnson, J.A. Winkelstein, and R.H. Yolken
  1985   Oral administration of human serum immunoglobulin in immunodeficient patients with viral gastroenteritis. J. Clin. Invest. 76:2362–2367.
Louhevaara, V., and J. Ilmarinen
  1985   Comparison of three field methods for measuring oxygen consumption. Ergonomics 28(2):463–470.
Lucia, A., S.J. Fleck, R.W. Gotshall, and J.T. Kearney
  1993   Validity and reliability of the COSMED K2 instrument. Int. J. Sports Med. 14:380–386.
Lukaski, H.C.
  1987a   Bioelectrical impedance analysis. Pp. 78–81 in Nutrition '87, O. Levander, ed. Bethesda, Md.: American Institute of Nutrition.
  1987b   Methods for the assessment of human body composition: Traditional and new. Am. J. Clin. Nutr. 46:537–556.
  1996   Biological indexes considered in the derivation of the bioelectrical impedance analysis. Am. J. Clin. Nutr. 64(3S):397S–404S.
Lukaski, H.C., and W.W. Bolonchuk
  1987   Theory and validation of the tetrapolar bioelectrical impedance method to assess human body composition. Pp. 49–60 in *In Vivo* Body Composition Studies, K.J. Ellis, S. Yasumura, and W.D. Morgan, eds. London: The Institute of Physical Sciences in Medicine.
Lusk, G.
  1928   The Elements of the Science of Nutrition, 4th ed. New York: Academic Press. Reprint: New York: Johnson Reprint Corp., 1976.
Lycke, N., T. Tsuji, and J. Holmgren
  1992   The adjuvant effect of *Vibrio cholerae* and *Escherichia coli* heat-labile enterotoxins is linked to their ADP-ribosyltransferase activity. Eur. J. Immunol. 22:2277–2281.
Lyons, A.B., and C.R. Parish
  1995   Are murine marginal-zone macrophages the splenic white pulp analog of high endothelial venules? Eur. J. Immunol. 25:3165–3172.
Ma, J.K-C., A. Hiatt, M. Hein, N.D. Vine, F. Wang, P. Stabila, C. van Dolleweerd, K. Mostov, and T. Lehner
  1995   Generation and assembly of secretory antibodies in plants. Science 268:716–719.
MacDonald, T.T.
  1982   Enhancement and suppression of Peyer's patch immune response by systemic priming. Clin. Exp. Immunol. 49:441–448.
Mackay, C.R.
  1991   Skin-seeking memory T-cells. Nature 349:737–738.
Mackay, C.R., W.L. Marston, L. Dudler, O. Spertini, T.F. Tedder, and W.R. Hein
  1992   Tissue-specific migration pathways by phenotypically distinct subpopulations of memory T-cells. Eur. J. Immunol. 22:887–895.
Mackie, R.R.
  1987   Vigilance research—are we ready for countermeasures? Hum. Factors 29(60):707–723.

Magnusson I., D.L. Rothman, L.D. Katz, R.G. Shulman, and G.I. Shulman
  1992   Increased rate of gluconeogenesis in Type II diabetes mellitus. A ^{13}C nuclear magnetic resonance study. J. Clin. Invest. 90:1323–1327.
Maitland, M.E., and A.R. Mandel
  1994   A client-computer interface for questionnaire data. Arch. Phys. Med. Rehabil. 75(6):639–642.
Manetti, R.
  1993   Natural killer cell stimulatory factor (interleukin 12 [IL-12]) induces T helper type 1 (TH$_1$)-specific immune responses and inhibits the development of IL-4-producing Th cells. J. Exp. Med. 177:1199–1204.
Manning, E.M.C., and A. Shenkin
  1995   Nutritional assessment in the critically ill. Crit. Care Clin. 11:603–634.
Mansfield, P.
  1977   Multi-planar image formation using NMR spin-echoes. J. Phys. Chem. 10:L55.
MAPW (Multicohort Analysis Project Workshop—Part I)
  1994   Immunologic markers of AIDS progression: Consistency across five HIV-infected cohorts. AIDS 8:911–921.
Marano, M.A., Y. Fong, L.L. Moldawer, H. Wei, S.E. Calvano, K.J. Tracey, P.S. Barie, K. Manogue, A. Cerami, G.T. Shires et al.
  1990   Serum cachectin/tumor necrosis factor in critically ill patients with burns correlates with infection and mortality. Surg. Gynecol. Obstet. 170:32–38.
Mariash, C.N., and J.H. Oppenheimer
  1983   Stimulation of malic enzyme formation in hepatocyte culture by metabolites: Evidence favoring a nonglycolytic metabolite as the proximate induction signal. Metabolism 33:545–552.
Marks, J.D., H.R. Hoogenboom, T.P. Bonnert, J. McCafferty, A.D. Griffiths, and G. Winter
  1991   By-passing immunization. Human antibodies from V-gene libraries displayed on phage. J. Mol. Biol. 222:16007–16010.
Martens, H., and T. Naes
  1989   Multivariate Calibration. New York: John Wiley & Sons.
Martin, A.D., L.F. Spenst, D.T. Drinkwater, and J.P. Clarys
  1990   Anthropometric estimation of muscle mass in men. Med. Sci. Sports Exerc. 22:729–733.
Martin, A.D., M.Z. Daniel, D. Drinkwater, and J.P. Clarys
  1994   Adipose tissue density estimated adipose lipid fraction and whole body adiposity in male cadavers. Int. J. Obes. 18:79–83.
Mason, H.S., D.M. Lam, and C.J. Arntzen
  1992   Expression of hepatitis B surface antigen in transgenic plants. Proc. Natl. Acad. Sci. USA 89:11745–11749.
Massimino, M.J., and T.B. Sheridan
  1994   Teleoperator performance with varying force and visual feedback. Hum. Factors 36(1):145–157.
Matarazzo, J.P.
  1992   Psychological testing and assessment in the 21st century. Am. Psychol. 47(8):1007–1018.
Matthews, D.E., and D.M. Bier
  1983   Stable isotopes for nutritional investigation. Annu. Rev. Nutr. 3:309–339.
Mattingly, J.A., and B.H. Waksman
  1978   Immunologic suppression after oral administration of antigen. I. Specific suppressor cells formed in rat Peyer's patches after oral administration of sheep erythrocytes and their systemic migration. J. Immunol. 121:1878–1883.

Matzinger, P.
1994   Tolerance, danger, and the extended family. Ann. Rev. Immunol. 12:991–1045.

Mays, M.Z.
1995   Impact of underconsumption on cognitive performance. Pp. 285–302 in Not Eating Enough, Overcoming Underconsumption of Military Operational Rations, B.M. Marriott, ed. A report of the Committee on Military Nutrition Research, Food and Nutrition Board, Institute of Medicine. Washington, D.C.: National Academy Press.

Mazanec, M.B., C.S. Kaetzel, M.E. Lamm, D. Fletcher, and J.G. Nedrud
1992   Intracellular neutralization of virus by immunoglobulin A antibodies. Proc. Natl. Acad. Sci. USA 89:6901–6905.

Mazanec, M.B., J.G. Nedrud, C.S. Kaetzel, and M.E. Lamm
1993   A three-tiered view of the role of IgA in mucosal defense. Immunol. Today 14:430–435.

Mazess, R.B., H.S. Barden, J.P. Bisek, and J. Hanson
1990   Dual-energy x-ray absorptiometry for total-body and regional bone-mineral and soft-tissue composition. Am. J. Clin. Nutr. 51:1106–1112.

Mazess, R.B., H.S. Barden, and E.S. Oldrich
1990b   Skeletal and body-composition effects of anorexia nervosa. Am. J. Clin. Nutr. 52:438–441.

Mazess, R., C.H. Chesnut III, M. McClung, and H. Genant
1992   Enhanced precision with dual-energy x-ray absorptiometry. Calcif. Tissue Int. 51:14–17.

Mazess, R.B., J. Bisek, J. Trempe, and S. Pourchot
1992   Effects of tissue thickness on body composition measurement using dual-energy x-ray absorptiometry. Annual Meeting of the American College of Sportsmedicine, May 1992.

McCabe, D.E., W.F. Swain, B.J. Martinell, and P. Christou
1988   Stable transformation of soybean (Glycine max) by particle acceleration. Bio/Tech. 6:923–926.

McConnell, H.M., J.C. Owicki, J.W. Parce, D.L. Miller, G.T. Baxter, H.G. Wada, and S. Pitchford
1992   The cytosensor microphysiometer: Biological applications of silicon technology. Science 257:1906–1912.

McCormick, B.A., S.P. Colgan, C. Delp-Archer, S.I. Miller, and J.L. Madara
1993   Salmonella typhimurium attachment to human intestinal epithelial monolayers: Transcellular signaling to subepithelial neutrophils. J. Cell Biol. 123:895–907.

McCormick, D.B.
1975   Metabolism of riboflavin. Pp. 153–198 in Riboflavin, R.R. Rivlin, ed. New York: Plenum Press.
1979   Some aspects of the metabolism of sulfur-containing heterocyclic cofactors: Lipoic acid, biotin, and 8α-(S-L-cysteinyl)-riboflavin. Pp. 423–434 in Natural Sulfur Compounds, D. Cavallini, G.E. Gaull, and V. Zappia, eds. New York: Plenum Press.
1989   Two interconnected B vitamins: Riboflavin and pyridoxine. Physiol. Rev. 69(4):1170–1198.

McCormick, D.B., and L.D. Wright
1970   The metabolism of biotin and its analogues. Pp. 81– 110 in Comprehensive Biochemistry, vol. 21, Metabolism of Vitamins and Trace Elements, M. Florkin and E.H. Stortz, eds. Amsterdam: Elsevier.

McCormick, D.B., and Z. Zhang
 1993 Cellular assimilation of water-soluble vitamins in the mammal: Riboflavin, B_6, biotin, and $C_{(43534B)}$. Proc. Soc. Exper. Biol. Med. 202:265–270.
McGandy, R.B., C.H. Barrows, Jr., A. Spanias, A. Meredith, J.L. Stone, and A.H. Morris
 1966 Nutrient intakes and energy expenditure in men of different ages. J. Gerontol. 21:581–587.
McGhee, J.R., J. Mestecky, M.T. Dertzbaugh, J.H. Eldridge, M. Hirasawa, and H. Kiyono
 1992 The mucosal immune system: From fundamental concepts to vaccine development. Vaccine 10:75–88.
McMahon, T.A., and G.C. Cheng
 1990 The mechanics of running: How does stiffness couple with speed? J. Biomech. 23:65–78.
McNeill, G. M.D. Cox, and J.P.W. Rivers
 1987 The Oxylog oxygen consumption meter: A portable device for measurement of energy expenditure. Am. J. Clin. Nutr. 45:1415–1419.
Meehan, C.D., L.A. Bove, and A.S. Jennings
 1992 Comparison of first-generation and second-generation blood glucose meters for use in a hospital setting. Diabetes Educ. 18(3):228–231.
Meijer, G.A., K.R. Westerterp, H. Koper, and F. Ten Hoor
 1989 Assessment of energy expenditure by recording heart rate and body acceleration. Med. Sci. Sports Exerc. 21:343–347.
Meiselman, H.L., and F.M. Kramer
 1994 The role of context in behavioral effects of foods. Pp. 137–157 in Food Components to Enhance Performance, An Evaluation of Potential Performance-Enhancing Food Components for Operational Rations, B.M. Marriott, ed. A report of the Committee on Military Nutrition Research, Food and Nutrition Board, Institute of Medicine. Washington, D.C.: National Academy Press.
Mendelson, Y., A.C. Clermont, R.A. Peura, and B.C. Lin
 1990 Blood glucose measurement by multiple attenuated total reflection and infrared absorption spectroscopy. IEEE Trans. Biomed. Eng. 37(5):458–465.
Merton, P.A.
 1954 Voluntary strength and fatigue. J. Physiol. 123:553–564.
Metcalf, J.A.
 1986 Laboratory Manual of Neutrophil Function. New York: Raven Press.
Metropolitan Life Insurance Company
 1937 Girth and death. Stat. Bull. 18:2–5.
Metzger, J.F., and G.E. Lewis, Jr.
 1979 Human-derived immune globulins for the treatment of botulism. Rev. Infect. Dis. 1:689–692.
Meyer G-J., H.H. Coenen, S.L. Waters, B. Langstrom, R. Contineau, K. Strijckmans, W. Vaalburg, C. Hallidin, C. Crouzel, B. Maziére, and A. Luxen
 1993 Quality assurance and quality control of short-lived radiopharmaceuticals for PET. Pp. 91–150 in Radiopharmaceuticals for Positron Emission Tomography, G. Stocklin and V.W. Pike, eds. Dordrecht, The Netherlands: Kluwer Academic Publishers.
Michalek, S.M., J.H. Eldridge, R. Curtiss III, and K.L. Rosenthal
 1994 Antigen delivery systems: New approaches to mucosal immunization. Pp. 373–380 in Handbook of Mucosal Immunology, P.L. Ogra, J. Mestecky, M.E. Lamm, W. Strober, J.R. McGhee, and J. Bienenstock, eds. Boston: Academic Press, Inc.

Michalek, S.M., N.K. Childers, and M.T. Dertzbaugh
    1995   Vaccination strategies for mucosal pathogens. Pp. 269–301 in Virulence Mecha-
            nisms of Bacterial Pathogens, 2nd ed., J.A. Roth, ed. Washington, D.C.: American
            Society for Microbiology.
Michie, H.R., K.R. Manogue, D.R. Spriggs, A. Revhaug, S. O'Dwyer, C.A. Dinarello, A.
        Cerami, S.M. Wolff, and D.W. Wilmore
    1988   Detection of circulating tumor necrosis factor after endotoxin administration. N.
            Engl. J. Med. 318:1481–1486.
Mitler, M.M.
    1988   Catastrophes, sleep and public policy: Consensus report. Sleep 11(1):100–109.
Mitta, D.A., and S.J. Packebush
    1995   Improving interface quality: An investigation of human-computer interaction task
            learning. Ergonomics 38(7):1307–1325.
Miyoshi, H., G.I. Schulman, E.J. Peters, M.H. Wolfe, D. Elahi, and R.R. Wolfe
    1988   Hormonal control of substrate cycling in humans. J. Clin. Invest. 81:1545–1555.
Mobilis
    1996a   Interview with General Magic's Jim White (Part I). Mobilis 2(3) URL
            http://www.volksware.com /mobilis/march.96/interv1.htm.
    1996b   Interview with General Magic's Jim White (Part II). Mobilis 2(4) URL
            http://www.volksware.com/mobilis/april.96/interv1.htm.
Mobley, J.A.
    1995   Biological warfare in the twentieth century: Lessons from the past, challenges for
            the future. Mil. Med. 160:547–553.
Moffat, A.S.
    1995   Exploring transgenic plants as a new vaccine source. Science 268:658–660.
Moldawer, L.L.
    1994   Biology of proinflammatory cytokines and their antagonists. Crit. Care Med.
            22:S3–S7.
Montoye, H.J.
    1971   Estimation of habitual physical activity by questionnaire and interview. Am. J.
            Clin. Nutr. 24:1113–1118.
Montoye, H.J., and H.L. Taylor
    1984   Measurement of physical activity in population studies: A review. Hum. Biol.
            56:195–216.
Montoye, H.J., R. Washburn, S. Servais, A. Ertl, J.G. Webster, and F.J. Nagle
    1983   Estimation of energy expenditure by a portable accelerometer. Med. Sci. Sports
            Exerc. 15:403–407.
Moody, D.L., J. Kollias, and E.R. Buskirk
    1969   The effect of a moderate exercise program on body weight and skinfold thickness
            in overweight college women. Med. Sci. Sports 1:75–80.
Moore, F.D.
    1963   The Body Cell Mass and Its Supporting Environment. London: W.B. Saunders.
    1966   Energy stores as revealed by body compositional study. Pp. 110–121 in Energy
            Metabolism and Body Fuel Utilization, with Particular Reference to Starvation and
            Injury, A.P. Morgan, ed. Proceedings of the Committee on Metabolism in Trauma
            of the U.S. Army Research and Development Command. Cambridge, Mass.:
            Harvard University Printing Office.
Moore, R.C.
    1995   Integration of speech with natural language understanding. Proc. Natl. Acad. Sci.
            USA 92(22):9983–9988.

Moore, R.J., K.E. Friedl, T.R. Kramer, L.E. Martinez-Lopez, R.W. Hoyt, R.E. Tulley, J.P. DeLany, E.W. Askew, and J.A. Vogel
  1992 Changes in soldier nutritional status and immune function during the Ranger training course. Technical Report No. T13-92. Natick, Mass.: U.S. Army Research Institute of Environmental Medicine.

Moore-Ede, M.C., F.M. Sulzman, and C.A. Fuller
  1982 The Clocks that Time Us. Physiology of the Circadian Timing System. Cambridge, Mass.: Harvard University Press.

Morikawa, Y., K. Tohya, H. Ishida, N. Matsuura, and K. Kakudo
  1995 Different migration patterns of antigen-presenting cells correlate with Th1/Th2-type responses in mice. Immunology 85:575–581.

Morris, P.G., D.J.O. McIntyre, R. Coxon, H.S. Bachelard, K.T. Moriarty, P.L. Greenhaff, and I.A. Macdonald
  1994 Nuclear magnetic resonance spectroscopy as a tool to study carbohydrate metabolism. Proc. Nutr. Soc. 53:335–343.

Morris, W., M.C. Steinhoff, and P.K. Russell
  1994 Potential of polymer microencapsulation technology for vaccine innovation. Vaccine 12:5–11.

Morrow, B.E., and R. Kucherlapati
  1995 Molecular genetic medicine. Pp. 556–561 in Molecular Biology and Biotechnology: A Comprehensive Desk Reference, R.A. Meyers, ed. New York: VCH Publishers.

Morrow, J.R., A.S. Jackson, P.W. Bradley, and G.H. Hartung
  1986 Accuracy of measured and predicted residual lung volume on body density measurement. Med. Sci. Sports Exerc. 18:647–652.

Moscovitz, H., F. Shofer, H. Mignott, A. Behrman, and L. Kilpatrick
  1994 Plasma cytokine determinations in emergency department patients as a predictor of bacteremia and infectious disease severity. Crit. Care Med. 22:1102–1107.

Mosmann, T.R., and S. Sad
  1996 The expanding universe of T-cell subsets: Th1, Th2 and more. Immunol. Today 17:138–146.

Mosskin, M., H. von Holst, M. Bergstrom, V.P. Collins, L. Ericksson, P. Johnstrom, and G. Norén
  1987 Positron emission tomography with ^{11}C-methionine and computed tomography of intracranial tumors compared with histopathologic examination of multiple biopsies. Acta Radiol. 28:673–681.

Mostov, K.E.
  1994 Transepithelial transport of immunoglobulins Annu. Rev. Immunol. 12:63–84.

Moulton, C.R.
  1923 Age and chemical development in mammals. J. Biol. Chem. 57:79–97.

Mowat, A.M.
  1994 Oral tolerance and regulation of immunity to dietary antigens. Pp. 185–201 in Handbook of Mucosal Immunology, P.L. Ogra, J. Mestecky, M.E. Lamm, W. Strober, J.R. McGhee, and J. Bienenstock, eds. Boston: Academic Press, Inc.

Mudd, S.H., J.D. Finkelstein, F. Irreverre, and L. Laster
  1965 Transsulfuration in mammals. Microassays and tissue distributions of three enzymes of the pathway. J. Biol. Chem. 240:4382–4392.

Muller, D.C., D. Elahi, J.D. Sorkin, and R. Andres
  1995 Muscle mass: Its measurement and influence on aging. The Baltimore Longitudinal Study of Aging. Pp. 60–62 in Nutritional Assessment of Elderly Populations: Measure and Function, I.H. Rosenberg, ed. New York: Raven Press.

Munro, H.N.
  1983   Metabolic basis of nutritional care in liver and kidney disease. Pp. 93–105 in Nutritional Support of the Seriously Ill Patient, R.W. Winters and H.L. Green, eds. New York: Academic Press, Inc.

Murphy, P.M.
  1995   Blood, sweat, and chemotactic cetaceans [commentary]. J. Leukocyte Biol. 57:438–439.

Nagy, K.A., and D.P. Costa
  1980   Water flux in animals: Analysis of potential errors in the tritiated water method. Am. J. Physiol. 238:R454–R465.

Nair, K.S., D. Halliday, and R.C. Creggs
  1988   Leucine incorporation into mixed skeletal muscle protein in humans. Am. J. Physiol. 254:E208–E213.

Nair, K.S., G.C. Ford, K. Ekberg, E. Fernqvist-Forbes, and J. Wahren
  1995   Protein dynamics in whole body and leg tissues in type I diabetic patients. J. Clin. Invest. 95:2926–2937.

Nathan, C., and M. Sporn
  1991   Cytokines in context. J. Cell Biol. 113:981–986.

Nautila, P., J. Knuuti, U. Ruotsalainen, V.A. Koivisto, E. Eronen, M. Teräs, J. Bergman, M. Haaparanta, L-M. Voipio-Pulkki, J. Viikari, T. Rönnemaa, U. Wegelius, and H. Yki-Järvomem
  1993   Insulin resistance is localized to skeletal but not heart muscle in type I diabetes. Am. J. Physiol. 264:E756–E762.

Neese, R.A., J-M. Schwartz, D. Faix, S. Turner, A. Letscher, D. Vu, and M.K. Hellerstein
  1995   Gluconeogenesis and intrahepatic triose phosphate flux in response to fasting or substrate loads. Application of the mass isotopomer distribution analysis technique with testing of assumptions and potential problems. J. Biol. Chem. 270:14452–14463.

Neutra, M.R., and J-P Kraehenbuhl
  1994   Cellular and molecular basis for antigen transport in the intestinal epithelium. Pp. 27–39 in Handbook of Mucosal Immunology, P.L. Ogra, J. Mestecky, M.E. Lamm, W. Strober, J.R. McGhee, and J. Bienenstock, eds. Boston: Academic Press, Inc.

Newman, R.W.
  1955   Skin-fold changes with increasing obesity in young American males. Hum. Biol. 27:53–64.

Newstead, C.G., W.R. Lamb, P.E. Brenchley, and C.D. Short
  1993   Serum and urine IL-6 and TNF-alpha in renal transplant recipients with graft dysfunction. Transplantation 56:831–835.

NIH (National Institutes of Health)
  1996   Technology Assessment Statement on Bioelectrical Impedance Analysis in Body Composition Measurement, 1994 December 12–14. Am. J. Clin. Nutr. 64(suppl.):524S–532S.

Nindl, B.C., K.E. Friedl, L.J. Marchitelli, R.L. Shippee, C. Thomas, and J.F. Patton
  1996   Fat placement in fit males and regional changes with weight loss. Med. Sci. Sports Exerc. 28:786–793.

Nord, R.H.
  1991   Soft tissue composition phantom for DXA. Osteoporos. Int. 1:203.

Nord, R.H., and R.K. Payne
  1990   Standards for body composition calibration in DEXA. Paper presented at the 2nd Annual Meeting of the Bath Conference on Bone Mineral Measurement, Bath, U.K.

NRC (National Research Council)
1986   Cognitive Testing Methodology, Proceedings of a Workshop Held on June 11–12, 1984. Committee on Military Nutrition Research, Food and Nutrition Board, Commission on Life Sciences. Washington, D.C.: National Academy Press.

Nyboer, J.
1959   Electrical Impedance Plethysmography. Springfield, Ill.: Charles C Thomas.

O'Halloran, T.V.
1993   Transition metals in control of gene expression. Science 261:712–725.

O'Malley, B.W., and O.M. Conneely
1992   Orphan receptors: In search of a unifying hypothesis for activation. Mol. Endocrinol. 6:1359–1361.

Ochs, H.D., S. Nonoyama, Q. Zhu, M. Farrington, and R.J. Wedgwood
1993   Regulation of antibody responses: The role of complement and adhesion molecules. Clin. Immunol. Immunopathol. 67(suppl. 2):S33–S40.

Office of Technology Assessment, U.S. Congress
1991   Biological rhythms: Implications for the worker. OTA-BA-463. Washington, D.C.: U.S. Government Printing Office.

Ogra, P.L., J. Mestecky, M.E. Lamm, W. Strober, J.R. McGhee, and J. Bienenstock, eds.
1994   Handbook of Mucosal Immunology. Boston: Academic Press, Inc.

Ohkawa, H., N. Ohishi, and K. Yagi 1983   Occurrence of riboflavinyl glucoside in rat urine. J. Nutr. Sci. Vitaminol. 29:515–522.

Okubo, K., N. Hori, R. Matoba, T. Niiyama, A. Fukushima, Y. Kojima, and K. Matsubara
1992   Large-scale cDNA sequencing for analysis of quantitative and qualitative aspects of gene expression. Nature Genetics 2:173–179.

Openshaw, P.J.M., E.E. Murphy, N.A. Hosken, V. Manio, K. Davis, and A. O'Garra
1995   Heterogeneity of intracellular cytokine synthesis at the single cell level in polarised T helper 1 and T helper 2 populations. J. Exp. Med. 182:1357–1367.

Oppenheimer, J.H., H.L. Schwartz, C.N. Mariash, W.B. Kinlaw, N.C. Wong, and H.C. Freake
1987   Advances in our understanding of thyroid hormone action at the cellular level. Endocr. Rev. 8:288–308.

Oppenheim, J.J., C.O.C. Zachariae, N. Mukaida, and K. Matsushima
1991   Properties of the novel proinflammatory supergene "intercrine" cytokine family. Ann. Rev. Immunol. 9:617–648.

Oritsland, N.A.
1990   Starvation survival and body composition in mammals with particular reference to *Homo sapiens*. Bull. Math. Biol. 52:643–655.

Orr, S., T.P. Hughes, C.L. Sawyers, R.M. Kato, S.G. Quan, S.P. Williams, O.N. Witte, and L. Hood
1994   Isolation of unknown genes from human bone marrow by differential screening and single-pass cDNA sequence determination. Proc. Natl. Acad. Sci. USA 91:11869–11873.

Orwoll, E.S., S.K. Oviatt, and J.A. Biddle
1993   Precision of dual-energy x-ray absorptiometry: Development of quality control rules and their application in longitudinal studies. J. Bone Miner. Res. 8:693–699.

Osborne, T.F.
1991   Single nucleotide resolution of sterol regulatory region in promoter for 3-hydroxy-3-methylglutaryl Coenzyme A reductase. J. Biol. Chem. 266:13947–13951.

Owen, R.L, and A.L. Jones
1974   Epithelial cell specialization within human Peyer's patches: An ultrastructural study of intestinal lymphoid follicles. Gastroenterology 66:189–203.

Owens, L., and D.E. Cress
  1985 Genotypic variability of soybean response to Agrobacterium strains harboring the Ti or Ri plasmids. Plant Physiol. 77:87–94.
Owicki, J.C., and J.W. Parce
  1992 Biosensors based on the energy metabolism of living cells: The physical chemistry and cell biology of extracellular acidification. Biosens. Bioelectron. 7:255–272.
Pace, N., and E.N. Rathbun
  1945 Studies on body composition. III. The body water and chemically combined nitrogen content in relation to fat content. J. Biol. Chem. 158:685–691.
Paffenbarger, R.S., R.T. Hyde, A.L. Wing, and C. Hsieh
  1986 Physical activity, all-cause mortality, and longevity of college alumni. N. Engl. J. Med. 314:605–613.
Palmiter, R.D., R.L. Brinster, R.E. Hammer, M.E. Trumbauer, M.G. Rosenfeld, N.C. Birnberg, and R.M. Evans
  1982 Dramatic growth of mice that develop from eggs microinjected with metallothionein-growth hormone fusion genes. Nature 300:611–615.
Papelis, Y.E.
  1994 Terrain modeling on high-fidelity ground vehicle simulators. Pp. 48–54 in 5th Annual Conference on Artificial Intelligence, Simulation and Planning in High Autonomy Systems. Los Alamitos, Calif.: Institute of Electrical and Electronics Engineers, Inc., Computer Society Press.
Papelis, Y.E., and S. Bahauddin
  1995 Logical modeling of roadway environment to support real-time simulation of autonomous traffic. Pp. 62–71 in Proceedings of the 1st Workshop on Simulation and Interaction in Virtual Environments. Iowa City, Iowa: Department of Computer Science, University of Iowa.
Pascale, L.R., T. Frankel, M.I. Grossman, S. Freeman, I.L. Faller, E.E. Bond, R. Ryan, and L. Bernstein
  1955 Changes in body composition of soldiers during paratrooper training. Technical Report 156. Denver, Colo.: Physiology Division, U.S. Army Medical Nutrition Laboratory.
Pascale, L.R., M.I. Grossman, H.S. Sloane, and T. Frankel
  1956 Correlations between thickness of skinfolds and body density in 88 soldiers. Hum. Biol. 28:165–176.
Patterson, R.
  1989 Body fluid determinations using multiple impedance measurements. IEEE Eng. Med. Biol. Mag. 3:16–18.
Patterson, R., C. Ranganathan, R. Engel, and R. Berkseth
  1988 Measurement of body fluid volume change using multisite impedance measurements. Med. Biol. Eng. Comput. 26:33–37.
Patterson, S.M., D.S. Krantz, L.C. Montgomery, P.A. Deuster, S. M. Hedges, and L.E. Nebel
  1993 Automated physical activity monitoring: Validation and comparison with physiological and self-reported measures. Psychophysiology 30(3):296–305.
Patton, J.F., M. Murphy, T. Bidwell, R. Mello, and M. Harp
  1991 Metabolic cost of military physical tasks in MOPP 0 and MOPP 4. Technical Report T95-9. Natick, Mass.: U.S. Army Research Institute of Environmental Medicine.
Patton, J.F., M. Murphy, T. Bidwell, R. Mello, and M. Harp
  1995 Metabolic cost of military physical tasks in MOPP 0 and MOPP 4. Technical Report T95-9, AD A294059. Natick, Mass.: U.S. Army Research Institute of Environmental Medicine.

Pedersen, H.C., J. Christiansen, and R. Wyndaele
  1983 Induction and *in vitro* culture of soybean crown gall tumors. Plant Cell Reports 2:201–204.
Peltola, H., A. Sittonen, H. Kyronseppa, I. Simula, L. Mattila, P. Oksanen, M.J. Kataja, and M. Cadoz
  1991 Prevention of travellers' diarrhoea by oral B-subunit/whole-cell cholera vaccine. Lancet 338(8778):1285–1289.
Pen Computing
  1996a Pen computers in healthcare. Pen Computing 3(9):18–35.
  1996b Pen computers in transportation. Pen Computing 3(10):18–33.
Penn, I-W., Z-M. Wang, K.M. Buhl, D.B. Allison, S.E. Burastero, and S.B. Heymsfield
  1994 Body composition and two-compartment model assumptions in male long distance runners. Med. Sci. Sports Exerc. 26:392–397.
Perrier Study of Fitness in America
  1979 Study No. S2813. New York: Louis Harris and Associates Inc.
Peuchant, E., C. Salles, and R. Jensen
  1987 Determination of serum cholesterol by near-infrared reflectance spectrometry. Anal. Chem. 59(14):1816–1819.
  1988 Value of a spectroscopic "fecalogram" in determining the etiology of steatorrhea. Clin. Chem. 34(1):5–8.
Phelps, M.E., J.C. Mazziotta, and H.R. Schelbert, eds.
  1986 Positron Emission Tomography and Autoradiography: Principles and Applications for the Brain and Heart. New York: Raven Press.
Pi-Sunyer, F.X., and K.R. Segal
  1992 Relationship of diet and exercise. Pp. 187–210 in Energy Metabolism—Tissue Determinants and Cellular Corollaries, J.M. Kinney and H.N. Tucker, eds. New York: Raven Press.
Pierce, N.F.
  1978 The role of antigen form and function in the primary and secondary intestinal immune responses to cholera toxin and toxoid in rats. J. Exp. Med. 148:195–206.
Pierce, N.S., and J.L. Gowans
  1975 Cellular kinetics of the intestinal immune response to cholera toxoid in rats. J. Exp. Med. 142:1550–1563.
Planas, A.M., C. Prenant, B.M. Mazoyer, D. Comar, and L. DiGiamberardino
  1992 Regional cerebral L-[^{14}C-*Methyl*]methionine incorporation into proteins: Evidence for methionine recycling in the rat brain. J. Cereb. Blood Flow Metab. 12:603–612.
Pocock, N.A., P.N. Sambrook, T. Nguyen, P. Kelly, J. Freund, and J.A. Eisman
  1992 Assessment of spinal and femoral bone density by dual x-ray absorptiometry: Comparison of Lunar and Hologic instruments. J. Bone Miner. Res. 7:1081–1084.
Pollitt, E.
  1995 Does breakfast make a difference in school? J. Am. Diet. Assoc. 95(10):1134–1139.
Pollock, M.L.
  1973 The quantification of endurance training programs. Exerc. Sport Sci. Rev. 1:155–188.
Powanda, M.C., and W.R. Beisel
  1982 Hypothesis: Leukocyte endogenous mediator/endogenous pyrogen/lymphocyte-activating factor modulates the development of nonspecific and specific immunity and affects nutritional status. Am. J. Clin. Nutr. 35:762–768.

Powell, K.E., and R.S. Paffenbarger
  1985   Workshop on epidemiologic and public health aspects of physical activity and exercise: A summary. Public Health Rep. 100:118–126.
Preston, T., and C. Slater
  1994   Mass spectrometric analysis of stable-isotope-labeled amino acid tracers. Proc. Nutr. Soc. 53:363–372.
Prieur, A.M., M.T. Kaufmann, C. Griscelli, and J.M. Dayer
  1987   Specific interleukin-1 inhibitor in serum and urine of children with systemic juvenile chronic arthritis. Lancet 2(8570):1240–1242.
Pritchard, J.E., C.A. Nowson, B.J. Strauss, J.S. Carlson, B. Kaymakci, and J.D. Wark
  1993   Evaluation of dual energy x-ray absorptiometry as a method of measurement of body fat. Eur. J. Clin. Nutr. 47:216–228.
Pruitt, J.H., E.M. Copeland, and L.L. Moldawer
  1995   Interleukin-1, interleukin-1 receptor antagonist and interleukin-1 receptors in sepsis, shock and the systemic inflammatory response syndrome. Shock 3:235–251.
Punt, J.A., and S. Singer
  1996   T-cell development. Pp. 157–175 in Clinical Immunology Principles and Practice, R.R. Rich, T.A. Fleisher, B.D. Schwartz, W.T. Shearer, and W. Strober, eds. Boston: Mosby.
Purcell, E.M., H.C. Torrey, and R.V. Pound
  1946   Resonance absorption by nuclear magnetic moments in a solid. Phys. Rev. 69:37–38.
Purcell, W.M., and C.K. Atterwill
  1994   Human placental mast cells as an *in vitro* model system in aspects of neuroimmunotoxicity testing. Hum. Exp. Toxicol. 13(6):429–433.
Quaim, S.M., J.C. Clark, C. Crouzel, M. Guillaume, H.J. Helmeke, B. Nebeling, V.W. Pike, and G. Stocklin
  1993   PET radionuclide production. Pp. 1–43 in Radiopharmaceuticals for Positron Emission Tomography, G. Stocklin and W.V. Pike, eds. Dordrecht, The Netherlands: Kluwer Academic Publishers.
Quiding-Jarbrink, M., M. Lakew, I. Nordstrom, J. Bachereau, E. Butcher, J. Holmgren, and C. Czerkinsky
  1995   Human circulating specific antibody-forming cells after systemic and mucosal immunizations: Differential homing commitments and cell surface differentiation markers. Eur. J. Immunol. 25:322–327.
Racette, S.B., D.A. Schoeller, A.H. Luke, K. Shay, J. Hnilicka, and R.F. Kushner
  1994   Relative dilution spaces of ^{2}H- and ^{18}O-labeled water in humans. Am. J. Physiol. 267 (30):E585–E590.
Raden, J.
  1917   On the determination of functions from their integrals along certain mainfolds. Math. Phys. Klasse. 69:262–277.
Rahelu, M., G.T. Williams, D.S. Kumararatne, G.S. Eaton, and J.S. Gaston
  1993   Human CD4+ cytolitic T cells kill antigen-pulsed target T cells by induction of apoptosis. J. Immunol. 150:4856–4866
Raichle, M.E., W.R.W. Martin, P. Herscovitch, M.A. Mintum, and J. Markham
  1983   Brain blood flow measured with intravenous $H_2^{15}O$. II. Implementation and validation. J. Nucl. Med. 24:790–798.
Ramsey, K.H., H. Schneider, R.A. Kuschner, A.F. Trofa, A.S. Cross, and C.D. Deal
  1994   Inflammatory cytokine response to experimental human infection with *Neisseria gonorrhoeae*. Ann. N.Y. Acad. Sci. 730:322–325.

Rathmacher, J.A., P.J. Flakoll, and S.L. Nissen
  1995   A compartmental model of 3-methylhistidine metabolism in humans. Am. J. Physiol. 269:E193–E198.
Rebar, E.J., and C.O. Pabo
  1994   Zinc finger phage: Affinity selection of fingers with new DNA-binding specificities. Science 263:671–673.
Rebuffe-Scrive, M., L. Enk, N. Crona, P. Lonroth, L. Ambrahmasson, U. Smith, and P. Björntorp
  1985   Regional human adipose tissue metabolism during the menstrual cycle, pregnancy, and lactation. J. Clin. Invest. 75:1973–1976.
Redmond, D.P., and F.W. Hegge
  1985   Observations on the design and specification of a wrist-worn human activity monitoring system. Behavior Research Methods, Instruments, and Computers 17(6):659–669.
Reed, L.J., and A.G. Love
  1932   Biometric studies on U.S. Army officers—Somatological norms, correlations, and changes with age. Hum. Biol. 4:509–524.
Reitan, R.M., and D. Wolfson
  1994   A selective and critical review of neuropsychological deficits and the frontal lobes. Neuropsychol. Rev. 4(3):161–198.
Renegar, K.B., and P.A. Small, Jr.
  1994   Passive immunization: Systemic and mucosal. Pp. 347–356 in Handbook of Mucosal Immunology, P.L. Ogra, J. Mestecky, M.E. Lamm, W. Strober, J.R. McGheee, and J. Bienenstock, eds. Boston: Academic Press, Inc.
Rennie, M.J.
  1994   Human skeletal and cardiac muscle proteolysis: Evolving concepts and practical applications. Pp. 23–48 in Organ Metabolism and Nutrition: Ideas for Future Critical Care, J.M. Kinney and H.N. Tucker, eds. New York: Raven Press.
Retzlaff, P., M. Butler, and R. Vanderploeg
  1992   Neuropsychological battery choice and theoretical orientation: A multivariate analysis. J. Clin. Psychol. 48(5):666–672.
Retzlaff, P.D., and M. Gibertini
  1994   Neuropsychometric issues and problems. Pp. 185–209 in Clinician's Guide to Neuropsychological Assessment, R.D. Vanderploeg, ed. Hillsdale, N.J.: Lawrence Erlbaum.
Reynolds, K.L., H.A. Heckel, C.E. Witt, J.W. Martin, J.A. Pollard, J.J. Knapik, and B.H. Jones
  1994   Cigarette smoking, physical fitness, and injuries in infantry soldiers. Am. J. Prev. Med. 10(3):145–150.
Ribeiro, R.A.
  1994   IL-8 causes *in vivo* neutrophil migration by a cell-dependent mechanism. Immunology 73:472–477.
Riggs, K.M., A. Spiro, K. Tucker, and D. Rush
  1996   Relationship of vitamin B_{12}, vitamin B_6, folate, and homocysteine to cognitive performance in the Normative Aging Study. Am. J. Clin. Nutr. 63(3):306–314.
Riley, M., J. McFarland, C.F. Stanford, and D.P. Nicholls
  1992   Oxygen consumption during corridor walk testing in chronic cardiac failure. Eur. Heart J. 13:789–793.
Rintala, E., K. Pulkki, J. Mertsola, T. Nevalainen, and J. Nikoskelainen
  1995   Endotoxin, interleukin-6 and phospholipase-A2 as markers of sepsis in patients with hematological malignancies. Scand. J. Infect. Dis. 27:39–43.

Rising, R., B. Swinburn, K. Larson, and E. Ravussin
   1991   Body composition in Pima Indians—validation of bioelectrical resistance. Am. J. Clin. Nutr. 53:594–598.

Ritz, P., P.G. Johnson, and W.A. Coward
   1994   Measurements of ^{2}H and ^{18}O in body water: Analytical considerations and physiological implications. Br. J. Nutr. 72:3–12.

Rizzo, M., G.S. Watson, D.V. McGehee, and T.A. Dingus
   1994a   Simulator driving and car crashes in aging and cognitively impaired drivers. J. Neurol. 241:526.
   1994b   Simulator driving and car crashes in Alzheimer's disease. Soc. Neurosci. Abstr. 20:439.

Roberts, S.B.
   1989   Use of doubly labeled water method for measurement of energy expenditure, total body water, water intake, and metabolizable energy intake in humans and small animals. Can. J. Physiol. Pharmacol. 67:1190–1198.

Robey, E., and J.P. Allison
   1995   T-cell activation: Integration of signals from the antigen receptor and costimulatory molecules. Immunol. Today 16:306–310.

Robinson, M.R., R.P. Eaton, D.M. Haaland, G.W. Koepp, E.V. Thomas, B.R. Stallard, and P.L. Robinson
   1992   Noninvasive glucose monitoring in diabetic patients: A preliminary evaluation. Clin. Chem. 38(9):1618–1622.

Rocken, M., and E.M. Shevach
   1996   Immune deviation—The third dimension of nondeletional T cell tolerance. Immunol. Rev. 149:175–194.

Roden, M., G. Perseghin, K.F. Petersen, J.H. Hwang, G.W. Cline, K. Gerow, D.L. Rothman, and G.I. Shulman
   1996   The roles of insulin and glucagon in the regulation of hepatic glycogen synthesis and turnover in humans. J. Clin. Invest. 97:642–648.

Rognum, T.O., K. Rodahl, and P.K. Opstad
   1982   Regional differences in the lipolytic response of the subcutaneous fat depots to prolonged exercise and severe energy deficiency. Eur. J. Appl. Physiol. 49:401–408.

Rogy, M.A., S.M. Coyle, H.S. Oldenburg, C.S. Rock, P.S. Barie, K.J. Van Zee, C.G. Smith, L.L. Moldawer, and S.F. Lowry
   1994   Persistently elevated soluble tumor necrosis factor receptor and interleukin-1 receptor antagonist levels in critically ill patients. J. Am. Coll. Surg. 178:132–138.

Romagnani, S.
   1991   Type 1 T-helper and Type 2 T-helper cells: Functions, regulation and role in protection and disease. Int. J. Clin. Lab. Res. 21:152–158.

Romano, R.A., and G.S. Watson
   1994   Assessment of capabilities—Iowa Driving Simulator. Technical Report No. FHWA-IR-94. Washington, D.C.: U.S. Department of Transportation Federal Highway Administration.

Rome, L.C.
   1992   Scaling of muscle fibers and locomotion. J. Exp. Biol. 168:243–252.

Rome, L.C., A.A. Sosnicki, and D.O. Goble
   1990   Maximum velocity of shortening of three fiber types from the horse soleus: Implications for scaling with body size. J. Physiol. (Lond.) 431:173–185.

Romijn, J.A., E.F. Coyle, J. Hibbert, and R.R. Wolfe
   1992   Comparison of indirect calorimetry and a new breath ^{13}C/^{12}C ratio method during strenuous exercise. Am. J. Physiol. 263(28):E64–E71.

Romijn, J.A., E.F. Coyle, L.S. Sidossis, A. Gastaldelli, J.F. Horowitz, E. Endert, and R.R. Wolfe
  1993 Regulation of endogenous fat and carbohydrate metabolism in relation to exercise intensity and duration. Am. J. Physiol. 265 (28):E380–E391.

Rose, R.C., D.B. McCormick, T-K. Li, L. Lumeng, J.G. Haddad, Jr., and R. Spector
  1986 Transport and metabolism of vitamins. Fed. Proc. 45:30–39.

Rosenberg, I.H., and J.W. Miller
  1992 Nutritional factors in physical and cognitive functions of elderly people. Am. J. Clin. Nutr. 55(6 suppl.):1237S–1243S.

Ross, R., and J. Rissanen
  1994 Mobilization of visceral and subcutaneous adipose tissue in response to energy restriction and exercise. Am. J. Clin. Nutr. 60:695–703.

Ross, R., L. Léger, R. Guardo, J. de Guise, and B.G. Pike
  1991 Adipose tissue volume measured by magnetic resonance imaging and computerized tomography in rats. J. Appl. Physiol. 70(5):2164–2172.

Ross, R., L. Léger, D. Morris, J. de Guise, and R. Guardo
  1992 Quantification of adipose tissue by MRI: Relationship with anthropometric variables. J. Appl. Physiol. 72:787–795.

Ross, R., K.D. Shaw, Y. Martel, J. de Guise, and L. Avruch
  1993 Adipose tissue distribution measured by magnetic resonance imaging in obese women. Am. J. Clin. Nutr. 57:470–475.

Ross, R., K.D. Shaw, J. Rissanen, Y. Martel, J. de Guise, and L. Avruch
  1994 Sex differences in lean and adipose tissue distribution by magnetic resonance imaging: Anthropometric relationships. Am. J. Clin. Nutr. 59:1277–1285.

Ross, R., H. Pedwell, and J. Rissanen
  1995a Effects of energy restriction and exercise on skeletal muscle and adipose tissue in women as measured by magnetic resonance imaging. Am. J. Clin. Nutr. 61:1179–1185.
  1995b Response of total and regional lean tissue and skeletal muscle to a program of energy restriction and resistance exercise. Int. J. Obes. 19(11):781–787.

Rossner, S., W.J. Bo, E. Hiltbrandt, W. Hinson, N. Karstaedt, P. Santago, W.T. Sobol, and J.R. Crouse
  1990 Adipose tissue determinations in cadavers—a comparison between cross-sectional planimetry and computed tomography. Int. J. Obes. 14:893–902.

Roth, E.M., D.D. Woods, and H.E. Pople
  1992 Cognitive simulation as a tool for cognitive task analysis. Ergonomics 35(10):1163–1198.

Rothman, D.L., I. Magnusson, L.D. Katz, R.G. Shulman, and G.I. Shulman
  1991 Quantitation of hepatic glycogenolysis and gluconeogenesis in fasting humans with ^{13}C NMR. Science 254:573–576.

Rothman, D.L., R.G. Shulman, and G.I. Shulman
  1992 ^{31}P nuclear magnetic resonance measurements of muscle glucose-6-phosphate. Evidence for reduced insulin-dependent muscle glucose transport or phosphorylation activity in non-insulin-dependent diabetes mellitus. J. Clin. Invest. 89:1069–1075.

Rothman, D.L., I. Magnusson, G. Cline, D. Gerard, C.R. Kahn, R.G. Shulman, and G.I. Shulman
  1995 Decreased muscle glucose transport/phosphorylation is an early defect in the pathogenesis of non-insulin-dependent diabetes mellitus. Proc. Natl. Acad. Sci. (USA) 92:983–987.

Rott, L.S., M.J. Briskin, D.P. Andrew, E.L. Berg, and E.C. Butcher
  1996   A fundamental subdivision of circulating lymphocytes defined by adhesion to mucosal addressin cell adhesion molecule-1. J. Immunol. 156:3727–3736.
Roubenhoff, R., and R.C. Rall
  1993   Humoral mediation of changing body composition during aging and chronic inflammation. Nutr. Rev. 51:1–11.
Roubenoff, R., J.J. Kehayias, B. Dawson-Hughes, and S.B. Heymsfield
  1993   Use of dual-energy x-ray absorptiometry in body composition studies: Not yet a "gold standard." Am. J. Clin. Nutr. 58:589–591.
Rubin, D.H., M.A. Eaton, and A.O. Anderson
  1986   Reovirus infection in adult mice: The virus hemagglutinin determines the site of intestinal disease. Microb. Pathogen. 1:79–87.
Ruedl, C., C. Rieser, N. Kofler, G. Wick, and H. Wolf
  1996   Humoral and cellular immune responses in the murine respiratory tract following oral immunization with cholera toxin or *Escherichia coli* heat-labile enterotoxin. Vaccine 14:792–798.
Rugeles, M.T., M. LaVia, J-M. Goust, J.M. Kilpatrick, B. Hyman, and G. Virella
  1987   Autologous RBC potentiate antibody synthesis by unfractionated human mononuclear cell cultures. Scand. J. Immunol. 26:119–127.
Rush, S., J.A. Abildskov, and R. McFee
  1963   Resistivity of body tissues at low frequencies. Circ. Res. 12:40–50.
Russell, C.M., D.F. Williamson, and T. Byers
  1995   Can the Year 2000 objective for reducing overweight in the United States be reached?: A simulation study of the required changes in body weight. Int. J. Obes. 19:149–153.
Russell, D.M., L.A. Leiter, J. Whitwell, E.B. Marliss, and K.N. Jeejeebhoy
  1983   Skeletal muscle function during hypocaloric diets and fasting: A comparison with standard nutritional assessment parameters. Am. J. Clin. Nutr. 37:133–138.
Russell, D.M., P.J. Prendergast, P.L. Darby, P.E. Garfinkel, J. Whitwell, and K.N. Jeejeebhoy
  1983   A comparison between muscle function and body composition in anorexia nervosa: The effect of refeeding. Am. J. Clin. Nutr. 38:229–237.
Russell, D.M., H.L. Atwood, J.S. Whittaker, T. Itakura, P.M. Walker, D.A.G. Mickle, and N. Jeejeebhoy
  1984   The effect of fasting and hypocaloric diets on the functional and metabolic characteristics of rat gastrocnemius muscle. Clin Sci. 67:185–194.
Sack, R.B.
  1980   Enterotoxigenic *Escherichia coli*: Identification and characterization. J. Infect. Dis. 142:279–296.
Sadeh, A., J. Alster, D. Urbach, and P. Lavie
  1989   Actigraphically based automatic bedtime sleep-wake scoring: Validity and clinical applications. J. Ambul. Monitor 2:209–216.
Sale, D.G., J.E. Martin, and D.E. Moroz
  1992   Hypertrophy without increased isometric strength after weight training. Eur. J. Appl. Physiol. 64:51–55.
Salgame, P., J.S. Abrams, C. Clayberger, H. Goldstein, J. Convit, R.L. Modlin, and B.R. Bloom
  1991   Differing lymphokine profiles of functional subsets of human CD4 and CD8 T cell clones. Science 254:279–282.
Santee, W.R., and R.W. Hoyt
  1994   Recommendations for meteorological data collection during physiological field studies. Technical Report T94-9. Natick, Mass.: U.S. Army Research Institute of Environmental Medicine.

Saris, W.H.M.
1986   Habitual physical activity in children: Methodology and findings in health and disease. Med. Sci. Sports Exerc. 18:253–263.

Sarraf, P., R.C. Frederich, E.M. Turner, G. Ma, N.T. Jaskowiak, D.J. Rivet III, J.S. Flier, B.B. Lowell, D.L. Fraker, and H.R. Alexander
1997   Multiple cytokines and acute inflammation raise mouse leptin levels: Potential role in inflammatory anorexia. J. Exp. med. 185:171–175.

Satlin, A., M.H. Teicher, H.R. Lieberman, R.J. Baldessarini, L. Volicer, and Y. Rheaume
1991   Circadian locomotor activity rhythms in Alzheimer's disease. Neuropsychopharmacology 5:115–126.

Sato, R., J. Yang, X. Wang, M.J. Evans, Y.K. Ho, J.L. Goldstein, and M.S. Brown
1994   Assignment of the membrane attachment, DNA binding, and transcriptional activation domains of sterol regulatory element-binding protein-1 (SREBP-1). J. Biol. Chem. 269:17267–17273.

Schedlowski, M., R. Jacobs, G. Stratman, S. Richter, A. Hadicke, U. Tewes, T.D. Wagner, and R.E. Schmidt
1992   Changes in natural killer cells during acute psychological stress. J. Clin. Immunol. 13:119–126.

Schelbert, R.R., and M. Schwaiger
1986   PET studies of the heart. Pp. 581–661 in Positron Emission Tomography and Autoradiography: Principles and Applications for the Brain and Heart, M. Phelps, J. Mazziotta, and H. Schelbert, eds. New York: Raven Press.

Scheltinga, M.R., D.O. Jacobs, T.D. Kimbrough, and D.W. Wilmore
1991   Alterations in body fluid content can be detected by bioelectrical impedance analysis. J. Surg. Res. 50:461–468.

Scherf, J., B.A. Franklin, C.P. Lucas, D. Stevenson, and M. Rubenfire
1986   Validity of skinfold thickness measures of formerly obese adults. Am. J. Clin. Nutr. 43:128–135.

Schmeichel, K.L., and M.C. Beckerle
1994   The LIM domain is a modular protein-binding interface. Cell 79:211–219.

Schmidt-Neilsen, K.
1984   Why is Animal Size So Important? Cambridge: Cambridge University Press.

Schneiders, P., and C. Reiners
1997   Changes in bone mineral density in male athletes [letter in response to Klesges et al., 1996, 276:226–230]. J. Am. Med. Assoc. 277(1):23–24.

Schoeller, D.A.
1988   Measurement of energy expenditure in free-living humans by using doubly labeled water. J. Nutr. 188:1278–1289.

Schoeller, D.A., and A. Coward
1990   The doubly labeled water method for measuring energy expenditure. Technical recommendations for use in humans. Practical consequences of deviations from the isotope elimination model. Pp. 166–190 in NAHRES-4, A Consensus Report by the IDECG Working Group, A.M. Prentice, ed. Vienna: IAEA.

Schoeller, D.A., and E. van Santen
1982   Measurement of energy expenditure in humans by doubly labeled water method. J. Appl. Physiol. 53(4):955–959.

Schoeller, D.A., E. van Santen, D.W. Peterson, W. Dietz, J. Jaspan, and P.D. Klein
1980   Total body water measurement in humans with ^{18}O and ^{2}H labeled water. Am. J. Clin. Nutr. 33:2686–2693.

Schoeller, D.A., R.F. Kushner, and P.J.H. Jones
1986   Validation of doubly labeled water for measuring energy expenditure during parenteral nutrition. Am. J. Clin. Nutr. 44:291–298.

Schonwetter,B.S., E.D. Stolzenberg, and M.A. Zasloff
  1995   Epithelial antibiotics induced at sites of inflammation. Science 267:1645–1648.
Schrader, C.E., A. George, R.L. Kerlin, and J.J. Cebra
  1990   Dendritic cells support production of IgA and other non-IgM isotypes in clonal microculture. Int. Immunol. 2(6):563–570.
Schutte, J.E., E.J. Townsend, J. Hugg, R.F. Shoup, R.M. Malina, and C.G. Blomqvist
  1984   Density of lean body mass is greater in blacks than in whites. J. Appl. Physiol. 56:1647–1649.
Schwan, H.P., and C.F. Kay
  1956   The conductivity of living tissues. Ann. N.Y. Acad. Sci. 65:1007–1013.
Schwan, H.P., and K. Li
  1953   Capacity and conductivity of body tissues at ultrahigh frequencies. Proceedings of
Seckinger, P., J.W. Lowenthal, K. Williamson, J.M. Dayer, and H.R. MacDonald
  1987   A urine inhibitor of interleukin-1 activity that blocks ligand binding. J. Immunol. 139:1546–1549.
Seckinger, P., K. Williamson, J.F. Balavoine, B. Mach, G. Mazzei, A. Shaw, and J.M. Dayer
  1987   A urine inhibitor of interleukin-1 activity affects both interleukin-1 alpha and -1 beta but not tumor necrosis factor alpha. J. Immunol. 139:1541–1545.
Seckinger, P., S. Isaaz, and J.M. Dayer
  1988   A human inhibitor of tumor necrosis factor alpha. J. Exp. Med. 167:1511–1516.
Segal, K.R., S. Burastero, A. Chun, P. Coronel, R.N. Pierson, and J. Wang
  1991   Estimation of extracellular and total body water by multiple-frequency bioelectrical-impedance measurement. Am. J. Clin. Nutr. 54:26–29.
Segal, K.R., B. Chatr-Aryamontri, and D. Guvakov
  1994   Validation of a new portable metabolic measurement system [abstract]. Med. Sci. Sports Exerc. 26(5):S54.
Segel, I.H.
  1968   Biochemical Calculations. How to Solve Mathematical Problems in General Biochemistry. New York: John Wiley & Sons.
Segura, R., and J.L. Ventura
  1988   Effect of L-tryptophan supplementation on exercise performance. Int. J. Sports Med. 9:301–305.
Seidell, J.C., C.J.C. Bakker, and K. van der Kooy
  1990   Imaging techniques for measuring adipose-tissue distribution—a comparison between computed tomography and 1.5-T magnetic resonance. Am. J. Clin. Nutr. 51:953–957.
Seidell, J.C., M. Cigolini, J. Chorzewska, B.M. Ellsinger, and G. Di Brase
  1990   Androgenicity in relation to body fat distribution and metabolism in 38-year-old women—The European Fat Distribution Study. J. Clin. Epidemiol. 43:21–34.
Selinger, A.
  1977   The body as a three-component system. Doctoral Dissertation. University of Illinois at Urbana-Champaign, Champaign, Ill.
Sergi, G., M. Bussolotto, P. Perini, I. Calliari, V. Giantin, A. Ceccon, F. Scanferla, M. Bressan, G. Moschini, and G. Enzi
  1994   Accuracy of bioelectrical impedance analysis in estimation of extracellular space in healthy subjects and in fluid retention states. Ann. Nutr. Metab. 38:158–165.
Settle, R.G., K.R. Foster, B.R. Epstein, and J.L. Mullen
  1980   Nutritional assessment: Whole body impedance and body fluid compartments. Nutr. Cancer 2:72–80.
Shanks, M.R., D. Cassio, O. Lecoq, and A.L. Hubbard
  1994   An improved polarized rat hepatoma hybrid cell line. J. Cell. Science 107:813–825.

Sharp, M.A., B.C. Nindl, K.A. Westphal, and K.E. Friedl
  1994 The physical performance of female Army basic trainees who pass and fail the Army body weight and percent body fat standards. Pp. 743–750 in Advances in Industrial Ergonomics and Safety VI, E. Agezadeh, ed. Washington, D.C.: Taylor and Francis.
Shay, N.F., and R.J. Cousins
  1993 Cloning of rat intestinal mRNAs affected by zinc deficiency. J. Nutr. 123(1):35–41.
Shephard, R.J.
  1968 Intensity, duration and frequency of exercise as determinants of the response to a training regimen. Int. Z. Angew Physiol. 28:272–278.
Shih, H-M., and H.C. Towle
  1992 Definition of the carbohydrate response element of the rat S_{14} gene. J. Biol. Chem. 267:13222–13228.
Shih, H-M., Z. Liu, and H.C. Towle
  1995 Two CACGTG motifs with proper spacing dictate the carbohydrate regulation of hepatic gene transcription. J. Biol. Chem. 270:21991–21997.
Shimokata, H., D.C. Muller, and R. Andres
  1989 Studies in the distribution of body fat. III. Effects of cigarette smoking. J. Am. Med. Assoc. 261:1169–1173.
Shipley, R.A., and R.E. Clark
  1972 Tracer Methods for *In Vivo* Kinetics. Theory and Applications. New York and London: Academic Press.
Shippee, R., K. Friedl, T. Kramer, M. Mays, K. Popp, E.W. Askew, B. Fairbrother, R. Hoyt, J. Vogel, L. Marchitelli, P. Frykman, L. Martinez-Lopez, E. Bernton, M. Kramer, R. Tulley, J. Rood, J. Delaney, D. Jezior, J. Arsenault, B. Nindl, R. Galloway, and D. Hoover
  1994 Nutritional and immunological assessment of Ranger students with increased caloric intake. Technical report T95-5. Natick, Mass: U.S. Army Research Institute of Environmental Medicine.
Shirreffs, S.M., and R.J. Maughan
  1994 The effect of posture change on blood volume, serum potassium and whole body electrical impedance. Eur. J. Appl. Physiol. 69:461–463.
Shirreffs, S.M., R.J. Maughan, and M. Bernardi
  1994 Effect of posture change on blood volume, serum potassium and body water as estimated by bioelectrical impedance analysis (BIA). Clin. Sci. (London) 87:21.
Shroff, K.E., K. Meslin, and J.J. Cebra
  1995 Commensal enteric bacteria engender a self-limiting humoral mucosal immune response while permanently colonizing the gut. Infect. Immun. 63:3904–3913.
Shulman, G.I., D.L. Rothman, T. Jue, P. Stein, R.A. DeFronzo, and R.G. Shulman
  1990 Quantitation of muscle glycogen synthesis in normal subjects and subjects with non-insulin-dependent diabetes by ^{13}C nuclear magnetic resonance spectroscopy. N. Engl. J. Med. 322:223–228.
Siconolfi, S.F., D.A. Coleman, and J. Staab
  1987 Determination of percent fat by hydrostatic weighing and functional residual capacity. Annual Meeting of the Eastern Region, American College of Sportsmedicine, 5 November.
Sidossis, L.S., A.R. Coggan, A. Gastaldelli, and R.R. Wolfe
  1995 Pathway of free fatty acid oxidation in human subjects. Implication for tracer studies. J. Clin. Invest. 95:278–284.

Sieber, B.J., J. Rodin, L. Larson, S. Ortega, N. Cummings, S. Levy, T. Whiteside, and R. Herberman
   1992   Modulation of human natural killer cell activity by exposure to uncontrollable stress. Brain Behav. Immunol. 6:141–156.
Sievanen, H., P. Oja, and I. Vuori
   1992   Precision of dual-energy x-ray absorptiometry in determining bone mineral density and content of various skeletal sites. J. Nucl. Med. 33:1137–1142.
Sim, G-K.
   1995   Intraepithelial lymphocytes and the immune system. Adv. Immunol. 58:297–343.
Simard, C.P., S.A. Spector, and V.R. Edgerton
   1982   Contractile properties of rat hind limb muscles immobilized at different lengths. Exp. Neurology 77:467–482.
Singh, H., J.H. LeBowitz, A.S. Baldwin, Jr., and P.A. Sharp
   1988   Molecular cloning of an enhancer binding protein: Isolation by screening of an expression library with a recognition site DNA. Cell 52:415–423.
Singh, M.V., S.B. Rawal, and A.K. Tyagi
   1990   Body fluid status on induction, reinduction and prolonged stay at high altitude of human volunteers. Int. J. Biometerorol. 34:93–97.
Siri, W.E.
   1961   Body composition from fluid spaces and density: Analysis of methods. Pp. 223–244 in Techniques for Measuring Body Composition, Proceedings of a Conference, Quartermaster Research and Engineering Center, Natick, Mass., January 22–23, 1959, J. Brozék and A. Henschel, eds. Washington D.C.: National Academy of Sciences/National Research Council.
Siscovick, D.S., R.E. LaPorte, and J.M. Newman
   1985   The disease-specific benefits and risks of physical activity and exercise. Public Health Rep. 100:180–188.
Sixma, T.K., S.E. Pronk, K.H. Kalk, E.S. Wartna, B.A.M. vanZanten, B. Witholt, and W.G. Hol
   1991   Crystal structure of a cholera toxin-related heat-labile enterotoxin from *E. coli*. Nature (London) 351:371–377.
Sjöström, L.
   1991   A computer-tomography based multicompartment body composition techniques and anthropometric predictions of lean body mass, total and subcutaneous adipose tissue. Int. J. Obes. 15(suppl. 2):19–30.
Sjöström, L., H. Kvist, A. Cederblad, and U. Tylen
   1986   Determination of total adipose tissue and body fat in women by computed tomography, ^{40}K, and tritium. Am. J. Physiol. 250:E736–E745.
Sjöström, L., M. Alpsten, B. Andersson, B-Å. Bengtsson, C. Bengtsson, P. Björtorp, I. Bosaeus, R.J. Brummer, B. Chowdhury, S. Edèn, I. Ernest, S. Holmäng, O. Isaksson, H. Kvist, L. Lapidus, B. Lasson, G. Lindstedt, S. Lindstedt, L. Lissner, L. Lönn, P. Marin, K. Stenlöf, and J. Töll
   1993   Hormones, body composition and cardiovascular risk. Pp. 223–273 in Methods on *In Vivo* Body Composition Assessment, K.J. Ellis and J. Eastman, eds. New York: Plenum Press.
Skov, L., O. Pryds, and G. Greisen
   1991   Estimating cerebral blood flow in newborn infants: Comparison of near infrared spectroscopy and 133-Xe clearance. Pediatr. Res. 30(6):570–573.
Slosman, D.O., J-P. Casez, C. Pichard, T. Rochat, F. Fery, R. Rizzoli, J-P. Bonjour, A. Morabia, and A. Donath
   1992   Assessment of whole-body composition with dual-energy x-ray absorptiometry. Radiology 185:593–598.

Smith, K., and M.J. Rennie
  1990   Protein turnover and amino acid metabolism in skeletal muscle. Ballière's Clin. Endocrinol. Metab. 4:461–498.
Smyth, M.J., and J.R. Ortaldo
  1993   Mechanisms of cytotoxicty used by human peripheral blood CD4+ and CD8+ T-cell subsets. The role of granule exocytosis. J. Immunol. 151:40–47.
Snead, D.B., S.J. Birge, and W.M. Kohrt
  1993   Age related differences in body composition by hydrodensitometry and dual-energy x-ray absorptiometry. J. Appl. Physiol. 74(2):770–775.
Snow-Harter, C., M. Bouxsein, B. Lewis, S. Charette, P. Weinstein, and R.
  1990   Muscle strength as a predictor of bone mineral density in young women. J. Bone Min. Res. 5:589–595.
Snyder, W.S., M.J. Cook, E.S. Nasset, L.R. Karhansen, G.P. Howells, and I.H. Tipton
  1975   Report of the Task Group on Reference Man. Oxford: Pergamon Press.
Soares, M.J., M.L. Sheela, A.V. Kurpad, R.N. Kulkarni, and P.S. Shetty
  1989   The influence of different methods on basal metabolic rate measurements in human subjects. Am. J. Clin. Nutr. 50:731–736.
Sobel, W., S. Rossner, B. Hinson, E. Hiltbrandt, N. Karstaedt, P. Santago, N. Wolfman, A. Hagaman, and J.R. Crouse III
  1991   Evaluation of a new magnetic resonance imaging method for quantitating adipose tissue areas. Int. J. Obes. 15:589–599.
Sohlström, A., and E. Forsum
  1995   Changes in adipose tissue volume and distribution during reproduction in Swedish women as assessed by magnetic resonance imaging. Am. J. Clin. Nutr. 61:287–295.
Sohlström, A., L-O. Wahlund, and E. Forsum
  1993   Adipose tissue distribution as assessed by magnetic resonance imaging and total body fat by magnetic resonance imaging, underwater weighing, and body-water dilution in healthy women. Am. J. Clin. Nutr. 58:830–838.
Sollenberger, R.L., and P. Milgram
  1993   Effects of stereoscopic and rotational displays in a three-dimensional path-tracing task. Hum. Factors 35(3):483–499.
Spangler, B.D.
  1992   Structure and function of cholera toxin and the related *Escherichia coli* heat-labile enterotoxin. Microbiol. Rev. 56:622–647.
Sparling, P.B., M. Millard-Stafford, L.B. Rosskopf, L.J. Dicarlo, and B.T. Hinson
  1993   Body composition by bioelectric impedance and densitometry in Black women. Am. J. Hum. Biol. 5:111–117.
Speakman, J.R., and P.A. Racey
  1986   Measurement of CO_2 production by the doubly labeled water technique. J. Appl. Physiol. 61:1200–1202.
Speakman, J.R., K.S. Nair, and M.I. Goran
  1993   Revised equations for calculating CO_2 production from doubly labeled water in humans. Am. J. Physiol. 264 (27):E912–E917.
Spear, D.H., J. Ericsson, S.M. Jackson, and P.A. Edwards
  1994   Identification of a 6-base pair element involved in the sterol-mediated transcriptional regulation of farnesyl diphosphate synthase. J. Biol. Chem. 269:25212–25218.
Spence, J.A., R. Baliga, and J. Nyboer
  1979   Changes during hemodialysis in total body water cardiac output and chest fluid as detected by bioelectric impedance analysis. Trans. Am. Soc. Artif. Intern. Organs 25:51–55.

Sprawls, P.
  1977   The Physical Principles of Diagnostic Radiology. Pp 101–117. Baltimore, Md.: University Park Press.
Sprenger, H., C. Jacobs, M. Nain, A.M. Gressner, H. Prinz, W. Wesemann, and D. Gemsa
  1992   Enhanced release of cytokines, interleukin-2 receptors, and neopterin after long-distance running. Clin. Immunol. Immunopathol. 63:188–195.
Spriggs, M.K.
  1996   One step ahead of the game: Viral immunomodulatory molecules. Annu. Rev. Immunol. 14:101–130.
Spurr, G.B., A.M. Prentice, P.R. Murgatroyd, G.R. Goldberg, J.C. Reina, and N.T. Christman
  1988   Energy expenditure from minute-by-minute heart-rate recording: Comparison with indirect calorimetry. Am. J. Clin. Nutr. 48:552–559.
Stager, J.M., A. Lindeman, and J. Edwards
  1995   The use of doubly labeled water in quantifying energy expenditure during prolonged activity. Sports Med. 19:166–172.
Stalnacke, C-G., B. Jones, B. Langstron, H. Lundquist, P. Malmborg, S. Sjoberg, and B. Larsson
  1982   Short-lived radionuclides in nutritional physiology. A model study with L-[Me-^{11}C]methionine in the pig. Br. J. Nutr. 47:537–545.
Stanney, K.M., and G. Salvendy
  1995   Information visualization: Assisting low spatial individuals with information access tasks through the use of visual mediators. Ergonomics 38(6):1184–1198.
Staten, M.A., W.G. Totty, and W.M. Kohrt
  1989   Measurement of fat distribution by magnetic resonance imaging. Invest. Radiol. 24:345–349.
Stavnezer, J.
  1995   Regulation of antibody production and class switching by TGF-beta. J. Immunol. 155:1647–1651.
Stegink, L.D., E.F. Bell, T.T. Daabees, D.W. Anderson, W.L. Zike, and L.T. Filer, Jr.
  1983   Factors influencing utilization of glycine, glutamate and aspartate in clinical products. Pp. 123–146 in Amino Acids—Metabolism and Medical Applications, G.B. Blackburn, J.P. Grant, and V.R. Young, eds. Boston: John Wright, PSG, Inc.
Stein, T.P., and M.D. Schluter
  1994   Excretion of IL-6 by astronauts during spaceflight. Am. J. Physiol. 266:E448–E452.
Steingrimsdottir, L., M.R. Greenwood, and J.A. Brasel
  1980   Effect of pregnancy, lactation, and a high-fat diet on adipose tissue in Osborne-Mendel rats. J. Nutr. 110:600–609.
Steinmetz, H.T., A. Herbertz, M. Bertram, and V. Diehl
  1995   Increase in interleukin-6 serum level preceding fever in granulocytopenia and correlation with death from sepsis. J. Infect. Dis. 171:225–228.
Stock, W., P.J. van der Heijden, and A.T.J. Bianchi
  1994   Conversion of orally induced suppression of the mucosal immune response to ovalbumin into stimulation by conjugating ovalbumin to cholera toxin or its B subunit. Vaccine 12:521–526.
Stocklin, G., and V.W. Pike, eds.
  1993   Radiopharmaceuticals for Positron Emission Tomography. Methodological Aspects. Dordrecht, The Netherlands: Kluwer Academic Publishers.
Stolarczyk, L.M., V.H. Heyward, V.L. Hicks, and R.N. Baumgartner
  1994   Predictive accuracy of bioelectrical impedance in estimating body composition of Native American women. Am. J. Clin. Nutr. 59:964–970.

Stoll, D., and S. Bourne
  1996 The National Advanced Driving Simulator: Potential applications to ITS and AHS research. Pp. 700–710 in Proceeding of the 6th Annual Meeting of the Intelligent Transportation Society. Washington D.C.: ITS America.
Storch, K.J., D.A. Wagner, J.F. Burke, and V.R. Young
  1988 Quantitative study, *in vivo*, of methionine cycle in humans using [methyl-^{2}H$_3$] and [1-^{13}C]methionine. Am. J. Physiol. 255:E322–E231.
Stouthard, J.M.L., J.A. Romijn, T. van der Poll, E. Endert, S. Klein, P.J.M. Bakker, C.H.N. Veenhof, and H.P. Sauerwein
  1995 Endocrinologic and metabolic effects of interleukin-6 in humans. Am. J. Physiol. 268:E813–E819.
Street, N., and T.R. Mosmann
  1991 Functional diversity of T lymphocytes due to secretion of different cytokine patterns. FASEB J. 5:171–177.
Stuart H.C., P. Hill, and C. Shaw
  1940 The growth of bone, muscle and overlying tissue as revealed by studies of roentgenograms of the leg area. Monogr. Soc. Res. Child Dev. V (no. 3, serial no. 26):1–190.
Stuart, G.W., P.F. Searle, H.Y. Chen, R.L. Brinster, and R.D. Palmiter
  1984 A 12-base pair DNA motif that is repeated several times in metallothionein gene promoters confers metal regulation to a heterologous gene. Proc. Natl. Acad. Sci. USA 81:7318–7322.
Study of the Military Services Physical Fitness
  1981 *See* U.S. Department of Defense, Office of the Assistant Secretary of Defense for Manpower, Reserve Affairs and Logistics, 1981.
Subramanyan, R., S.C. Manchanda, J. Nyboer, and M.L. Bhatia
  1980 Total body water in congestive heart failure. A pre and post treatment study. J. Assoc. Physicians India 28:257–262.
Sugden, P.H., and S.J. Fuller
  1991 Regulation of protein turnover in skeletal and cardiac muscle. Biochem. J. 273:21–27.
Sun, J-B., J. Holmgren, and C. Czerkinsky
  1994 Cholera toxin B subunit: An efficient transmucosal carrier-delivery system for induction of peripheral immunological tolerance. Proc. Natl. Acad. Sci. USA 91:10795–10799.
Suter, P.M., S. Suter, E. Girardin, P. Roux Lombard, G.E. Grau, and J.M. Dayer
  1992 High bronchoalveolar levels of tumor necrosis factor and its inhibitors, interleukin-1, interferon, and elastase, in patients with adult respiratory distress syndrome after trauma, shock, or sepsis. Am. Rev. Respir. Dis. 145:1016–1022.
Svanborg, C., W. Agace, S. Hedges, R. Lindsedt, and M.L. Svensson
  1994 Bacterial adherence and mucosal cytokine production. Ann. N.Y. Acad. Sci. 730:162–181.
Svendsen, O.L., J. Haarbo, B.L. Heitmann, A. Gotfredsen, and C. Christiansen
  1991 Measurement of body fat in elderly subjects by dual-energy x-ray absorptiometry, bioelectrical impedance, and anthropometry. Am. J. Clin. Nutr. 53:1117–1123.
Svendsen, O.L., J. Haarbo, C. Hassager, and C. Christiansen
  1993 Accuracy of measurements of body composition by dual-energy x-ray absorptiometry *in vivo*. Am. J. Clin. Nutr. 57:605–608.
Swain, S.L., G. Huston, S. Tonkonogy, and A. Weinberg
  1991 Transforming growth factor-β and IL-4 cause helper T-cell precursors to develop into distinct effector helper cells that differ in lymphokine secretion pattern and cell surface phenotype. J. Immunol. 147:2991–3000.

Szeto, E.G., D.E. Carlson, T.B. Dugan, and J.C. Buchbinder
  1987   A comparison of nutrient intakes between a Fort Riley contractor-operated and a Fort Lewis military-operated garrison dining facility. Technical Report T2-88. Natick, Mass.: U.S. Army Research Institute of Environmental Medicine.
Taube, G.
  1995   Epidemiology faces its limits. Science 269:164–169.
Taylor, C.R.
  1992   Cost of running springs. In Physiological Adaptations in Vertebrates: Respiration, Circulation, and Metabolism, S. Wood, R. Weber, A. Hargens, and R. Millard, eds. New York: Dekker.
Taylor, C.R., K. Schmidt-Neilsen, and J.L. Raab
  1970   Scaling of the energetic cost of running to body size in mammals. Am. J. Physiol. 219:1104–1107.
Taylor, C.R., A. Shkolnik, R. Dmi'el, D. Bahrav, and A. Borut
  1974   Running in cheetahs, gazelles, and goats: Energy cost and limb configuration. Am. J. Physiol. 227:848–850.
Taylor, C.R., N.C. Heglund, T.A. McMahon, and T.R. Looney
  1980   Energetic cost of generating muscular force during running: A comparison of large and small animals. J. Exp. Biol. 86:9–18.
Taylor, C.R., N.C. Heglund, and G.M.O. Maloiy
  1982   Energetics and mechanics of terrestrial locomotion. I. Metabolic energy consumption as a function of speed and body size in birds and mammals. J. Exp. Biol. 97:1–21.
Taylor, R., T.B. Price, L.D. Katz, R.G. Shulman, and G.I. Shulman
  1993   Direct measurement of change in muscle glycogen concentration after a mixed meal in normal subjects. Am. J. Physiol. 265:E224–E229.
Tedner, B., L.E. Lins, H. Asaba, and B. Wehle
  1985   Evaluation of impedance technique for fluid-volume monitoring during hemodialysis. Int. J. Clin. Monit. Comp. 2:3–8.
Teicher, M.H., J.M. Lawrence, N.I. Barber, S. Finkelstein, H.R. Lieberman, and R.J. Baldessarini
  1986   Altered locomotor activity in neuropsychiatric patients. Prog. Neuropsychopharmacol. Biol. Psychiatry 10:755–761.
Teicher, M.H., J.M. Lawrence, N.I. Barber, S.P. Finklestein, H.R. Lieberman, and R.J. Baldessarini
  1988   Altered circadian activity rhythms in geriatric patients with major depression. Arch. Gen. Psychiatry 45:913–917.
Ter-Pogossian, M.M., M.E. Raichle, and B.E. Sobel
  1980   Positron-emission tomography. Sci. Am. 243:171–181.
Terry, R.B., M.L. Stefanick, W.L. Haskell, and P.D. Wood
  1991   Contributions of regional adipose tissue depots to plasma lipoprotein concentrations in overweight men and women: Possible protective effects of thigh fat. Metabolism 40:733–740.
Tessari, P., S. Inchiostro, B. Biolo, E. Vincent, and L. Sabadin
  1991   Effects of acute systemic hyperinsulinemia on forearm muscle proteolysis in healthy man. J. Clin. Invest. 88:27–33.
Tessari, P., S. Inchiostro, M. Zanett, and R. Barazzoni
  1995   A model of skeletal muscle kinetics measured across the human forearm. Am. J. Physiol. 269:E127–E136.

Thomas, C.D., K.E. Friedl, M.Z. Mays, S.H. Mutter, R.J. Moore, D.Z. Jezior, C.J. Baker-Fulco, L.J. Marchitelli, R.T. Tulley, and E.W. Askew
  1995   Nutrient intakes and nutritional status of soldiers consuming the Meal, Ready-to-Eat (MRE XII) during a 30-day field training exercise. Technical Report No. T95-6. Natick, Mass.: U.S. Army Research Institute of Environmental Medicine.
Thomas, E.V., and D.M. Haaland
  1990   Comparison of multivariate calibration methods for quantitative spectral analysis. Anal. Chem. 62:1091–1099.
Thomasset, A.
  1962   Bio-electrical properties of tissue impedance measurements. Lyon Med. 207:107–118.
Thompson, K.S., and H.C. Towle
  1991   Localization of the carbohydrate response element of the rat L-type pyruvate kinase gene. J. Biol. Chem. 266:8679–8682.
Thorne, D.P., and T.D. Lockwood
  1993   Four proteolytic processes of myocardium, one sensitive to thiol reactive agents and thiol protease inhibitor. Am. J. Physiol. 265:E10–E19.
Tiplady, B.
  1992   Continuous attention: Rationale and discriminant variation of a test designed for use in psychopharmacology. Behavior Research Methods, Instruments, and Computers 24(1):16–21.
Todd, I.C., D. Wosornu, I. Stewart, and T. Wild
  1992   Cardiac rehabilitation following myocardial infarction. Sports Med. 14:243–259.
Tomkins, G.M.
  1975   The metabolic code. Science 189:760–763.
Tothill, P., A. Avenell, J. Love, and D.M. Reid
  1994a Comparisons between Hologic, Lunar and Norland dual-energy x-ray absorptiometers and other techniques used for whole-body soft tissue measurements. Eur. J. Clin. Nutr. 48:781–794.
Tothill, P., A. Avenell, and D.M. Reid
  1994b Precision and accuracy of measurements of whole-body bone mineral: Comparisons between Hologic, Lunar and Norland dual-energy x-ray absorptiometers. Br. J. Radiol. 67:1210–1217.
Tothill, P., and R.H. Nord
  1995   Limitations of dual-energy x-ray absorptiometry [letter]. Am. J. Clin. Nutr. 61:398–399.
Tran, Z.V., and A. Weltman
  1988   Predicting body composition of men from girth measurements. Hum. Biol. 60:167–175.
Trautman, E., M.A. Trautman, and P. Moskal
  1995   Preferred viewing distances for handheld and structurally fixed displays. Ergonomics 38(7):1385–1394.
Tremblay, A., J-P. Despres, C. Leblanc, C.L. Craig, B. Ferris, T. Stephens, and C. Bouchard
  1990   Effect of intensity of physical activity on body fatness and fat distribution. Am. J. Clin. Nutr. 51:153–157.
Trinchieri, G.
  1993   Interleukin-12 and its role in the generation of TH1 cells. Immunol. Today 14:335–338.
Trumbo, P.R., M.A. Banks, and J.F. Gregory III
  1990   Hydrolysis of pyridoxine-5'-β-D-glucoside by a broad-specificity β-glucosidease from mammalian tissues. Proc. Soc. Exp. Biol. Med. 195:240–246.

Tryon, W.W.
   1991   Activity Measurement in Psychology and Medicine. New York: Plenum Press.
Tsunemitsu, H., M. Shimizu, T. Hirai, H. Yonemichi, T. Kudo, K. Mori, and S. Onoe
   1989   Protection against bovine rotaviruses in newborn calves by continuous feeding of
           immune colostrum. Nippon Juigaku Zasshi 51:300–308.
Tugwood, J., I. Issemann, R.G. Anderson, K.R. Bundell, W.L. McPheat, and S. Green
   1992   The mouse peroxisome proliferater activated receptor recognizes a response ele-
           ment in the 5' flanking sequence of the rat acyl CoA oxidase gene. EMBO J
           11:433–439.
Turnage, J.J., R.S. Kennedy, M.G. Smith, D.R. Baltzley, and N.E. Lane
   1992   Development of microcomputer-based mental acuity tests. Ergonomics
           35(10):1271–1295.
Tzankoff, S.P., and A.H. Norris
   1977   Effect of muscle mass on age-related BMR changes. J. Appl. Physiol. 43:1001–
           1006.
U.S. Congress, House
   1992   Gender Discrimination in the Military. Hearing before the Defense Policy Panel,
           Committee on Armed Services, July 29–30. 102d Congress, 2d Session. Washing-
           ton, D.C.: U.S. Government Printing Office.
U.S. Department of Defense. Office of the Assistant Secretary of Defense for Manpower,
           Reserve Affairs and Logistics
   1981   Study of the Military Services Physical Fitness. April 3. Washington D.C.
U.S. Department of the Army
   1986   Army Regulation 600-9. "The Army Weight Control Program." September 1.
           Washington, D.C.
   1992   U.S. Army field manual FM 21-20. "Physical Fitness Training." September 30.
           Washington, D.C.
Underdown, B.J., and J. Mestecky
   1994   Mucosal immunoglobulins. Pp. 79–97 in Handbook of Mucosal Immunology, P.L.
           Ogra, J. Mesteck, M.E. Lamm, W. Strober, J.R. McGhee, and J. Bienenstock, eds.
           Boston: Academic Press, Inc.
Urban, R.J., Y.H. Bodenburg, C. Gilkison, J. Foxworth, A.R. Coggan, R.R. Wolfe, and A.
           Ferrando
   1995   Testosterone administration to elderly men increases skeletal muscle strength and
           protein synthesis. Am. J. Physiol. 269:E820–E826.
USACDEC/USARIEM (U.S. Army Combat Developments Experimentation Center and U.S.
           Army Research Institute of Environmental Medicine)
   1986   Combat Field Feeding System-Force Development Test and Experimentation
           (CFFS-FDTE). Technical Report CDEC-TR-85-006A. Vol. 1, Basic Report; vol. 2,
           Appendix A; vol. 3, Appendixes B through L. Fort Ord, Calif.: U.S. Army Combat
           Developments Experimentation Center.
Vallee, B.L., J.E. Coleman, and D.S. Auld
   1991   Zinc fingers, zinc clusters, and zinc twists in DNA-binding protein domains. Proc.
           Natl. Acad. Sci. USA 88:999–1003.
Vallera, D.A., M.G. Bissell, and W. Barron
   1991   Accuracy of portable blood glucose monitoring. Effect of glucose level and pran-
           dial state. Am. J. Clin. Pathol. 95(2):247–252.
van Dale, D., and W.H.M. Saris
   1989   Repetitive weight loss and weight regain: Effects on weight reduction, resting
           metabolic rate, and lipolytic activity before and after exercise and/or diet treat-
           ment. Am. J. Clin. Nutr. 49:409–416.

van der Poll, T., S.E. Calvano, A. Kumar, C.C. Braxton, S.M. Coyle, K. Barbosa, L.L. Moldawer, and S.F. Lowry 1995
  Endotoxin induces downregulation of tumor necrosis factor receptors on circulating monocytes and granulocytes in humans. Blood 86:2754–2759.
van der Pouw-Kraan, T., R. deJong, and L. Aarden
  1993   Development of human TH$_1$ and TH$_2$ cytokine responses: The cytokine production profile of T cells is dictated by the primary *in vitro* stimulus. Eur. J. Immunol. 23:1–5.
Van Loan, M.D., and P.L. Mayclin
  1992a Body composition assessment: Dual-energy x-ray absorptiometry (DEXA) compared to reference methods. Eur. J. Clin. Nutr. 46:125–130.
  1992b Use of multi-frequency bioelectrical impedance analysis for the estimation of extracellular fluid. Eur. J. Clin. Nutr. 46:117–124.
van Marken Lichtenbelt, W.D., K.R. Westerterp, L. Wouters, and S.C. Luijendijk
  1994   Validation of bioelectrical-impedance measurements as a method to estimate body-water compartments. Am. J. Clin. 60:159–166.
van Mechelen, W.
  1992   Running injuries. A review of the epidemiological literature. Sports Med. 14:320–335.
Van Zee, K.J., T. Kohno, E. Fischer, C.S. Rock, L.L. Moldawer, and S.F. Lowry
  1992   Tumor necrosis factor soluble receptors circulate during experimental and clinical inflammation and can protect against excessive tumor necrosis factor alpha *in vitro* and *in vivo*. Proc. Natl. Acad. Sci. USA 89:4845–4849.
Vaughan, L., F. Zurlo, and E. Ravussin
  1991   Age and energy expenditure. Am. J. Clin. Nutr. 53:821–825.
Vettorazzi, C., C. Barillas, and O. Pineda
  1987   A model for assessing body composition in amputees using bioelectric impedance analysis. Fed. Proc. 46:1186.
Villa, M.L., E. Ferrario, F. Bergamasco, F. Bozzetti, L. Cozzaglio, and E. Clerici
  1991   Reduced natural killer cell activity and IL-2 production in malnourished cancer patients. Br. J. Cancer 63:1010–1014.
Virella, G., ed.
  1993   Introduction to Medical Immunology, 3d ed. New York: Marcel Dekker.
Virella, G., and B. Hyman
  1991   Quantitation of anti-tetanus and anti-diphtheria antibodies by enzymoimmunoassay: Methodology and applications. J. Clin. Lab. Anal. 5:43–48.
Virella, G., H.H. Fudenberg, K.U. Kyong, J.P. Pandey, and R.M. Galbraith
  1978   A practical method for quantitation of antibody responses to tetanus and diphtheria toxoids in normal young children. Zeitschrift fur Immunitatsforschung 155:80–86.
Virella, G., M.T. Rugeles, B. Hyman, M. La Via, J.M. Goust, M. Frankis, and B.E. Bierer
  1988   The interaction of CD2 with its LFA-3 ligand expressed by autologous erythrocytes results in enhancement of B cell responses. Cell. Immunol. 116:308–319.
Virella, G., T. Thompson, and R. Haskill-Stroud
  1990   A new quantitative Nitroblue Tetrazolium Reduction Assay based on kinetic colorimetry. J. Clin. Lab. Anal. 4:86–89.
Virella, G., K. Fourspring, B. Hyman, R. Haskill-Stroud, L. Long, I. Virella, M. La Via, A.J. Gross, and M. Lopes-Virella
  1991   Immunosuppressive effects of fish oil in normal human volunteers: Correlation with the *in vitro* effects of eicosapentanoic acid on human lymphocytes. Clin. Immunol. Immunopathol. 61:161–176.

Virella, G., C. Patrick, and J.M. Goust
  1993   Diagnostic evaluation of lymphocyte functions and cell-mediated immunity. Pp.
         291–306 in Introduction to Medical Immunology, 3d ed., G. Virella, ed. New
         York: Marcel Dekker.
Visser, M., P. Deurenberg, and W.A. Van Staveren
  1995   Multi-frequency bioelectrical impedance for assessing total body water and extra-
         cellular water in the elderly. Eur. J. Clin. Nutr. 49:256–266.
Vogel, J.A.
  1992   Obesity and its relation to physical fitness in the U.S. military. Armed Forces Soc.
         18:497–513.
Vogel, J.A., and J.P. Crowdy
  1979   Aerobic fitness and body fat of young British males entering the Army. Eur. J.
         Appl. Physiol. 40:73–83.
Vogel, J.A., and K.E. Friedl
  1992a Army data: Body composition and physical capacity. Pp. 89–103 in Body Com-
         position and Physical Performance, Applications for the Military Services, B.M.
         Marriott and J. Grumstrup-Scott, eds. A report of the Committee on Military Nu-
         trition Research, Food and Nutrition Board, Institute of Medicine. Washington,
         D.C.: National Academy Press.
  1992b Body fat assessment in women—Special considerations. Sports Med. 13:245–269.
Vogel, J.A., J.W. Kirkpatrick, P.I. Fitzgerald, J.A. Hodgdon, and E.A. Harman
  1988   Derivation of anthropometry-based body fat equations for the Army's weight con-
         trol program. Technical Report T17-88. Natick, Mass.: U.S. Army Research Insti-
         tute of Environmental Medicine.
Vogel J.A., K.E. Friedl, and P.I. Fitzgerald
  1990   Generalized prediction of body fat in young U.S. females. Med. Sci. Sports Exerc.
         22 (suppl.):S672.
von Behring, E., and S. Kitasato
  1890   On the acquisition of immunity against diphtheria and tetanus in animals. Deutsch.
         Med. Wochenschr. 16:1113–1114.
von Bezold, A.
  1857   Untersuchungen uber die vertheilung von Wasser, organischer Materie und
         anorganischen Verbindungen im Thierreiche. Zeitschrift fur Wissenschaftlische
         Zoologie, 8:487–524.
Waage, A., T. Espevik, and J. Lamvik
  1986   Detection of tumour necrosis factor-like cytotoxicity in serum from patients with
         septicaemia but not from untreated cancer patients. Scand. J. Immunol. 24:739–
         743.
Waage, A., A. Halstensen, and T. Espevik
  1987   Association between tumour necrosis factor in serum and fatal outcome in patients
         with meningococcal disease. Lancet 1(8529):355–357.
Waage, A., P. Brandtzaeg, A. Halstensen, P. Kierulf, and T. Espevik
  1989   The complex pattern of cytokines in serum from patients with meningococcal sep-
         tic shock. Association between interleukin-6, interleukin-1, and fatal outcome. J.
         Exp. Med. 169:333–338.
Walker, N., D.E. Meyer, and J.B. Smelcer
  1993   Spatial and temporal characteristics of rapid cursor-positioning movements with
         electromechanical mice in human-computer interaction. Hum. Factors 35(3):431–
         458.
Walker, R.I.
  1994   New strategies for using mucosal vaccination to achieve more effective immuniza-
         tion. Vaccine 12(5):387–400.

Walmsley, B., J.A. Hodgson, and R.E. Burke
  1978   Forces produced by the medial gastrocnemius and soleus muscles during locomotion in freely moving cats. J. Neurophysiol. 41:1203–1216.
Wang Z. M., S. Heshka, and S.B. Heymsfield
  1993   Application of computerized axial tomography in the study of body composition: Evaluation of lipid, water, protein, and mineral in healthy men. Pp. 343–344 in Human Body Composition: *In Vivo* Methods, Models, and Assessment, K.J. Ellis and J.D. Eastman, eds. New York: Plenum Press.
Wang, X., M.R. Briggs, X. Hua, C. Yokoyama, J.L. Goldstein, and M.S. Brown
  1993   Nuclear protein that binds sterol regulatory element of low density lipoprotein receptor promoter. II. Purification and characterization. J. Biol. Chem. 268:14497–14504.
Wang, X., R. Sato, M.S. Brown, X. Hua, and J.L. Goldstein
  1994   SREBP-1, a membrane-bound transcription factor released by sterol-regulated proteolysis. Cell 77:53–62.
Wang, Z.M., R.N. Pierson, Jr., and S.B. Heymsfield
  1992   The five-level model: A new approach to organizing body-composition research. Am. J. Clin. Nutr. 56: 19–28.
Wang, Z.M., S. Heshka, R.N. Pierson, Jr., and S.B. Heymsfield
  1995   Systematic organization of body composition methodology: Overview with emphasis on component-based methods. Am. J. Clin. Nutr. 61: 457–465.
Wannemacher, R.W., Jr., H.L. DuPont, R.S. Pekarek, M.C. Powanda, A. Schwartz, R.B. Hornick, and W.R. Beisel
  1972   An endogenous mediator of depression of amino acids and trace metals in serum during typhoid fever. J. Infect. Dis. 126:77–86.
Ward, L.C., I.H. Bunce, B.H. Cornish, B.R. Mirolo, B.J. Thomas, and L.C. Jones
  1992   Multi-frequency bioelectrical impedance augments the diagnosis and management of lymphoedema in post-mastectomy patients. Eur. J. Clin. Invest. 22:751–754.
Waterlow, J.C.
  1995   Whole-body protein turnover in humans—past, present and future. Annu. Rev. Nutr. 15:57–92.
Waterlow, J.C., P.J. Garlick, and D.J. Millward
  1978   Protein Turnover in Mammalian Tissues and in the Whole Body. Amsterdam: North-Holland Publishers.
Watson, C.A.
  1977   Near infrared reflectance spectrophotometric analysis of agricultural products. Anal. Chem. 49:835a–840a.
Watson, G.S.
  1995   Simulator effects in a high-fidelity driving simulator. Pp. 124–138 in Proceedings of the 1995 Driving Simulation Conference. Sophia-Antipolis, France: Neuf Associes.
Webb, A.R., L.A. Newman, M. Taylor, and J.B. Keogh
  1989   Hand grip dynamometry as a predictor of postoperative complications: Reappraisal using age-standardized grip strengths. J. Parenter. Enteral. Nutr. 13:30–33.
Webster, J.B., D.F. Kripke, S. Messin, D.J. Mullaney, and G. Wyborney
  1982   An activity-based sleep monitor system for ambulatory use. Sleep 5:389–399.
Weinstein, C.J.
  1995   Military and government applications of human-machine communication by voice. Proc. Natl. Acad. Sci. USA 92(22):10011–10016.

Weinstein, P.D., and J.J. Cebra
  1991   The preference for switching to IgA expression by Peyer's patch germinal center B-cells is likely due to the intrinsic influence of their microenvironment. J. Immunol. 147:4126–4135.
Weinstein, P.D., P.A. Schweitzer, J.A. Cebra-Thomas, and J.J. Cebra
  1991   Molecular genetic features reflecting the preference for isotype switching to IgA expression by Peyer's patch germinal center B-cells. Int. Immunol. 3:1253–1263.
Weinstein, P.D., A.O. Anderson, and R.G. Mage
  1994   Rabbit IgH sequences in appendix germinal centers: VH diversification by gene conversion-like and hypermutation mechanisms. Immunity 1:647–659.
Weinstein, P.D., R.G. Mage, and A.O. Anderson
  1994   The appendix functions as a mammalian bursal equivalent in the developing rabbit. Adv. Exp. Med. Biol. 355:249–254.
Weits, T., E.J. van der Beek, M. Wedel, and B.M. Ter Haar Romeny
  1988   Computed tomography measurement of abdominal fat deposition in relation to anthropometry. Int. J. Obes. 12:217–225.
Welle, S.
  1990   Two-point vs. multipoint sample collection for the analysis of energy expenditure by use of the doubly labeled water method. Am J. Clin. Nutr. 52:1134–1138.
Welle, S., C. Thornton, R. Jozefowicz, and M. Statt
  1993   Myofibrillar protein synthesis in young and old men. Am. J. Physiol. 264:E693–E698.
Wellens, R., W.C. Chumlea, S. Guo, A.F. Roche, N.V. Reo, and R.M. Siervogel
  1994   Body composition in white adults by dual-energy x-ray absorptiometry, densitometry, and total body water. Am. J. Clin. Nutr. 59:547–555.
Westerterp, K.R., F. Brounds, W.H.M. Saris, and F.T. Hoor
  1988   Comparison of doubly labeled water with respirometry at low- and high-acitivity levels. J. Appl. Physiol. 65(1):53–56.
Westerterp, K.R., G.A.L. Meijer, E.M.E. Janssen, W.H.M. Saris, and F. ten Hoor
  1992   Long-term effect of physical activity on energy balance and body composition. Br. J. Nutr. 68:21–30.
Westphal, K.A., N. King, K.E. Friedl, M.A. Sharp, T.R. Kramer, and K.L. Reynolds
  1995   Health, performance, and nutritional status of U.S. Army women during basic combat training. Technical Report T95-99. Natick, Mass.: U.S. Army Research Institute of Environmental Medicine.
Whitby, L.G.
  1952   Riboflavinyl glucoside: A new derivative of riboflavin. Biochem. J. 50:433–438.
White, J.W., and M. Wolraich
  1995   Effect of sugar on behavior and mental performance. Am. J. Clin. Nutr. 62(1 suppl.):242S–249S.
White, R.F., and S.P. Proctor
  1992   Research and clinical criteria for the development of neurobehavioral test batteries. J. Occup. Med. 34(2)140–148.
White, R.F., F. Gerr, R.F. Cohen, R. Green, M.D. Lezak, J. Lyberger, J. Mack, E. Silbergeld, J. Valciukas, and W. Chappell
  1994   Criteria for progressive modification of neurobehavioral batteries. Neurotoxicol. Teratol. 16(5):511–524.
WHO (World Health Organization)
  1985   Energy and protein requirements. Report of a joint FAO/WHO/UNU Expert Committee. WHO Technical Report Series 724. Geneva, Switzerland: World Health Organization.

Wilkinson, R.T.
  1968   Sleep deprivation: Performance tests for partial and selective sleep deprivation. Pp. 28–43 in Progress in Clinical Psychology, B.F. Reiss and L.A. Abt, eds. New York: Grune and Stratton.
Williams, L.M., P.E. Ballmer, L.T. Hannah, I. Grant, and P.J. Garlick
  1994   Changes in regional protein synthesis in rat brain and pituitary after systemic interleukin 1-ß administration. Am. J. Physiol. 267:E915–E920.
Williams, I.M., A.J. Picton, S.C. Hardy, A.J. Mortimer, and C.N. McCollum
  1994   Cerebral hypoxia detected by near infrared spectroscopy. Anaesthesia 49(9):762–766.
Willson, R.L.
  1989   Zinc and iron in free radical pathology and cellular control. Pp. 147–172 in Zinc in Human Biology, C.F. Mills, ed. New York: Springer-Verlag.
Wilmore, J.H., R.N. Girandola, and D.L. Moody
  1970   Validity of skinfold and girth assessment for predicting alterations in body composition. J. Appl. Physiol. 29:313–317.
Wilmore, J.H., P.A. Vodak, R.B. Parr, R.N. Girandola, and J.E. Billing
  1980   Further simplification of a method for determination of residual lung volume. Med. Sci. Sports Exerc. 12:216–218.
Wilpon, J.G.
  1995   Voice-processing technologies—their application in telecommunications. Proc. Natl. Acad. Sci. USA 92(22):9991–9998.
Wing, R.R., J.A. Vasquez, and C.M. Ryan
  1995   Cognitive effects of ketogenic weight-reducing diets. Int. J. Obes. Relat. Metab. Disord. 19(11):811–816.
Winter, G., A.D. Griffiths, R.E. Hawkins, and H.R. Hoogenboom
  1994   Making antibodies by phage display technology. Ann. Rev. Immunol. 12:433–455.
Withers, R.T., and C.T. Ball
  1988   A comparison of the effects of measured, predicted, estimated and constant residual volumes on the body density of female athletes. Int. J. Sports Med. 9:24–28.
Withers, R.T., D.A. Smith, B.E. Chatterton, C.G. Schultz, and R.D. Gaffney
  1992   Comparison of four methods of estimating the body composition of male endurance athletes. Eur. J. Clin. Nutr. 46:773–784.
Wolcdge, R.C., N.A. Curtin, and E. Homsher
  1985   Energetic Aspects of Muscle Contraction. London: Academic Press.
Wolfe, R.R.
  1992   Radioactive and Stable Isotope Tracers In Biomedicine: Principles and Practice of Kinetic Analysis. New York: Wiley-Liss.
Wolfe, R.R., and E.J. Peters
  1987   Lipolytic response to glucose infusion in human subjects. Am. J. Physiol. 252(15):E189–E196.
Wolfe, R.R., E.J. Peters, S. Klein, O.B. Holland, J. Rosenblatt, and H. Gary, Jr.
  1987   Effect of short-term fasting on the lipolytic responsiveness in normal and obese human subjects. Am. J. Physiol. 252:E189–E196.
Wolpaw, J.R., and D.J. McFarland
  1994   Multichannel EEG-based brain-computer communication. Electroencephalogr. Clin. Neurophysiol. 90(6):444–449.
Wong, Y.W., P.H. Kussie, B. Parhami-Seren, and M.N. Margolies
  1995   Modulation of antibody affinity by an engineered amino acid substitution. J. Immunol. 154:3351–3358.

Wright, S.
  1995   Turning the other cheeks: Insights into the cost of locomotion from running back-
          wards. Cambridge, Mass.: Harvard University Press.
Wu, H., W-P.Yang, and C.F. Barbas III
  1995   Building zinc fingers by selection: Toward a therapeutic application. Proc. Natl.
          Acad Sci. USA 92:344–348.
Wu, H-Y., and M.W. Russell
  1994   Comparison of systemic and mucosal priming for mucosal immune responses to a
          bacterial protein antigen given with or coupled to cholera toxin (CT) B subunit,
          and effects of pre-existing anti-CT immunity. Vaccine 12(3):215–222.
Wurtman, R.J.
  1994   Effects of nutrients on neurotransmitter release. Pp. 239–261 in Food Components
          to Enhance Performance, An Evaluation of Potential Performance-Enhancing Food
          Components for Operational Rations, B.M. Marriott, ed. A report of the Committee
          on Military Nutrition Research, Food and Nutrition Board, Institute of Medicine.
          Washington, D.C.: National Academy Press.
Wurtman, R.J., and M.C. Lewis
  1991   Exercise, plasma composition, and neurotransmission. Med. Sports Sci. 32:94–
          109.
Wyatt, J.S.
  1993   Near-infrared spectroscopy in asphyxial brain injury. Clin. Perinatol. 20(2):369–
          378.
Xu-Amano, J., H. Kiyono, R.J. Jackson, H.F. Staats, K. Fujihashi, P.D. Burrows, C.O. Elson,
          S. Pillai, and J.R. McGhee
  1993   Helper T cell subsets for immunoglobulin A responses: Oral immunization with
          tetanus toxoid and cholera toxin as adjuvant selectively induces Th2 cells in mu-
          cosa associated tissues. J. Exp. Med. 178:1309–1320.
Yamamoto, I., N. Muto, E. Nagato, T. Nakamura, and Y. Suzuki
  1990   Formation of a stable L-ascorbic acid α-glucoside by mammalian α-glucosidease-
          catalyzed transglucosylation. Biochem. Biophys. Acta 1035:44–50.
Yamamura, M., K. Uyemura, R.J. Deans, K. Weinberg, T.H. Rea, B.R. Bloom, and R.L.
          Modlin
  1991   Defining protective response to pathogens: Cytokine profiles in leprosy lesions.
          Science 254:277–279.
Yan, C., J.H. Resau, J. Hewetson, M. West, W.L. Rill, and M. Kende
  1994   Characterization and morphological analysis of protein-loaded poly(lactide-co-
          glycolide) microparticles prepared by water-in-oil-in-water emulsion technique. J.
          Controlled Release 32:231–241.
Yang, J., R. Sato, J.L. Goldstein, and M.S. Brown
  1994   Sterol-resistant transcription in CHO cells caused by gene rearrangement that trun-
          cates SREBP-2. Genes Dev. 8:1910–
1919.
Yang, L-Y., A. Kuksis, J.J. Myher, and G. Steiner   1996   Contributions of *de novo*
          fatty acid synthesis to very low density lipoprotein triacylglycerols: Evidence
          from mass isotopomer distribution analysis of fatty acids synthesized from
          [^{2}H$_6$]ethanol. J. Lipid Res. 37:262–274.
Yarasheski, K.E., J.A. Campbell, K. Smith, M.J. Rennie, J.O. Halloszy, and D.M. Bier
  1992   Effect of growth hormone and resistance exercise on muscle growth in young men.
          Am. J. Physiol. 262:E261–E267.

Yarasheski, K.E., K. Smith, M.J. Rennie, and D.M. Bier
1992   Measurement of muscle protein fractional synthetic rate by capillary gas chromatography-combustion-isotope ratio mass spectrometry. Biol. Mass Spectrom. 21:486–490.

Yarasheski, K.E., J.J. Zachwieja, and D.M. Bier
1993   Acute effects of resistance exercise on muscle protein synthesis rate in young and elderly men and women. Am. J. Physiol. 265:E210–E214.

Yasumoto, K., H. Tsuji, and H. Mitsuda
1977   Isolation from rice bran of a bound form of vitamin B_6 and its identification as 5'-O-(β-D-glucopyranosyl)-pyridoxine. Agric. Biol. Chem. 41:1061–1067.

Yoshiya, I., Y. Shimada, and K. Tanaka
1980   Spectrophotometric monitoring of arterial oxygen saturation in the finger tip. Med. Biol. Eng. Comp. 18:27–32.

Young, H.A., P. Ghosh, J. Ye, J. Lederer, A. Lichtman, J.R. Gerard, L. Penix, C.B. Wilson, A.J. Melvin, M.E. McGurn, D.B. Lewis, and D.D. Taub
1994   Differentiation of the T helper phenotypes by analysis of the methylation state of the IFN-β gene. J. Immunol. 153:3603–3610.

Young, J.C.
1995   Exercise prescription for individuals with metabolic disorders. Practical considerations. Sports Med. 19:43–54.

Young, V.R.
1970   The role of skeletal and cardiac muscle in the regulation of protein metabolism. Pp. 585–674 in Mammalian Protein Metabolism, H.N. Munro, ed. New York: Academic Press.

Young, V.R.
1992   Macronutrient needs in the elderly. Nutr. Rev. 50:454–462.

Young, V.R., and A.E. El-Khoury
1995   The notion of the essentiality of amino acids, revisited, with a note on the indispensable amino acid requirements of adults. Pp. 191–232 in Amino Acid Metabolism and Therapy in Health and Nutritional Disease, LC. Cynober, ed. Boca Raton, Fla.: CRC Press.

Young, V.R., and H.N. Munro
1978 $N^τ$-methylhistidine (3-methylhistidine) and muscle protein turnover: An overview. Fed. Proc. 37:2291–2300.

Young, V.R., J.S. Marchini, and J. Cortiella
1990   Assessment of protein nutritional status. J. Nutr. 120:1496–1502.

Young, V.R., Y-M. Yu, and M. Krempf
1991   Protein and amino acid turnover using the stable isotopes 15N, ^{13}C and ^2H as probes. Pp. 17–72 in New Techniques in Nutritional Research, R.G. Whitehead and A. Prentice, eds. San Diego: Academic Press.

Yu, Y-M., D.A. Wagner, E.E. Tredgett, J.A. Walaszewski, J.F. Burke, and V.R. Young
1990   Quantitative role of splanchnic region in leucine metabolism: L-[1-^{13}C,^{15}N]leucine and substrate balance studies. Am. J. Physiol. 259:E36–E50.

Zachariah, T., S.B. Rawal, S.N. Pramanik, M.V. Singh, S. Kishnani, H. Bharadwaj, and R.M. Rai
1987   Variations in skinfold thickness during de-acclimatisation and re-acclimatisation to high altitude. Eur. J. Appl. Physiol. 56:570–577.

Zamir, O., P-O. Hasselgren, S.L. Kunkel, J. Frederick, T. Higashiguchi, and J.E. Fischer
1992   Evidence that tumor necrosis factor participates in the regulation of muscle proteolysis during sepsis. Arch. Surg. 127:170–174.

Zamir, O., P-O. Hasselgren, W. O'Brien, R.C. Thompson, and J.E. Fischer
1992 Muscle protein breakdown during endotoxemia in rata and after treatment with interleukin-1 receptor antagonist (IL-Ira). Ann. Surg. 216:381–385.

Zawel, L., and D. Reinberg
1993 Initiation of transcription by RNA polymerase II: A multistep process. Prog. Nucleic Acids Res. Mol. Biol. 44:67–108.

Zhang, R.G., M.L. Westbrook, S. Nance, B.D. Spangler, G.G. Shipley, and E.M. Westbrook
1995 The three-dimensional crystal structure of cholera toxin. J. Mol. Biol. 251:563–573.

Zhang, Z., and D.B. McCormick
1992 Uptake and metabolism of N-(4'-pyridoxal)amines by isolated rat liver cells. Arch. Biochem. Biophys. 294:394–397.

Zhang, Z., J.F. Gregory III, and D.B. McCormick
1993 Pyridoxine-5'-β-D-glucoside competitively inhibits   uptake of vitamin B6 into isolated rat liver cells. J. Nutr. 123:85–89.

Zierath, J.R., and H. Wallberg-Henriksson
1992 Exercise training in obese diabetic patients. Sports Med. 14:171–189.

Zilberg, N.J., D.S. Weiss, and M.J. Horowitz
1982 Impact of events scale: A cross-validation study and some empirical evidence supporting a conceptual model of stress response syndromes. J. Consult. Clin. Psychol. 50:407–414.

Zillikens, M.C., and J.M. Conway
1991 Estimation of total body water by bioelectrical impedance analysis in Blacks. Am. J. Hum. Biol. 3:25–32.

Zuntz, N.
1897 Über den Stoffverbauch des Hundes bei Muskelarbeit. Arch. Gesamte Physiol Menschen Tiere 68:191–211.

Zurlo, F., K. Larsen, C. Bogardus, and E. Ravussin
1990 Skeletal muscle metabolism is a major determinant of resting energy expenditure. J. Clin. Invest. 86:1423–1427.

Index

This index is organized in sections according to the part of the book covered.

I

COMMITTEE SUMMARY AND RECOMMENDATIONS

Adenosine triphosphate (ATP), 16
Anthropometric measurements, 2,
   7, 8, 9, 12, 19, 52, 53, 54, 66,
   67
   fat mass, 6, 12, 13
   See also BMI; CAT; Dual-
      energy x-ray absorptiometry;
      MRI
Antibodies, 2, 25, 27, 30–32, 61–
   63, 66–67, 68
   cloning of, 31–32
   production of, 25–26, 32
   See also CDR; Immune function;
      Polymerase chain reaction;
      Vaccines and vaccination

Army Regulations, 7, 12
BC. *See* Body composition
   assessment
BIA. *See* Bioelectric impedance
   analysis (BIA)
BIS. *See* Bioimpedance
   spectroscopy (BIS)
BMD. *See* Bone mineral density
   (BMD)
BMI. *See* Body mass index (BMI)
Bioelectric impedance analysis
   (BIA), 9, 12, 13, 52, 53, 54,
   66, 67
Bioimpedance spectroscopy (BIS),
   9, 52

II

THE CURRENT ARMY PROGRAM AND ITS FUTURE NEEDS

III

TECHNIQUES OF BODY COMPOSITION ASSESSMENT

IV

TRACER TECHNIQUES FOR THE STUDY OF METABOLISM

V

AMBULATORY TECHNIQUES FOR MEASUREMENT OF ENERGY EXPENDITURE

VI

MOLECULAR AND CELLULAR APPROACHES TO NUTRITION

VII

ASSESSMENT OF IMMUNE FUNCTION

VIII

FUNCTIONAL AND BEHAVIORAL MEASURES OF NUTRITIONAL STATUS